UNIVERSITY OF ROCHESTER LIBRARIES
3 9087 01830363 8

D1560847

Clinical Diagnostic Immunology: Protocols in Quality Assurance and Standardization

Clinical Diagnostic Immunology: Protocols in Quality Assurance and Standardization

Edited By

ROBERT M. NAKAMURA, MD
Chairman Emeritus
Department of Pathology
Scripps Clinic and Research Foundation
La Jolla, California

C. LYNNE BUREK, PhD, ABMLI
Assistant Professor
Department of Pathology
Johns Hopkins University
Baltimore, Maryland

LINDA COOK, PhD
Section Head
Clinical Immunology
Lahey Hitchcock Clinic
Burlington, Massachusetts

JAMES D. FOLDS, PhD
Professor of Microbiology, Immunology, and Pathology
The University of North Carolina School of Medicine
Director
William McLendon Clinical Laboratories
Chapel Hill, North Carolina

John L. Sever, MD, PhD
Professor of Pediatrics, Obstetrics and Gynecology, Microbiology, and Immunology
The George Washington University Medical Center
Children's National Medical Center
Washington, District of Columbia

b

Blackwell
Science

© 1998 by Blackwell Science, Inc.

Editorial Offices:
350 Main Street, Malden, MA 02148-5018, USA
Osney Mead, Oxford OX2 0EL, England
25 John Street, London WC1N 2BL, England
23 Ainslie Place, Edinburgh EH3 6AJ, Scotland
54 University Street, Carlton, Victoria 3053, Australia

Other Editorial Offices:
Blackwell Wissenschafts-Verlag GmbH
Kurfürstendamm 57
10707 Berlin, Germany

Blackwell Science KK
MG Kodenmacho Building
7–10 Kodenmacho Nihombashi
Chuo-ku, Tokyo 104, Japan

Distributors

USA
Blackwell Science, Inc.
Commerce Place
350 Main Street
Malden, Massachusetts 02148
(Telephone orders: 800-215-1000 or 781-388-8250;
fax orders: 781-388-8270)

Canada
Login Brothers Book Company
324 Saulteaux Crescent
Winnipeg, Manitoba
Canada, R3J 3T2
(Telephone orders: 204-224-4068)

Australia
Blackwell Science Pty, Ltd.
54 University Street
Carlton, Victoria 3053
(Telephone orders: 03-9347-0300;
fax orders: 03-9349-3016)

Outside North America and Australia
Blackwell Science, Ltd.
c/o Marston Book Services, Ltd.
P.O. Box 269
Abingdon
Oxon OX14 4YN
England
(Telephone orders: 44-01235-465500;
fax orders: 44-01235-465555)

All rights reserved. No part of this book may be reproduced in any form or by any electronic or mechanical means, including information storage and retrieval systems, without permission in writing from the publisher, except by a reviewer who may quote brief passages in a review.

First published 1998

Acquisitions: Christopher Davis
Production: Ellen Samia
Manufacturing: Lisa Flanagan
Typeset by Best-set Typesetter Ltd., Hong Kong
Printed and bound by Braun-Brumfield, Inc.
Printed in the United States of America
98 99 00 01 5 4 3 2 1

The Blackwell Science logo is a trade mark of Blackwell Science Ltd, registered at the United Kingdom Trade Marks Registry

Library of Congress Cataloging-in-Publication Data
Clinical diagnostic immunology/ [edited by]
Robert M. Nakamura, James D. Folds.
p. cm.
Includes bibliographical references and index.
ISBN 0-86542-518-3
1. Immunodiagnosis. 2. Immunodiagnosis—Quality Control.
3. Immunodiagnosis—Standards. I. Nakamura, Robert M., 1927– .
II. Folds, James D.
[DNLM: 1. Immunologic Tests—methods. 2. Immunologic Techniques.
3. Immunologic Tests—standards. QY 250 C6405 1998]
RB46.5.C526 1998
616.07′56—dc21
DNLM/DLC 98-21394
for Library of Congress CIP

For further information on Blackwell Science, visit our website:
www.blackwell-science.com

QY
250
C641
1998

Contents

PART III 83

Recommendations for Quality Assurance, Quality Control, and Standardization of Humoral Analytes

Linda Cook, editor

PART IV 125

Quality Assurance, Quality Control, and Standardization in Cellular and Tissue Assays

C. Lynne Burek, Robert M. Nakamura, editors

PART V 195

Recommendations for Quality Assurance and Standardization of Laboratory Procedures for Evaluation of Diseases Mediated by Immune Mechanisms

C. Lynne Burek, editor

Preface

This book is sponsored and written mostly by members of the Association of Medical Laboratory Immunologists (AMLI). The royalties will go to further the efforts of the Standards Committee of the AMLI.

What is the mission of AMLI?

The organization was founded in 1987 and consists of immunologists, physicians, laboratory scientists, and technologists who are interested in clinical diagnostic immunology.

The mission statement from the AMLI bylaws is as follows:

> "The purpose of the Association is to unite basic and clinical scientists who have developed expertise in diagnostic laboratory immunology, its subspecialties and related sciences, in order to: (1) facilitate the interchange of ideas and information among workers in the field; and (2) promote and encourage excellence in research, development, and delivery of immunologic laboratory services in health-related areas and thus contribute to the health and welfare of the public."

The chapters in this book on Quality Assurance and Standardization were selected to inform laboratory scientists and technologists about:

1. The impact and consequences of the many changes in health care delivery systems and the clinical laboratories.
2. Current concepts of quality assurance to provide helpful information for *prospective* real-time quality control on many individual analytes.
3. The current and future role of the clinical immunology laboratory scientist.
4. The impact of emerging technologies, governmental regulations, and advances in therapy.
5. Numerous recommendations in the quality control, standardization, and assays of many different analytes performed in the diagnostic immunology laboratory.

The majority of assays in the clinical immunology laboratory are the CLIA '88 high complexity category. The laboratory scientist will perform various humoral and cellular immune tests as well as nucleotide tests needed for the evaluation and monitoring of immune mediated diseases.

The book was designed to provide important information to each and every clinical laboratory scientist and be kept as a reference guide.

"In the field of observation, chance favors only the mind that is prepared."

Louis Pasteur

This book should help the readers to improve the performance of their respective immunology laboratories and prepare for the major changes in the future.

We would like to thank and acknowledge the help and encouragement of Christopher Davis, Executive Editor of Blackwell Science. Also, we thank all the authors for their excellent contributions which make this book the "state-of-the-art in quality assurance and standardization in clinical diagnostic immunology".

R.M.N.
C.L.B.
L.C.
J.D.F
J.L.S.

Contributors

Thomas S. Alexander, PhD
Assistant Professor of Clinical Immunology and Pathology
Northeastern Ohio Universities College of Medicine
Rootstown, Ohio
Immunologist
Department of Pathology
Summa Health System
Akron, Ohio

Theodore D. Anderson, MFS
Department of the Army
Armed Forces Institute of Pathology
Washington, District of Columbia

Mark E. Astill
Assistant Vice President
Manager, Research and Development
Associated and Regional University Pathologists
ARUP Laboratories, Inc.
Salt Lake City, Utah

Linda L. Baum, PhD
Associate Professor of Microbiology and Immunology
Finch University of Health Sciences
The Chicago Medical School
Chicago, Illinois

Joseph A. Bellanti, MD
Professor of Pediatrics and Microbiology
Director
The International Center for Interdisciplinary Studies of Immunology
Georgetown University School of Medicine
Washington, District of Columbia

C. Lynne Burek, PhD, ABMLI
Assistant Professor
Department of Pathology
Johns Hopkins University
Baltimore, Maryland

David F. Carney, PhD
Assay Development Scientist
Scripps Reference Laboratory of the Scripps Research Institute
San Diego, California

A. Betts Carpenter, MD, PhD
Marshall University School of Medicine
Huntington, West Virginia

Yiping Chen, DDS
University of Pittsburgh Medical Center
Pittsburgh, Pennsylvania

Neil T. Constantine, PhD
Associate Professor
University of Maryland School of Medicine
Director
Clinical Immunology
University of Maryland Medical Systems
Institute of Human Virology
Baltimore, Maryland

Linda Cook, PhD
Section Head
Clinical Immunology
Lahey Hitchcock Clinic
Burlington, Massachusetts

Daniel C. Edelman, PhD
Department of Pathology
University of Maryland Medical Systems
Baltimore, Maryland

Garth D. Ehrlich, PhD
Allegheny University of the Health Sciences
Center for Geonomic Sciences
Pittsburgh, Pennsylvania

Constance Emmett
Senior Scientist
T Cell Sciences, Inc.
Needham, Massachusetts

A. Farhoudi, MD
Professor of Pediatrics
Head, Immunology and Allergy
Children's Hospital
Iran
Visiting Professor, Immunology
Royal Victoria Hospital
Montreal, Quebec
Canada

Howard A. Fields, MD
Department of Health and Human Services
Public Health Service
Centers for Disease Control and Prevention
Atlanta, Georgia

Mildred K. Fleetwood, PhD, ABMLI
Department of Laboratory Medicine
Geisinger Clinic
Danville, Pennsylvania

Mary Ann Fletcher, MD
Professor of Medicine, Microbiology, and Immunology
University of Miami School of Medicine
Director
The E.M. Papper Clinical Immunology Laboratory
Miami, Florida

James D. Folds, PhD
Professor of Microbiology, Immunology, and Pathology
The University of North Carolina School of Medicine
Director
William McLendon Clinical Laboratories
Chapel Hill, North Carolina

Kimberly Foster
Chiron Diagnostics, Inc.
Walpole, Massachusetts

Teryl K. Frey, PhD
Professor
Department of Biology
Georgia State University
Atlanta, Georgia

Thomas Gahm, PhD
Vice President and Director of Image Research and Development
AutoCyte, Inc.
Elon College, North Carolina

Patricia C. Giclas, PhD
Director
Diagnostic Complement Laboratory
NJC Clinical Laboratories
Associate Faculty Member
Department of Pediatrics
Allergy and Immunology Division

National Jewish Center for Immunology and Respiratory Medicine
Immunology Department
University of Colorado Health Science Center
Denver, Colorado

Alice Gilman-Sachs, PhD
Associate Professor of Microbiology and Immunology
Finch University of Health Sciences
The Chicago Medical School
Chicago, Illinois

Wayne W. Grody, MD, PhD
Associate Professor
Divisions of Molecular Pathology and Medical Genetics
Departments of Pathology and Laboratory Medicine and Pediatrics
UCLA School of Medicine
Los Angeles, California

Robert G. Hamilton, PhD, DABMLI
Associate Professor of Medicine
Division of Allergy and Clinical Immunology
Johns Hopkins University School of Medicine
Reference Laboratory for Dermatology, Allergy, and Clinical Immunology
Baltimore, Maryland

E. Nigel Harris, Mphil, MD, DM
Dean and Professor of Medicine
Morehouse School of Medicine
Atlanta, Georgia

Nick S. Harris, PhD, ABMLI
IGeneX, Inc.
Reference Laboratory
Palo Alto, California

Jørgen Henrichsen, MD
Division of Microbiology
Statens Serum Institute
Copenhagen, Denmark

W. Edward Highsmith, Jr., PhD
Assistant Professor of Pathology
University of Maryland at Baltimore
Director
Molecular Diagnostics Laboratory
University of Maryland Medical Systems
Baltimore, Maryland

Wayne R. Hogrefe, PhD
Director, Research and Development
MRL Reference Laboratory
MRL Diagnostics
Cypress, California

Henry A. Homburger, MD
Professor of Laboratory Medicine and Pathology
Mayo Medical School
Consultant
Division of Clinical Biochemistry and Immunology
Mayo Clinic and Mayo Foundation
Rochester, Minnesota

Charles A. Horwitz, MD
Professor of Pathology
University of Minnesota Medical School
Pathologist
Abbott Northwestern Hospital
Minneapolis, Minnesota

Dorlinda Varga House, MD
Fellow in Pediatric Endocrinology and Diabetes
Departments of Pathology, Laboratory Medicine, Immunology, and Pediatrics
University of Florida
Gainesville, Florida

Karen James, PhD
Laboratory Management Consultant
Immunology Consultant
Vilas, North Carolina

Josef V. Kadlec, SJ, MD, PhD
Department of Pediatrics and Microbiology-Immunology

The International Center for
Interdisciplinary Studies of
Immunology
Georgetown University School of Medicine
Washington, District of Columbia

David F. Keren, MD
Clinical Professor of Pathology
The University of Michigan
Medical Director
Warde Medical Laboratory
Ann Arbor, Michigan

Vijay Kumar, PhD, FACB
Departments of Microbiology and
Dermatology
SUNY
University at Buffalo
President and CEO
IMMCO Diagnostics, Inc.
Buffalo, New York

Stephen B. Lambert
Unit Chief
Hepatitis Reference Laboratory
Department of Health and Human
Services
Public Health Service
Centers for Disease Control and
Prevention
Atlanta, Georgia

Sandra A. Larsen, PhD
Treponernal Pathogenesis and Immunology
Branch
Department of Health and Human
Services
Public Health Service
Centers for Disease Control and Prevention
Atlanta, Georgia

Julie Leana-Cox
Department of Pathology
University of Maryland Medical Systems
Baltimore, Maryland

Daisy R. Lee, MD
Department of Pathology
Grady Memorial Hospital
Atlanta, Georgia

Raphaël Marcelpoil, PhD
Assistant Professor
Université Joseph Fourier
Grenoble, France
Senior Software Engineer
AutoCyte, Inc.
Elon College, North Carolina

Gerald C. Miller, PhD
Chief of Immunology, Flow Cytometry, and
Microbiology
Regional Medical Laboratory, Inc.
Tulsa, Oklahoma

Bryan Millett
Senior Scientist
T Cell Sciences, Inc.
Needham, Massachusetts

William E. Morrill, BS
Research Microbiologist
Department of Health and Human
Services
Public Health Service
Centers for Disease Control and Prevention
Atlanta, Georgia

Ray B. Nagle, MD, PhD
Department of Pathology
University of Arizona Health Sciences
Center
Tucson, Arizona

Masamichi Nakamura, PhD
Postdoctoral Research Fellow
Departments of Pathology, Laboratory
Medicine, Immunology, and Pediatrics
University of Florida
Gainesville, Florida

Robert M. Nakamura, MD
Chairman Emeritus
Department of Pathology
Scripps Clinic and Research Foundation
La Jolla, California

Kevin L. Nellis, BS, MT(ASCP)
Technical Coordinator
Laboratories of Pathology
University of Maryland Medical Systems
Baltimore, Maryland

David E. Normansell, PhD
Professor
Department of Pathology and Microbiology
University of Virginia Health Sciences Center
Charlottesville, Virginia

Nora C. Nugent, BA, CHS
Department of Laboratory Medicine
Geisinger Clinic
Danville, Pennsylvania

Maurice R.G. O'Gorman, MD
Department of Pediatrics
Northwestern University Medical School
The Children's Memorial Hospital
Diagnostic Immunology Laboratory
Chicago, Illinois

C. Kirk Osterland
Thorp Professor of Medicine
McGill University
Director
Clinical Immunology
Royal Victoria Hospital
Montreal, Quebec
Canada

Helene Paxton, MS, MT (ASCP)
Integrated Diagnostics, Inc.
Baltimore, Maryland

Stephen M. Peters, PhD
Department of Pediatrics and Microbiology-Immunology
Georgetown University School of Medicine
Washington, District of Columbia

Silvia S. Pierangeli, PhD
Assistant Professor of Microbiology and Immunology
Director, Antiphospholipid Standardization Laboratory
Morehouse School of Medicine
Atlanta, Georgia

Herbert F. Polesky, MD
Director
Memorial Blood Centers of Minnesota
Minneapolis, Minnesota

Harry E. Prince, PhD
Associate Director, Immunology
MRL Reference Laboratory
MRL Diagnostics
Cypress, California

M. Rajadhyaksha, PhD
Departments of Microbiology and Dermatology
SUNY
University at Buffalo
IMMCO Diagnostics, Inc.
Buffalo, New York

Rhonda K. Roby, MPH
PE Applied Biosystems
Foster City, California

Katherine M. Scott, MD
Department of Pathology
University of Arizona Health Sciences Center
Tucson, Arizona

John L. Sever, MD, PhD
Professor of Pediatrics, Obstetrics and Gynecology, Microbiology, and Immunology
The George Washington University Medical Center
Children's National Medical Center
Washington, District of Columbia

Sanford A. Stass, MD, PhD
Department of Pathology
University of Maryland Medical Systems
Baltimore, Maryland

Theresa A. Steeper, MD
Assistant Professor of Pathology
University of Minnesota Medical School
Pathologist
Abbott Northwestern Hospital
Minneapolis, Minnesota

Elizabeth R. Unger, MD, PhD
Department of Pathology
Grady Memorial Hospital
Atlanta, Georgia

Victor W. Weedn, MD, JD
Department of the Army
Armed Forces Institute of Pathology
Washington, District of Columbia

Theresa L. Whiteside, PhD
Professor of Pathology and Otolaryngology
Director
UPCI Immunologic Monitoring and Diagnostic Laboratory
University of Pittsburgh Cancer Institute
Pittsburgh, Pennsylvania

Lorraine W. Wilson
Associated and Regional University Pathologists
ARUP Laboratories, Inc.
Salt Lake City, Utah

William E. Winter, MD
Professor
Departments of Pathology, Laboratory Medicine, Immunology, Pediatrics, and Molecular Genetics and Microbiology
Section Chief
Departments of Pathology and Laboratory Medicine
Medical Director, Clinical Chemistry
University of Florida
Gainesville, Florida

Yingze Zhang, MS
Research Associate
Division of Rheumatology and Clinical Immunology
Department of Medicine
University of Pittsburgh
Pittsburgh, Pennsylvania

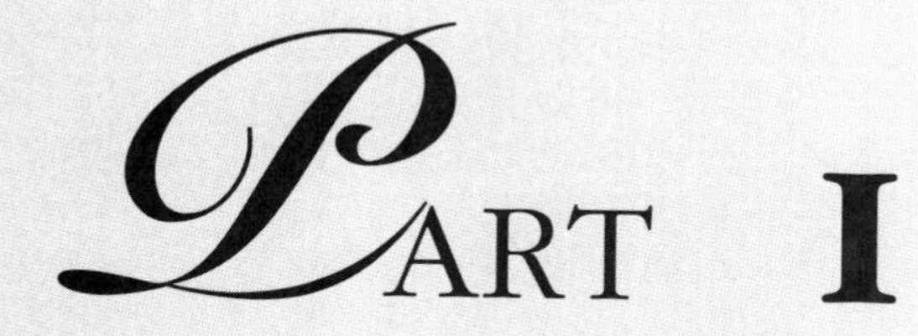

Current and Future Role of the Clinical Immunology Laboratory

JAMES D. FOLDS, EDITOR

CHAPTER 1

What Is Clinical and Laboratory Immunology?

JOSEPH A. BELLANTI
JOSEF V. KADLEC
STEPHEN M. PETERS

The remarkable development of basic immunology during the past 50 years has been accompanied by a parallel development of the application of new knowledge to the study of human diseases. Thus, in the 1970s was born the new discipline of clinical immunology, which can be defined as the application of the principles of basic immunology to the clinical investigation, diagnosis, and treatment of patients with immunologically mediated diseases. In a similar way, the evolving discipline of clinical immunology stimulated the development of modern basic immunology. The discovery of agammaglobulinemia, for example, by Bruton in 1952 (1) triggered the whole evolution of our understanding of T-cell, B-cell, and antigen-presenting cells. Similarly, the study of human myeloma disorders characterized by monoclonal expansion of cells and cell products (e.g., immunoglobulin G and E myeloma proteins) opened the way for an understanding of the basic structure, function, and genetic regulation of antibody molecules.

Accompanying the growth of clinical and basic immunology was the development of yet another new discipline, laboratory immunology, which is involved with the performance and interpretation of laboratory tests that evaluate immunologic function in patients with immunologically mediated diseases. Thus, the development of clinical and laboratory immunology proceeded simultaneously and they represent an interdependent and interrelated two-way process that links the patient's clinical signs and symptoms of disease with physicians who care for these individuals and laboratory testing by specialized laboratories that perform the test procedures.

Understandably, owing to the rapid expansion of these new and exciting disciplines, a wide variety of individuals were attracted from both clinical and basic science backgrounds. Over the years, many attempts have been made to define the specialists and subspecialists from medicine as well as the identity of basic science immunologists who function in both these disciplines of clinical and laboratory immunology (2). Both non-MD basic and clinical scientists and MD clinicians claim some competence in these fields and have contributed greatly to the development of these disciplines. This also has unfortunately led to some difficulty in definition, particularly for the clinical immunologists and their role in this whole developing field. This confusion has derived from the many issues related to board certification, licensure and regulation of laboratories, and reimbursement charges, which are continually evolving. These issues are described elsewhere in this book.

A model for an operational definition of clinical and laboratory immunology is shown in **Figure 1-1**. For ease of discussion, the immune response can be viewed as the interaction of three domains: 1) the *external environment*, which contains all of the foreign configurations that eventually activate and stimulate the immune system; 2) the *internal environment*,

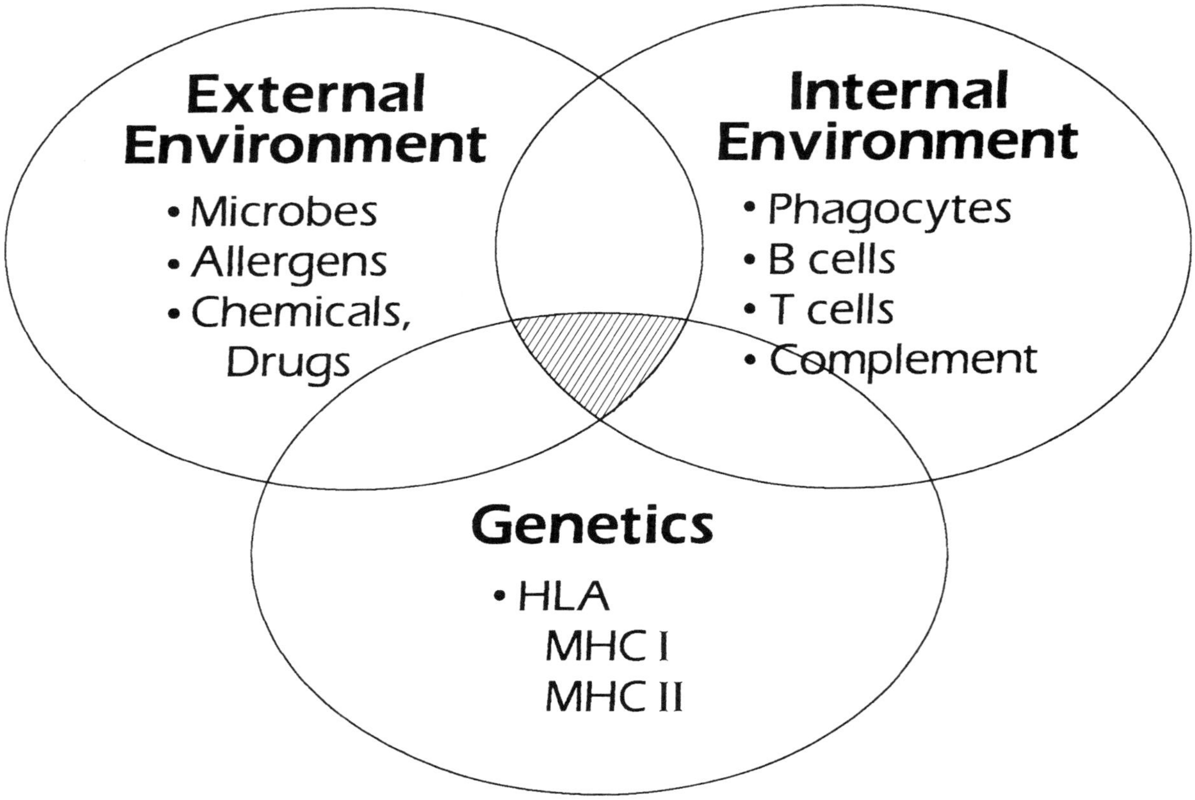

FIGURE 1-1

Schematic representation depicting the immune response (*shaded area*) as the net interaction of the three domains of external and internal environments and the genetic endowment that controls the response. HLA, human leukocyte antigen; MHC, major histocompatibility complex.

TABLE 1-1

Clinical Applications of Immunology

Domain	Components	Clinical Manifestations
External environment	Microbes, allergens, chemicals, drugs	Infectious diseases, allergies
Internal environment	Phagocytes, B cells, T cells, complement	Allergic diseases, immunodeficiencies, lymphoproliferative diseases, autoimmune diseases, malignancy
Genetics	HLA (MHC I, MHC II)	Transplantation (solid organs and bone marrow), disease susceptibility

HLA, human leukocyte antigen; MHC, major histocompatibility complex.

which contains the cells and cell products of the immune system that respond to this vast array of foreign configurations; and 3) the *genetic endowment*, which controls the whole array of the immune response. Shown in **Table 1-1** are the clinical applications of immunology, which are based on the interaction of these three major domains.

TABLE 1-2
Clinical Applications of Immunology

A. Diseases of immunodeficiency: patients who present with recurrent infections
   1. Primary (B-cell, T-cell, phagocytic cell, complement deficiency)
   2. Secondary [malnutrition, human immunodeficiency virus (acquired immunodeficiency virus), and other viral infections]
B. Diseases of overexpression of immune function
   1. Allergy: genetic predisposition to allergens; infections trigger allergic attacks
   2. Autoimmune diseases
   3. Lymphoproliferative diseases and tumor immunity
      a. B cell: multiple myeloma
      b. T cell: leukemias, lymphomas
C. Immunoprophylaxis and immunotherapy
   1. Use of vaccines: immunoprophylaxis
   2. Use of sera and gamma globulin: immunotherapy (classic)
   3. Transplantation of cells: immunotherapy
   4. New expansion of immunotherapy with products of the immune system available through molecular biology, e.g., cytokines (interferons, interleukins, hematopoietic growth factors) and gene therapy

TABLE 1-3
The Methodologies Comprising Laboratory Immunology

Electrophoresis and immunoelectrophoresis, immunofixation, immunodiffusion applied to serum, urine, and spinal fluid
Nephelometry and fluorometry
ELISA and radioimmunoassay
Direct and indirect immunofluorescence and immunohistochemistry
Measurement of complement components and their activities
Flow cytometry and production of monoclonal antibodies
Lymphocyte functional assays
Evaluation of chemotaxis, phagocytosis, and microbicidal activity
HLA typing
Techniques of molecular biology, PCR

The Content of Clinical and Laboratory Immunology

The fields of clinical and laboratory immunology evolved from the study of clinical entities, which include the immunologically mediated diseases which are listed in **Tables 1-2** and **1-3**. These vary from the allergic and infectious diseases, the autoimmune disorders, malignancies, and the immunodeficiencies to the emerging applications of immunotherapy, which range from the classic use of gamma globulin and vaccines to the more modern applications of immunology relating to transplantation and gene therapy (3).

The Interrelationships of Clinical Immunology and Laboratory Immunology

It is obvious from this discussion that individuals trained in both the clinical disciplines of immunology and laboratory immunology are required to carry out the functions of these respective fields. Shown in **Table 1-3** are the various methodologies comprising laboratory immunology (3). It is expected that both the clinical and laboratory immunologist understand these procedures, which are required both for their proper utilization and their performance and interpretation. These include electrophoresis and immunoelectrophoresis, nephelometry and fluorometry, enzyme-linked immunosorbent assay (ELISA) and radioimmunoassay, the use of immunofluorescence, the measurement of complement components, flow cytometry, lymphocyte proliferation assays, evaluation of chemotaxis, phagocytosis and microbicidal activity, human leukocyte antigen (HLA) typing, and techniques of molecular biology. Specialized training in these fields is required for both PhD and MD specialists who are interested in these diagnostic areas.

Some clinical immunologists may also wish to function as directors of laboratories of immunology, and graduate training in this field will also be required; this is described below. The clinical skills that the clinical immunologist should develop are shown in **Table 1-4**. These include the ability to interpret tests, as well as the ability to modulate the immune system by a variety of techniques, ranging from plasmapheresis to the administration of immunoglobulins or cytokines; the use of cytotoxic drugs; gene therapy; and the administration of antigens, allergens, venoms, and peptides. Examples of these include the use of plasmapheresis for the removal of the undesirable effects of myeloma proteins, which lead to increased viscosity, or the use of FK506, an inhibitor of calcineurin-linked T-cell proliferation in the prevention of graft versus host disease (GVH) by T cells. Conversely, these clinical skills may be applied in situations in which it is necessary to supplement a missing component, that is, the use of immunoglobulins. The most contemporary example of reconstitution is gene therapy, which could lead to a more durable and permanent cure of these disorders.

Although laboratory immunologists may lack the clinical training necessary for the management of patients with immunologically mediated diseases, they nevertheless contribute greatly in their role as the directors of diagnostic laboratories and in the performance and interpretation of laboratory procedures that measure immune function. The laboratory immunologist needs to participate in discussions of clinical cases with management and the clinical immunologist needs to communicate with the laboratory immunologist concerning the ever-changing clinical needs of patients, which will result in modification of existing laboratory tests or the development of new test procedures required for the management of these clinical cases. Thus, there exists a mutually beneficial bidirectional relationship between the laboratory immunologist and the clinical immunologist that is crucial in these rapidly developing fields to provide optimal patient care.

TABLE **1-4**

Clinical Skills of the Clinical Immunologist

The ability to interpret specialized tests in the context of a patient consultation

The ability to modulate the immune system by
- Plasmapheresis or plasma exchange
- The adminstration of immunoglobulins, purified or recombinant proteins such as antienzymes, or inhibitors of activated complement components
- The administration of interferons, other cytokines, and monoclonal antibodies

Application of cytotoxic drugs

Gene therapy

Administration of antigens, allergens, venoms, and peptides

The Certifying Mechanisms

It is apparent from this discussion that the vast degree of heterogeneity of activities of laboratory and clinical immunologists requires correspondingly a broad spectrum of training and certifying mechanisms offered by various certifying specialty boards which coordinate and unify these efforts. For example, the American Board of Medical Specialists of the American Society for Microbiology, that is, the American Board of Medical Laboratory Immunology (ABMLI); and the Association of Clinical Chemists. Shown in **Table 1-5** are some of the certifying pathways for laboratory immunologists and clinical immunologists and the number of diplomats who have been certified over 10-year periods.

The Impact of Health Care Reform on the Evolving Disciplines of Clinical Immunology and Laboratory Immunology

It has become apparent in recent years that the restructuring of health care has had important implications in the disciplines of clini-

TABLE **1-5**

Certifying Pathways for Individuals Interested in Laboratory and Clinical Immunology

Certifying Board	Group Certified	No. of Diplomats (yr)
ABAI	MDs trained in allergy and immunology, additional training in CDLI	174 (1994)
ABPATH*	Certificates of added qualifications in immunopathology	45 (1995)
AB Dermatology*	Certificates of added qualifications in dermatologic/diagnostic and laboratory immunology	58 (1993)
ABMLI	MD and non-MD immunologists	147 (1996)

ABAI, American Board of Allergy and Immunology; ABPATH, American Board of Pathology; ABMLI, American Board of Medical Laboratory Immunology; CDLI, Clinical Diagnostic and Laboratory Immunology.
*No longer provide certifying examinations.

cal immunology and laboratory immunology. These have included issues related to reimbursement of clinical services as well as laboratory procedures, the drastic curtailment of tests, and the assignment of laboratory testing to regional/commercial laboratories dictated in part by the increasing number of health maintenance organizations (HMOs), which collectively have created tremendous tensions and difficulties in the ordering and performance of these tests. These issues are described more fully in another section of this book, but it is important that they be identified, and it is hoped that they will be resolved in the near future.

REFERENCES

1. Bruton OC. Agammaglobulinemia. Pediatrics 1952;9:722–728.
2. Bellanti JA. Allergy and clinical immunology: An interdisciplinary concept. Ann Allergy 1978;41: 129–135.
3. Bloch KJ. What is a clinical immunologist? Pediatr Clin North Am 1994;41:591–596.

CHAPTER 2

The Anatomy and Organization of a Modern Clinical Immunology Laboratory

DAVID E. NORMANSELL

The clinical immunology laboratory is an important component of the modern suite of clinical laboratories. **Table 2-1** lists the areas of expertise of the laboratory. Although the workload may constitute only about 5% of that of all of the clinical laboratories, the number of different tests involved may easily exceed 25% of the total panel offered by the laboratories. Because of this diversity of tests, the technical staff must be of a high caliber and extremely versatile. In addition, rigorous proficiency and quality assurance programs must be in place.

Laboratory Design and Overall Organization

The laboratory should be divided into areas, each with its focal theme and the appropriate equipment. The nerve center of the laboratory is the specimen receipt and processing area, which should be located at or near the entrance. If the specimens have passed through a central departmental receiving facility, each should be bar-coded and need only be processed (centrifuged, aliquotted, etc.) and taken to a specific work area, or to appropriate storage, ready for analysis. If, however, the specimens are brought directly to the laboratory, they must first be accessed (entered into the computer system and bar-coded) and then processed. Accession is the most important part of the procedure; it ensures that the specimens are appropriate for the tests ordered (correct tubes and volume), that tests are properly ordered in the main computer (correct history number, test on the departmental panel), and that all necessary patient information has been obtained.

A specimen storage area, containing refrigerators, freezers (−20° and −80°C), and liquid nitrogen storage, should be adjacent to the receiving area. All samples are received and stored in this area before analysis; there must be no possibility of a sample being brought directly to a specific bench from outside the laboratory and bypassing accession. This is essential to eliminate any "lost" or "unknown" specimens, and to make sure that all tests are properly ordered. The receipt and processing area should also contain an inquiry desk, to handle all requests for information, results, and so forth, and to prevent interruption of the bench technologists.

Specific laboratory areas should fan out from the receiving area, in such a way as to maximize efficiency. The three main areas are immunochemistry, including analyses for allergy, immunodeficiency, and tumor markers; serology and autoimmunity; and flow cytometry and tissue typing.

It is useful to have a database of all immunology results. This is achieved by downloading the day's immunology results from the department computer at a set time each day. A freestanding immunology computer is updated each day and backed up weekly. Since the department computer saves results for only 3

TABLE **2-1**

Clinical Immunology Areas of Expertise

Immunochemistry
- Identification and quantitation of normal and abnormal proteins in body fluids
- Response to specific immunogens
- Reactivity to specific allergens
- Tumor antigen levels and immune responses to these antigens

Serology and autoimmunity
- Detection of antibodies to infectious organisms
- Estimation of viral load
- Detection of immune responses to self antigens

Flow cytometry and tissue typing
- Identification and enumeration of cells in blood and tissues
- Ploidy analysis
- Immune responses in transplantation therapy
- Cell sorting
- Detection of MHC antigens
- Detection of preformed antibodies to MHC antigens

TABLE **2-2**

Immunochemistry

Protein chemistry
- SPE, UPE
- Specific protein levels:
  - IgG, IgA, IgM, K, L, C3, C4, RF, Alb, Pre-Alb, Mic-Alb, Hpt, Tf, AAT, Apo A, Apo B, Ce, CRP, C1 inh
- IFE, IEF, OCB, B2-Tf, Cryos
- IgD, sIgA, IgG and IgA subclasses
- Specific antibody titers

Allergy and immunodeficiency
- IgE, RAST

Tumor markers
- PSA-1, CEA

SPE, serum protein electrophoresis; UPE, urine protein electrophoresis; K, kappa light chains; L, lambda light chains; C3, C4, complement components; RF, rheumatoid factors; alb, serum albumin; Pre-Alb, prealbumin; Mic-Alb, microalbumin; Hpt, haptoglobin; Tf, transferrin; AAT, α_1-antitrypsin; Apo A, apolipoprotein A-1; Apo B, apolipoprotein B-100; Ce, ceruloplasmin; CRP, C-reactive protein; C1 inh, C1 esterase inhibitor; IFE, immunofixation electrophoresis; IEF, isoelectric focusing; OCB, oligoclonal bands; B2-Tf, B_2-transferrin; Cryos, cryoglobulins; RAST, radioallergosorbent test; PSA-1, prostate-specific antigen-1; CEA, carcinoembryonic antigen.

months, the laboratory database enables technologists to review *all* previous immunology results on a given patient. The minimal work needed to maintain the database results saves both the time and money expended on unnecessary repeats of previous tests.

Immunochemistry

Analysis of physiologically important plasma proteins in various body fluids is performed at this bench. Many routine and special tests are done here (**Table 2-2**), but the emphasis is on quantitation of individual proteins and detection of anomalous immunoglobulins.

Protein Chemistry

The bench is organized around an analyzer (such as the Beckman Array) and an electrophoresis and densitometer station (such as the Beckman Paragon System). About 30 linear feet of bench space is usually adequate, together with a sink and a small clean area for silver staining. The key to the efficient operation of this bench is the use of a flow diagram such as that in **Figure 2-1**. For patients with suspected immunoglobulin anomalies, a low-cost screening test, serum protein electrophoresis (SPE) or urine protein electrophoresis (UPE), is first performed, and further tests follow as necessary. This protocol ensures that expensive tests such as immunofixation are performed only when indicated. Careful documentation of patient results in a database is essential; once the identity of a patient's monoclonal gammopathy has been established, it is not necessary to reidentify the monoclonal protein in subsequent serum samples. Certain specialty tests, such as the detection of oligoclonal immunoglobulin G (IgG) bands in cerebrospinal fluid or beta-2 transferrin in leakage fluid, may be requested. However, unless these tests are needed on a stat basis, or are ordered at a sufficient volume to justify setting them up inhouse, they should be sent to a specialty or reference laboratory.

Allergy and Immunodeficiency

Some of the appropriate laboratory tests for these areas (e.g., IgE and other immunoglobulin levels, protein electrophoresis, etc.) are performed in the immunochemistry area, while others, such as lymphocyte phenotypes and lymphocyte responses to mitogens and antigens, are performed in the flow cytometry area. Other tests may be needed, such as those to

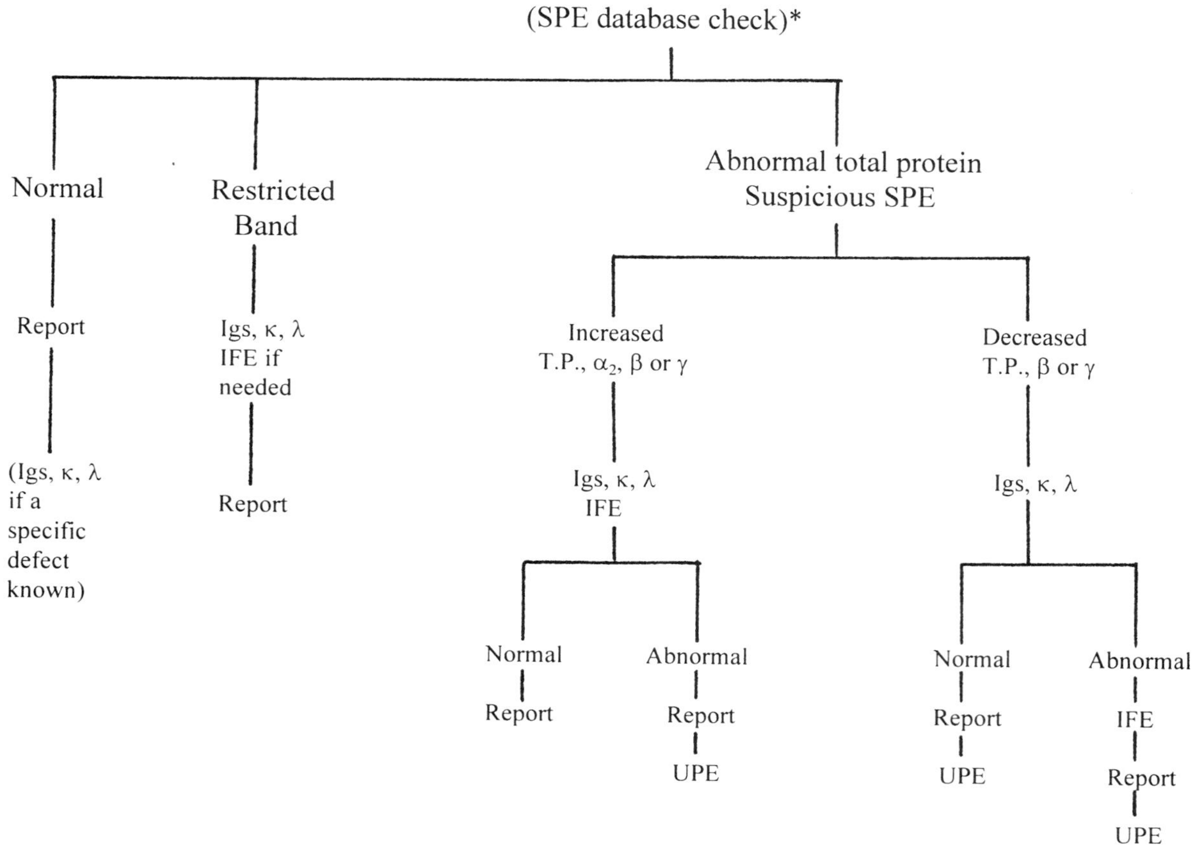

FIGURE 2-1

Complete protein workup. *, computerized database of previous test results; SPE, serum protein electrophoresis; α, β, γ, alpha, beta, gamma regions of SPE; TP, total protein; Igs κ, λ, immunoglobulins IgG, IgA, IgM plus kappa and lambda light-chain quantitation; IFE, immunofixation electrophoresis; UPE, urine protein electrophoresis. (Reproduced by permission from Normansell DE. The principles and practice of diagnostic immunology. New York: VCH Publishers, 1994:25.)

detect specific allergic responses and to determine responses to specific immunizations, but it is more likely that these will be sent to a reference laboratory. It may also be necessary to determine IgG or IgA subclass levels, or total or subclass specific responses to immunizations. Again, unless there is a large number of requests for these specific tests, they should be sent to a reference laboratory.

Tumor Markers

Assays for tumor antigens such as prostate specific antigen (PSA-1) and carcinoembryonic antigen (CEA) are often included in the immunology workload. These assays are performed by enzyme immunoassay (EIA) on instruments such as the TOSOH (TOSOH Medics Inc., Foster City, California) for PSA-1 or the AxSym (Abbott Diagnostics, Abbott Park, Illinois) for CEA. Since these instruments are often located in the special chemistry section of the core chemistry laboratory, the immunology laboratory may need to assign only specimen preparation space in the accessioning area. However, it is now common to group special chemistry with the immunology laboratory, because of the similarity of many of the procedures used. In this case, the special chemistry area will need about 20 linear feet of bench space, and about 150 square feet of floor space for the instruments.

Serology and Autoimmunity

This bench performs the majority of the tests in the laboratory, from routine rapid plasma reagin tests (RPRs) for syphilis and antinuclear antibodies (ANAs) for autoimmunity, to immunoblots for antibody to human immunodeficiency virus (HIV). Although it is common to use different methods for each of these tests (**Table 2-3**), and to have separate areas for HIV and hepatitis virus antibodies, for classic serology, and for autoimmune studies, much of this work can now be accomplished by enzyme immunoassay (EIA), with considerable savings in space, effort, and money. A single bench of about 20 feet is sufficient for this area, with two small extra workstations for RPRs and for immunoblots, and a darkroom or dark area for immunofluorescence. The workhorse is a microplate analyzer capable of performing fully EIAs using 96-well microplates. Analyzers available commercially, for purchase or on a reagent rental basis, with alternatives for different laboratory workloads, include the Access and Procession Analyzers (Sanofi Diagnostics/Pasteur, Chaska, Minnesota) and the Labotech Analyzer (Biochem Immunosystems, Allentown, Pennsylvania). EIAs are relatively simple tests, straightforward and accurate, whereas non-EIA tests are labor intensive and subjective. Eventually, as suitable substrates become available, all the non-EIA tests will be converted to EIAs, to take advantage of automation.

One problem faced by many immunology laboratories is that of persuading clinical rheumatologists to accept an EIA panel as an appropriate ANA test. Many institutions are locked into the sequence of an indirect immunofluorescent screening test followed by either an anti-deoxyribonucleic acid (DNA) test on a *Crithidia luciliae* substrate or modified Farr assay for the detection of anti-double-stranded DNA, or by a double diffusion test to detect antibodies to saline extractable nuclear antigens (anti-ENA). These extremely subjective tests should be replaced with a multiantigen EIA panel run on one of the automated microplate analyzers mentioned above. Suitable EIA panel antigens for ANAs are offered by several companies, including Diamedix, GenBio, Incstar, Inova Diagnostics, Sanofi Diagnostics/Pasteur, and Tri-Delta Diagnostics. Some of these companies also carry extensive serology EIA panels.

The newest requirement of the serology bench is to provide estimates of viral load in cases of infection with hepatitis C virus or with HIV. These assays should be performed in a separate work space, either as part of a molecular diagnosis laboratory or as a separate segment of the immunology laboratory.

Flow Cytometry and Tissue Typing

Flow cytometry identifies and enumerates cells in blood and tissue. Its uses are listed in **Table**

TABLE **2-3**

Serology and Autoimmunity

Serology
- Hepatitis viruses
- HIV, HIV immunoblots
- Toxo (IgM and IgG), Rub (IgM and IgG), CMV
- HSV (IgM and IgG), VZV, treponemal tests
- Fungal antibodies
- Viral load

Autoimmunity
- ANA screen and follow-up
- Antithyroid antibodies
- Anti-GBM, ANCA

HIV, human immunodeficiency virus; Toxo, *Toxoplasma gondii*; Rub, rubella (German measles); CMV, cytomegalovirus; HSV, herpes simplex virus; VZV, varicella zoster virus (chickenpox); ANA, antinuclear antibody; GBM, glomerular basement membrane; ANCA, antineutrophil cytoplasmic antibody.

TABLE **2-4**

Flow Cytometry and Tissue Typing

Flow cytometry
- Phenotyping
  - Blood, bone marrow, fluids, biopsy tissue, cells
- Ploidy
- CD4:CD8 ratios
- CD3 enumeration in transplantation
- Detection of anti-CD3 antibodies
- Cell sorting

Tissue typing
- Microcytotoxicity
- Crossmatching
- Flow cytometric crossmatching
- Antigen gene nucleotide sequencing

CD, cluster of differentiation.

2-4. If the laboratory is concerned only with analysis of specimens, and not sorting, one or two benchtop flow cytometers will be sufficient. However, if the laboratory is involved with the isolation and analysis of stem cells, a higher-level flow cytometer is needed. Both Becton Dickinson and Coulter supply models for either purpose. Flow cytometers designed for cell sorting are floorstanding and require a high level of expertise from the operator. Some flow cytometers require access to all sides of the instrument, and some also have specific utility requirements. For maximum productivity, three color staining (4 if possible) of cell surface antigens (termed CD for clusters of differentiation) should be standard. The instruments should be linked into a computer network so that appropriate data can be stored on an optical drive. The average laboratory requires about 20 feet of bench space for sample preparation, slide preparation and staining, centrifuges, computer equipment, and data management. Space is also needed for a safety hood for teasing of biopsy samples.

Phenotyping studies should be performed only after consultation with a Pathology resident, to keep antibody profiles to a minimum. As the number of recognized CD antigens increases, the phenotyping workload will increase. To control this, laboratory staff should attend hematology or flow cytometry rounds, at which recent patient results, and the appropriateness and usefulness of the markers ordered, are discussed with residents, fellows, and attending physicians.

Specialized tests, such as the detection of blocking antibodies to anti-CD3 antibody (used to prevent rejection of a transplanted organ), and the analysis of blood products for stem cells, may be requested, and some flow cytometer laboratories are responsible for reticulocyte counting. The laboratory may also be involved in the preparation of cell populations by cell sorting. Sorting, especially sterile sorting, requires exceptional expertise, and is probably not practical for the average flow cytometer laboratory. However, if the technical expertise is available, there is no reason why it cannot be done.

The immunology laboratory often includes a tissue typing service, which involves identification of the major histocompatibility complex (MHC) class I and II antigens on recipient and potential donor cells, and the detection of antibodies to these antigens. For solid organ transplants, the classical serologic determination of MHC antigens by microcytotoxicity is sufficient. About 20 feet of bench space is needed, together with a sterile hood, incubators, refrigerators and freezers, and centrifuges. Access to a fluorescent microscope and a computer network hookup are also required. When immunocompetent tissue such as bone marrow is to be transplanted, the classical serologic specificities are not adequate, and the nucleotide sequences of the antigen coding genes must be obtained, either by polymerase chain reaction or by direct sequence analysis. These procedures are best left to a separate molecular diagnosis laboratory. Occasionally, mixed lymphocyte culture will be needed; this requires a separate, lockable clean room, with 10 feet of bench space, a sterile hood, cell washing and harvesting equipment, a scintillation counter, and isotope storage facilities.

Crossmatching is the detection in the recipient of antibodies that are reactive with the potential donor cells, and that generally cause graft rejection. The standard crossmatch procedure uses microcytotoxicity, and will detect all but the very lowest levels of antibody. Very low levels of antibody do not affect a primary organ transplant, but can cause rejection of a second transplant in the patient. In this situation, a flow cytometric crossmatch is performed to detect recipient antibodies bound to donor lymphocytes. This assay is 10 to 100 times more sensitive than the serologic procedure.

Hours of Operation and Staffing

In general, the laboratory will be a daytime operation. For the small number of stat procedures, for example, disease testing on potential transplant donors, it is sufficient that technologists are available for call-back during off hours.

Each of the three major areas (immunochemistry, serology and autoimmunity, flow cytometry and tissue typing) should have a supervisor who is responsible for one or more senior technologists, each of whom is in turn responsible for one or more technologists. Because of the number and complexity of tests associated with the laboratory, the technologists need, and must maintain, a high level of technical expertise. This is achieved by a pyramidal structure of responsibility coupled with appropriate cross-training. All technologists should be registered medical technologists, and preferably should have spent one or more years in another division of the clinical laboratories, such as blood bank or chemistry, before joining the immunology laboratory. Cross-training is achieved by having the senior technologists and supervisors in each area spend 2 to 3 weeks per year in each of the other two areas, and by rotating technologists to a different area every 2 to 3 months. After the initial training, all technologists and supervisors should be able to fill in on any of the benches, as needed. The goal is to have a laboratory staffed with cooperating technologists, who, if their own work is finished, will go and help at another bench without having to be asked or directed. Since they are cross-trained, they know how much can be done in each area and can tell when another technologist is struggling under a heavy workload and needs help.

Adequate turnaround time must be achieved whatever the sample load, and therefore the technologists must work well together. Because of this need for close cooperation, recruiting should be a whole laboratory operation; potential technologists should talk to everyone, and everyone should have a say in whether a position is offered. To support morale, it is useful to have a brief laboratory meeting each day, at which each technologist notes any changes, difficult analyses, problems, and so forth, that could affect the laboratory operation. A longer, more general meeting should be held weekly to cover such areas as safety, personnel issues, or problems that might affect all of the laboratories.

Technologists at all levels should attend annual retraining sessions for universal precautions and infection control, fire safety, chemical hygiene, and radiation safety (if needed).

Proficiency Testing and Inspections

Because the results generated by the laboratory are frequently used as a basis for diagnosis and therapy, they must be correct and consistent with other results. To maintain standards in the laboratory it is essential that the laboratory participate in proficiency programs, such as those run by the College of American Pathologists (CAP). These programs provide specimens to be analyzed by the usual procedures in the laboratory. For the proficiency programs to be of any use, the samples must be analyzed as part of a routine run; it is not correct to assign them to the best technologist, or to analyze them more than once and report a consensus result. The purpose of these tests is to determine the effectiveness of the routine runs, by comparing the results obtained with those obtained by others and by selected reference laboratories. This is the only way that the laboratory can determine whether its analyses are providing the correct answers. If results are outside the accepted range, the reason must be found. This is especially important for those tests that contain subjective judgment, such as the interpretation of electrophoresis patterns, where bias may creep in unnoticed. These testing services can also be used to check on the sensitivity of detection of low positives, especially in serology. Although these proficiency tests are expensive, they are the only independent assessment of accuracy and proficiency.

For tests that are not covered by any of these services, other arrangements must be made. One option is to have some samples reanalyzed by another reputable laboratory; another is to select a number of known positive and negative samples and to have someone outside the laboratory code them to make up a proficiency panel for analysis.

The College of American Pathologists also has a program for inspecting and certifying laboratories. Most hospitals require at least a Joint Commission on Accreditation of Health Care Organizations (JCAHO) inspection, but, depending on the services offered by the laboratory, they may also be subject to Health Care Financing Administration (HCFA) and Food and Drug Administration (FDA) inspections. A CAP inspection is an exhaustive analysis of how the laboratory operates. The inspecting team looks at all aspects of the procedures used (whether the reagents are within the shelf life period, whether proper quality controls are included in each run, whether appropriate procedures are detailed for dealing with out-of-range controls, what the laboratory performance has been with proficiency surveys), and at all facets of laboratory safety and training.

Conclusion

The disciplines covered in a modern immunology laboratory overlap considerably, so that results obtained in one area can, and should, be coordinated with those from other areas. One example is a patient whose peripheral blood contains plasmacytoid lymphocytes consistent with Waldenström's macroglobulinemia (by flow cytometry). The serum of this patient may contain a monoclonal spike, usually IgM kappa, by SPE. Another example is the correlation of HIV serology with the CD4:CD8 ratio, and the absolute number of CD4 cells. The coordination of results from different benches is the key to providing accurate results efficiently, and at minimum expense.

CHAPTER 3

The Clinical Laboratory Improvement Act (CLIA) of 1988 and Its Impact on the Immunology Laboratory

KAREN JAMES

History of Laboratory Regulation by the Federal Government

CLIA '67

The original Clinical Laboratory Improvement Act of 1967 (CLIA '67) (1) was intended to regulate and license laboratories involved in interstate commerce where specimens to be tested had crossed state boundaries and were, therefore, outside of control or regulations of state(s) that had developed laboratory licensure or regulations within their state. CLIA '67 did not apply to most hospital laboratories, which, at that time, were not generally performing more than 100 referral tests in interstate commerce per year. A few major medical centers, located in proximity to state boundaries and accepting esoteric testing across state lines, were subject to CLIA '67. Independent commercial laboratories were subject to CLIA '67 regulations not only for interstate commerce but also to receive Medicare or Medicaid reimbursement for testing required to meet Medicare conditions of participation. CLIA '67 regulations primarily specified the credentials (education and experience) required of laboratory testing personnel, supervisors, and directors. The author was responsible for a CLIA '67 licensed hospital laboratory in the late 1970s and found the CLIA '67 regulations to be appropriate and not significantly different from the accreditation guidelines for College of American Pathologists (CAP) accreditation at that time.

CLIA '67 Final Rules

In 1987, several local and national media stories sensationalized a number of horrible (and perhaps preventable) deaths that resulted from poor laboratory practices, primarily involving Papanicolaou (Pap) smears. Since the news stories originated with an NBC affiliate in Washington, DC, members of Congress were immediately aware of the issues. In October 1988, Congress passed CLIA '88 to amend and expand on regulations in effect as CLIA '67. To allow time for committees to thoroughly evaluate the needs for additional laboratory regulation, publication of the new regulations, time for comments, review of comments, and possible revisions based on the comments, Congress stipulated in CLIA '88 an interim set of regulations known variously as the March 14, 1990

Final Rule; CLIA '67 Revisions; or CLIA '67 Final Rules (2).

The CLIA '67 Final Rules immediately applied to all hospital laboratories' requirements for proficiency testing, personnel requirements for technical supervisors and laboratory directors, and requirements for patient test management, quality control, quality assurance, and cytology testing. The CLIA '67 Final Rules also allowed the Department of Health and Human Services (HHS) or its delegate(s) to conduct unannounced inspections of any laboratory at any time during its hours of operation. By far, the most disturbing aspect of the implementation of CLIA '67 Final Rules was the threat of sanctions. Failure to comply with federal regulations could result in severe enforcement procedures that could close the laboratory by limiting or revoking its CLIA certificate, denying Medicare reimbursement for laboratory testing, and/or imposing costly monetary penalties.

TABLE 3-1

Factors Considered in Test Complexity Categories

The degree of risk of harm to the patient if the test is performed incorrectly
The type of tests performed by a laboratory
The degree of independent judgment involved in running the test
The amount of interpretation required to issue a test result
The difficulty of the calculations required to issue a test result
The calibration and quality control requirements of the instruments used in performing the test
The type of training required to operate the instruments used to obtain test results
Any other factors the Dept of Health and Human Services (HHS) considers relevant

SOURCE: US Dept of Health and Human Services, Health Care Financing Administration. Regulations implementing the Clinical Laboratory Improvement Amendments of 1988: proposed rule. Federal Register May 21, 1990;55:20896–20959 (HSQ-176).

CLIA '88

CLIA '88 extended the regulatory scope to *all* laboratory testing, including physicians' office laboratories, clinics, and anywhere else that diagnostic testing is performed (including mobile cholesterol screenings). All CLIA regulations supersede state regulations wherever CLIA requirements are more stringent; however, if state regulations are more stringent, they become the standard. In recognizing the need for ongoing assessment and assignment of complexity category, Congress established the Clinical Laboratory Improvement Advisory Committee (CLIAC). The CLIAC is composed primarily of individuals involved in the provision of laboratory services, use of laboratory services, development of laboratory testing devices or methodologies, and others as approved by the HHS. CLIAC has four subcommittees: cytology; personnel; proficiency testing, quality control, and quality assurance; and test categorization, and is an ongoing advisory board.

Quality Standard Regulations of CLIA '88

Test Complexity Categories

Test complexity categories were designed to consider the factors listed in **Table 3-1** (3). The original categories of test complexity were waivered, moderate complexity, and high complexity. Subsequent to receiving and analyzing comments about test complexity, two more categories have been developed to meet the needs of various laboratories: physician-performed microscopy (PPM) (4), which exempts specific tests performed by physicians and other primary care professionals, and a subcategory of moderate complexity tests termed *accurate and precise technology (APT)* (5).

Certificate of Waiver Tests

Certificate of waiver tests were originally defined in the regulation as simple laboratory examinations and procedures that 1) are cleared by the Food and Drug Administration (FDA) for home use, 2) employ methodologies that are so simple and accurate as to render the likelihood of erroneous results negligible, or 3) pose no reasonable risk of harm to the patient if the test is performed incorrectly. Nine tests were originally defined in the waivered category: dipstick or tablet reagent urinalysis, fecal occult blood, ovulation tests, urine pregnancy tests, erythrocyte sedimentation rate, hemoglobin by copper sulfate, blood glucose by monitoring devices cleared by the FDA for home use, spun hematocrit, and hemoglobin by a self-contained, single analyte instrument. In 1993, CLIAC determined that the criteria for waivered tests should

TABLE **3-2**

Revised Criteria for Waivered Tests

1. Uses direct unprocessed specimens; requires no specimen manipulation before analysis or analyst intervention during analysis.
2. Provides direct readout of results. Quantitative tests must be fully automated while qualitative tests are limited to simple reagent-impregnated devices that produce only a positive or negative result.
3. Contains failsafe mechanisms that render no results when the results are outside of the reportable range or when the test system malfunctions.
4. Requires no invasive test system troubleshooting, or electronic or mechanical maintenance.
5. Contains instructions written at a comprehensive level no higher than 7th grade.

SOURCE: US Dept of Health and Human Services, Health Care Financing Administration. LIA program; categorization of waived tests: proposed rule. Federal Register September 13, 1995;60:47534–47543 (HSQ-225-P).

be better defined and that a process for considering additional tests in the waivered category should be developed. In late 1994, the Centers for Disease Control (CDC) submitted guidelines that can be used to verify the accuracy and precision of testing devices and to demonstrate that the test meets the statutory criteria for waiver, to all manufacturers of moderate-complexity tests (6). The revised criteria for waivered tests are listed in **Table 3-2**. Since the publication of the revised criteria (7), several additional tests have been granted waived status: cholesterol, triglyceride, high-density lipoprotein (HDL) cholesterol, fructosamine, glycosylated hemoglobin, antigens and antibodies to *Helicobacter pylori*, and group A streptococcus from the throat only. For a current list of the tests and manufacturers for waived tests see www.cdc.gov/phppo/dls/waived.htm.

Provider-Performed Microscopy

Provider-performed microscopy (PPM) (4) procedures include wet mounts, potassium hydroxide (KOH) preparations for fungi, pinworm examinations, fern tests, postcoital direct examinations of vaginal or cervical mucus, and urine sediment. Procedures must meet specifications that include 1) examination performed by a physician, 2) procedure classified as moderately complex, 3) primary instrument is the microscope, 4) specimen is labile and delay could compromise the accuracy of the test, 5) no control materials are available, and 6) limited specimen processing is required.

Moderate- and High-Complexity Tests

Moderate- and high-complexity test listings are in a state of almost constant change. Most manufacturers are striving to get their test systems reclassified to moderate complexity. **Table 3-3** shows the most recent (February 1996) criteria for classifying tests as either moderate or high complexity (8). The Public Health Service periodically publishes a list of moderate- and high-complexity tests in the *Federal Register* in a notice with opportunity for comments (7). For new commercial test systems, assays, or examinations, the manufacturer, as part of its 510(k) and premarket approval (PMA) application to the FDA will submit supporting data for device/test categorization. The FDA will determine the complexity category, notify the manufacturers, and inform the Health Care Financing Administration (HCFA) and Center for Disease Control and Prevention (CDC). The Food and Drug Administration will confer with the CDC when categorizing previously uncategorized new technology or if the FDA receives a request for change in categorization from a manufacturer. For test systems, assays, or examinations that are not commercially available, a laboratory or professional group can submit a written request for categorization to the Public Health Service (PHS). If a laboratory test system, assay, or examination does not appear in the lists of tests in the *Federal Register* notices, it is considered to be a test of high complexity until it is formally reviewed.

Accurate and Precise Technology Tests

The accurate and precise technology (APT) (5) tests subcategory is being proposed to encourage manufacturers to produce accurate, easy-to-use test systems for physicians and laboratories to improve test quality and enhance patient care. The HHS believes that many highly accurate, simple, easy-to-use test systems that are currently categorized as moderate complexity could be eligible for less stringent requirements, and laboratories that perform such tests should be provided financial and regulatory relief through a reduction in the CLIA require-

TABLE 3-3

Test Categorization Criteria

Using these seven criteria for categorizing tests of moderate or high complexity, each specific laboratory test system, assay, and examination will be graded for level of complexity by assigning scores of 1, 2, or 3 within each criteria. These scores will be totaled. Test systems, assays, or examinations that receive scores of 12 or less will be ategorized as moderate complexity, while those that receive scores above 12 will be categorized as high complexity.

1. Knowledge
   - Score 1
     A. Minimal scientific and technical knowledge is required to perform the test.
     B. Knowledge required to perform the test can be obtained through on-the-job instruction.
   - Score 3
     C. Specialized scientific and technical knowledge is essential to perform preanalytic, analytic, or postanalytic phases of the testing.
2. Training and experience
   - Score 1
     A. Minimal training is required for preanalytic, analytic, and postanalytic phases of the testing process; and
     B. Limited experience is required to perform the test.
   - Score 3
     C. Specialized training is essential to perform preanalytic, analytic, or postanalytic phases of the testing process; or
     D. Substantial experience may be necessary for analytic test performance.
3. Reagents and materials preparation
   - Score 1
     A. Reagents and materials are generally stable and reliable; and
     B. Reagents and materials are prepackaged, or premeasured, or require no special handling, precautions, or storage conditions.
   - Score 3
     C. Reagents and materials may be labile and may require special handling to assure reliability; or
     D. Reagents and materials preparation may include manual steps such as gravimetric or volumetric measurements.
4. Characteristics of operational steps
   - Score 1. Operational steps are either automatically executed (such as pipetting, temperature monitoring, or timing of steps) or are easily controlled.
   - Score 3. Operational steps in the testing process require close monitoring or control, and may require special specimen preparation, precise temperature control, or timing of procedural steps, accurate pipetting, or extensive calculations.
5. Calibration, quality control, and proficiency testing materials
   - Score 1
     A. Calibration materials are stable and readily available;
     B. Quality control materials are stable and readily available; and
     C. External proficiency testing materials, when available, are stable.
   - Score 3
     D. Calibration materials, if available, may be labile;
     E. Quality control materials may be labile or not available; or
     F. External proficiency testing materials, if available, may be labile.
6. Test system troubleshooting and equipment maintenance
   - Score 1
     A. Test system troubleshooting is automatic or self-correcting, or clearly described or requires minimal judgment; and
     B. Equipment maintenance is provided by the manufacturer, is seldom needed, or can easily be performed.
   - Score 3
     C. Troubleshooting is not automatic and requires decision-making and direct intervention to resolve most problems; or
     D. Maintenance requires special knowledge, skills, and abilities.
7. Interpretation and judgment
   - Score 1
     A. Minimal interpretation and judgment are required to perform preanalytic, analytic, and postanalytic processes; and
     B. Resolution of problems requires limited independent interpretation and judgment.
   - Score 3
     C. Extensive independent interpretation and judgment are required to perform preanalytic, analytic, or postanalytic processes; and
     D. Resolution of problems requires extensive interpretation and judgment.

SOURCE: US Dept of Health and Human Services, Health Care Financing Administration. CLIA program; interpretive guidelines—laboratories: 493.17 test categorization by criteria. Available on the World Wide Web: http://www.os.dhhs.gov:80.

ments, primarily less frequent (random) inspections and fewer personnel requirements. The three primary differences between moderate-complexity categorized tests and APT tests are that field studies must 1) demonstrate that individuals with no formal laboratory training can correctly perform the test, 2) confirm that study participants are able to read and interpret test end points with the same precision as laboratory professionals, and 3) confirm that the performance of study participants is essentially the same as that of laboratory professionals when samples are tested at or near the cutoff and at sufficient distance above and below the cutoff to confirm precision at all analytical decision points. The APT testing category has not been implemented as of 1998. Comments received by HCFA regarding the proposed APT category have not been supportive.

Proficiency Testing Requirements

Proficiency testing (PT) is mandated by CLIA '88 as a method to externally evaluate the quality of a laboratory's performance. PT requirements were phased in to allow time for newly regulated laboratories to learn the PT process without penalties for errors until 1995. There are six specialties of PT, most of which have subspecialties. A list of the HCFA-approved proficiency testing programs is found in **Table 3-4**. Each PT shipment is to include five samples for each analyte or test and the laboratory must participate in three testing events per year. The minimum passing score (subject to change) is 80% with the exception of ABO and D(Rho) typing and compatibility testing, where 100% is required. Failure of any PT event requires documentation of corrective action. A laboratory that fails two consecutive or two out of three testing events will be subject to sanctions for the specialty, subspecialty analyte, or test.

Patient Test Management

Each laboratory that performs APT, moderate-complexity, or high-complexity testing must employ and maintain a system that provides for proper patient preparation; proper specimen collection, identification, preservation, transportation, and processing; and accurate reporting of results. This system must assure optimum patient specimen integrity and positive identification throughout the preanalytic, analytic, and postanalytic processes and must meet the standards as they apply to the testing performed. Standards for issuing corrected reports and retaining original reports are also included.

TABLE 3-4

HCFA-Approved Proficiency Testing Programs (1997)

Accutest
American Academy of Family Physicians
American Academy of Pediatrics
American Association of Bioanalysts
American Proficiency Institute
American Society of Internal Medicine—Medical Laboratory Evaluation
American Thoracic Society
College of American Pathologists—Excel
College of American Pathologists—Surveys
California Thoracic Society
Idaho Bureau of Laboratories
State of Maryland (cytology only)
New Jersey Department of Health
New York State Department of Health
Ohio Department of Health
Pacific Biometrics Research Foundation
Commonwealth of Pennsylvania
Puerto Rico Department of Health
Solomon Park Research Institute
Wisconsin State Laboratory of Hygiene

Quality Control

An overview of the standards for quality control of high-complexity tests is found in **Table 3-5**. Moderate-complexity test requirements for quality control (QC) standards 493.1201 to 493.1218 are less stringent and primarily include following the manufacturer's requirements as cleared by the FDA *unless* the laboratory has modified the test system in any way, in which case the standards for high-complexity tests apply. Standard 493.1219 specifies how to issue and maintain corrected reports, does apply to moderate-complexity testing, and will also apply to APT testing when results of control and calibration materials fail to meet the laboratory's established criteria for acceptability or when errors in reported patient test results are detected. Additionally, specific QC conditions for specialties and subspecialties are included in regulations 493.1223 to 493.1285.

Personnel Standards

There are no personnel standards for waivered tests. For moderate-complexity and APT testing,

TABLE 3-5

Quality Control Requirements for High-Complexity Testing

493.1201 The laboratory must establish and follow written quality control procedures for monitoring and evaluating the quality of the analytical testing process of each method to assure the accuracy and reliability of patient test results and reports.
493.1203 The laboratory will be in compliance if it meets all applicable quality control requirements and follows manufacturer's instructions when using products cleared by the FDA as meeting the CLIA requirements of general quality control detailed in subsequent sections. In addition, the laboratory must comply with requirements that are unique to the laboratory facility and cannot be met by manufacturer's instructions.
493.1202 Standard; Facilities
493.1203 Standard; Test methods, equipment, instrumentation, reagents, materials, and supplies.
493.1211 Standard; Procedure Manual.
493.1213 Standard; Establishment and verification of method performance specifications.
493.1215 Standard; Equipment maintenance and function checks.
493.1217 Standard; Calibration and calibration verification procedures.
493.1218 Standard; Control procedures.
493.1219 Standard; Remedial actions.
493.1204 Standard; Quality control records.

personnel qualifications are defined similarly for the laboratory director, a technical consultant, and a clinical consultant. For both moderate-complexity and APT testing, the minimum standards for testing personnel are a high school diploma and "appropriate training," but the definition of appropriate training for APT testing is limited to training for the specific APT test(s) to be performed, while the personnel qualifications for moderate-complexity testing are broader.

The personnel qualifications for high-complexity testing are more stringent, and include board certification in the specific subspecialty for the laboratory director; technical supervisor qualifications that range from a minimum of a Bachelor of Science degree to doctoral level or board-certified pathologist depending on the subspecialty; clinical consultant and general supervisors who have a minimum of a BS (unless grandfathered); and testing personnel who have at least an Associate's degree or have completed a nondegreed clinical laboratory training program.

Cytology Requirements

The regulations for cytology contain very specific standards, primarily because concern for Pap smear analysis was a major catalyst behind the passage of CLIA '88. Cytology regulations are aimed at individuals as well as laboratories. Proficiency testing for cytology was required in the regulations, but has yet to be accomplished, primarily because of the general unavailability of sufficient glass slides for individual testing. HCFA received 400 comments on computer-based cytology PT programs, but as of 1998 is still evaluating the options. Cytology quality control has been implemented, establishing workload limits, result reporting and confirmation, error detection, slide retention, and comparison of cytology results with clinical information and histopathology results. Cytology personnel standards are the most rigorous, requiring certification for cytotechnologists and technical supervisors. (Certification of testing personnel is not required for any other specialty.)

Inspections

Unannounced inspections by HHS or its designee are specified to assess compliance with all parts of the regulations. Most states with laboratory licensure laws have been granted "deemed status," as have CAP, the Joint Commission on Accreditation of Healthcare Organizations (JCAHO), and the Commission on Office Laboratory Accreditation (COLA).

Enforcement Procedures for Laboratories (9)

Sanctions

In order to ensure the accuracy and reliability of laboratory testing, HCFA may impose sanctions against laboratories for failure to comply with CLIA '88 regulations. Three types of sanctions may be imposed if a laboratory has a "condition level deficiency": intermediate, principal, or civil action. The statute grants broad powers to HCFA to quickly suspend or limit a laboratory's CLIA certificate *and* Medicare payments when deficiencies pose immediate jeopardy to patient care or to the public health. Intermediate sanctions include directing the laboratory to take corrective action within specific time frames. HCFA may require the laboratory to submit the names of its clients to the state survey agency, and may mandate that the state agency notify all clients of the laboratory's deficiencies. It may require the state agency to monitor the laboratory to ensure that it makes the required improvements (the laboratory being assessed the costs of monitoring). Intermediate sanctions may also include the suspension of payment by Medicare for individual tests or for the entire specialty. Additionally, civil monetary penalties can be assessed, with the amount dependent upon the seriousness of the deficiency. Principal sanctions that might be imposed in the case of noncompliance that is determined to pose immediate jeopardy to patients or the public health would include suspension, limitation, or revocation of the laboratory's CLIA '88 certificate. HCFA can also enjoin a laboratory or a person who had owned or operated a laboratory whose CLIA '88 certificate had been revoked from owning or operating a laboratory within 2 years of that revocation.

Laboratory Registry

Once a year, HCFA will publish a list of laboratories 1) on which intermediate sanctions have been imposed showing corrective action taken to achieve compliance; 2) that have had their CLIA certificates suspended, limited, or revoked; 3) that have been excluded from Medicare or Medicaid and the reason for the exclusion; 4) that have had their CLIA certificates suspended, limited, or revoked; and 5) that have been convicted of fraud and abuse activities. HCFA's Laboratory Registry will include a list of persons convicted of violating CLIA requirements and all appeals and hearing decisions.

Applications and User Fees

Certificate Requirements and Application Process

There are currently five types of certificates: 1) *certificate of waiver*, 2) *certificate for PPM procedures*, 3) *registration certificate* to be issued as an interim document to all laboratories that apply for certification as moderate- or high-complexity laboratories, 4) *certificate* issued to laboratories performing moderate- or high-complexity testing that have complied with applicable requirements but whose accreditation has not been verified through on-site inspection, and 5) *certificate of accreditation* issued to laboratories that have met the standards of an accreditation program for moderate- or high-complexity testing approved by HCFA. Laboratories that perform only waived tests must obtain a certificate of waiver, PPM procedures a certificate for PPM, or certificates for any combination of these tests. Laboratories in which moderate- or high-complexity tests are performed must obtain a registration certificate of compliance, valid for a maximum of 2 years, unless they have a state license from a state that is exempt from CLIA '88 regulations. Every laboratory must apply for the appropriate certificate and some may apply for more than one certificate. After being issued a certificate, the laboratory must notify HCFA within 30 days of changes in ownership, name, location, or management personnel, and within 6 months of any change in testing.

Fees

CLIA '88 mandates that laboratories must pay all costs involved in administering the program. Each certificate application must include fees that are assessed and payable biennially. Fees are also assessed for determining compliance (inspections). Effective January 1, 1998, fees were increased and range from $150 every two years for a certificate of waiver to $7940 biennially for a registration certificate for a high-volume laboratory (10). According to HCFA, the increase is needed to eliminate a shortfall in program funds (the CLIA statute requires the program be self-financed). Follow-up visits or complaint inspections will result in fees to pay the costs involved, unless on inspection the complaint was determined not to be justified.

Impact on Immunology Laboratories

Immunology testing must first be defined before the impact of CLIA '88 regulations on the field can be discussed. Review of the *Survey Procedures and Interpretive Guidelines for Laboratories and Laboratory Services* (11), the manual used by CLIA surveyors, indicates that the federal government is defining immunology as Current Procedure Terminology (CPT) codes 86000 to 86849, which includes autoimmune and infectious disease serology [encompassing hepatitis and human immunodeficiency virus (HIV) testing], specific protein analysis, leukocyte function assays, flow cytometry (which can also be found under cytopathology in the CPT coding book), and histocompatibility testing. Although other tests can be included in any given immunology laboratory (e.g., endocrinology or therapeutic drug monitoring), and some of the above tests are more often performed in other laboratories (e.g., hepatitis and HIV testing), for purposes of this discussion immunology is defined as CPT codes 86000 to 86849.

TABLE 3-6

General Immunology Analytes for Which Proficiency Testing Is Required

Alpha-1 antitrypsin
Alpha-fetoprotein (tumor marker)
Antinuclear antibody
Antistreptolysin O—quantitative
Anti–human immunodeficiency virus (HIV)
Complement C3
Complement C4
Hepatitis markers (HB_sAg, anti-HBc, HB_eAg)
IgG, IgA, IgM, IgD, IgE
Infectious mononucleosis
Rheumatoid factor
Rubella

SOURCE: National Technical Information Service. US Dept of Commerce. Survey procedures and interpretive guidelines for laboratory services. PB92-14674.

Test Complexity Categories

The majority of immunology tests were classified as high complexity. The few moderate-complexity tests included pregnancy tests, certain methods for doing specific protein quantitations, allergen-specific immunoglobulin E (IgE) screening systems, dipstick, or closed reagent systems for performing infectious disease serology, including HIV and hepatitis. Because every manufacturer is "retooling" its systems to be moderately complex, the list of moderate-complexity tests increases each time they are published in the *Federal Register*. The most current list of tests and instruments by complexity is available on the World Wide Web (8). The list can be easily downloaded, converted to a format comfortable for the user, and searched. Laboratorians have come to rely on vendor sales representatives to provide information about test complexity. Anyone who wishes to verify vendor claims can obtain the information published in the *Federal Register* at many libraries or can download the information from the World Wide Web at the Government Printing Office's web site: http://www.access.gpo.gov. Additional information about laboratory regulations can be obtained from the web site: http://www.clianet.org, sponsored by the American Association of Clinical Chemistry (AACC)/ Dade Diagnostics.

Proficiency Testing

The primary impacts of the CLIA '88 quality standard on immunology laboratories are the added cost of proficiency testing and the lack of availability of proficiency testing for many analytes tested in the immunology laboratory. Standard 493.837 specifies that proficiency testing be evaluated for the general immunology analytes listed in **Table 3-6**. Most immunology laboratories make every effort to subscribe to proficiency testing programs that include every test performed in their laboratory. It is also important to "share" proficiency testing materials with other laboratory sections that may be performing tests included in that subscription, to save the expense of multiple subscriptions, but also for record-keeping purposes. For example, if the CLIA certificate shows that the laboratory performs alpha-fetoprotein (AFP) tumor markers, but proficiency test results are not included with the remainder of the subscription because that test has been moved to a new instrument in chemistry, an inspector could incorrectly conclude that PT results for that analyte have not been submitted. Not submitting results for an analyte is unsatisfactory performance that results in a score of 0 for the testing event. If this happens twice, the laboratory is subject to sanctions.

Quality Control

Quality control for moderate- or high-complexity tests that use commercially available test systems must follow the manufacturer's specifications for instruments or assays cleared by the FDA as meeting the CLIA requirements for general quality control. If any part of the

TABLE 3-7

CLIA Requirements for General Quality Control that Must be Met for any Test Not Previously Cleared by the FDA

- The laboratory must document the evaluation of
  - Instrument and reagent stability.
  - Operator variance in determining the number, type, and frequency of testing calibration or control materials.
- Test performance must be monitored using calibration materials or control materials or a combination thereof.
- For qualitative tests, the laboratory must include a positive and negative control with each run of patient specimens.
- For quantitative tests, the laboratory must include at least two samples of different concentrations of either calibration materials, control materials, or a combination thereof not less often than once each run of patient specimens.
- For electrophoretic determinations, at least one control sample must be used in each electrophoretic cell and the control sample must contain fractions representative of those routinely reported in patient specimens.
- Each day of use, the laboratory must evaluate the detection phase of direct antigen systems using an appropriate positive and negative control material. When the direct antigen system includes an extraction phase, the system must be checked each day of use using a positive control.
- If calibration materials and control materials are not available, the laboratory must have an alternative mechanism to assure the validity of patient test results.
- Control samples must be tested in the same manner as patient samples.
- Statistical parameters (e.g., mean and standard deviation) must be determined through repetitive testing for each lot of control or calibration material.
- Control results must meet the laboratory's criteria for acceptability before patient test results are reported. (This implies that the laboratory must establish criteria for acceptability.)
- Reagent and supply checks must be performed; e.g., fluorescent stains must be checked for positive and negative reactivity at each time of use.

SOURCE: National Technical Information Service. US Dept of Commerce. Survey procedures and interpretive guidelines for laboratories and laboratory services. PB92-146174.

manufacturer's instructions cannot be met due to unique conditions in the laboratory, the entire list of QC regulations that apply to non-FDA cleared products must be verified and validated. For each method that is developed inhouse, is a modification of a manufacturer's test procedure, or is a method that has not been cleared by the FDA as meeting the CLIA requirements for general quality control, the laboratory must evaluate all of the parameters defined in **Table 3-7**. A more detailed presentation is found in Chapter 9, Method Validation and Verification for High-Complexity and Inhouse (Home Brew) Diagnostic Immunology Tests.

Personnel Standards

If any high-complexity testing is performed in the laboratory, the laboratory director must be an MD or Doctor of Osteopathy (DO) with 1 year of laboratory training during residency or 2 years of experience directing or supervising high-complexity testing, *or* be a PhD with certification in one of the laboratory specialties (e.g., American Board of Medical Laboratory Immunology). Before the enactment of CLIA, immunology testing was often under the direction of MDs with medical board certifications in rheumatology, infectious disease, or hematology/oncology. Individuals who are board certified in medical specialties other than clinical pathology can direct moderate-complexity testing, which is a primary reason why vendors are rapidly developing test systems and instruments for moderate-complexity testing. The laboratory director is responsible for the overall operation and administration of the laboratory, including the employment of personnel who are competent to perform test procedures and to record and report test results promptly, accurately, and proficiently, and for assuring compliance with the applicable regulations. The laboratory director must be accessible to the laboratory to provide onsite, telephone, or electronic consultation as needed. Many other specific duties of a laboratory director of high-complexity testing can be found in standard 493.1445.

For moderate-complexity testing, the CLIA regulations specify that in addition to a medical license and board certification, the laboratory director must have had laboratory training or experience consisting of at least 1 year directing or supervising nonwaivered laboratory testing or 20 continuing medical education credit hours in laboratory practice. According to CLIA regulations, the laboratory director of a moderate-complexity laboratory is not required to be an MD or DO; with appropriate education and experience, individuals with a PhD, MS, or even BS degree qualify to be laboratory directors. PhD laboratory directors of moderate-complexity testing must have either board certification or 1 year of experience directing or supervising nonwaivered laboratory testing. Individuals with MS degrees must have a year of laboratory training and a year of supervisory experience to be qualified as a laboratory director. Persons with BS degrees must have 2 years of laboratory training and 2 years of supervisory experience to be qualified as directors of laboratories in which moderate-complexity testing is performed.

CLIA regulations require that laboratories in which moderate-complexity testing is performed have a technical consultant. The purpose of this personnel qualification is to require that laboratories directed by nonpathologist physicians have access to a clinical laboratory scientist to ensure that the work performed in nonpathology laboratories meets the standards set forth in the regulations. The qualifications of a technical consultant are similar to those of a laboratory director.

In practice, most nonpathology immunology laboratories have been consolidated into pathology laboratories, employing the nonpathologist physicians as clinical consultants in their specialties. The responsibilities of a clinical consultant are to provide clinical consultation, to assist in ensuring that the appropriate tests are ordered and that test result reports include pertinent information required for specific patient interpretation, and to be available for consultation by other physicians regarding the interpretation of test results.

High-complexity testing requires a technical supervisor. The laboratory director can function as the technical supervisor in all areas of the laboratory except histocompatibility and clinical cytogenetics *if* that person is a pathologist who is board certified in both clinical and anatomic pathology. In the subspecialties of cytology, histocompatibility, cytogenetics, and immunohematology, the technical supervisor must be at the doctoral level. In most other subspecialties (chemistry, microbiology, hematology, immunology), the technical supervisor can have a BS with 4 years of laboratory training or experience. The technical supervisor is not required to be onsite at all times, but must be accessible. The technical supervisor is responsible for selection of appropriate test methodology, establishment and verification of test performance characteristics, participation in proficiency testing commensurate with the services provided, and establishment and monitoring of a quality control program, resolving technical problems and so forth, as specified in standard 493.1451.

The laboratory must have one or more general supervisors to provide day-to-day supervision of testing personnel and reporting of test results. A general supervisor must be onsite at all times and may have minimum qualifications of an Associate's degree with 2 years of training or experience. In most immunology laboratories, all qualified staff are listed as general supervisors to ensure that a general supervisor is present onsite at all times that testing is being performed.

Until September 1, 1997, the minimum requirement for testing personnel for high-complexity testing was a high school diploma with documentation of appropriate training in laboratory sciences. Since that date, the minimum qualifications for testing personnel have been an Associate's degree; Department of Health, Education and Welfare (HEW) certification; or 10 years of laboratory experience before January 1, 1968, or possession of a current license in a state that requires personnel licensure. In the author's experience, CLIA personnel standards have had little or no impact on immunology laboratories.

Reimbursement Issues

Technically, reimbursement issues are not part of the CLIA '88 laboratory regulations. Since these issues are not covered elsewhere in this book, they are addressed briefly here. Medicare and Medicaid, as well as many other third-party carriers, base reimbursement on the CPT code assigned to each test. In the author's experience as a laboratory management consultant, often CPT codes are assigned by staff in the financial departments of hospitals with little or no input from laboratory professionals. If there is an exact match in the hospital's charge master test description to the CPT code description, the coding is often correct but still may not be appropriate to legitimately optimize reimbursement. In the area of immunology, many tests have separate CPT codes for screening versus titering a semiquantitative test such as antinuclear antibodies (ANA), antistreptolysin O (ASO), cold agglutinins, rheumatoid factor, or syphilis serology. Additionally, there are two codes that could be used for ANA: 86038 Antinuclear antibodies (ANA) or 86255 Fluorescent antibody; screen, each antibody. In many states, the reimbursement for these two codes is different. The CPT coding book indicates that for Antinuclear antibodies by fluorescent technique, use 86255, 86256 (titer). For many immunology tests, separate charges should be established for each antigen tested (complement, counterimmunoelectrophoresis) or antibody tested (immunofluorescent assay (IFA), antibody to extractable nuclear antigen, flow cytometry for each cell surface marker). Although many of the antibodies to infectious agents have unique CPT code listings, there are "catchall" CPT codes for those not yet assigned: 86313 Immunoassay for infectious agent antigen, qualitative or semiquantitative; multiple step method; 86315 . . . ; single step method (reagent strip); 86317 Immunoassay for infectious agent antibody, quantitative, not elsewhere specified; 86318 Immunoassay for infectious agent antibody, qualitative or semiquantitative, single step method (e.g., reagent strip). To add confusion, alpha-fetoprotein (AFP) and carcinoembryonic antigen (CEA) are coded in the chemistry section of the CPT coding book, but other tumor antigens are to be coded: 86316 Immunoassay for tumor antigen (e.g., cancer antigen 125), each. It is imperative that the laboratory director or technical supervisor of the immunology laboratory review the CPT coding assignments on a yearly basis when the new book is available, and correct the codes if necessary to optimize reimbursement.

The other reimbursement issue that must be addressed in this book for the sake of completeness is the evolving nature of HCFA requirements to reimburse for a test. The National Correct Coding Initiative (NCCI), effective January 1, 1996, specifies that every laboratory test must be justified by an ICD-9 (diagnosis) code or written documentation that justifies the medical necessity for ordering that test. Screening tests are not reimbursed by HCFA, only tests specifically ordered for diagnostic purposes. Although the greatest impact has been on chemistry tests ordered as profiles (now disallowed), the regulations also apply to immunology profiles. Most hospital information systems have insufficient provision for capturing a diagnosis code for each test, and physicians must be re-educated to provide it. The law was reversed, effective January 1, 1998, to require the physician to provide medical information when ordering the test (12).

The impact of the NCCI on immunology laboratories is that all profiles should be considered to be "unbundled"; that is, one should only offer single tests for which the physician must make a clinical judgment regarding the medical necessity and provide a diagnosis code or written description. Alternatively, a single entry level test should be offered followed by additional tests only if indicated, with those follow-up tests coded in response to the results of the initial test, for example, ANA for a suspected diagnosis of systemic lupus erythematosus (SLE) with follow-up tests only if the ANA is positive. However, if the laboratory does reflexive testing based on previous test results, the tests subsequently ordered and charged must be accompanied by appropriate ICD-9 codes. This is certainly a conundrum since managed care organizations often request that laboratories develop reflexive testing to expedite diagnosis and treatment versus HCFA refusing to pay for any testing not accompanied by an appropriate ICD-9 code. The laboratory is caught in the middle, losing revenue whether or not it does the testing. HCFA requirements would seem to be in direct contrast to the managed care environment where payors want testing done efficiently to expedite diagnoses and treatment of patients.

REFERENCES

1. Clinical Laboratory Improvement Act of 1967. Pub L No. 90–174. Regulations found at 42 CFR part 74 implement section 353 of the Public Health Service Act.
2. US Dept of Health and Human Services, Health Care Financing Administration. Laboratory requirements: CLIA '67 final rule and regulations. Federal Register March 14, 1990;55:9538–9610 (HSQ-146-FC).

3. US Dept of Health and Human Services, Health Care Financing Administration. Regulations implementing the Clinical Laboratory Improvement Amendments of 1988: proposed rule. Federal Register May 21, 1990;55:20896–20959 (HSQ-176).
4. US Dept of Health and Human Services, Health Care Financing Administration. Regulations implementing physician-performed microscopy: proposed rule. Federal Register April 24, 1995; 60:20035–20051 (HSQ-216-FC).
5. US Dept of Health and Human Services, Health Care Financing Administration. CLIA program; categorization and certification requirements for a new category of moderate complexity testing: accurate and precise technology: proposed rule. Federal Register September 15, 1995;60:47981–47998 (HSQ-222-P).
6. US Dept of Health and Human Services, Health Care Financing Administration. CLIA Program; categorization of waived tests: proposed rule. Federal Register September 13, 1995;60:47534–47543 (HSQ-225-P).
7. US Dept of Health and Human Services, Health Care Financing Administration. CLIA program; notice of addition of test systems to the waived category: proposed rule. Federal Register July 8, 1996;61:35736–35762.
8. US Dept of Health and Human Services, Health Care Financing Administration. CLIA program; interpretive guidelines—laboratories: 493.17 test categorization by criteria. Available to download in several formats from the World Wide Web: http://www.cdc.gov/phppo/dls/testcat.htm.
9. US Dept of Health and Human Services, Health Care Financing Administration. Medicare program: Medicare and Laboratory Certification Program: enforcement procedures for laboratories: final rule. Federal Register February 28, 1992;57:7218–7243 (HSQ-179).
10. US Dept of Health and Human Services Health Care Financing Administration. CLIA program; notification of fee increase. Federal Register August 29, 1997;62:45815–45821.
11. National Technical Information Service. US Dept of Commerce. Survey procedures and interpretive guidelines for laboratories and laboratory services. 1992:PB92-146174.
12. Balanced Budget Act of 1997. Conference Report to Accompany H.R. 2015. 1997 Section 4317:18.

CHAPTER 

Clinical Immunology Laboratory of the Future

JAMES D. FOLDS

Clinical Immunology and the Clinical Immunology Laboratory

For the last several decades, a considerable effort has been directed at the elusive definition of the discipline of clinical immunology (1,2). Clinical immunology crosses many disciplines of medicine but it is possible to separate, at least to some extent, the practice of clinical immunology into either a medical specialty or a laboratory-based practice, the clinical or diagnostic immunology laboratory. In the medical-based practice, clinical immunologists deal with the study of patients who have disordered immune systems or diseases that require immunologic manipulations. In the laboratory-based practice, the clinical laboratory immunologist is involved in laboratory studies that employ immunologic techniques in the study of disease or evaluate the immune system of patients suspected of having an immunologic disorder. In some cases, the clinical immunologist sees patients and is also responsible for the diagnostic immunology laboratory. In other medical centers, the laboratory may be directed by an MD or PhD with specialized training in immunology. This chapter focuses on the future of the clinical immunology laboratory.

The clinical immunology laboratory and the type and scope of testing performed there vary from institution to institution. **Table 4-1** lists the general categories of laboratory sections found in a modern clinical immunology laboratory (3,4). Probably very few, if any, hospital laboratories offer this broad range of tests in a single clinical immunology laboratory. The actual diagnostic tests provided in the immunology laboratory will vary according to the size and type of hospital and the expertise available within the medical center. In general, most modern clinical immunology laboratories perform infectious disease serology, autoimmune antibody testing, immunochemistry, or basic quantitation of immunoglobulins and complement components C3 and C4 and cellular immunology testing. Cellular immunology testing may include immunophenotyping of blood cells taken from patients with leukemia or lymphoma and possibly lymphocyte subsets from patients with human immunodeficiency virus type 1 (HIV). Assays for lymphocyte, neutrophil, and natural killer cell function can also be carried out within the immunology laboratory. Although histocompatibility testing and allergy testing can be considered in the repertoire of the immunology laboratory, these tests are often performed in other parts of the pathology department or in other departments within the medical center. Molecular diagnosis or molecular pathology is expected to have a major impact on clinical laboratories as well as the diagnostic immunology laboratory. Diagnostic testing using molecular techniques is now offered in many clinical immunology laboratories.

Pressure for Change in the Clinical Immunology Laboratory

Clinical immunology laboratories are components of hospital laboratories and are subject to the same pressures that impact all of medicine and health care in general (5). These constraints

TABLE 4-1

Components of an Idealized Clinical Immunology Laboratory

Infectious disease serology
Autoimmunity testing
Cellular immunology
Flow cytometry
Histocompatibility testing
Immunochemistry
Immunopathology
Allergy testing
Radioimmunoassay
Molecular diagnosis

or forces include new forms of payment for health care services and managed care, cost containment initiatives, governmental regulations, development of point-of-care or bedside testing, and newer and more comprehensive instrumentation and molecular diagnosis. Each of these factors is expected to change the structure and function of the clinical immunology laboratory.

There is a clear and inevitable need for change in laboratory medicine services, and clinical immunology laboratories will be in the forefront of these changes. The driving force is the need to decrease the cost per test to a small fraction of what the cost is today. This will happen by a number of different means from consolidation of laboratory services and the more widespread use of automated instrumentation to the simple elimination of laboratory tests. Ultimately, the changes will be due to the need to decrease the cost per test for laboratory services.

Changes in methods of payment for health care from a fee-for-service format to a prepaid format that started in the early 1980s have had a major impact on health care services and in the provision of clinical laboratory services. In this payment format, health care providers are given a predetermined fee to provide health care for an individual. This fee is usually all inclusive and, with some exceptions, does not provide separate fees for diagnostic tests that may be ordered. The prepaid format requires that the health care provider determines which laboratory tests and other ancillary services are necessary for the care of the patient. Further efforts to reduce the cost of health care through competition and control of utilization will continue to impact health care. As the payment for patient care shifts even further to a capitation per case and per diem payment for inpatient care, the demand will continue for the laboratories to be more efficient and less costly.

Governmental regulations through the Clinical Laboratory Improvement Act of 1967 and the Clinical Laboratory Improvement Amendment of 1988 have impacted all laboratory testing of human specimens. The regulations clearly stipulate personnel requirements for various test categories and mandate interlaboratory proficiency programs and inspection programs by both governmental agencies and professional organizations such as the College of American Pathologists. These regulations add scrutiny to the quality of the tests offered, the location where the tests are offered, and the utilization of the laboratory tests and expected outcomes.

Newer, simpler and more mobile instrumentation is integral to a trend to move testing closer to the patient. This so-called "point-of-care" or "near-patient" testing is important in many types of laboratory services and is resulting in an unprecedented decentralization of the laboratory. In most cases, the point-of-care tests are performed by nonlaboratory personnel but the laboratories are still responsible for the testing. Currently, point-of-care testing does not involve immunology tests but it will in the future. Instrumentation now under development may permit point-of-care immunologic testing for the detection of bacterial or viral antigens and antibodies. Instrumentation for measuring absolute lymphocyte numbers in peripheral blood and that does not require specially trained technologists is available now. It is expected that instruments of this type will permit absolute lymphocyte subset determinations in the clinics near where HIV patients are seen.

Technology and new and more automated instrumentation are playing an important role in changing the immunology laboratory. Instruments under development will use increasingly sensitive detectors that can be modified to detect and quantitate a much broader range of analytes including those that are traditionally performed in the immunology laboratory. For example, the Abbott Diagnostics AXSYM system is capable of performing an extensive menu of tests that includes testing for thyroid function, cancer markers, and therapeutic drug monitors as well as hepatitis antigens and antibodies. This menu is expected to grow and to include many other analytes. This instrumentation, as well as those under development by other manufacturers, may be capable of providing rapid, sensitive, and specific methods to measure analytes previously performed in the immunology laboratory. If more tests are performed on a single instrument, the use of expensive reagents will be less, thereby decreasing the cost. This trend will produce pressure to move laboratory testing to areas of the laboratory where the instruments are located. The tests previously performed in the immunology laboratory may be moved to another laboratory section such as the chemistry or hematology laboratory.

Flow cytometry is another technology that has extensive possibilities for the immunology laboratory. Currently, flow cytometry is used primarily for immunophenotyping of lymphocytes, but newer applications of functional assays for neutrophils and natural killer cells are becoming accepted in many laboratories. More recently, flow cytometry applications have been directed toward detection of intracellular cytokines, detection of bacteria in body fluids, antimicrobial sensitivity testing, and human leukocyte antigen (HLA) crossmatching for transplantations. It is easy to see how tests and assays may flow both into and out of the immunology laboratory depending upon where these tests can be performed more rapidly, more efficiently, and less expensively.

Use of molecular biology techniques is relatively widespread in clinical laboratories (6). These methods are becoming standardized and semiautomated. Molecular methods, in addition to many research purposes, are applicable to a broad range of diagnostic tests. These tests can detect genetic abnormalities and tumor cells, monitor minimal residual disease in cancer patients, and detect infectious agents in body fluids. Molecular biology methods are having a profound impact on the diagnosis of HIV infection by tracking HIV disease progression and evaluating the efficacy of new chemotherapeutic agents. Until recently, the most reliable marker for HIV disease progression was the enumeration of the CD4-positive subset of T lymphocytes by flow cytometry. The availability of the polymerase chain reaction (PCR) and related methods permits the quantitation of viral load in the infected patient. This new method is useful in monitoring the effectiveness of therapy for HIV infection. A PCR-based amplification method [nucleic acid sequence base amplification (NASBA)] is used for the detection of HIV in infants. This is an important advancement in the early detection of HIV infection in infants born to mothers with immunologic evidence of HIV infection. These newer molecular approaches may decrease the need for CD4 enumeration for following HIV infection and thereby decrease the use of the clinical immunology laboratory. This new technology will offer other opportunities for growth of the immunology laboratory.

Overall, these forces for change will be important in shaping the future of the diagnostic immunology laboratory as well as in the discipline of clinical immunology.

The Clinical Immunology Laboratory of the Future

As a result of the pressures listed previously, the clinical immunology laboratory of the future will take on a very different look. The combination of efforts toward cost containment, enlightened test utilization, and new and more versatile instrumentation will lead to diagnostic immunologic tests being performed in areas outside the traditional immunology laboratory. Many serologic tests for infectious disease agents or antibodies, or both, will be performed on a universal analyzer using sensitive fluorescence or chemiluminescent assays. These tests can be done on random-access instruments that are capable of performing tests for drugs, tumor markers, or other analytes in a rapid, cost-efficient manner. It is possible that some of the autoantibody testing and allergy testing currently performed in the immunology laboratory may be moved to the chemistry laboratory or core laboratory facility and performed on specialized analyzers that are already available. The necessity to decrease cost and effectively and efficiently use instrumentation will drive testing into areas of the laboratory where the most versatile instrumentation is available.

Many of the tests in cellular immunology are already performed on flow cytometers that permit three- or four-color analysis. These instruments are frequently located in the immunology laboratory but also may be found in the hematology laboratory or the anatomic pathology laboratories. To justify the cost, these instruments must be available for all testing that is suitable for flow cytometric analysis, including ploidy analysis, reticulocyte assays, HLA crossmatching for transplantation, and possibly for detection of microorganisms, and/or antibiotic susceptibility testing. As these instruments are further developed with more automation and more sophisticated computers and software, flow cytometry will become a more important component of the clinical laboratory.

Molecular diagnosis using various methods for amplification of nucleic acids will also have a major impact on the clinical immunology laboratory. Many of the tests currently performed in the immunology laboratory are prime candidates for molecular biology approaches. To test for the presence of a microorganism by molecular probes may be less expensive than to test for antigens of a microorganism or antibodies directed against it. It may be more timely to look for the presence of the pathogen rather than the immune response directed against the microbial antigens. Automated methods for nucleic acid amplification will increase the usefulness and timeliness of molecular testing, and this will also increase the scope of the methods that are useful in the clinical laboratory.

In this new format for laboratory services, immunology testing may be performed at multiple workstations throughout the main diagnostic laboratory. Quality control may be centralized and performed by individuals who are not necessarily trained as immunologists but who actually have more technology- and instrumentation-based training.

To provide better and more useful data for clinicians, the new generation of laboratory information systems will be capable of providing current data on patients as well as retrieving archival data. This will permit the assimilation of immunologic data from multiple testing sites into a more effective format. The possibility of presenting data in graphic form will make it easier for both the laboratory director and the physician to follow the progress of the patient.

The Role of the Laboratory Director in the Clinical Immunology Laboratory of the Future

The duties of the director of the clinical immunology laboratory will also change in the future. The same pressures that require change in the laboratory will change the role of the laboratory director. These changes will require retraining for both the immunology laboratory director and the technologist. As the diagnostic immunology laboratory tests are moved to new instrumentation and potentially into other sections of the clinical laboratory, the director must provide technical expertise to multiple areas of the clinical laboratory. This may require the director to learn more about new instrumentation and its clinical usefulness in immunology testing and patient care. The director will be responsible for collating and managing patient test results from different sources and preparing useful interpretative reports. This responsibility will become the most important role for the director. Newer and more flexible laboratory information systems should make the collection of data and development of reporting formats possible. The director will be expected to provide professional direction for testing in different laboratory sections and to consult with physicians, trainees, and technologists on issues of interpretation and appropriate use of the immunology laboratory.

Another important and potential new role for the immunology laboratory director will involve managing the utilization of immunology laboratory tests. As the laboratory moves from being a revenue-generating resource to a cost-containment center, it is in the best interest of the laboratorians to work with the physicians and the continuous quality improvement (CQI) teams to develop useful algorithms for appropriate laboratory usage. It is also beneficial to the physicians and the hospital administration to provide necessary testing for the management of the patient. This interaction between the laboratory director, CQI teams, and the physicians will provide important leadership opportunities for the laboratory directors and for better patient care.

The immunology laboratory director must become involved in the selection of instrumentation and testing formats to give reliable and effective immunologic diagnostic services. Opportunities will also become available to develop new reporting formats that contain sequential data and provide data for monitoring therapy.

Summary

The clinical immunology laboratory of the future may not be an identifiable entity; rather it may be a concept or virtual laboratory where the laboratory director finds many of the areas and tests for which he or she is responsible scattered throughout the clinical laboratory. The role of the director will be to assimilate data, develop interpretative reports, monitor utilization, and serve as a technical director in multiple sections of the clinical laboratory. Cost containment, governmental regulations, and newer instrumentation will dictate these changes. These changes will be made possible through the effective use of improved laboratory information systems and by more interaction between the clinicians treating the patients and the laboratorians responsible for diagnostic services.

REFERENCES

1. Rich RR. Whither clinical immunology? J Immunol 1995;55:4992–4995.
2. Clinical immunology—guidelines for organization, training and certification: memorandum from a WHO/IUIS/IAAC1 meeting. Bull WHO 1994;72:543–551.
3. Gaur S, Kesarwala H, Gavai M, et al. Clinical immunology and infectious disease. Pediatr Clin North Am 1994;41:745–777.
4. Hamilton R. The clinical immunology laboratory of the future. Clin Chem 1994;40:2186–2192.
5. Nakamura R, Bylund D. Factors influencing changes in the clinical immunology laboratory. Clin Chem 1994;40:2193–2204.
6. Sever J. Major technological advances affecting clinical and diagnostic immunology. Clin Diag Lab Immunol 1997;4:1–3.

CHAPTER 5

Impact of the Health Care Revolution and Future Role of the Clinical Immunology Laboratory

ROBERT M. NAKAMURA

During the last 20 years, revolutionary advances have been made in the knowledge of diseases mediated by primary or secondary immune mechanisms.

The clinical immunology laboratory is concerned with laboratory tests for the diagnosis and monitoring of diseases mediated by primary or secondary immune mechanisms. The disease categories mediated by immune mechanisms are shown in **Table 5-1**.

The clinical immunology laboratory is also concerned with laboratory tests for the following (1):

1. Infections
2. Acquired immunodeficiency syndrome (AIDS)
3. Retroviral disease
4. Lymphoreticular malignancies
5. Immunogenetics
6. Immunotoxicology
7. Immunopharmacology

Immunotoxicology is a discipline concerned with the effect of foreign substances on host immune mechanisms. These foreign substances can induce susceptibility to infections and tumors in the host. Immunopharmacology is concerned with various humoral mediators involved in immune recognition and end-stage immunologic response (2). These mediators include cytokines, growth factors, interferons, adhesion molecules, and so forth.

The diagnostic immunology laboratory is very much concerned with the newer deoxyribonucleic acid (DNA) and ribonucleic acid (RNA) molecular assays, which are essential for diagnosis, evaluation, and monitoring of therapy of the many diseases mediated by immune mechanisms.

In this chapter, the new health care changes and their impact on the diagnostic clinical immunology laboratory are discussed, as well as the nature and use of clinical laboratory tests. The factors that will influence the future of clinical laboratory tests are listed in **Table 5-2**.

Uses and Characteristics of Clinical Laboratory Tests

The various uses of laboratory tests are listed in **Table 5-3**. The most frequently performed tests are those requested by physicians to make decisions in therapy and monitor the course of disease. Thus, high-volume clinical laboratory tests are those that are necessary for medical care and are used in therapeutic decisions or routine screening, have a rapid assay time and turnaround, and are adaptable to automation (3).

The usefulness of a new clinical laboratory

TABLE 5-1

Categories of Diseases Mediated by Immune Mechanisms

Immunodeficiency diseases
Autoimmune diseases
Allergic diseases
Neoplastic diseases
Transplantation and histocompatibility

TABLE 5-2

Major Factors that Influence the Future of Clinical Laboratory Tests

Governmental regulations
Health care economics
Advances in technology
Advances in therapy

TABLE 5-3

Uses of Clinical Laboratory Tests

Diagnosis of diseases
Early detection and screening of diseases
Genetic classification of diseases
Prognostic markers
Therapeutic decisions
Monitoring and evaluation of therapy

test is how well it differentiates diseased persons as diseased and unaffected persons as unaffected (4).

Diagnostic Versus Evaluation Tests

Diagnostic tests are concerned with the current status of the person being tested. A good diagnostic test will provide an answer to the question: Does the person have the disease now? Also, the diagnostic test should give results that are reproducible over a period of time (4).

On the other hand, *evaluation* tests are concerned with measuring changes in the clinical status or disease activity. A good evaluative test will help determine if a patient's disease status has improved or become worse over a period of time. The evaluative test should be sensitive to change (4,5).

For example, the indirect immunofluorescent microscopy (IFM) test for nuclear and cytoplasmic antibodies is useful for diagnostic evaluation of systemic lupus erythematosus (SLE) or for ruling out the possibility of SLE in the differential diagnosis. However, the IFM test for nuclear cytoplasmic antibodies is a poor evaluative test to monitor disease activity of SLE, since changes in IFM test titer over time correlate poorly with other measures of disease activity.

A laboratory test that may not be important or necessary today may become important in the future when a new therapeutic drug or modality is discovered. For example, oncogene mutation assays, which are often used for clinical investigations, will become useful and important when therapeutic agents that can interfere with activation of oncogenes and prevent tumor become available (1).

Governmental Regulation and Health Care Reform

The evolving changes that are rapidly proceeding in health care are being driven by the need to reduce *costs*. During the 1970s and 1980s, the rate of increase of health care costs did not stop the increases in the cost of living.

The changes in the health care industry have been largely driven by technologic and therapeutic advances and demographic shifting. The state and federal governments are seeking to impose a complex regulatory structure on the health care industry and service delivery system. The new proposals are initiatives to limit cost.

Currently, laboratory charges are approximately 5% of health care billings. There has been a rapid emergence of "managed care." The managed care providers wish to reduce laboratory payments to 1% of health care billings (6).

There are numerous governmental regulations that are attempting to reduce costs and still impose strict regulations to maintain quality control performance standards.

The clinical laboratory is one of the most regulated areas of patient care. The passage of Medicare legislation in 1965 and the implementation of the Clinical Laboratory Improvement Act (CLIA) in 1967 stimulated the development of interlaboratory proficiency survey programs and formal inspection programs by state and federal agencies as well as private organizations such as the College of American Pathologists. Under CLIA '88, regulation has been expanded to physicians' office laboratories and all other sites that involve laboratory testing for humans. The personnel requirements for various test categories have

TABLE 5-4

Criteria for Test Category of Analytes in Immunology

Moderate Complexity	High Complexity
Manual procedures with limited steps	Manual procedures with multiple steps
Automated procedures not requiring operator intervention during analytic process	Immunoassay methods requiring microscopic evaluation
	Radioimmunoassays
	Gel-based immunochemical procedures
	Electrophoresis
	Nucleotide amplification

been defined and the specific responsibilities of the laboratory director and supervisor have been delineated.

Under CLIA '88, many of the analytes in the immunology specialty are classified in both the moderate- and high-complexity categories. The characteristics used to classify the test procedures for these analytes are listed in **Table 5-4** (7). The new regulations and changing health care environment will decrease the demand for per-patient utilization of highly complex and esoteric immunology laboratory tests.

Health Care Economics

The high cost of health care is constantly being addressed today by government and health care providers and the payors (insurance companies).

To help address the current problems, many managed care programs have been developed. The payment for health care has shifted from fee-for-service to prepaid capitation or capitation per case and per diem payment for inpatient hospital services (1,6).

What Is Managed Care?

Peterson and Hilborne (8) have defined managed care as anything that alters or interferes with the traditional autonomous decisions regarding a patient's care that occur between a patient and a physician. The physician's role is changing from one of patient's advocate to one in which the patient's needs and desires are balanced against the need for cost control.

A health maintenance organization (HMO) is a government-qualified prepaid health plan organization and is the model for a managed care health delivery system.

What Is Managed Competition?

By this system, the government sets the rules for the minimum benefits package and establishes criteria for competition, with the goal of a market-based approach to improve access and contain costs in the health care reform program.

Managed competition is expected to encourage health care providers and insurance companies to form alliances, joint ventures, and partnerships to expand and improve current HMOs. The new health care organizations will provide employers with a health plan with a fixed premium and will compete by contract on price, quality, patients' outcomes, and patients' satisfaction (9).

Role of the Clinical Laboratory in Managed Care

Clinical laboratories of the future must comprehend the financial arrangement between clinicians and hospitals and work with the clinicians to increase efficiency, productivity, and reduction of inappropriate testing. In the new managed care plans, the clinical laboratory becomes a cost center, and resources must be carefully managed. Any test performed is a net expenditure; there is no increase in incremental revenue from additional esoteric test ordering since no payment is made per test.

Much of the reimbursement for clinical laboratory tests in the future will be made on a contract basis. Thus, for many hospital laboratories, the charge for a particular test will be reimbursed at a fixed specific amount regardless of the actual cost to produce a particular test result (10).

The clinical laboratory professionals will redefine their role in managed care and must become integral players in the management of patients' care. The clinical laboratory provides important clinical information for an effective mandated care program (8,10).

The clinical laboratory will also be involved in central and near-patient testing, with major efforts focused on patient management, quality improvement, and assessment of the outcome of patient care (8,10).

Immunology Laboratories

In the future, there will be different types of immunology laboratories: acute care (hospital laboratories), primary reference laboratories, and secondary reference laboratories. These will be geared to provide different tests, depending on turnaround time requirements for diagnostic and therapeutic evaluation. The highly complex tests that do not require a rapid turnaround time will be decentralized and performed in the reference laboratories. Centralization of tests will offer advantages of cost effectiveness and higher volume. A secondary reference laboratory can perform the more esoteric low-volume tests.

Advances in Technology

The new technologic advances that are likely to bring about many changes in the immunology laboratory are shown in **Table 5-5**. Some of these advances are discussed below.

Recombinant DNA Technology

Recombinant DNA technology has led to the development of many new applications in clinical immunology and medicine. Many nucleotide probe assays have been developed for diagnosis and monitoring of infectious diseases, genetic diseases, immune-mediated diseases, and cancer. The Human Genome Project is likely to progress rapidly, and already gene therapy has become a reality (1). Many new laboratory tests will be needed to evaluate and monitor the immune diseases treated with gene therapy (11,12).

TABLE **5-5**

Technological Advances that Influence the Future of Immunology Laboratories

Design of antibodies (combined monoclonal and recombinant DNA technology)
Rapid, automated solid phase and homogeneous immunochemical assay instruments
DNA/RNA probe tests and amplification systems, such as PCR
Synthetic peptides
Biosensors
Supercomputers with image storage and retrieval
Cellular immune assays, cytokines, adhesion molecules

Synthetic Peptide Technology

With the advances in recombinant DNA technology, DNA can be cloned and sequenced easily, rapidly, and accurately. The translation of nucleotide sequences into amino acid sequences has become commonplace (3). Since the amino acid sequences of many proteins are in computer programs, one can obtain the unique specific peptide structures of a virus, protein, hormone, and so forth. The peptide can be selected for its hydrophilic, hydrophobic, and antigenic properties and a specific monoclonal antibody can be produced. A monoclonal antibody to a specific peptide can then be produced.

Numerous peptides have been identified as neurotransmitters and brain hormones. Besides medical therapeutic uses, the synthetic peptides are helpful in developing specific diagnostic assay kits for use in infectious and many other diseases. Synthetic peptide immunoassays have been developed to detect human immunodeficiency virus (HIV) and especially to identify specific infections caused by HIV-1 and HIV-2 subspecies (13).

Biosensors

Biosensors can be defined as devices consisting of a synergistic combination of biochemistry and microelectronics that simplify biochemical and chemical analysis on a micro or macro scale (14,15). Some biosensors do not contain an immobilized biologic material, for example, gas sensory electrodes.

There are four main types of biosensors (14): 1) small handheld devices, 2) the bench-type analyzer or multisample automated analyzer, 3) flow devices (bioreactors) for online monitoring of continuous processes, and 4) the continuous in vivo or implanted monitor. The trend today is toward miniaturization of biosensors. In the future, data from small biosensors used at the point of care will be sent to central laboratory computers by wireless means.

Supercomputers

Computers of the future will report laboratory data by graphics with retrieval of previous data on the same patient. Thus, trends and changes in the specific analyte will readily be seen by the clinician. Future reports will be in a consultative format with interpretative information, and many of the immunology laboratory tests will help monitor the innovative complex forms of therapy and will require reporting of information beyond the level of the specific analyte (3).

Besides interpretative profiling of laboratory tests, the technology will allow extensive image storage and retrieval and transmission of pictures and data. This will have an impact in the area of anatomic pathology with image analysis and immunohistochemical analyses.

Today, a wide variety of computational chemistry and computer molecular modeling techniques are used for optimization of drug design (16). The use of computers in designing drugs will speed the progress of development of new therapeutic drugs in the future.

Cellular Immune Assays, Cytokines, and Adhesion Molecules

Cellular Immune Assays

Technologic instruments will be developed so that cellular marker assays will become routine in most hospital laboratories. These cellular markers and receptor assays will be necessary for evaluation of diseases and monitoring the future therapeutic modalities. Flow cytometry and image analyzers will be common instruments in an immunology laboratory (1).

Cytokines

Considerable advances in cellular immunology have been achieved through various in vitro studies of isolated lymphocytes or macrophages under very defined conditions. These studies have shown that all stages of development, growth, proliferation, and activation are regulated and influenced by the intracellular elaboration of numerous cytokines. Cytokines are signaling molecules involved in communication between cells. These are polypeptide products of activated cells that influence the state of activation, proliferation, and differentiation (2).

Cytokines are releasing during the effector phase of cellular stimulation and are important in translating immune recognition. A particular cytokine produced by one cell type may affect the production of cytokines by other cell types. The various types of cytokines are involved in immunoregulation and hematopoietic blood development. Several have been cloned and are being used for therapeutic purposes.

Interferons

Interferon (IFN) was discovered more than 30 years ago by Isaacs and Lindenmann (17), who observed that virus-infected cell cultures produced a protein that reacted with cells to render them resistant to infection by many viruses. The three major IFN classes present in mammalian species are leukocyte IFN-alpha, fibroblast IFN-beta, and immune IFN-gamma. The IFNs are one of the body's natural responses to microbes, tumors, and antigens, and induce antiviral, antimicrobial, and immunomodulatory activities.

Cell Adhesion Molecules

Four families of cell adhesion molecules (CAM) have been identified (18):

1. *Immunoglobulin supergene family* (19): ICAM (intercellular adhesion molecules) and VCAM (vascular CAM) on endothelial cells. This group of adhesion molecules is involved in cell-cell adhesion required for inflammation. The members are characterized by the presence of one or more immunoglobulin superfamilies, VCAM-1 and ICAM-1, and are ligands for leukocyte integrins.
2. *Selectins.* Selectins are a recently described family of adhesion proteins that appear on endothelial cells, platelets, and leukocytes (19). They have various numbers (2 to 9) of complementary regulatory repeats, an epithelial growth factor–like domain, and an amino terminal lectin domain. One known member is L-selectin, a lymphocyte homing receptor. The natural ligands of selectins are the carbohydrate moieties of glycoproteins to which they bind via N-terminal lectin domains.
3. *Cadherins* (20). Present on most cells, cadherins are a molecular family that is essential for the calcium-dependent process of cell-cell adhesion.
4. *Integrins.* Integrins can be divided into three groups on the basis of their binding properties (21,22): 1) cell-cell adhesion molecules, 2) those that bind to basement membranes, and 3) those that bind to matrix proteins of

inflammation, wound healing, and development. Integrins are important in tumor progression of many epithelial cancers and melanomas (23).

Recently, two unrelated cases of congenital defects in adhesion molecules have been reported, resulting in leukocyte adhesion deficiency with a clinical history of recurrent bacterial infections (24). In these cases, the neutrophils have severe adhesion and motility defects.

Criteria for Evaluation of Diagnostic Technology

Most new diagnostic technologies have not been adequately assessed to determine whether their application improves health (25). Guyatt et al (26) have presented guidelines to evaluate diagnostic technologies to determine the range of possible uses, diagnostic accuracy, impact on the health care provider, therapeutic impact, and impact on patient outcome. The criteria are listed in **Table 5-6**.

Advances in Therapy

High-volume immunology laboratory tests are needed to monitor therapy and to make medical treatment decisions. Many advances have been made in the therapy of immunologically mediated diseases, some of which are discussed below.

TABLE 5-6

Criteria for Evaluation of Diagnostic Technology

Technologic capability: The ability of the technology to perform to specifications in a laboratory setting has been demonstrated.
Range of possible uses: The technology promises to provide important diagnostic information in a number of clinical situations.
Diagnostic accuracy: The technology provides information that allows health care workers to make a more accurate assessment regarding the presence and severity of disease.
Impact on health care providers: The technology allows health care workers to be more confident of their diagnoses and thereby decreases their anxiety and increases their comfort.
Therapeutic impact: The therapeutic decisions made by health care providers are altered as a result of application of the technology.
Patient outcome: Application of the technology results in benefit to the patient.

SOURCE: Guyatt GH, Tuguell PX, Feeny DH, et al. A framework for clinical evaluation of diagnostic techniques. Can Med Assoc J 1986;134:587–594.

Therapeutic Immunosuppression in Autoimmune Diseases and Transplantation

With nonspecific immunosuppressive treatments of autoimmune disease, there are different levels of interaction (27,28): corticosteroids, which suppress autoimmune reactions and reduce inflammation; chemical immunosuppressive drugs, such as cyclophosphamide; and cyclosporins and FK506. The newer and future therapeutic modalities involve T-cell vaccination; monoclonal antibodies to CD3, CD4, T-cell receptors (TcR), and class II major histocompatibility center (MHC) molecules; and peptide therapy for blocking of antigen to MHC molecules (**Table 5-7**).

The specific targets of the therapeutic agents in autoimmune disease involve immune recognition and antigen processing. The normal immune system recognizes invading foreign molecules by three different types of recognition structures: immunoglobulins, TcR, and glycoprotein products of the MHC (29). The first two types are found only on lymphocytes, whereas the MHC glycoproteins (class I) are present on the surface of all nucleated cells of the body. Each of the fully developed lymphocytes expresses a specific and unique immunoglobulin or TcR, whereas all of the cells of the same host express the same MHC gene products (30).

Cell Adhesion Molecules and Therapeutic Modalities

Different classes of therapeutics are being developed to treat a wide variety of diseases: CAM expression blockers, which prevent the

TABLE 5-7

Newer Therapeutic Modalities in Autoimmune Diseases

T-cell vaccination
Monoclonal antibodies to CD3, CD4, T-cell receptors
Class II (MHC) monoclonal antibodies
Peptide therapy for blocking antigen to MHC molecules

production of CAM and its expression on cell surfaces; CAM binding blockers, which bind to cell surface CAMs and block binding to receptors or ligands; anti-CAMs, including anti-CAM antibodies, soluble CAM proteins, or peptide analogs; and CAM-ligand analogs, which promote cell-matrix adhesions (18).

Interferon Therapy

Recent advances have led to Food and Drug Administration approval of five clinical indications for IFNs. IFN-alpha is approved for the treatment of hairy cell leukemia, condyloma acuminatum, Kaposi's sarcoma in acquired immunodeficiency syndrome (HIV), and hepatitis C. Also, IFN-gamma has been approved as an immunomodulatory treatment of chronic granulomatous disease (31).

Promising clinical results with IFNs have been reported for basal cell carcinoma, chronic myelogenous leukemia, cutaneous squamous cell carcinoma, early HIV infection, hepatitis B, and laryngeal papillomatosis (31). One would anticipate that future therapies and uses of IFNs can be combined with other agents such as cytokines and hormones, and other therapeutic methods such as radiation and surgery.

Multiple sclerosis is a common neurologic disease and the present consensus is that damage to the nervous system results from immunologic processes (32). Various experimental modes of immunosuppression and new therapies for autoimmune disorders are being studied in cases of multiple sclerosis. IFN-beta 1b was effective in cases of relapsing-remitting multiple sclerosis (32).

Gene Therapy

Gene therapy in human diseases has been proved successful. The first attempts to treat two children with adenosine deaminase immunodeficiency and an adult woman with familial hypercholesterolemia are proving effective (33). In October 1992, on the second anniversary of therapy, both girls whose deficiencies were treated with gene therapy demonstrated functioning immune systems. Currently, approximately 17 biotechnology companies are directly involved in gene therapy work (34).

Gene therapy can be a curative therapy for certain genetic diseases with monogenic disorders of metabolism. Also, gene therapy can be aimed at treating acquired diseases by delivering novel therapeutic proteins, such as cytokines, in cases of cancer (35).

Cancer Gene Therapy in Humans

Genes that encode tumor necrosis factor (TNF) or IL-2 have been transferred into tumor cells in the hope that secretion of these cytokines will stimulate a tumor-specific immune response that results in tumor destruction at other sites or that will allow collection of tumor-infiltrating lymphocytes from adjacent lymphoid tissue (35).

Immunotherapy in Cancer

Over the past several years, cancer immunotherapy has undergone many innovative strategies with periods of optimism and disappointments.

The current immunotherapy strategies include 1) active specific immunotherapy (36), involving treatment of cancer patients with tumor vaccines; 2) active nonspecific immunotherapy with cytokines, involving the use of cytokines such as IL-2; 3) adaptive immunotherapy (lymphokine-activated killer cells and tumor-infiltrating lymphocytes); and 4) chemoimmunotherapy.

More recently, an effective approach has been discovered to treat a certain number of patients with melanoma (37). The gene MAGE-1 (melanoma antigen-1) encodes an MHC class I human leukocyte antigen (HLA)-A1–restricted epitope that is recognized by cytotoxic T lymphocyte (CTL) isolated from HLA-A1–positive patients. MAGE-1 is expressed in high amounts in 40% of melanomas as well as other tumors and in low amounts in melanocytes and other tissues. It can be used in appropriate form (peptide, transfected antigen-presenting cells, retroviral vector, or naked DNA) to develop a vaccine that may be effective in more than the 10% of patients with melanoma who carry HLA-A1.

Novel Anticancer Agents

An early step in maturation of the *ras* oncogene is the transfer of the farnesyl group from farnesyl diphosphate, a cellular chemical used to synthesize cholesterol, to the protein by the enzyme farnesyltransferase (38). The mature *ras* protein then moves to the cell's inner membrane edge, and the farnesyl group is the molecular hook to attach the mature *ras* protein. Several groups have discovered compounds that will inhibit the attachment and block the farnesyl group of the ras protein and restore normal growth patterns to cells that express a *ras* oncogene (38).

Future Perspectives and Conclusions

In the future, the immunology laboratory will provide tests on a disease-oriented basis, rather than by assay methodology. The laboratorian will perform the humoral and cellular immune tests as well as the nucleotide tests needed for the evaluation and monitoring of immune-mediated diseases.

Also, the future immunology laboratorian will perform complex assays to help monitor the new therapeutic options. The laboratory scientists will work closely with the clinicians and provide interactive consultative information. There will be a trend toward 1) centralization of complex immunologic and nucleotide probe assays, which may require a 1-day turnaround time or longer; 2) decentralization of tests, which are important for monitoring of critical care patients in intensive care, heart, or transplantation surgery; and 3) decentralization of high-volume tests to alternative sites such as the patient's bedside or the physician's office. The tests that are urgently needed for medical treatment decisions will be rapidly transferred when the biosensors become available.

Most of us agree that the major factors that will influence the future of the immunology laboratory will be government regulations, economics of health care, technology, and advances in therapy. New diagnostic technologies should be used to provide a better understanding of disease processes with the prospect of more effective treatments.

However, there are many ethical issues in genetic testing and screening (39). A negative aspect of new technologic developments is that some health care providers may be tempted to use new diagnostic tests to serve their own economic and administrative purposes. However, new diagnostic techniques can also be used to predict late-onset genetic diseases and behavioral disorders, thus reflecting the strategies of the health care providers to reduce costs, minimize the risk of malpractice suits, and plan for the efficient use of health care resources (40).

In the future, there will be a focus on preventive medicine. This will place emphasis on predictive tests to screen for data that will identify important population phenotypes that represent risk factors (5,41). One can foresee application of tests to identify genes in patients predisposed to autoimmune diseases.

Autoimmune diseases (AID) are usually revealed at a late stage of their natural history, and immunointervention is only used when all other treatments have failed. This should be changed in the future by the early prediction of disease onset using genetic tests and immunologic markers. Early identification of patients at risk will allow intervention with autoantigen-specific therapy. Experimental models of spontaneous AID show that, at these early stages, the autoimmune response is much more sensitive to immunointervention than in the late stages, when immunosuppression is presently applied in human diseases (41). It is also obvious that such early intervention prevents the occurrence of the irreversible lesions that characterize advanced autoimmune diseases (5,41).

The discovery of immunologic tests that allow prediction, early diagnosis, or prognosis of AID is a matter of intensive research. The most spectacular progress has been achieved in insulin-dependent diabetes mellitus (IDDM) (42), in which islet cell autoantibodies can be found several years before the onset of clinical disease (as defined by insulin requirement). The quality of prediction is sufficient to enable recognition of future diabetics with a reliability that approaches greater than 80%. It remains true, however, that some diabetics never show the presence of islet cell antibodies (ICAs: GAD, IA2, ICA-69 antibodies) whatever the antibody assay used and that some ICA+ subjects fortunately never become diabetic. One can assume that the inclusion of a T-cell assay would improve the quality of prediction inasmuch as the disease is apparently exclusively mediated (41).

REFERENCES

1. Nakamura RM, Bylund DJ. Factors influencing change in the clinical immunology laboratory. Clin Chem 1994;40:2193–2204.
2. Burrell R, Flaherty DK, Sauers LJ. Toxicity of the immune system—a human approach. New York: Van Nostrand Reinhold, 1992.

3. Nakamura RM, Bylund DJ. New developments in clinical laboratory molecular assays. J Clin Lab Anal 1992;6:73–83.
4. Ward MM. Evaluative laboratory testing. Assessing tests that assess disease activity. Arthritis Rheum 1995;38:1555–1563.
5. Osterland CK. Laboratory diagnosis and monitoring in chronic systemic autoimmune diseases. Clin Chem 1994;40:2146–2153.
6. Young DS, Bruns DE, Doumas BT, Valdes R. The future of clinical chemistry and its role in healthcare: a report of the Athena Society. Clin Chem 1996;42:96–101.
7. Abbott DB, Homburger HA. HHS categorization of CLIA tests systems in laboratory immunology. Clin Immunol Newsletter 1993;13:9–11.
8. Peterson P, Hilborne LH. Facing managed care's challenge to pathology. Am J Clin Pathol 1993; 99(suppl):S3-S6.
9. Cohen C. View from Washington—reimbursement and regulatory trends. Am J Clin Pathol 1993;99(suppl):S17-S21.
10. Skootsky SA, Oye RK. The changing relationship between clinicians and the laboratory medicine specialist in the managed care era. Am J Clin Pathol 1993;99(suppl):S7-S11.
11. Anderson WF. Human gene therapy. Science 1992;256:808–813.
12. Mulligan RD. The basic science of gene therapy. Science 1993;260:926–932.
13. Smith RS, Parks DE. Synthetic peptide assays to detect human immunodeficiency virus types 1 and 2 in seropositive individuals. Arch Pathol Lab Med 1990;114:254–258.
14. Gronow M. Biosensors. Trends Biochem Sci 1984;9:336–340.
15. Rechnitz GA. Biosensors. Chem Eng News 1988;66:24–36.
16. Dixon JS. Computer-aided drug design: getting the best results. Trends Biotechnol 1992;10: 357–363.
17. Isaacs A, Lindenmann J. Virus inference I: the interferon. Proc R Soc Lond [Biol] 1957;147: 258–267.
18. Sherman-Gold R. Companies pursue therapies based on complex cell adhesion molecules. Genet Eng News 1993;7(July 6):14.
19. Cronstein BN, Weissmann G. The adhesion molecules of inflammation. Arthritis Rheum 1993;36:147–157.
20. Takeichi M. Cadherins: a molecular family important in selective cell-cell adhesion. Annu Rev Biochem 1990;59:237–252.
21. Ruoslahti E, Pierschbacher MD. New perspectives in cell adhesion: RGD and integrins. Science 1987;238:491–497.
22. Cheresh DA. Structural and biologic properties of integrin-mediated cell adhesion. Clin Lab Med 1992;12:217–236.
23. Albeda SM. Role of integrins and other cell adhesion molecules in tumor progression and metastasis. Lab Invest 1993;68:4–17.
24. Etzioni A, Frydman M, Pollack S, et al. Brief report: recurrent severe infections caused by a novel leukocyte adhesion deficiency. N Engl J Med 1992;327:1789–1792.
25. Berger ML, Hillman HL, Bryan R, et al. Economic analysis of health care technology: a report on principles. Ann Intern Med 1995;122:61–70.
26. Guyatt GH, Tuguell PX, Feeny DH, et al. A framework for clinical evaluation of diagnostic techniques. Can Med Assoc J 1986;134:587–594.
27. Bach JF. Monoclonal antibodies and peptide therapy in autoimmune diseases. New York: Marcel Dekker, 1993.
28. Hoffman ES. Immunosuppressive therapy for autoimmune diseases. Ann Allergy 1993;70:263–274.
29. Nakamura MC, Nakamura RM. Contemporary concepts of autoimmunity and autoimmune diseases. J Clin Lab Anal 1992;6:275–289.
30. Rose NR. The concept of autoimmunity and autoimmune disease. In: Krawitt EL, Wiesner RH, eds. Autoimmune liver diseases. New York: Raven, 1993:1–20.
31. Baron S, Tyring SK, Fleischmann R, et al. The interferons—mechanisms of action and clinical applications. JAMA 1991;266:1375–1383.
32. Sibley WA, Ebers GC, Panitch HS, Reder AT. 1FND multiple sclerosis study group. Interferon beta 1b is effective in relapsing-remitting multiple sclerosis. 1. Clinical results of a multicenter, randomized, double-blind, placebo-controlled trial. Neurology 1993;43:655–661.
33. Thompson L. At age 2, gene therapy enters a growth phase. Science 1992;258:744–746.
34. Dodet B. Commercial prospects for gene therapy—a company survey. Trends Biotechnol 1993;11:182–189.

35. Sikora K. Gene therapy for cancer. Trends Biotechnol 1993;11:197–201.

36. Livingston P. Active specific immunotherapy in the treatment of patients with cancer. Immunol Allergy Clin North Am 1991;11:401–423.

37. Boon T. Teaching the immune system to fight cancer. Sci Am 1993;268:82–89.

38. Travis J. Novel anti-cancer agents move closer to reality. Science 1993;260:1877–1878.

39. Durfey SJ. Ethics and the human genome project. Arch Pathol Lab Med 1993;117:466–469.

40. Nelken D, Taneredi L. Dangerous diagnostics—the social power of biological information. New York: Basic Books, 1989.

41. Bach JF. Predictive medicine in autoimmune diseases: from the identification of genetic predisposition and environmental influence to precocious immunotherapy. Clin Immunol Immunopathol 1994;72:156–161.

42. Palmer JD. Predicting IDDM (insulin dependent diabetes mellitus) use of humoral markers. Diabetes Rev 1993;1:104–115.

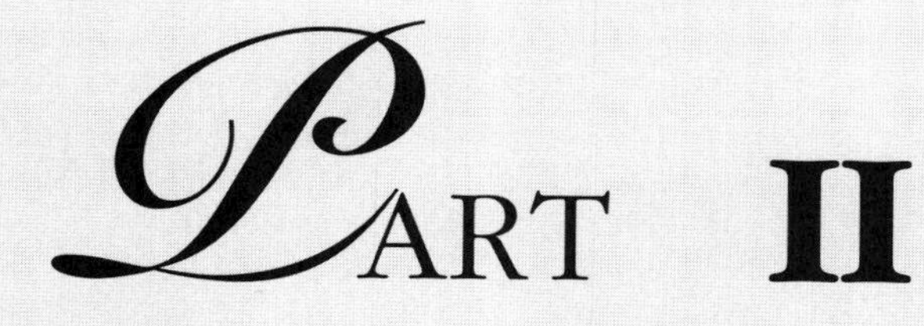

Part II

Present Concepts of Quality Assurance, Quality Control, and Standardization

LINDA COOK, EDITOR

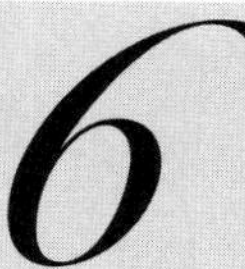

CHAPTER 6

Principles of Quality Assurance and Quality Control in the Clinical Immunology Laboratory

LINDA COOK

The primary goal of all clinical diagnostic laboratory testing should be to generate accurate and reproducible laboratory test results. All activities performed to monitor the quality of laboratory testing are referred to as quality control (QC). The most common aspect of quality control in the laboratory has a focus on the technical aspects of the testing process. A second, much broader aspect of quality in laboratory testing has been referred to as quality assurance (1). Quality assurance encompasses quality control but also refers to the myriad of other components of the entire process, such as physician ordering practices, response to laboratory data, clarity of reports and interpretive statements, appropriateness of testing methods, and continuing education efforts. Current management strategies as described in quality circles, total quality management (TQM), and continuous quality improvement (CQI) programs, which focus on all aspects of testing, can also be applied in clinical immunology laboratories to improve testing systems (2–4). Each clinical immunology laboratory should establish its quality program by applying quality control principles to all aspects of its service. The program should include the following key elements:

A. Personnel
  1. Acceptable hiring practices and verification of credentials
  2. New employee training programs and documentation
  3. Continual monitoring of testing performance (competence)
  4. Continuing education
  5. Training in performance of new testing procedures
  6. Continual compliance with all laboratory safety regulations and yearly review
  7. Thorough and effective computer training and subsequent competence

B. Instrumentation
  1. Selection of appropriate instrumentation based on testing to be done, required turnaround times, instrument performance, and test characteristics
  2. Comprehensive training provided by instrument manufacturers
  3. Thorough training of all technologist staff
  4. Continuous performance of acceptable preventive maintenance procedures for all instruments, including pipets, centrifuges, water baths, and so forth
  5. Preventive maintenance at periodic intervals
  6. Ongoing validation of correct function of instrument computer interfaces

C. Test procedures
  1. Selection of new test methods
     a. Comparison with accepted methods and results
     b. Documentation of evaluation procedures
     c. Linearity and recovery studies

2. Continuous validation of all purchased reagents
3. Checks of inhouse prepared reagents
4. Periodic calibrations and validation of acceptable calibrations of instruments
5. Validation of acceptable standard curves at accepted intervals
6. Daily performance of quality control checks with appropriate materials
7. Negative controls, positive controls, and controls with established values as appropriate
   a. Blind replicate testing (within run)
   b. Control materials run blinded
   c. Samples run on previous runs rerun blinded
8. Periodic review of all quality control results
9. Review of patient data for normal range and technical failures
10. Comparison of patient data to previous data where available
11. Maintenance and verification of computer functions (analysis software on plate readers, QC ranges and calculations in instrument and lab computers)
12. Proficiency testing
13. Interlaboratory testing validation for assays where Clinical Laboratory Improvement Act/College of American Pathologists (CLIA/CAP) approved proficiency testing is not available

D. External issues
1. Physician interactions
   a. Establishment of effective communication lines with laboratory personnel
   b. Involvement during initial test evaluations
   c. Continuous educational efforts at rounds and conferences
   d. Monitoring of verbal and written questions from physicians and support staff
   e. Effective discussion of unusual patients and laboratory data
   f. Establishment of alert laboratory values, and clearly defined procedures for follow-up and notification to physicians
   g. Clearly defined policies for additional follow-up testing when medically indicated
2. Nursing staff and other personnel interactions
   a. Maintenance of laboratory procedures within nursing manuals
   b. Effective communication of sample collection and identification requirements
3. Computers
   a. Test definition and ordering strategies
   b. Computer monitoring of patient and quality control data
   c. Validation of instrument-computer interfaces
   d. Validation and periodic monitoring of computer calculations
   e. Maintenance of computer result failure checking (normal ranges, technical failures, delta checking of repetitive patient samples)
   f. Clear, complete, and prompt reporting of results
   g. Routine monitoring for computer entry errors
   h. Simple and rapid methods for modification of results
4. Patient samples
   a. Sample collection, identification, storage, and handling procedures
   b. Criteria for acceptable samples, sample rejection policies

As can been seen by the previous list, a large number of systems need to be established and maintained in order to perform all these aspects correctly and to ensure testing quality. Since many of these issues are common to all clinical laboratories, the systems are frequently established and monitored by personnel with laboratory-wide quality control and safety responsibilities. However, there are a variety of unique aspects to immunology testing that require different quality assurance strategies than those found routinely in chemistry or hematology laboratories. Some of these are test specific, others are quality control related, and some are educational in nature.

Test-Specific Issues

Immunoassay methods currently used in autoimmune and infectious diseases are very complex and inherently more variable than other laboratory tests. A number of factors significantly contribute to this variability. First, the clinically important epitopes for most of the antigens used have not been well defined. The antigens used for routine test kits, with a few exceptions, are large macromolecular complexes that contain a variety of antigenic sites in which the three-dimensional structure may be of critical importance. The antigen complexities lead to major differences in the reactivity of the antigen substrates with serum samples from patients who present with the same clinical symptoms. This antigenic variation also leads to significant differences in results obtained from different manufacturers' kits. This is demonstrated in **Figure 6-1**, in which the amount of rheumatoid factor as determined by two different methods is compared. This lack of agreement between methods is commonly seen with many clinical immunology tests, and results in significant difficulties during initial evaluations of new tests and during changes to testing methods. Thus, new test evaluations and methodology changes require the parallel testing of large numbers of samples and close clinical correlation and resolution of discrepant results.

A second major factor that contributes to test variability is the complex nature of the antibodies to be measured. They are polyclonal and a mixture of immunoglobulins (Ig) G, A, M, and E. The antibodies are very heterogeneous and the affinity and avidity of the individual antibodies may be significantly different depending on the testing conditions. This makes the assays very time, temperature, pH, and buffer concentration dependent. When the assays are performed on automated instrumentation, where the conditions are carefully controlled, within run coefficients of variation (CVs) in the range of 3% to 4% can be obtained. Between run CVs are usually in the 4% to 6% range for most nephelometry assays. Between run CVs can be monitored by the routine running of a patient sample on a subsequent run as an additional control. Results from this type of control can be found in **Figure 6-2**, which contains quality control data generated from routine runs of IgG quantitation by neph-

FIGURE **6-1**

Results from comparison testing of 80 positive rheumatoid factor samples with two different manufacturers' reagents by nephelometry. Results are shown as IU/mL.

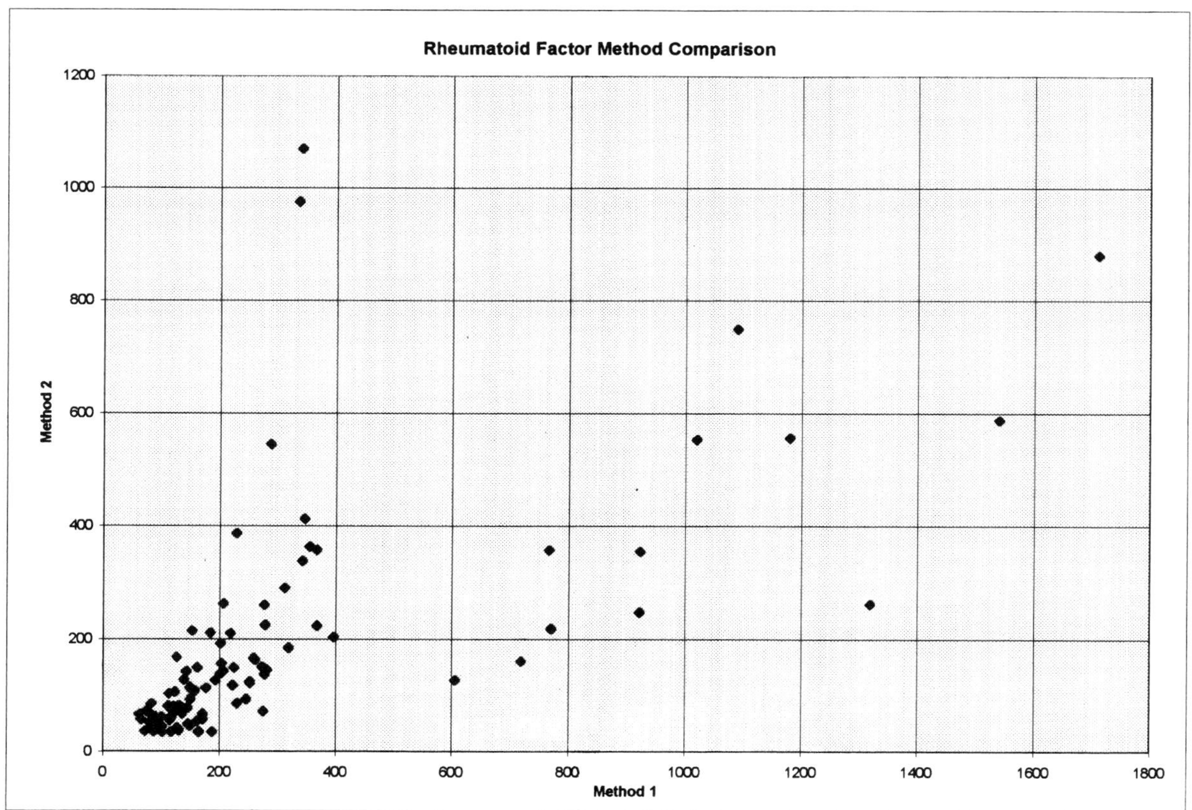

elometry. The figure was generated from data gathered over 36 runs in which a patient sample with a result in the normal range was pulled and run on a subsequent run, after which the two results were compared to determine the percent difference. As the figure shows, frequently the second value was more that 5% higher or lower than the initial value even though the positive and negative controls were within range for each of the runs.

In contrast to the reasonable reproducibility found with nephelometric assays, CVs obtained for manual enzyme-linked immunosorbent assay (ELISA) testing are usually in the range of 10% to 20%. Both between run and within run variation are especially high (50% or more) at the low end of the standard curve for most ELISA assays, which unfortunately is usually the critical cutoff point for interpretation of the majority of ELISA assays. Even with the best testing methods available, significant variation in patient results can be seen.

Also contributing to immunoassay variability is the heterogeneous nature of the antibody because of the mixture of antibody classes present. This is a source of variation because the specific antibodies measured in each test are distributed in the IgA, IgM, IgE, IgG, and subclasses of IgG and IgA and this distribution can vary with each patient. Significantly different results, especially for assays that measure only a single class of antibody, can be seen because of this variation in antibody mixtures. Because of the heterogeneous nature of the antibodies present in most patient sera, reagent manufacturers must rigorously produce and characterize secondary detection antibody reagents to ensure that they are broadly reactive enough to detect all the appropriate antibodies but not cross-react with undesired antibodies.

A third source of variation in the tests is the presence in the serum from normal individuals of low levels of antibodies that react with the majority of autoimmune and infectious disease

FIGURE 6-2

Results are from IgG quantitations run on 36 different runs. Each data point represents a single sample with an IgG level within the normal range that is saved and rerun on the next run. The plotted value percent difference is the initial run value divided by the repeat value ×100.

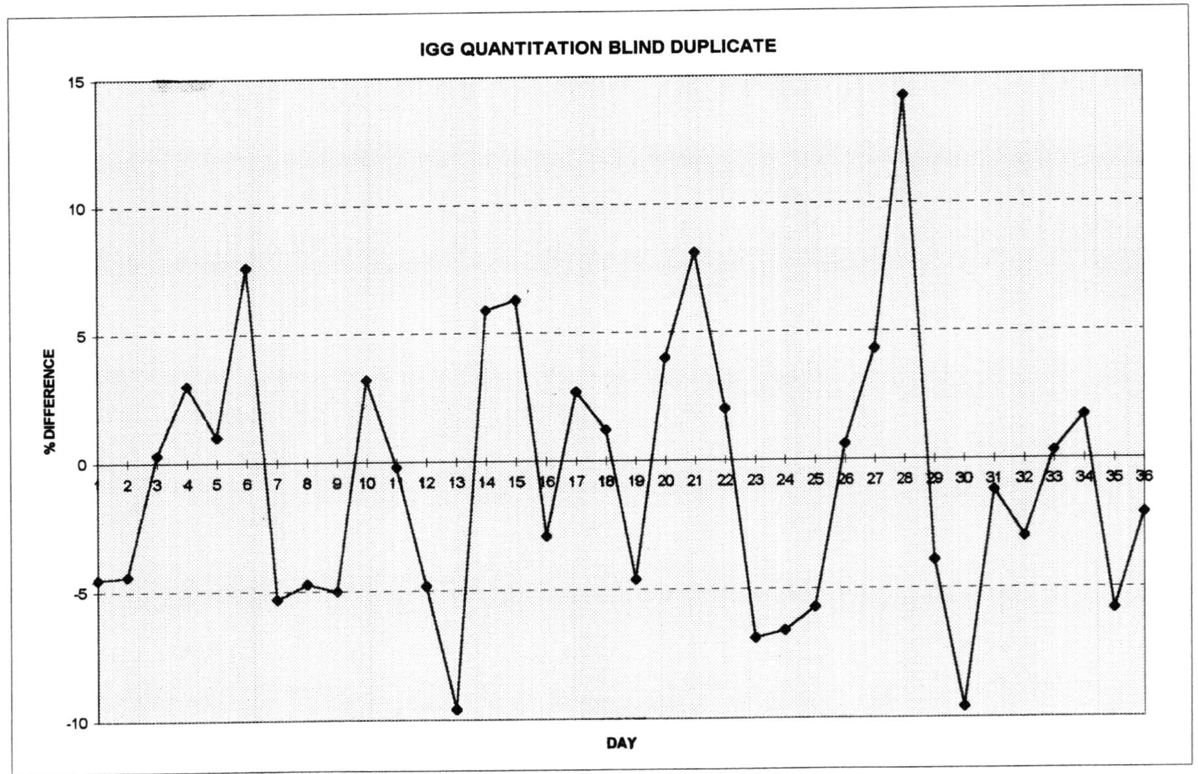

antigens. For most serologic tests, the major question to be answered is whether the presence or absence of antibody indicates exposure to the infectious disease agent or the production of autoantibodies that are reactive with self-antigens. The challenge for reagent manufacturers is to create testing conditions in which there is a clear cutoff between positive and negative results such that the test is 100% specific and sensitive. Since this challenge is rarely met, in most clinical testing situations, the test selected is either very specific or very sensitive, but rarely both. Therefore, the selection of the best testing methods and reagents must be at least partially based on the patient population that will routinely be tested. For many immunologic tests, the most sensitive assay is not always the best assay because of the high rate of "false-positive" results that these assays have. This is particularly true in assays that are less disease specific, such as tests for rheumatoid factor, antinuclear antibodies, infectious mononucleosis, and non-treponemal syphilis (RPR, VDRL).

The measurement of antibody quantity can be especially difficult for assays in which high levels of antibody may be present. Most ELISA immunoassays that use colorimetric substrates have a linear measuring range of 0.3 to 3.5 OD (optical density) when measured by a spectrophotometer. This results in a linear measuring range of about 1.0 to 1.5 logs; however, actual antibody quantities in patient serum may vary by 3 to 4 logs. Most commercial ELISA assays are designed to measure in the range of lower patient values, and a significant number of samples that contain high levels of antibodies are above the measuring range. This is a problem for a significant number of patient samples with many of the immunoassay methods routinely used. It is a major issue when testing for IgE, rheumatoid factor (RF), antiribonucleoprotein (RNP), antithyroid peroxidase, and antithyroglobulin antibodies, in which situations many patients may have very high levels of the antibody being measured.

For some reagent kits, the manufacturers recommend retesting all samples that give results above the top standard point at several additional dilutions, while for other kits it is recommended only to report values as greater than the top standard. Because the assays are frequently nonlinear at higher dilutions and because the kit manufacturers differ in their recommended methods, patient samples that contain very high levels of antibody can give significantly different results when tested with a variety of commercial kits. The problem of high antibody levels is less significant in ELISA assays that utilize fluorescent or chemiluminescent substrates because the detection instruments (fluorometers and luminometers) are capable of broader linear measuring ranges of 3 to 4 logs. Unfortunately, the use of these newer substrates and instruments is not widespread and is currently restricted to a only a few manufacturers and a few automated immunoassay instruments. Patient samples with high levels of antibodies are also problematic for radioimmunoassay (RIA), radial immunodiffusion (RID), and nephelometric methods, which rely on precipitation at approximately equal antigen-antibody concentrations, because antigen excess (the "hook effect") can cause significant errors in the measurement of high antibody levels.

Quality Control Materials

In general, good quality control materials are not readily available for the majority of clinical immunology tests. The exceptions to this are the multilevel QC materials available for most serum quantitations performed by nephelometry, for which assayed and unassayed multilevel controls as well as linearity verification materials are available from several manufacturers. Most other Food and Drug Administration (FDA) approved test kits on the market for clinical diagnostic assays have a negative and positive control only. Positive controls included in the kits are frequently low in antibody quantity and run near the cutoff point. Because low values are the most variable points for most methods, the established ranges for these controls usually have broad ranges (15–50%). The high variability of these low controls leads to insensitivity of the controls to significant changes in standard curve values and incorrect patient results.

High positive controls that have lower CVs and validate the higher parts of the standard curves are rarely included in reagent kits. High positive controls can be produced from pools of previously positive patient samples but the inhouse production of these controls is often not simple. Difficulties may include a very low percent of patient samples with high results, insufficient sample volume, the expenses necessary to validate the lack of infectious agents in the sample (i.e., hepatitis B and C, human immunodeficiency virus), and the technologist time and expense related to aliquotting samples and establishing acceptable QC ranges. Because of the effort that is involved in producing these controls, it is important to try to produce at least a year's worth of control if possible in order to standardize and stabilize the control materials as much as possible. In spite of the difficulties with the production of inhouse quality control materials, it is important to include high-level controls for all tests. These should include titer controls for latex and hemagglutination assays, intensity controls at various levels for fluorescent assays, and both high- and low-level controls for most EIA assays (5). Additional more specific information concerning controls that are necessary for each test can be found in each of the individual sections of this book and also in a variety of National Committee for Clinical Laboratory Standards (NCCLS) documents.

Analysis of quality control materials in immunology is frequently complicated by the lack of nonnormal distribution of the data. This is especially true for the establishment of normal ranges for many assays, including RF, IgE, virtually all assays in which the normal range is less than the test cutoff level, and the percentage data generated by flow cytometry. Very few laboratory information systems have statistical packages that calculate control or normal range data for nonnormal distributed data. When establishing normal and quality control ranges, care must be taken to evaluate the data for normal distribution, and when assays have results with nonnormal distribution the normal and control ranges should be calculated by statistical software that has nonnormal statistical calculation capability.

Standard Levy-Jennings charts can be used for review of quality control values (6). Most laboratory information systems and the majority of new automated immunoassay instruments generate Levy-Jennings charts from quality control data entered on a daily basis. When using Levy-Jennings charts as part of the periodic review of quality control results, two major differences seen with immunoassays should be kept in mind. First, since some tests may be done only once or twice a week, it is important to review 2 or 3 months worth of data. This is critical since shifts and trends in quality control values are very difficult to detect when fewer than 12 to 15 data points are present. Second, for assays in which the data have a nonnormal distribution, the Levy-Jennings statistical analysis which assumes a normal distribution can be used but the acceptable ranges should be set at the 5% to 95% points rather than at the mean +/− 2 standard deviation (SD). This will allow the generation of Levy-Jennings charts with the data points plotted correctly, but most acceptable data points will be in the lower half of the range whenever the data has a chi-square distribution. An example of data displayed in this manner is in **Figure 6-3** where the percent of B cells present in normal control samples is plotted over 150 days. For this data set, the acceptable range was set at 6% to 22% even though the mean of the data was 12%. As in this example, the mean calculated by the statistical software will not be correct. When reviewing these data over shorter time periods, a calculated mean that is lower than the middle of the range set for the Levy-Jennings chart should not be mistaken for a downward shift in the control or normal range for that test. Alternatively, the data can be analyzed with commercially available statistical software which will analyze nonnormal data and print adjusted Levy-Jennings plots. This software is rarely available on most laboratory computer systems.

Statistical analysis is also available from at least one commercial source (StatLIA, Brendan Scientific, Oak Park, Michigan), which will allow the comparison of ELISA data between runs. The software is capable of storing raw optical density data on standards and controls for up to 20 runs per test, and then using these data to analyze subsequent runs to determine the reproducibility of optical density values for all points on the standard curve and all control values. The package reviews all the data, determines on a statistical basis whether the run is acceptable, and when the data are unacceptable determines the most likely problems that are present on the run. Extensive use of statistical packages such as this may lead to a decrease in the variability of EIA control and patient test results.

Quality Assurance for Diagnostic Immunology

Quality assurance of immunology testing involves a large variety of aspects. Many of them are common to all laboratory sections and a variety of tests. Some of the issues that are unique to the immunology laboratory are the difficulties of establishing normal ranges, the lack of standardized tests, and the related nature of many of the assays.

Setting normal ranges can be complex for a variety of tests. For assays in which normal is the absence of antibody, for example, RF, ANA, and IgE, samples with low antibody levels do not have a normal distribution such that the 95% cutoff level should be used as the negative/positive cutoff point for these assays. This means that a large number (>50) of normal samples should be used to determine the normal range and that both age- and sex-matched ranges are frequently required. If the cutoff is set too low, a high number of normal samples can incorrectly be interpreted as positive. This is especially true for some of the autoimmune assays, where positive antinuclear and antithyroid autoantibodies can be seen in low titers in as many as 20% to 30% of women over the age of 50. Since few kit manufacturers supply age- and sex-adjusted ranges for their assays, it is important for each laboratory to carefully determine normal ranges for the population that is routinely tested.

Most immunoassays used for diagnostic testing are not sufficiently standardized to allow comparison of results between vendors (7). Recently, a new standard was developed by the International Federation of Clinical Chemistry (IFCC) that contains immunoglobulin and some serum proteins (8). Standards or reference materials are also available from the Centers for Disease Control (CDC) or the World Health Organization (WHO) for some infectious disease tests and some antinuclear antibodies (ANAs). Thyroid antibodies and thyroglobulin reference material are available from the European Community Bureau of Reference (BCR), and anticardiolipin standards from the Louisville APL Diagnostic Laboratories (see Chapter 7 and the chapters that contain details of the individual assays for complete information). When assays are not standardized, care must be taken when assay methods are changed to compare

FIGURE **6-3**

Results are from 150 days of testing in which normal individuals, one per day, were drawn and the percent of B cells determined.

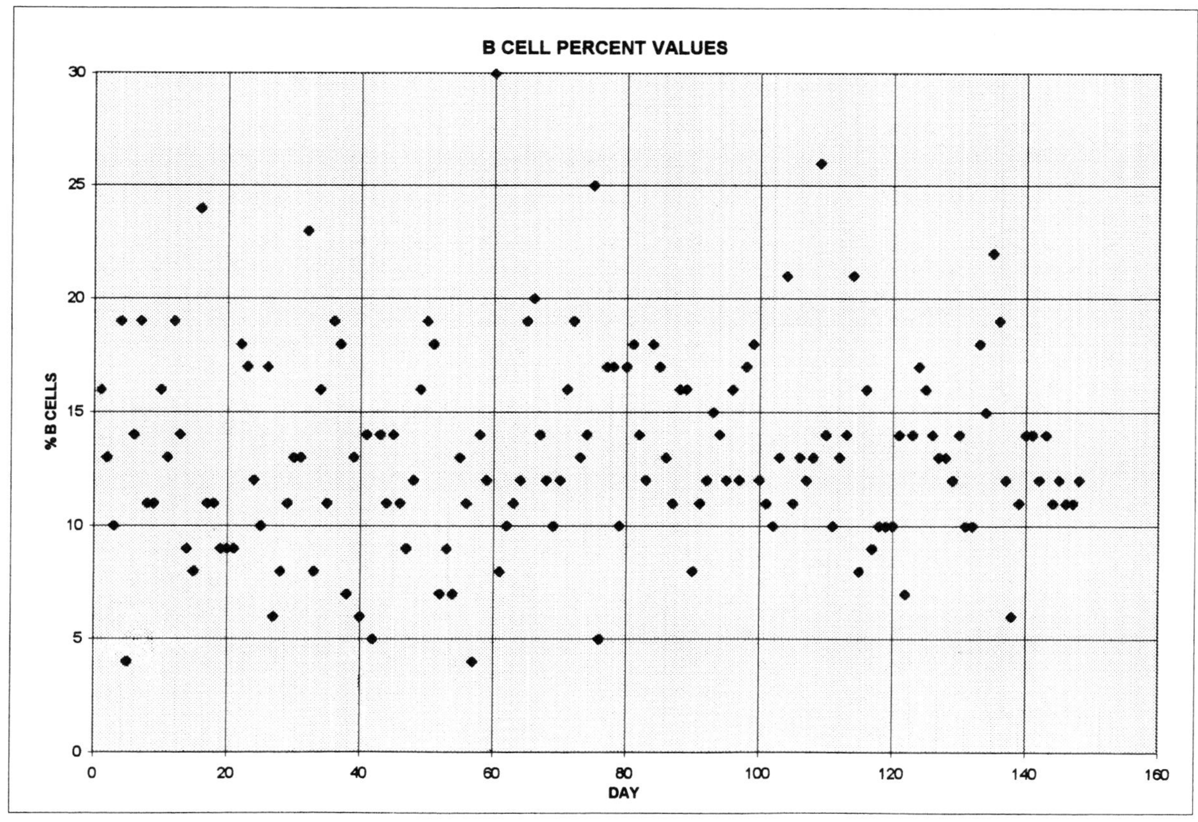

the results and communicate changes to the physicians who use the test results. Summary results from CAP and other proficiency testing services can be useful to evaluate results obtained from different methods.

Results from a large number of immunology tests can be correlated to ensure the quality of the test result. For example, if the pattern for a positive ANA is carefully determined, the most likely antibodies present can be determined. The pattern can therefore be used either to determine the most useful follow-up EIA assays for SS-A, SS-B, Sm, RNP, Scl-70, or double-stranded deoxyribonucleic acid (ds-DNA) antibodies, or correlation of the pattern with the EIA assay can be used to determine the acceptability of the EIA assay results. Other useful tests that can be correlated to improve the results are

1. Protein electrophoresis with immunoglobulin quantitations
2. IgG, IgA, and IgM levels with kappa and lambda levels
3. Fluorescent anti-neutrophil cytoplasmic antibodies (ANCA) with proteinase 3 (PR3), myeloperoxidase (MPO), and elastase EIA assays
4. ds-DNA with C3, C4, and CH50 levels (C3 and C4 with CH50)
5. Thyroglobulin with antithyroglobulin levels

Quality Assurance Monitors

The quality of test results in the clinical immunology laboratory can also be improved by the routine monitoring of test results

FIGURE 6-4

Results are the percent of samples with positive ANA results tallied on a monthly basis over a 5-year period.

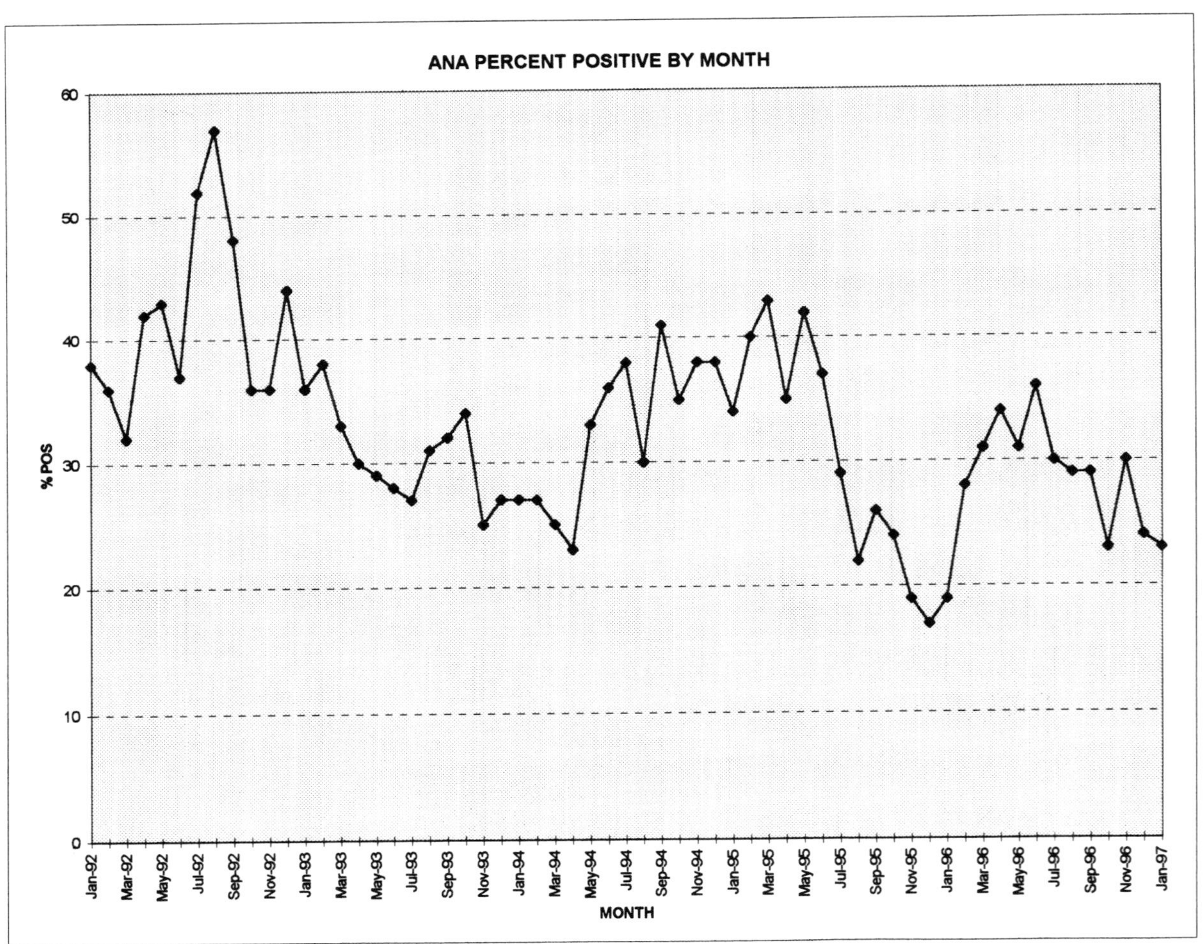

obtained for key assays. The assays to be monitored should be selected based on either their high volume or significant clinical value. Effective monitoring strategies can be designed that are simple but powerful. An example of a simple and effective monitoring strategy is the monthly determination of the percent of positive ANAs. Data from 4 years of ANA testing at the Clinical Immunology Laboratory of the Lahey Hitchcock Clinic is shown in **Figure 6-4**. Tracking changes in the percent positives has easily demonstrated changes in the ANA substrate (2 times), the fluorescent microscope sensitivity (once), contamination in the buffers (2 times), and an increase in the number of new technologists performing and overinterpreting the test results. Monitoring of the ANA test results on a monthly basis has helped to ensure consistent results over a long time period. In addition to ensuring the quality of the results, the use of this ANA monitor has helped to reduce the cost of ANA testing. This cost savings can be seen in the laboratory, where it reduces the number of unnecessary titrations, as well as in the clinic, where it reduces the number of unnecessary referral visits by patients who do not have clinical disease but have low titered positive ANAs.

Similar strategies can be designed that monitor results from a wide variety of immunoassays. These monitors can be an effective part of the overall quality assurance program for diagnostic immunology laboratories.

REFERENCES

1. Howanitz PJ, Howanitz JH. Quality control for the clinical laboratory. Clin Lab Med 1983;3:541–552.
2. Howanitz PJ, Howanitz JH. Quality assurance. In: Rose NR, deMacario EC, Folds JD, et al, eds. Manual of clinical laboratory immunology. 5th ed. Washington, DC: ASM Press, 1997:1180–1190.
3. Berwick DM. Continuous improvement as an ideal in health care. N Engl J Med 1989;320:53–56.
4. Sewell DL, Schifman RB. Quality assurance: quality improvement, quality control, and test validation. In: Murray PD, Baron EJ, Pfaller MA, et al, eds. Manual of clinical microbiology. 6th ed. Washington, DC: ASM Press, 1995:55–67.
5. Westgard JO. Planning statistical quality control procedures. In: Rose NR, DeMacario EC, Folds JD, et al, eds. Manual of clinical laboratory immunology. 5th ed. Washington, DC: ASM Press, 1997:1191–1200.
6. Levy S, Jennings ER. The use of control charts in the clinical laboratory. Am J Clin Pathol 1950;20: 1059–1066.
7. Feldkamp CS, Carey JL. Standardization of immunoassay methodologies. In: Rose NR, DeMacario EC, Folds JD, et al, eds. Manual of clinical laboratory immunology. 5th ed. Washington, DC: ASM Press, 1997:1168–1179.
8. Wicher J, et al. New international reference preparation for proteins in human serum (RPPHS). Clin Chem 1994;40:934–938.

CHAPTER 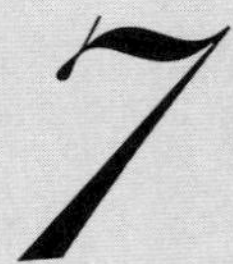

National and International Reference Preparations for the Clinical Diagnostic Immunology Laboratory

ROBERT M. NAKAMURA

Several organizations are involved in standards and reference preparations for use in clinical diagnostics. National organizations include the National Committee for Clinical Laboratory Standards (NCCLS), College of American Pathologists (CAP), Centers for Disease Control (CDC), Arthritis Foundation, American Association of Clinical Chemists (AACC), and Biological Response Modifier's Program of the National Cancer Institute.

International organizations that are involved in preparations of reference materials are the World Health Organization (WHO), National Institute of Biological Standards and Control of the United Kingdom, International Union of Immunological Societies (IUIS), United Kingdom External Quality Assessment Schemes for Autoimmune Serology and Special Immunochemistry (UK NEQAS), International Laboratory for Biological Standards of the Netherlands, Community Bureau of Reference (BCR; Belgium), and International Federation of Clinical Chemistry (IFCC).

The College of American Pathologists prepared a document entitled *Standards, Reference Materials, and Method—A Practical Guide to the Medical Laboratory*. The last edition by CAP was in 1984. However, the NCCLS, in cooperation with CAP and their National Reference System for Clinical Laboratory (NRSCL) Council, was responsible for the publication in January 1994 of NCCLS Document NRSCL 12-P Vol 14 No. 1, *Sourcebook of Reference Methods, Materials, and Related Information for the Clinical Laboratory; Proposed Guideline*. In this sourcebook, information has been compiled on methods and materials that are useful in the general clinical laboratory.

In this chapter, we discuss some of the available reference materials that may be useful in the clinical diagnostic laboratory. The available reference material for infectious disease serology is not included in this chapter. Other useful reference materials and calibrators may be included in chapters that discuss specific assays.

Definitions and Nomenclature (1–3)

WHO International Standards (to each of which an international unit has been assigned) are for biologic substances that member states have agreed to subject to national control of quality and to express their potency in international units or their equivalents.

WHO International Reference Preparations (to which international units may or may not be assigned) are biologic substances that are provided as a service but for which national control of quality has not been agreed on as obligatory.

WHO International Reference Reagents (of high specificity) are for qualitative use in identification. *National Standards* have designated units calibrated in terms of WHO International Standards or International Reference Preparations.

WHO Reference Laboratories Working Standards (international or national) are often of the same material as the WHO International or the National Standards and have units directly related to these.

Other standards (e.g., manufacturers' standards, research laboratory standards) may have provisional units designated by the source laboratory if no units exist.

The International Standards Organization (ISO) has added the following definitions:

> *Reference material (RM):* A material or substance, one or more properties of which are sufficiently well established to be used for the calibration of an apparatus or for the verification of a measurement method. A reference material is intended to transfer the value of a measured quantity (physical, chemical, biologic, technologic) between one place and another. It may be in the form of a pure or mixed gas, liquid, or solid, or even a simple manufactured object.
>
> *Certified reference material (CRM):* An RM accompanied by, or traceable to, a certificate stating the property value(s) concerned, issued by an organization that is generally accepted as technically competent.

Once specifications for a standard or reference material have been established, a pool of sufficient material should be collected. The minimal number of ampules of the pool should be 4000 for an international standard or reference preparation (4). It is generally agreed that for worldwide use and ease of transportation, a standard should be lyophilized.

Four principal criteria should be satisfied before a preparation can be defined as a biologic reference material (5):

1. The preparation should be as pure as possible.
2. The preparation should be stable.
3. The preparation should have specific activity.
4. Specific activity should be definable, where possible in units.

Units of Measurements: Definition and Continuity

The assignment of international units (IU) as applied to biologic materials is completely arbitrary. For any given substance an international unit is *continuous* and represents the same amount of activity with each succeeding standard. This is ensured by comparing the new standard with the old again in an international collaborative assay and by assigning unitage to the new standard. By expressing the activity of a new standard in terms of that of the old standard, the activity of one unit of the material remains the same even though the weight of dried material that contains this activity in the new standard is likely to be different (6).

International units have been assigned to initial reference preparations for immunoglobulins. The international unit of immunoglobulin (Ig) G has by definition the same activity as 0.8147 mg of the dry powder present in an ampule of the International Research Standard for human serum immunoglobulins G, M, and A. Of course, we would not try to weigh out this amount, but we would reconstitute the total contents of the ampule in a suitable volume of diluent in the knowledge that this volume now contains 100 units of IgG. An international unit of IgE, on the other hand, has the same activity as is present in 0.006562 mg of the dry powder in an ampule of the International Reference Preparation of human serum IgE. In accepting the arbitrary nature of units it must also be accepted that just as there is no relationship between units of length and mass, there is no relationship between the unit of a specific antigen or antibody and the unit of a second different antigen or antibody (6).

Reference Preparations for Autoantibodies to Nuclear and Intracellular Antigens

International Reference Preparations

In 1971, Anderson et al (7) reported on a collaborative international study of a proposed research standard for antinuclear factor 66/233 (homogeneous). This material was adopted by WHO and IUIS as an International Reference Preparation. Each ampule was defined to contain 100 IU. After dilution of the contents in 1 mL, a concentration of 100 IU/mL is obtained.

This International Reference Preparation, WHO 1064 [antinuclear factor 66/233 (homogeneous)], can be obtained from the Central Laboratory of the Netherlands, Red Cross Blood Transfusion Service, Plesmanlaan, 125, Amsterdam, Netherlands.

Antinuclear Antibody (ANA; Homogeneous WHO 66/233)

Holborow et al (3,7,8) have recommended the use of the WHO International Reference Preparation 66/233 as follows:

> If the determined end point of the WHO standard 66/233 is 1:160 in a particular laboratory, the end point dilution contains 1/160 × 100 IU/mL = 0.625 IU/mL. (The undiluted 66/233 contains 100 IU/mL.)

For another laboratory with another system, the end point might represent less or more IU/mL of ANA activity. The differences among laboratories and systems may be nullified by expressing results of test sera in IU/mL calculated by multiplying the reciprocals of their dilutions at their titration end points by the number of units of activity present in the reference preparation at its titration end point in the particular laboratory.

The WHO 66/233 standard has been available since 1970. However, the use of the standard is not widespread. There are several reasons, expressed as follows:

1. WHO serum 66/233 is probably an inappropriate reference for speckled or other patterns of nuclear fluorescence.
2. The ANA titer is dependent on the total antibody content and antibody avidity. These sera with similar total amounts of antibody but varying avidity may give different end points.
3. WHO 66/233 contains mostly IgG ANA and is thus best used in comparison of test sera that contain ANA activity of the IgG class.
4. Many laboratories use the immunofluorescent microscopy (IFM)-ANA as a screening test for ANA. Quantitative results are often obtained by testing one or two serum dilutions, that is, 1:20 and 1:160, indicating the intensity of fluorescence (3).

Feltkamp et al (9) have done a collaborative laboratory study with the use of WHO 66/233. The study showed an improvement of interlaboratory comparability for the homogeneous fluorescence pattern when the common reference standard was used. Molden et al (10) showed that IFM-ANA tests can be monitored with the use of Arthritis Foundation (AF)/CDC reference sera of defined antibody specificities.

WHO/IUIS IgM Class ANA (HL)

A freeze-dried batch of ANA-positive serum was pooled from six patients with systemic lupus erythematosus (11,12). The ampule contains 100 arbitrary units of ANA activity as lyophilized serum. The end point is the highest dilution showing the minimal nuclear staining distinguishable from a negative reaction.

WHO Immunofluorescent Conjugate Standards

The first chairman of the IUIS immunofluorescence committee was Professor Astrid Fagraeus (3). This committee, established in 1971, was instrumental in developing two WHO/IUIS international fluorescein-conjugated antibody preparations and a reference serum containing ANA of IgM class (HL).

The above preparations—fluorescein isothiocyanate (FITC)-labeled sheep antihuman Ig (480010), FITC-labeled sheep antihuman IgM (anti-mu chain), and IgM class ANA (HL)—are available from the WHO Immunology Unit, Geneva, Switzerland (11,12).

Fluorescein Isothiocyanate-Conjugated Antihuman Immunoglobulin International Standard (WHO/IUIS 480010)

FITC-conjugated antibodies to human immunoglobulins are used in IFM-ANA test methods. The quality of the conjugate is extremely important for accurate diagnostic results. The Medical Research Council of the United Kingdom assembled a working party to define the specifications of the preparation, conjugation, and characterization of fluorescent conjugates (13). Subsequently, the IUIS standardization committee encouraged development of the sheep antihuman Ig conjugate 480010 and helped conduct an international collaborative study with the WHO reference standard 66/233.

The sheep antihuman Ig conjugate (480010) was submitted to the WHO Expert Advisory Panel on Biological Standardization as an International Standard. It was accepted as an International Standard by WHO and IUIS. Each ampule of 0.5 mL of 480010 is defined to contain 100 IU or 200 IU/mL. The preparation can be obtained from WHO Immunology Unit, Unit 1211, Geneva 28, Switzerland (3).

The quality of the conjugate is based on the specificity and potency performance. The conjugate 480010 was prepared from an antiserum raised by immunization with human IgG and human $F(ab)_2$, which resulted in strong anti-IgG and good reactivity with IgM and IgA. The conjugate reacts with heavy and light chains of IgG and with the light chains of IgM and IgA.

The potency of the conjugates is assessed by their presence in a chessboard titration of dilutions of conjugates against dilutions of the same middle layers of serum on a tissue substrate. A good conjugate should give a constant titer for the middle layer of serum over a wide range of conjugate dilutions. The constant end point dilution of the middle layer in the *plateau titer* and the highest conjugate dilution at which the plateau titer is maintained is the *plateau end point* of the conjugate (14). The working dilution of a conjugate is at least twice the concentration at the plateau end point.

In the same way, standard preparations of FITC-conjugated anti-IgM and FITC-conjugated anti-IgG have been prepared and accepted by WHO and IUIS. Both standards contain 100 IU per ampule.

WHO Standard for Antibodies to Double-Stranded Deoxyribonucleic Acid

In 1988, Dr. TEW Feltkamp and coworkers (12,15), from the Netherlands, developed the first International Standard for antibodies to double-stranded deoxyribonucleic acid (dsDNA) antibodies, coded Wo/80. The Wo/80 sera were obtained after recalcification of plasma taken from a patient with systemic lupus erythematosus. Vials were filled with 500 μL serum and lyophilized. The specimens contained no other autoantibodies in measurable quantities (15).

Methods of Assay and Evaluation

The Wo/80 serum vials were tested in eight laboratories by the immunofluorescence technique on *Crithidia lucidiae* (15). The titers varied between 1/20 and 1/640 (mean 1/160). In seven laboratories, the FARR assay for DNA antibodies with the Amersham kit (Amersham International, Buckinghamshire, United Kingdom) was performed on the Wo/80 specimen. At a dilution of 1:40, a mean binding percentage of about 50% was observed. After reconstitution with 500 μL distilled water, the vials were labeled to contain 100 IU/500 μL or 200 IU/mL.

The Wo/80 and other WHO standards can be requested from Central Laboratory of the Netherlands, Red Cross Blood Transfusion Service, Plesmanlaan, 125, Amsterdam, Netherlands (11). Another address given for the same institution is Department of Reagents CLB, PO Box 9190, 1006 AD Amsterdam, Netherlands (16).

AF/CDC Reference Sera for Autoantibodies to Nuclear and Intracellular Antigens

In 1980, the Arthritis Foundation in the United States, in collaboration with the Centers for Disease Control, established a Committee on Antinuclear Antibody Serology (17–19). The charge of the committee was as follows:

1. Establish a repository of ANA reference sera to be made available to researchers and clinical laboratories in the United States and other foreign countries.
2. The ANA reference reagents will serve as primary reference standards defining ANA specificities and be used by clinical laboratories to define their own secondary reference reagents.

In 1982, the AF/CDC reference preparations were prepared and assayed by the methods listed in **Table 7-1** by a committee on Antinuclear Antibody Serology of the Arthritis Foundation, 3400 Peachtree Road NE, Atlanta, GA 30326. The five reference sera provided reference reagents for antinuclear antibodies defined in the following terms:

1. Three patterns of fluorescent antinuclear antibodies: homogeneous/rim pattern and two different speckled nucleoplasmic patterns
2. Four different antinuclear antibodies identified by immunodiffusion analysis: antibodies to native DNA, SS-B/La, nuclear ribonucleoprotein (RNP), and Sm

TABLE 7-1

ANA Reference Sera Established by AF/CDC in 1982*

Assay	Method	Assay Readout	Specificities of Reference Sera: CDC1 FANA and Anti-nDNA	CDC2 FANA and Anti-SS-B/La	CDC3 FANA Only	CDC4 Anti-nRNP Only	CDC5 Anti-Sm Only
ANA	Immunofluorescence microscopy (IFM-ANA)	Pattern titer	H/R 1:5:512 (1:160–1:640)	Sp 1:160 (1:80–1:320)	Sp 1:320 (1:180–1:640)		
Anti-nDNA	Millipore filter	% DNA bound	74% (64–82%)				
	FARR	DNA bound	85% (75–95%)				
	Crithidia	Titer	1:90 (1:180–1:320)				
ANA-SS-B/La	Immunodiffusion	Titer		1:40 (1:16–1:80)			
ANA-nRNP	Immunodiffusion	Titer				1:64 (1:32–1:80)	
Anti-Sm	Immunodiffusion	Titer					1:64 (1:32–1:64)

FANA, fluorescence ANA; H/R, homogeneous/rim; Sp, speckled pattern.

*Results show the median value with range of values.

SOURCE: Tan EM, Fritzler MJ, McDougal JS, et al. Reference sera for antinuclear antibodies. I. Antibodies to native DNA, Sm, nuclear RNP, and SS-B/La. Arthritis Rheum 1982;25:1003–1005; and McDougal JS, Kennedy S, McDuffie FC. Standards and quality assurance for immunologic tests: standards and reference materials for autoantibodies to nuclear antigens. In: Rippey JH, Nakamura RM, eds. Diagnostic immunology: technology assessment and quality assurance. Skokie, IL: College of American Pathologists, 1983:147–155.

The bank of reference reagents at the AF/CDC laboratory was expanded to include five more reference ANAs (18,19), which were processed and analyzed as the first five reagents described above. The reference reagents were made available in 1988 and are described in **Table 7-2**.

As of June 30, 1994, a total of 1598 laboratories from 58 different countries have received AF/CDC ANA reference sera (MG Byrd, AF/CDC ANA Reference Laboratory, CDC Immunology Branch, Atlanta, GA, personal communication, 1994).

In October 1992, the AF/CDC committee on antinuclear antibody serology in the United States was reorganized and is now called the IUIS-ANA subcommittee. Participating organizations in the IUIS-ANA subcommittee include the CDC (Atlanta), Arthritis Foundation (Atlanta), WHO, ILAR (International League Against Rheumatism), and the European League Against Rheumatism (11,20,21).

The AF/CDC reference preparations have been of great value to researchers and clinical laboratories. The reference sera from the AF/CDC Laboratory with defined specificities

TABLE 7-2

Reference Antinuclear Antibodies (ANA) Available from AF/CDC ANA Reference Laboratory from 1988

Reagent	Immunologic Features
AF/CDC1	Homogeneous-pattern ANA (doubles as antinative DNA)
AF/CDC2	Anti-La (SS-B)
AF/CDC3	Speckled-pattern ANA
AF/CDC4	Anti-U1 RNP (U1 small nuclear RNP)
AF/CDC5	Anti-Sm (U1, U2, U5, U4/6 small nuclear RNP)
AF/CDC6	Nucleolar-pattern ANA
AF/CDC7	Anti-Ro (SS-A)
AF/CDC8	Centromere-pattern ANA
AF/CDC9	Anti-Scl-70 (DNA topoisomerase 1)
AF/CDC10	Anti-Jo-1 (histidyl-transfer ribonucleic acid synthetase)

SOURCE: McDougal JS, Kennedy S, McDuffie FC. Standards and quality assurance for immunologic tests: standards and reference materials for autoantibodies to nuclear antigens. In: Rippey JH, Nakamura RM, eds. Diagnostic immunology: technology assessment and quality assurance. Skokie, IL: College of American Pathologists, 1983:147–155; and Tan EM, Feltkamp TEW, Alarcón-Segovia D, et al. Reference reagents for antinuclear antibody. Arthritis Rheum 1988;31:1331. Letter.

were used for standardization of the indirect immunofluorescence test for ANA (IFM-ANA). The AF/CDC area with defined specificities for ds-DNA, SS-B/La, nRNP, and Sm nucleoli were reacted to the commonly used IFM-ANA substrates, mouse kidney sections, KB, and HEp-2 tissue culture cells. The use of reference sera for IFM-ANA testing was recommended (10,22,23).

College of American Pathologists Reference Serum for Anti-SS-A/Ro Antibodies

In 1991, the College of American Pathologists Standards Committee in cooperation with the CAP Immunology Resource Committee prepared a monospecific reference serum that contained only anti–SS-A/Ro nuclear antibody (24). The College of American Pathologists reference preparation (lot #C103BG) has an assigned value of positive immunodiffusion precipitin antibody to SS-A/Ro and the positive range of titer is 1:4 to 1:32. This reference serum should be used to test IFM-ANA substrate cell lots for the presence of the SS-A/Ro antigen. In addition, the monospecific anti-SS-A/Ro reference serum can be used for specific identification of unknown anti-SS-A/Ro by immunodiffusion analyses.

CAP reference preparation (lot #C103BG) for anti–SS-A/Ro can be obtained from College of American Pathologists, 325 Waukegan Road, Northfield, IL 60093-2750.

Reference Preparations for Serum Proteins

The WHO, with various collaborating organizations, has developed reference preparations for IgG, IgA, IgM, and IgE (25,26), which were initially expressed in international units (6).

In the late 1970s, Dr. Charles Reimer et al (26) prepared a reference material for human serum proteins. This material was lyophilized in vaccine vials and became the CDC/USNRP (United States National Reference Preparation), which in turn became the WHO Reference Preparation for Six Human Serum Proteins (WHO 6HSP) (27). International units were arbitrarily assigned to WHO 6HSP for six proteins (albumin, α_1-antitrypsin, ceruloplasmin, α_2-macroglobulin, transferrin, and the C3 component of complement).

In collaboration with CDC, CAP produced a series of reference preparations for serum proteins (RPSP-1 to RPSP-4) and assigned mass units (28,29). During the process of preparation of RPSP-1 to RPSP-3, a "drift of values" was assigned, since values were assigned by consensus against the preceding reference material.

RPSP-4 was assigned values similar to those of final and currently accepted reference preparations for protein in human serum (RPPHS). This project was a collaborative effort of BCR/IFCC/and CAP.

Reference Preparations for Proteins in Human Serum

The CAP/BCR/IFCC Reference Preparation for Proteins in Human Serum was prepared from pooled human serum (obtained from 364 healthy donors) that had been clarified to eliminate lipoprotein. It contains sodium azide (1.0 g/liter), benzamidine chloride (0.157 g/liter), and aprotinin (80,000 IU/liter) as preservatives (29,30). After microfiltration and filling, the material was freeze-dried, resulting in a mean weight of 71.8 mg lyophilizate per vial with a mean residual moisture of 0.57%.

The intended use of the product was for standardization of the 14 serum proteins listed in **Table 7-3**.

Assigned Values

The concentrations of the 14 proteins contained in this material have been assigned using existing international and national reference preparations and purified proteins (29,30).

The mass/volume values for IgA, IgG, IgM, complement C3, complement C4, albumin, α_2-macroglobulin, haptoglobin, and ceruloplasmin have been assigned from the CDC's USNRP (120575/C); for C-reactive protein (CRP), from the WHO's first International Standard for Human C-Reactive Protein (85/506); and for prealbumin (transthyretin), α_1-antitrypsin, α_1-acid glycoprotein (orosomucoid), and transferrin, from highly purified proteins. For α_1-antitrypsin, α_1-acid glycoprotein (orosomucoid), and transferrin, values based on the USNRP are also given for comparison purposes.

International units for IgA, IgG, and IgM have been assigned from the WHO International Reference Preparation for Human Serum Immunoglobulins (67/86); for C3, albumin, α_2-macroglobulin, and ceruloplasmin, from the WHO International Reference Preparation for

TABLE 7-3

Analyte	Assigned Value (g/liter)	95% Confidence Interval (g/liter)	International Units (IU/mL)	95% Confidence Interval (IU/mL)
IgA	1.96	1.92–2.00	125	(122.4–127.6)*
IgG	9.68	9.58–9.78	117	(115.8–118.2)
IgM	0.797	0.774–0.820	105	(102–108)
Complement C3	1.091	1.064–1.118	89	79–99
Complement C4	0.151	0.146–0.156	60	(58–62)
Albumin	39.7	38.9–40.5	97	93–101
α_1-antitrypsin	1.206	1.195–1.217	91	87–95
α_1-acid glycoprotein	0.656	0.651–0.661	NA	
α_2-macroglobulin	1.64	1.59–1.69	79	75–83
Haptoglobin	0.893	0.884–0.902	NA	
Transferrin	2.45	2.39–2.51	100	96–104
Ceruloplasmin	0.205	0.194–0.216	67	57–77
Prealbumin	0.243	0.225–0.261	NA	
C-reactive protein	0.0392	0.0373–0.0411	0.0392	0.0373–0.0411

NA, not applicable (no WHO reference available).

*Values in parentheses are calculated, using the uncertainty for g/liter; separate SDs were not done for IUs.

SOURCE: Johnson AM. A near international reference preparation for proteins in human serum. Arch Pathol Lab Med 1993;117:29–31; and Whicher JT, Ritchie RF, Johnson AM, et al. New international reference preparation for proteins in human serum (RPPHS). Clin Chem 1994;40:934–938.

Six Human Serum Proteins (4/2); and for C4, from the WHO first Reference Preparation for Complement Components (5/4).

The values for prealbumin (transthyretin), α_1-antitrypsin, α_2-acid glycoprotein (orosomucoid), and transferrin have been assigned from purified proteins because the values in the USNRP are now different from those currently accepted by the scientific community or, in the case of prealbumin, were never established.

Value transfer is based on the linear relationship of several dilutions of the reference material in which the overall regression is used to determine the ratio of concentrations between them. The slope of regression is then used to assign the value for the proteins. The value assignment was undertaken by collaborating laboratories in Europe, Japan, and the US. The methods employed were nephelometry and turbidimetry, analyzed by a variety of instruments (29,30).

CAP/BCR/IFCC (RPPHS) can be ordered from College of American Pathologists, 325 Waukegan Road, Northfield, IL 60093-2750; telephone: (847) 446-8800; FAX: (847) 446-3563; *or* Community Bureau of Reference (BCR), Commission of the European Community, 200 Rue de la Loi, 1049 Brussels, Belgium; telephone: (32,2) 235 31 15; Telex: 21877 COMEU B; FAX: (32,2) 235 80 72.

Other Available Reference Preparations

WHO Standard for C-reactive protein (CRP) 1986 (85/506)

WHO International Reference human serum for smooth muscle (antiactin) antibody WHO 106

WHO 1066-human rheumatoid arthritis serum (rheumatoid factor)

These are available from International Laboratory for Biological Standards, Central Laboratory of the Netherlands, Red Cross Blood Transfusion Service, Plesmanlaan, 125, Amsterdam, Netherlands (11,16).

Autoantibodies

64/2 First British Standard for rheumatoid arthritis serum, human
64/93 Antithyroglobulin serum, human
66/387 Antithyroid microsome serum, human
67/183 Primary biliary cirrhosis serum, human
90/656 Cardiolipin antibody

These are available from National Institute of Biological Standards and Control, Blanche Lane, South Mimms, Potters Bar, Herts EN6 30G, United Kingdom (16).

Antiphospholipid Antibodies

Antiphospholipid antibody standards studied at different workshops can be obtained from E. Nigel Harris, M. Phil., MD, Division of Rheumatology, Department of Medicine, University of Louisville, Louisville, KY 40292; current address: Dean, Morehouse School of Medicine, 720 Westview Drive Southwest, Atlanta, GA 30310-1495 (31,32).

The problems of assay standards for anticardiolipin and phospholipid antibodies are discussed in another section of this book.

Reference Reagents for Human Cytokines

Biological Response Modifiers Program (NCI), the Division of Microbiology and Infectious Diseases (NIAID), and the National Institute for Biological Standards and Control (United Kingdom) have made available reference reagents for murine and human cytokines. The reagents are available in small amounts (approximately 1 μg/sample) for use in the calibration of in vitro bioassays and inhouse standards only and are not to be used for experimental purposes.

Human Reference Reagents Currently Available

IFN-α	IL-1-α	IL-4	IL-8	G-CSF	TGF-β_1
IFN-β	IL-1-β	IL-5	IL-9	GM-CSF	TNF-α
IFN-γ	IL-2	IL-6	IL-10	M-CSF	TNF-β
	IL-3	IL-7	LIF	SCF	RANTES

To obtain these reagents, contact Dr. Craig W. Reynolds, Biological Response Modifiers Program, NCI-FCRDC, Building 1052, Room 253, Frederick, MD 21702-1201; FAX: (301) 846-5429. Shipments will be made collect express. Please allow 3 to 4 weeks for delivery.

Whiteside (33) has written an excellent review on cytokine measurements and interpretation of cytokine measurements in human disease.

Summary and Future Perspectives

There has been considerable progress in standardization of procedures and available reference preparations. Of course, standards and reference preparations comprise only a part of any quality assurance and improvement program. The ultimate goal of standardization is for various clinical laboratory test results to be interchangeable and for an exchange of data to be done with confidence.

With the development of more rapid and sensitive assays, there will be a need for the continuous development of new reference preparations that will be adaptable to the new assay methods. For example, a future generation of reference preparations and standards will be needed that will demonstrate specific antibody reactivity on sensitive assays such as enzyme-linked immunosorbent assay (ELISA). These types of reference preparations are currently being developed by the Standards Committee of the Association of Medical Laboratory Immunologists (AMLI) chaired by Dr. Betts Carpenter. In addition, efforts should be made toward the characterization and standardization of the specific antigen preparations that may be natural or of recombinant technology origin.

One can foresee that new reference preparations will be needed and become available to address the new nucleotide molecular assays in the clinical laboratory.

REFERENCES

1. Batty I. Standards and quality control in clinical immunology. In: Thompson RA, ed. Techniques in clinical chemistry. 2nd ed. Oxford: Blackwell, 1981:306–324.
2. Holborow EJ, Johnson GD, Chantler S. Use of international reference preparations for immunofluorescence. In: Wick G, Traill KN, Schwanenstein K, eds. Immunofluorescence technology: selected theoretical and clinical aspects. New York: Elsevier Biomedical, 1982: 1–10.
3. Holborow EJ, ed. Standardization in immunofluorescence. Oxford: Blackwell, 1970.
4. Outschoorn AS, Bangham DR, Evans DG, et al, eds. Guidelines for the preparation and establishment of reference materials and reference reagents for biological substances. WHO Expert Committee on Biological Standardization, 29th report, Geneva, 1978.
5. Perkins FT. The establishment and use of biological standards. In: Dumonde DC, Steward MW, eds. Laboratory tests in rheumatic diseases: standardization in laboratory and clinical practice. Baltimore: University Park Press, 1979:73–79.

6. Batty I. Standardization of immunological reagents. In: Dumonde DC, Steward MW, eds. Laboratory tests in rheumatic diseases: standardization in laboratory and clinical practice. Baltimore: University Park Press, 1979:81–91.
7. Anderson SE, Addison IE, Dixon HG. Antinuclear factor serum (homogeneous): an international collaborative study of the proposed research standard 66/233. Ann NY Acad Sci 1971;177:337–345.
8. Johnson GD, Chantler S, Batty I, Holborow EJ. Use and abuse of international reference preparations in immunofluorescence. In: Dumonde DC, Steward MW, eds. Laboratory tests in rheumatic diseases: standardization in laboratory and clinical practice. Baltimore: University Park Press, 1979:93–100.
9. Feltkamp TEW, Klein F, Janssens MBJA. Standardization of the quantitative determination of antinuclear antibodies (ANAs) with a homogeneous pattern. Ann Rheum Dis 1988;47:906–909.
10. Molden DP, Nakamura RM, Tan EM. Standardization of the immunofluorescence test for autoantibody to nuclear antigens (ANA): use of reference sera of defined antibody specificity. Am J Clin Pathol 1984;82:57–66.
11. Feltkamp TEW. Standards and reference preparations. In: van Venrooij WJ, Maini RN, eds. Manual of biological markers of diseases. Norwell, MA: Kluwer Academic, 1993;pA11:1–12.
12. Feltkamp TEW. Standards for ANA and anti-DNA. Clin Rheumatol 1990;9(suppl):74–81.
13. Working party recommendations on the characterization of antisera as reagents. Immunology 1971;20:1.
14. Beutner EH, Kumar V, Krasny SA, Chorzelski TP. Defined immunofluorescence in immunodermatology. In: Beutner EH, Chorzelski TP, Kumar V, eds. Immunopathology of the skin. 3rd ed. New York: Wiley, 1987:3–40.
15. Feltkamp TEW, Kirkwood TBL, Maini RN, Aarden LA. The first international standard for antibodies to double-stranded DNA. Ann Rheum Dis 1988;47:740–746.
16. Ward AM. United Kingdom external quality assessment scheme for autoimmune serology and special chemistry. Department of Immunology, PO Box 894, Sheffield S5 7YT, United Kingdom, 1995–1996.
17. Tan EM, Fritzler MJ, McDougal JS, et al. Reference sera for antinuclear antibodies. I. Antibodies to native DNA, Sm, nuclear RNP, and SS-B/La. Arthritis Rheum 1982;25:1003–1005.
18. McDougal JS, Kennedy S, McDuffie FC. Standards and quality assurance for immunologic tests: standards and reference materials for autoantibodies to nuclear antigens. In: Rippey JH, Nakamura RM, eds. Diagnostic immunology: technology assessment and quality assurance. Skokie, IL: College of American Pathologists, 1983:147–155.
19. Tan EM, Feltkamp TEW, Alarcón-Segovia D, et al. Reference reagents for antinuclear antibodies. Arthritis Rheum 1988;31:1331. Letter.
20. Tan EM. International cooperative activities in standardization of antinuclear antibodies. In: van Venrooij WJ, Maini RN, eds. Manual of biological markers of diseases. Norwell, MA: Kluwer Academic, 1993;pA1:1–5.
21. Kalden JR. WHO/IUIS standardization programme. Clin Exp Rheumatol 1992;10:513–514.
22. Nakamura RM, Bylund DJ, Tan EM. Current status of available standards for quality improvement of assays for detection of autoantibodies to nuclear and intracellular antigens. J Clin Lab Anal 1994;8:360–368.
23. Charles PJ, van Venrooij WJ, Maini RN. The consensus workshops for the detection of autoantibodies to intracellular antigens in rheumatic diseases: 1989–1992. Clin Exp Rheumatol 1992;10:507–511.
24. Bylund DJ, Nakamura RM. Importance of detection of SS-A/Ro autoantibody in screening immunofluorescence tests for autoantibodies to nuclear antigens. J Clin Lab Anal 1991;5:212–218.
25. Taylor RN, Huong AY, Fulford KM, et al. Quality control for immunologic tests. HEW Publication No. (CDC) 79–8376, 1979.
26. Reimer CB, Smith SJ, Hannon WH, et al. Progress towards international reference standards for human serum proteins. J Biol Stand 1978;6:133–138.
27. WHO Expert Committee on Biological Standardization, 29th report. Technical Report Series 626. Geneva: WHO, 1978:19.
28. Reimer CB, Smith SJ, Wells TW, et al. Collaborative calibration of the U.S. National and the College of American Pathologists reference preparations for specific serum proteins. Am J Clin Pathol 1982;77:12–19.

29. Johnson AM. A new international reference preparation for proteins in human serum. Arch Pathol Lab Med 1993;117:29–31.

30. Whicher JT, Ritchie RF, Johnson AM, et al. New international reference preparation for proteins in human serum (RPPHS). Clin Chem 1994;40: 934–938.

31. Harris EH. The second international anticardiolipin standardization workshop/The Kingston Anti-phospholipid Antibody Study (KAPS) group. Am J Clin Pathol 1990;94:476–484.

32. Harris EH. Anticardiolipin wet workshop report. Fifth International Symposium on Antiphospholipid Antibodies. Am J Clin Pathol 1994;101:616–624.

33. Whiteside T. Cytokine measurements and interpretation of cytokine assays in human disease. J Clin Immunol 1994;14:327–339.

CHAPTER 8

Proficiency Testing Surveys in Clinical Diagnostic Immunology

HENRY A. HOMBURGER

The term *proficiency testing* refers to the process whereby many different laboratories analyze identical aliquots of the same test specimens and report their results to a central location. The reported results are analyzed statistically, the data for all participants are summarized, and the summarized data are returned to each of the participants. In this way, each participating laboratory can determine whether its test results agree with the consensus defined statistically by results reported from all other laboratories. Over the years, various terms have been used to refer to the process of proficiency testing described above, including interlaboratory comparison testing, external quality control programs, and interlaboratory surveys.

Organized proficiency testing programs in laboratory medicine have existed for more than 60 years. The first program, begun in 1935, was overseen by the United States Public Health Service and evaluated syphilis serology testing (1). Since that time, several professional societies, including the College of American Pathologists, the American Association of Clinical Chemists, and the American Association of Blood Banks, as well as various state and federal agencies and several for-profit organizations have developed proficiency testing programs to which individual laboratories can subscribe. These programs now offer surveys for virtually all analytes tested in clinical laboratories. A separate listing of agencies and organizations that offer proficiency testing programs in laboratory immunology is found in **Table 8-1**.

As originally conceived, participation in proficiency testing programs was voluntary and served an educational function. However, with increasing regulation of clinical laboratories by government, enrollment and acceptable performance on proficiency testing surveys have become mandatory for accreditation as stipulated in the Clinical Laboratory Improvement Amendments (CLIA) of 1988 (2). Recently, the criteria for acceptable performance on proficiency surveys were explicitly defined for many analytes in regulations set forth in the *Federal Register*, February 28, 1992 (3) (see below).

Description of Interlaboratory Proficiency Programs in Laboratory Immunology

Proficiency surveys in laboratory immunology can be broadly classified into two categories: those that include primarily "regulated" analytes and those that include primarily "unregulated" analytes. Regulated analytes include those clinical tests performed in most laboratories for which acceptable performance is defined by current Department of Health and Human Services (HHS) regulations (3) (**Table 8-2**). Many tests for commonly measured analytes and most newer technologies in laboratory immunology are not regulated at this time (**Table 8-3**).

As currently mandated, proficiency testing programs for regulated analytes must include at least three mailings a year with at least five challenges per analyte per mailing. Acceptable performance is defined for each analyte by the criteria shown in Table 8-2. Overall performance for an analyte is defined as "acceptable"

TABLE **8-1**

Providers of Proficiency Testing Surveys in Laboratory Immunology and Related Disciplines

Proficiency Provider	**Analytes**
American Association of Bioanalysts	Regulated analytes in immunology and immunohematology; syphilis serology
American Academy of Family Physicians	Regulated analytes [antinuclear antibody (ANA), infectious mononucleosis, rheumatoid factor, immunoglobulin E (IgE), rubella, antistreptolysin O (ASO)]; syphilis serology; immunohematology (ABO group, RhD) type and antibody detection
American Academy of Pediatrics	Infectious mononucleosis
Accutest	Regulated analytes (ANA and rubella); syphilis serology
American Proficiency Institute	Regulated analytes [α_1-antitrypsin, ANA, anti–human immunodeficiency virus (HIV)-1, infectious mononucleosis, rheumatoid factor, rubella, immunoglobulins A, G, M, E]; syphilis serology; immunohematology
American Society of Internal Medicine–Medical Laboratory Evaluation	Regulated analytes (ASO, ANA, C3, C4, infectious mononucleosis, rheumatoid factor, rubella, IgE); syphilis serology; immunohematology (ABO, RhD) type and antibody detection
College of American Pathologists	Regulated analytes (all); syphilis serology; immunohematology; unregulated analytes: autoantibodies, including SS-A, SS-B, Sm, ribonucleoprotein (RNP), smooth muscle, mitochondria, thyroid, antineutrophil cytoplasmic antibodies (ANCA), glomerular basement membrane (GBM); diagnostic allergy; infectious disease serology, including anti-hepatitis B cmv antigen (Hb_cAg), *B. burgdorferi*, delta hepatitis, anti-cytomegalovirus (CMV), cryptococcal Ag, anti–HIV-2, anti-Hepatitis A virus (HAV); flow cytometry, including lymphocyte immunophenotyping, DNA analysis, and lymphoma/leukemia analysis
Idaho Bureau of Laboratories	Regulated analytes (infectious mononucleosis, rheumatoid factor, rubella); syphilis serology
New Jersey Department of Health	Regulated analytes (ANA, ASO, infectious mononucleosis, rheumatoid factor, rubella); syphilis serology; immunohematology
New York State Department of Health	Regulated analytes (all); syphilis serology; immunohematology
Ohio Department of Health	Regulated analytes (infectious mononucleosis); syphilis serology; immunohematology [ABO, Rh(D) type]
Puerto Rico Department of Health	Regulated analytes (all); syphilis serology; immunohematology
Wisconsin State Laboratory of Hygiene	Regulated analytes (all); syphilis serology; immunohematology

if a laboratory obtains an acceptable grade on four of the five challenges in each mailing. If a laboratory fails to obtain acceptable performance for an analyte in two successive mailings or in two of three consecutive mailings, that laboratory is designated as having "unsuccessful analyte status." In the event that a laboratory is found to have unsuccessful analyte status, remedial proficiency testing with acceptable performance is required to reinstate the laboratory in good standing.

While the above-mentioned grading criteria seem straightforward, the entire process of grading results reported for regulated analytes in laboratory immunology is, in practice, more complicated. As outlined in the CLIA regulations, proficiency challenges for regulated analytes must include specimens that span the ranges of analyte concentrations commonly encountered in clinical situations. Target values for grading the results on such specimens are determined by a process of consensus, with consensus defined either by results obtained in selected "referee" laboratories or by results reported from at least 90% of all participating laboratories. Given the wide range of analytic sensitivities of different immunologic techniques and the systematic differences that often

TABLE **8-2**

Regulated Analytes in General Immunology

Analyte or Test	**Criteria for Acceptable Performance**
α_1-antitrypsin	Target value ± 3 SD
α_1-fetoprotein (tumor marker)	Target value ± 3 SD
Antinuclear antibody	Target value ± 2 dilutions or positive or negative*
Antistreptolysin	Target value ± 2 dilutions or positive or negative*
Anti–human immunodeficiency virus	Reactive or nonreactive
Complement C3	Target value ± 3SD
Complement C4	Target value ± 3SD
Hepatitis (Hb_sAg and Hb C, Hb_eAg)	Reactive (positive) or nonreactive (negative)
IgA	Target value ± 3SD
IgE	Target value ± 3SD
IgG	Target value ± 25%
IgM	Target value ± 3SD
Infectious mononucleosis	*Target value ± 2 dilutions or positive or negative
Rheumatoid factor	*Target value ± 2 dilutions or positive or negative
Rubella	*Target value ± 2 dilutions or immune or nonimmune or positive or negative

*Quantitative criteria not currently used for ANA, ASO, rheumatoid factor, or rubella. Grading is based upon qualitative results only. Grading for infectious mononucleosis also is based on qualitative results, as no quantitative data are collected from participants.

exist between methods because of differences in standardization and calibration of the methods, it is often impossible to define a single acceptable consensus value for grading all participants' results. Some providers of proficiency surveys have dealt with this problem by defining target values based upon the consensus of results reported by "peer groups" of laboratories that use identical reagents and instruments. In this way, participants are not inadvertently penalized for results that may be systematically biased when compared to other laboratories that use different methods (4). In some instances, for example, specimens that contain low concentrations of an analyte, variations among reagents and instruments within and between peer groups can be extreme and it may not be possible to determine consensus target results. In these situations, it is common practice not to grade any of the results for a particular challenge. This solution has been accepted by regulatory agencies; however, as described below, if proficiency surveys do not contain a significant number of challenging specimens, the overall value of the survey to participants is greatly diminished.

In respect to the use of proficiency results to identify poorly performing laboratories, there is an inherent limitation in the process that can be defined in terms of cost effectiveness. If the goal of the regulatory process is to identify as many "poor performers" as possible, then the range of acceptable results should be narrowly defined about the target mean (the so-called true value). If one assumes that poor performers are a small minority of all the participants, the grading process will lead to a large number of good laboratories obtaining unacceptable results. In other words, the predictive value of an unacceptable result for identifying a poor performer is low. In this situation, the entire process must then be repeated in an attempt to cull out those participants that really do need to take remedial measures to improve the quality of their testing. Ultimately such a process requires a large bureaucracy, is inefficient, and is costly for all concerned. In laboratory immunology, it is clear that the grading criteria for regulated analytes are not particularly stringent (see Table 8-2), and the vast majority of participating laboratories have little difficulty in obtaining acceptable results.

As was noted previously, many of the analytes commonly measured in immunology laboratories are in the unregulated category (see Table 8-3). Participation in proficiency testing programs for these analytes is not required for accreditation if the challenges are not formally evaluated by the proficiency provider, and the decision by a laboratory to participate in

TABLE **8-3**

Additional Analytes in Laboratory Immunology for Which Proficiency Testing Is Available

Analyte or Test	**Evaluation Criteria***
Protein analytes	
Ceruloplasmin	Not graded
C-reactive protein	90% participant consensus
Haptoglobin	Not graded
Kappa : lambda ratio	Not graded
Serum human chorionic gonadotropin (HCG)	90% participant consensus
IgD	Not graded
IgG subclass proteins	Not graded
Prealbumin	Not graded
Specific antibodies and autoantibodies	
Anticardiolipin antibodies	Not graded
Antineutrophil cytoplasmic antibodies	Not graded
Anti-DNA antibodies	90% participant consensus by method (neg/pos)
Anti-GBM antibodies	Not graded
Antimicrosomal antibodies	90% participant consensus (neg/normal/pos/abnormal)
Antimitochondrial antibodies	90% participant consensus (normal/abnormal)
Anti-RNP antibodies	90% participant consensus (normal/abnormal)
Anti-Sm antibodies	90% participant consensus (normal/abnormal)
Anti-Sm/RNP antibodies (for those laboratories that cannot distinguish between RNP and Sm/RNP)	90% participant consensus (normal/abnormal)
Anti–smooth-muscle antibodies	90% participant consensus (normal/abnormal)
Antithyroglobulin antibodies	90% participant consensus (neg/normal/pos/abnormal)
Anti–SS-A antibodies	Not graded
Anti–SS-B antibodies	Not graded
Anti-*B. burgdorferi*	Not graded
Flow cytometry	
Lymphocyte immunophenotyping	Not graded
DNA content analysis	Not graded
Lymphoma and leukemia analysis	Not graded
Diagnostic allergy	
Allergen-sepcific IgE antibodies	Not graded
Viral antigens and antibodies	
Anti-delta	90% participant consensus
Anti-HAV (IgM and total)	90% participant consensus
Anti-Hb_s	90% participant consensus
Hb_cAg	90% participant consensus
Anti–HIV-2	90% participant consensus
Anti–HCV (Hepatitis C virus)	90% participant consensus
Cryptococcal Ag	90% participant consensus
Anti-CMV	90% participant consensus

*These grading criteria are defined by the proficiency provider and are not established by regulatory agencies.

proficiency testing for unregulated, ungraded analytes is based on the perception that the survey provides valuable information to the participant. The pool of results reported by laboratories to proficiency providers does indeed constitute a large database that provides a powerful tool for real-time assessment of the overall state of the art in laboratory immunology. The results also enable individual laboratories to measure their performance against other laboratories that use the same methods (reagents and instruments) or closely related analytic systems. The value of participating in such voluntary programs is illustrated in the following examples from the laboratory immunology surveys of the College of American Pathologists. It is commonplace in laboratory medicine that tests for new analytes are requested by physicians based on the results of published clinical investigations. Clinicians often assume that the methods available in clinical laboratories perform the same as published methods and well enough to make the results useful for medical decision making. Accordingly, the results of proficiency surveys are useful to laboratorians to decide whether particular tests are likely to provide medically useful results and whether they should offer these tests in their own laboratories. Results of recent surveys of tests for antiphospholipid antibodies illustrate this point (5). Despite the fact that several commercial methods are now approved by the Food and Drug Administration (FDA) to measure these antibodies in patients' sera, the results of proficiency surveys show large quantitative differences from method to method and significant disagreement between methods even when results are examined qualitatively, that is, when measurements are used to determine the simple presence or absence of detectable antibodies (**Table 8-4**). In this situation, a laboratory may elect not to perform the test onsite, and might prefer instead to send specimens to an outside laboratory that has an established assay of proven usefulness in clinical practice.

Results of proficiency surveys are also useful to point out problems with newer technologies that may occur sporadically among a subset of laboratories. Such is the case with results reported recently to the College of American Pathologists for the Flow Cytometry Survey (6) (**Fig. 8-1**). These results show that while many laboratories can accurately estimate the S-phase fraction of aneuploid cells tested for deoxyribonucleic acid (DNA) content, some laboratories consistently overestimate or underestimate the percentages of cells in S phase. In this case, the proficiency results suggest that some laboratories have a problem with the linearity of responses measured by their instruments. While these results do not reveal a fundamental problem with all instrument systems, they do show a clinically significant problem with results produced by a subset of participants. Consequently, participants whose

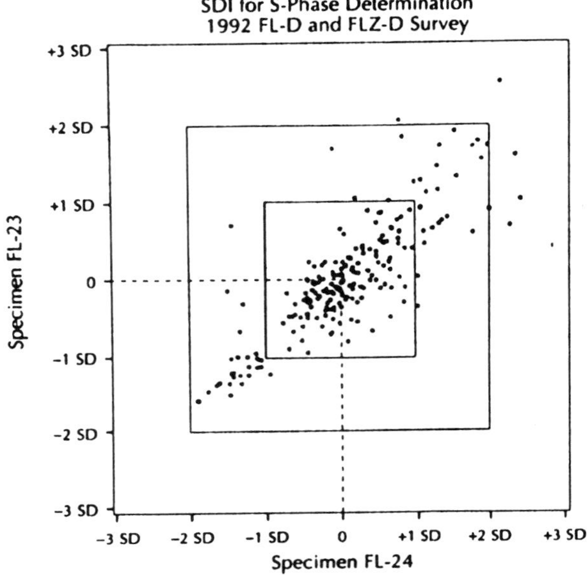

FIGURE **8-1**

Youden plot of paired participant S-phase responses for the 1992 FL-D Survey. This illustrates the observation that some laboratories consistently gave responses above or below the mean value for S phase (15.0 and 27.7 in this example). SDI indicates SD interval (5.95 and 10.88 in this example).

TABLE **8-4**

Interlaboratory Variability in Measurements of Anticardiolipin Antibodies

Specimen; No. of Laboratories	Positive/Negative Consensus	aCl-Ab Levels (mean, SD, CV)
A; 32	100% (pos)	64.5, 10.6, 16.4 (GPL) 19.7, 2.8, 14.2 (MPL)
B; 92	94% (pos)	41.0, 12.4, 30.4 (GPL) 22.3, 9.3, 41.5 (MPL)
C; 140	95.7% (pos)	48.0, 15.4, 32.2 (GPL) 33.6, 13.3, 39.6 (MPL)
D; 84	56% (neg)	12.3, 3.9, 31.4 (GPL) 9.0, 2.6, 29.0 (MPL)
E; 51	94.1% (pos)	28.3, 3.7, 13.0 (GPL) 16.9, 3.0, 18.0 (MPL)

CV, coefficient of variation; GPL = unit of measurement of IgG anticardiolipin antibodies; MPL = unit of measurement of IgM anticardiolipin antibodies.

data accurately reflect the composition of the test specimens serve as a useful benchmark for those laboratories that report biased results.

Limitations of Proficiency Testing in Laboratory Immunology

Proficiency testing is useful to participants for purposes of internal quality assurance and is required for accreditation and certification. Nevertheless, it is self-evident to laboratorians that proficiency testing is but one element in a comprehensive quality assurance program (7,8). Other elements discussed elsewhere in this volume are daily quality control activities, use of appropriate standards and reference materials, personnel requirements and training, and laboratory inspection activities. As part of an overall program of quality assurance, proficiency surveys reveal important information about the accuracy of results reported for clinical analytes by providing a benchmark of results reported by peer laboratories. Proficiency surveys are of little value in determining the precision (reproducibility) of results reported daily by clinical laboratories. For some analytes, use of proficiency results as a benchmark for accuracy of results obtained on clinical specimens is limited by dissimilarities between proficiency samples and actual clinical specimens. For example, samples in the aforementioned DNA Flow Cytometry Survey are comprised of neoplastic cell lines in tissue culture medium, whereas clinical laboratories customarily make measurements of DNA content on sections of deparaffinized surgical specimens. It follows that the results obtained on DNA survey samples may not be a totally reliable indicator of the ability of a laboratory to obtain accurate results on patients' specimens.

Survey samples are also subject to so-called matrix effects (9). Matrix effects occur when analytes present in the matrix of the proficiency sample interact with one another or with extraneous constituents of the sample, for example, stabilizers added to preserve the specimen to produce results with some analytic methods that are systematically biased when compared with results obtained on actual patients' specimens. In laboratory immunology, matrix effects are of particular concern in surveys of specific antibodies, for example, in syphilis serology and in testing for autoantibodies where care must be taken by the proficiency provider to pretest the samples using a variety of different analytic methods. In some instances, it is necessary to obtain specimens from single donors to avoid producing samples that give biased results with some analytic methods.

A further limitation on the usefulness of proficiency results is the relative infrequency of testing of proficiency samples and the length of time required to process data and report results to participants. This limitation is overcome in part by the development by some providers of proficiency surveys of so-called survey-validated reference materials. These reference materials are prepared from large pools of survey materials that are identical in composition to proficiency samples. The reference materials have assigned concentrations for various analytes that are determined by analyzing the results reported by participants on aliquots mailed in previous survey cycles. Survey-validated reference materials may, therefore, be used more frequently as independent, internal quality control specimens or as secondary standards. In this way, a laboratory can monitor both the accuracy and precision of its results by using a single material. An important advantage of survey-validated reference materials is that the assigned concentrations are often method specific and are based on results generated by a large number of independent laboratories.

Future Developments in Proficiency Testing

With increased emphasis placed on the results of proficiency surveys for regulated analytes by accrediting agencies and with widespread consolidation of clinical laboratories occurring throughout the health care delivery system, providers of proficiency programs will be called on to improve the logistics of their services to participants. It is likely that proficiency testing soon will be available on an analyte-by-analyte basis, so-called menu ordering, with participants able to order proficiency samples for only those analytes that they perform onsite. It is also likely that electronic media will be used by survey participants and providers to report results and receive graded responses more expeditiously. At the same time, one can anticipate an expanded array of new voluntary proficiency programs designed to evaluate the performance of emerging technologies and new analytes in laboratory immunology. This is particularly likely for molecular techniques since these methods will certainly play an important role in evaluating patients with immunodeficiency diseases and neoplasms of immunocompetent cells. These programs will follow on the rich tradition of concern for quality that originally prompted physicians and scientists in laboratory immunology to initiate proficiency testing of clinical laboratories.

REFERENCES

1. Belk WP, Sunderman FW. A survey of the accuracy of chemical analyses in clinical laboratories. Am J Clin Pathol 1947;17:853–861.
2. Revision of laboratory regulations: final rule with request for comments. Federal Register 1990;55: 9538–9610.
3. Rules and Regulations. Federal Register February 28, 1992;57:7156–7157.
4. Tholen DW. Reference values and participating means as targets in proficiency testing. Arch Pathol Lab Med 1993;117:885–889.
5. Homburger HA, Paton ML. Interlaboratory comparison of immunoassays for anti-cardiolipin antibodies: results of the College of American Pathologists' S2 Survey. Presented at the Sixth International Symposium on Antiphospholipid Antibodies, Leuven, Belgium, September 14–17, 1994.
6. Coon JS, Paxton H, Lucy L, Homburger HA. Interlaboratory variation in DNA flow cytometry. Arch Pathol Lab Med 1994;118:681–685.
7. Rippey JH. Quality control in the diagnostic immunology laboratory. Pathologist 1983;37: 252–253.
8. Rippey JH, Williamson WE. The overall role of a proficiency testing program. Arch Pathol Lab Med 1988;112:340–342.
9. Kaufmann HW, Gochman N. College of American Pathologists Conference XXIII on matrix effects and accuracy assessment in clinical chemistry. Report of Working Group on Method Development. Arch Pathol Lab Med 1993;117:427–428.

CHAPTER 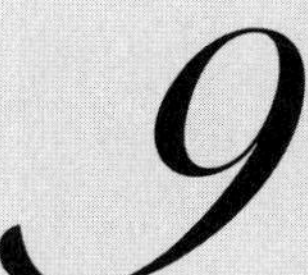

Method Validation and Verification for High-Complexity and Inhouse (Home Brew) Diagnostic Immunology Tests

HELENE PAXTON

The fiscal and regulatory environment since the inception of the new Clinical Laboratory Improvement Act (CLIA) '88 (1) creates a unique and complex situation for the diagnostic immunology laboratory, bringing new diagnostic tests to the institution for use in the laboratory diagnosis of new clinical entities or emerging diseases, or both. This also applies to new diagnostic technologies that were not previously available such as ribonucleic acid (RNA) and deoxyribonucleic acid (DNA) probes with old analytes, as well as new disease markers. What factors must a laboratory consider and be aware of before initiating a test validation protocol?

A Historical Perspective

Validation of laboratory tests is usually the domain of the diagnostic test manufacturer, which operates under the jurisdiction of the Food and Drug Administration (FDA). Under the current Health Care Financing Administration (HCFA) guidelines for laboratories and the final rule of CLIA '88 and later amendments, most tests performed by laboratories and doctors' offices fall in the waived or moderate-complexity category. These tests require little validation and their specific validation or quality control (QC) requirements are defined by the manufacturer. Laboratories may accept these specifications for their QC program. Most of the necessary requirements are carefully documented by the manufacturers in the package insert as part of the QC procedures defined in the method and as part of the marketing clearance. In these tests, the role of the laboratory is to meet the quality control monitoring rules as well as the proficiency testing requirements defined in the regulations for waived and *unmodified* moderate-complexity assays. Occasionally, a moderately complex assay will be modified and will, as a result, need to follow the same rules as the higher-complexity assays that have not been FDA cleared and are considered "home brews." Under CLIA, three government agencies have taken the responsibility for laboratory testing: the FDA, the Centers for Disease Control and Prevention (CDC), and the HFCA. The overlapping and sometimes conflicting roles of these agencies in clinical testing and certification are often confusing and can be in conflict, especially with regard to reimbursement for tests. Originally, the Department of Health and Human Services (HHS) had envisioned that laboratories would only be under the rule of HCFA with the CLIA '88 rule. Because of overwhelming public criticism and congressional pressure, the HCFA had to share this function with the FDA and CDC.

The diagnostic laboratory may often be confused as to the level of validation that a new test requires as well as the category into which it falls with regard to CLIA. Most manufacturers in the United States provide reagents to the laboratory in kits that have been cleared for use by the FDA and classified by the CDC as to complexity level. The FDA clearance usually takes the form of a premarket approval (PMA) and/or a 510(k) mechanism of "substantial equivalence" to a product or method that is already on the market. This approach, complex in its requirements, determines the "safety, effectiveness, and potential for patient risk" of a device being placed in commercial distribution. This determination places the device in a specific regulatory class (21CFR, section 513, 21 USC 360c).

The regulatory class determines the stringency of good manufacturing practices (GMP) and the level of control that must be administered by the manufacturer to assure performance of that device. Class I and class I exempt devices are very low risk and include items such as tongue depressors or tests such as sedimentation rate. Many of the class I diagnostic tests fall in the waived category according to CLIA. A class II device is more complex and includes tests such as antinuclear antibody (ANA) assay. These tests may fall into a CLIA moderate-complexity (level 1) or high-complexity (level 2) category based on test methodology. A dipstick enzyme immunoassay ANA test is moderate in complexity. An ANA immunofluorescent antibody (IFA) test is a high-complexity test, but the risk of the device has not changed and therefore it remains a class II device by FDA classification. CLIA is more concerned with operator intervention and potential for error, whereas the FDA is concerned with a device's potential risk. Class I and II devices can be cleared by the 510(k) process [section 510(k) 21 USC 360(k) and 21CFR, part 807] if a previous device measuring the same analyte exists in the marketplace (2). A class III device is defined as any test not in commercial distribution before May 22, 1976; a new analyte not classified as to its device category; a device that represents a potential risk to the patient if the test fails and the patient is misdiagnosed; or a test that is defined as a new analyte or an old test performed by a new technology. Many immunology tests fall into the latter category. This is also true for the new genetic tests. Class III devices are expensive and costly to put through a PMA process. The new genetic tests have undetermined implications in patient management and future disease processes. The potential financial impact for public health and insurance liability is unknown. This will not be a simple regulatory process for the consumer or the manufacturer.

Manufacturers are faced with the dilemma of getting a product to market as quickly as possible versus spending large sums of money in the validation of yet unproved tests. Often the manufacturer depends on the marketplace as well as the peer-reviewed literature to determine the clinical utility of the tests and places the reagents in a "*research use only*" (RUO) category to remove some of the cost burdens while clinical utility is being defined externally.* Further, tests that are cleared and on the market for a specific "*intended use*" that are used by laboratories for an "*off label use*" and are then marketed by laboratories to have certain diagnostic and patient management utility as well as implications for treatment now fall into the inhouse or "home brew" category. It is the laboratory's responsibility to validate and determine clinical ranges as well as to determine the test's appropriate clinical use and its effect on patient management. A recent example of this was the combination of ANA and Epstein-Barr virus (EBV) antibody profiles combined with flow cytometry T-cell subset panels in the clinical diagnosis of "chronic fatigue syndrome." The ANA and the EBV test are in this combined profile panel being used for other applications than their *cleared, intended use.* This action

* A new compliance guide (CPG) published by the FDA January 5, 1998 encourages manufacturers to develop certification programs for RUOs to prevent improper commercialization of the nonapproved tests (3). This new CPG version has not yet gone into effect pending a comment period. The CPG does not cover the analyte specific reagents (ASR) (4) recently published. This CPG will affect the availability of the RUOs for clinical use and will have strong regulatory action for high risk products that have not moved to regulatory clearance in the required time frame.

places those specific test applications in a home brew category. If a reference laboratory advertises that these tests have diagnostic properties and performs tests across state lines without performing the validation studies, it is in violation of FDA laws and *can* be investigated and sanctioned by the FDA.

Definition of Inhouse or "*Home Brew*" Tests

The CLIA rule under subpart K *mandates that tests that are defined as home brew are the responsibility of the diagnostic laboratory to validate and that all QC parameters apply. It is important to note that the CLIA regulations do not provide for product control as defined by the FDA*; that is, product performance and stability parameters are part of the GMP criteria. Moderate- and high-complexity tests that were cleared by the FDA and in use by the laboratory before September 1, 1994, do not have to have the supporting evidence of their verification and validation. Tests added to the laboratory menu after this date must meet the new validation and QC requirements. Noncleared home brew or modified tests must have validation records independent of the date of their inception in the laboratory. To further complicate matters, the National Committee for Laboratory Standards (NCCLS), a fourth regulatory body and a private organization, has added a level of complexity as to the definition of a *new test or procedure requiring validation*—a change in methodology, a change in bodily fluids, moving from a manual to automated method, and so forth (5,6). A recent example with important implications of the justification for this was a change in methodology for detecting Sjogren's A antibody from an Ouchterlony gel technique to one being performed by an enzyme-linked immunosorbent assay (ELISA). This methodology change completely altered the prevalence numbers and implications for the presence or absence of this antibody in certain populations (M. Reichlin, personal communication).

Another important factor in the validation of immunologic tests is that many of the standards and references were defined historically by chemistry methods and do not readily apply to immunologic assay measurements or genetic tests. Further, defined sample sets are more difficult to procure than are bodily fluids such as urine and serum used in chemistry assays. Therefore, how does a laboratory bring a new test to its institution?

The subpart K section states that the laboratory must meet all applicable standards 493-1203 to 493-1223 (HCFA, 45CFR, part 405), which include facilities, reagents, procedure manuals, method performance, limitations, and so forth. The laboratory is urged to review the specific details of those standards before initiation of a validation protocol is undertaken.

How to Validate and Verify a *Home Brew Test* and *High-Complexity Test*

This discussion will concentrate on the validation and verification of test and methodology (493-1225 to 493-1285) that must be met "*unless an alternative procedure specified in the manufacturer's protocol has been cleared by the FDA as meeting certain CLIA requirements for quality control, or HCFA approves an equivalent procedure specified in Appendix C of the State Operations Manual* (HCFA Pub. 7), which to date has not occurred for most high-complexity cleared tests (7).* Few specific guidelines exist in the regulations for how validations are to be accomplished. There are no consensus documents. Additionally, the number of specimens and the adequacy of sampling are not discussed in the rules.

Three steps must be performed before a validation of method can occur. The first step is to define the test's *intended use or clinical utility*. When a manufacturer clears a kit through the FDA *for in vitro diagnostic use*, it must state for exactly what purpose the kit is to be used. If the test is used for any other purpose, it falls outside its labeling and must be revalidated by the user, and the laboratory must

* Originally the FDA was to approve QC procedures or guidelines determined by the manufacturer and the laboratories would be able to use or develop their own QC in high-complexity assays (493-1223 guidelines). This has never occurred and, in a meeting held in Atlanta on September 24 to 25, 1996 (8), at the CDC convened by the CDC and CLIAC committee, it was stated that the FDA did not have the resources to do this specific provision of the CLIA rule except as it applied to the clearance of a kit or reagents through the PMA/510(k) process. Therefore, laboratories are still left to their own validation methods.

accept the responsibility for validation. Once the laboratory defines the clinical use of the test being proposed, the second step is the design of the appropriate validation protocol. In the third and most critical step, the laboratory must have established that all the reagents (493-1241b) to be used in the protocol are (see also Table 9-1)

1. *Reliably available.* Has the laboratory been able to source the active ingredients from more than one supplier, or is there an alternate source if the first source fails?
2. *Stable: The laboratory has performed the necessary stability studies to ensure that the analytes will not break down, changing the analytic range over time.* Reagent instability studies must go through actual shelf-life studies for the length of the intended stability or anticipated outdate of active ingredients. Accelerated shelf-life studies can be used but require real-time validation in addition.
3. *Consistent: The lot numbers of the same analyte will not give different values.* A minimum of three lots must be tried in the method.
4. *Defined-known sampling parameters and sample type.* The specimen type and patient requirements need to be defined, as do storage and shipment requirements, if applicable. If the laboratory is modifying a current kit that is already in commercial distribution, many of these parameters have already been defined and need not be repeated by the laboratory unless the reagents have been modified in any manner.*

Further, if a laboratory uses a moderate-complexity or a high-complexity test by definition and this kit is cleared for market by the FDA, the laboratory only has to meet the QC requirements and demonstrate that the expected patient ranges are appropriate for their specific patient population and match those published in the package insert. It does not have to repeat steps 1 through 4 listed above, but it does need to obtain the appropriate quality control reagents and standards suggested in the package insert for QC.

TABLE 9-1

Requirements for Reagent Validation

Definition of stability of analyte
Definition of accuracy and precision parameters
Definition of analyte specificity
Definition of lot-to-lot consistency—minimum 3 lots
Definition of reliability of supply
Definition of analyte cross-reactivity
Definition of analytic method
Definition of reference material (if applicable)
Definition of proper sample type for study

Defining the Working Protocol

Upon satisfactory completion of the above conditions intended use, design of validation protocol and definition of reagents these parameters are then incorporated into the *working protocol.* Items to be considered in the development of a "kit" protocol or method are the following:

1. The method should be tested using multiple sites with common lots of reagents or patients should be obtained from a geographically diverse area.

2. Comparison should be made to another well-established method specific for that analyte. In immunology this may be difficult, as other methodologies may not exist. Validation may also mean measuring the absence of that specific analyte in certain populations. One example is the polymerase chain reaction (PCR) methods, which, because of their unique sensitivity, may not have comparable methods other than culture. If culture is not viable, clinically well-documented samples must be available to validate the PCR assay.

* Any modification of the manufacturer's reagent such as dilution or working range will require that the laboratory re-establish the stability of the reagent(s). If a laboratory is either synthesizing or purchasing what are now described as analyte-specific reagents (ASRs) [which is a new category of reagents by FDA (21CFR parts 809 and 864, Final Rule, 1997), which allows *certain reagents to be placed in commercial distribution with only their scientific designation and no data or intended use descriptions*], the definition of stability and analytic range by the laboratory will be made more difficult as manufacturers are, in this proposed rule, not allowed to give or publish this information. The goal of the ASR rule is to provide reagents that should have more consistency than ones produced by nonmanufacturing entities (university laboratories, etc.), as they will be produced in controlled conditions (GMP) and will be more reliable than an RUO, which does not have to be produced under GMP.

3. Large numbers of these samples must be used to determine sensitivity as well as specificity. Specificity must be defined with well-characterized panels or sera or samples that are known to cross-react with the analyte of interest. This is not easy to do in a small institution and, therefore, the requirement of test validation and verification is that it should be done across several laboratories or multiple patient referral centers. The use of several laboratories has the advantage of assuring a cross section of patient samples and serves as a means for establishing proficiency testing for that analyte, a requirement for QC.

4. The appropriate clinical range of the analyte must be established by the laboratory defining the test. Again, this requires a large number of well-characterized sera or samples and definition of the population that is being served. A *normal range* may not be appropriate if the analyte is not present in the general population in normal conditions. In this case, the threshold of significance and reference range must be defined. Standard preparations should be used, if available, for comparison. In immunology these standards are relatively rare (9).

When the laboratory has defined the raw materials or reagents to be used in the test methodology, the *intended use* for this test, and the *clinically significant ranges* (although these may need modifications), it is now ready to *perform* the validation protocol. As in any clinical trial, the documentation of the *processes* is critical to the success of the study. This is often referred to as *good clinical practice* (10). The laboratory must design the study to include (see also Table 9-2)

1. A well-versed investigator or expert(s)
2. Defined patient populations
3. A clearance from an Institutional Review Board (IRB), including patient consent form where appropriate
4. Definition of the clinical sites
5. Definition of support personnel and equipment
6. Definition of appropriate statistical support: the number of samples needed to meet the sensitivity and specificity requirements necessitated by the test
7. Appointment of a clinical trial monitor by the laboratory to make sure that all aspects of the test protocol are being followed and that the equipment and reagents being used are performing appropriately
8. Definition of the statistical methods to be used for analysis

TABLE 9-2
Study Design

Defined investigator and expert(s)
Defined patient population
Defined sampling parameters
Clearance from Institutional Review Board (IRB)/defined patient consent forms
Defined clinical sites/if not other laboratories, cooperating physicians obtaining sample sets
Defined support personnel and equipment
Approved patient data forms
Defined statistical parameters for sensitivity and specificity
Defined number of samples for power of study
Defined clinical trial monitor
Defined audit trial
Summary of trial data/modification of method/final procedure
Laboratory director must define interpretation of test results and definition of clinical ranges
Defined limitations
Definition of disclaimer to be used if ASR reagents are used
Defined references

Further, it is recommended that the test samples remain blinded to those performing the testing especially if they are referenced against another method, so that bias is not introduced. At the end of the trial, the data are then analyzed by the appropriate statistics. Further, patient report forms, test result forms, quality control parameters, and deviations from the protocol during the course of the study must all be documented and reported; then, these must be audited by the quality assurance officer of the laboratory.

The *good clinical practice* requirements are complex and may seem excessive for simple changes or modifications to a particular test. In each case, the laboratory director must decide to what extent a clinical study must be carried, to support the subpart K regulation. Upon completion of the clinical study, the data should be summarized, any changes to the kit method documented, reporting units defined, a QC scheme defined, participation in a Proficiency Testing (PT) program initiated, the normal range defined (if appropriate), the proper clinical interpretations for the test agreed to, and all other subpart K standards met. All validation records must be available to the laboratory inspector. The laboratory director is responsible for detailing the new method and its application to the clinical faculty and others who order the test. The laboratory must maintain surveillance statistics for the new analyte and make appropriate corrections to the clinical range as needed. The clinical ranges should be defined by populations if the analyte is age, sex, and/or ethnicity specific. Appropriate interpretative guidelines are needed and the level of authority for patient result release should be defined. It is also the laboratory's responsibility to train the staff in specimen collection, handling, and transport for the appropriate laboratory performance of the test.

Additionally, the laboratory director must define the American Medical Association's Current Procedural Terminology (CPT) billing codes to be used as well as any disclaimers that must accompany the test results on patient reports.*

Reimbursement Issues

If a test is a home brew and has been validated to the satisfaction of subpart K of the CLIA rule, it should be eligible for reimbursement through HCFA (Medicare and Medicaid). FDA approval is not necessarily needed for reimbursement, although this point is subject to interpretation. HCFA considers *safety and effectiveness* of a procedure when determining part A and B (of Medicare) reimbursement. Anything considered to be for research or investigational use by HCFA is typically not reimbursed by Medicare. (The ASR proposed rule will be problematic for reimbursement as it requires a disclaimer.) FDA clearance is usually required for reimbursement by HCFA, *but* FDA clearance does not necessarily guarantee reimbursement (11). It is also clear that many flow cytometry tests that are still under RUO are being reimbursed for certain defined diagnostic conditions, as they have become the standard of practice, which is in conflict with the above stated (usual) policy. The new FDA RUO CPG is an attempt to control these issues. The reimbursement rules are often interpreted differently by the states, and tests must be individually negotiated on a state-by-state basis by the provider. If an FDA cleared test is available for a specific analyte, as compared to a home brew test, Medicare does require the use of that test for reimbursement [Social Security Act {42USC} 1395y(a)(1)(A)](11). Laboratories that are involved in tissue staining with immunohistochemistry reagents and in performing flow cytometry should be in constant contact with their local HCFA office to monitor reimbursement issues. It is strongly suggested that laboratorians maintain close vigilance over the recent actions of the FDA with regard to the new ASR rule and the new CPG guideline, as well as other pending actions, to monitor their potential impact on their practice of laboratory medicine.

It is clear that the home brew tests being used must demonstrate safety and effectiveness and cannot be considered experimental for reimbursement, and that they therefore require extensive validation as mandated under CLIA subpart K before being used in patient care. The suggestions made in this chapter should help laboratories meet the necessary requirements.

REFERENCES

1. Health Care Financing Administration; HHS 42CFR, part 405, Clinical Laboratory Improvement Amendments of 1988, Final Rule. Federal Register 57, No. 40, February 28, 1992.
2. HHS 21CFR, section 510(k) 360(k), and 21CFR, part 807.
3. Compliance policy guide (CPG) draft. Commercialization of in vitro diagnostic devices (IVDs) labeled for research use only or investigational use only. Subchapter 300, January 5, 1998.
4. HHS 21CFR, parts 809 and 864. ASR Final Rule; Federal Register, 62, No. 225, Friday, November 21, 1997.
5. Jaros M. Guidelines for evaluating and introducing new clinical tests. Clin Immunol Newsletter 12, No. 3, 1992.
6. National Committee for Clinical Laboratory Standards. Glossary and guidelines for procedures, reagents and reference materials; approved

* The ASR rule specifically defines that any "home brew" test must state the following: "This test was developed and its performance characteristics determined by (laboratory name). It has not been cleared or approved by the U.S. Food and Drug Administration." 62 Fed. Reg. at 62259. This applies to ASRs produced within the laboratory's domain even if not distributed to others.

guideline. NCCLS pub. DL1-A. Villanova, PA: NCCLS, 1986.

7. HHS, HCFA state operations manual. Pub.7, May 1993.
8. CDC-CLIAC Conference on Quality Control Issues, Atlanta, GA, Sept. 24–25, 1996.
9. Batty I. Standards and quality control in clinical immunology. In: Thompson RA, ed. Techniques in clinical immunology. Blackwell Scientific Publications, Oxford, England, 1977:219–236; 1977.
10. DeSain C. The master plan: introducing a new series on documentation basics that support good clinical practice guidelines. Eugene, OR, BioPharm, June 1993.
11. Heller, MA. Guide to medical device regulation. Washington, DC, Thompson Publishing Group, 1993:1230–1231.

CHAPTER 10

Improvement of Effectiveness of Immunologic Tests

GERALD C. MILLER

Clinical laboratory immunology has grown and will continue to expand and evolve in the analytic phase; more importantly, however, the preanalytic and postanalytic responsibilities have expanded even more dramatically. The majority of evaluations of the components of the antibody-mediated immune response, the cell-mediated immune response, the complement system, and the phagocytic system for the sake of resolving clinical problems in serology, autoimmunity, immunodeficiency, immunophenotyping, cancer immunology, transplantation, and so forth, have been in close association with clinical specialists who have ordered the evaluations and understood the complex nature of the tests and, more importantly, how to interpret the results.

The dynamics of patient care have changed significantly. One important change has been the appointment by third-party payers of physicians who act as "gatekeepers" to manage patients and, most specifically relevant to us, patients with immunologic problems. "Gatekeeper physicians" may have, through no fault of theirs, a very limited knowledge base, background, or training in diseases associated with abnormalities of the immune system. Our responsibility as an immunologist has expanded dramatically because of the changes in medicine, but our number one focus must remain the patient and doing the "right thing right" for the patient (1).

The dynamics of medicine have now changed, with significantly increased demands on the clinical laboratory immunologist (CLI), who is now required but should also be readily accepting of responsibility to educate physicians in short 60- to 90-second phone conversations, guidance in test selection, and appropriate specimen collection and interpretation of the results generated. The CLI must now grasp the opportunity to take on even more responsibility in the supporting role to physicians and most specifically the gatekeeper physicians.

Not only have the dynamics of medicine required more direct involvement in the practice of medicine but also involvement in the efficient and cost-effective administration of the laboratory. Those who demand equal or even higher quality of testing with a reduction in costs are patients, practitioners, third-party payers, and, of course, the administrators to whom we answer.

The task ahead is almost overwhelming but the opportunities are phenomenal if we are up to the challenge. Each of us is at a point in our career of clinical laboratory immunology where we must choose one of three choices (2); no, one of four choices. Those choices are: 1) Change the system, an impossibility in the present-day dynamics of medicine, although there are those who will try; 2) leave the profession, each of us has invested a lifetime of effort to fulfill goals to do something we feel as a call in our lives; and 3) change our perspective and evolve with the dynamics of the present changes with a positive approach. Change is difficult but we are trained as scientists and should welcome the opportunity to experiment in our practice of immunology and develop positive perspectives in our approach to the dynamics of the changes in medicine that have, are, and will continue to influence our way of doing clinical laboratory immunology. And yes, the fourth choice is: Go insane, be unhappy, be frustrated because we are not willing to make any of the first three choices and therefore we choose the fourth choice by omission. If we choose either 1, 2, or 4, then the remaining remarks will be of little value, but if we choose choice 3, then the rest of the chapter holds some suggestions of direction for some positive approaches in dealing with the ever-changing field of clinical laboratory immunology.

Our first step in implementing the third choice is to understand that we are a service industry with a goal to do the "right thing right" for the benefit of the patient (1). In attaining this goal in the present-day environment, we commit ourselves to *availability, communication, cooperation, mutual respect, and trust* with physicians, physician assistants, nursing staff, administrators, and others. Each of us must make ourselves *available*, first and foremost, in order to *communicate* regarding patient care, personnel problems, cost-cutting measures, and so forth, and then *cooperate* in implementing the measures to which we had a direct, indirect, or no part in the decision. The decision may have been for test selection or it may have been an administrative decision. Out of these kinds of interactions develop *mutual respect and trust,* opening the door for future interaction. As relationships develop based on trust and mutual respect, the demands and difficulty of the questions will intensify for the CLI. Immunology is an abstract science for many physicians and we, being trained and well versed in the field, provide a viable source of immunologic information without threatening the physician with the loss of the patient to another practice.

Regardless of our demeanor with physicians and their staff and administrators, we have the responsibility of providing quality results. *Quality* is an elusive term and difficult to define (1). *Quality assurance* is working very diligently to guarantee the quality, and presumably the best we can achieve will be provided (3). *Active quality assurance* indicates that our laboratory is in the constant process of improving our reliability and the efficiency by which it is implemented. Quality assurance is reinforced by proficiency programs (4) but most importantly by the results we report and their confirmation of clinical diagnosis or direction, or both, in the differential tree toward diagnosis (1).

Quality control implies that whoever is given the responsibility for the direction of that laboratory has the authority to establish the level of quality that will be provided. *Quality* is an active process of detecting and correcting defects by establishing limits of acceptable performance of each test (3,4). Experience will demonstrate that one of the best avenues of quality control is feedback from the physician who has utilized a reported result with a patient with whom he or she is very familiar clinically. This goes back to availability, communication, cooperation, mutual respect, and trust, and back to a relationship with those who utilize the results. A clinical immunology laboratory must produce quality results to survive but it must also be cost effective and well managed (5,6). A CLI should know the monthly fixed costs and variable costs and watch for trends of increased overhead. The best example of a fixed cost is labor. Labor should be tracked on a monthly basis and on a cost-per-test basis. The direct labor (DL) cost per test is calculated as (5):

$$\text{DL} = \text{salary/hr} \times 1\,\text{hr/60 min} \times \text{no. min/test}$$

The costs of running a laboratory are variable primarily because of supplies. Supply costs can be viewed as total dollars per month for supplies; however, a very effective way of monitoring supply costs is determining the cost per test of all tests performed that month as compared to previous months. The cost per test is calculated as (5):

$$\text{Cost/test} = \text{Rgt cost for mo} + \text{assoc supplies/mo total test volume}$$

This result can give you a benchmark from which to gauge the financial management of supplies from month to month. Again, one should watch for trends over a 3- to 4-month period. If we, as CLI, "manage the pennies, the dollars will take care of themselves."

Coding is an important part of our responsibility as Director or Chief of a clinical immunology laboratory. Jaros (5) has done an excellent job of summarizing test coding. Incorrect coding can bring nothing but grief. On the one side of incorrect coding, charges of fraud can be brought, while the other side can bring incorrect reimbursement. Third-party payers and the government are quick to notify a laboratory if they suspect incorrect coding that stimulates overpayment; however, it would be very unusual for them to notify a laboratory of miscoding that would initiate underpayments.

It is important for us as CLI to take the time to acquaint ourselves with Current Procedural Terminology (4th ed; CPT-4), International Classification of Disease (9th revision) Clinical Modification (ICD-9-CM), and Diagnosis-Related Groups (DRG) codings. The CPT-4 is the standard, systematic listing and coding of medical procedures and services performed. The ICD-9-CM is used to classify the diagnosis or reason for the medical treatment. It is recommended in all clinical settings but mandated for the reporting of diagnosis and diseases to all United States Public Health Service and Health Care Financing Administration (HCFA) programs and most third-party payers. It is supported by the utilization and mix of procedures identified by CPT-4 codes. Therefore, it is absolutely imperative that the laboratory submit all appropriate CPT-4 codes for each test performed. Many times there will be more than one CPT-4 code for doing one evaluation; for example, a CD4 count by flow cytometry will generate more than one CPT-4 code.

The DRGs are groups of ICD-9-CM codes that are also supported by diagnoses, procedures, complications, morbidities, signs and symptoms, and discharge status. The fixed reimbursements of Medicare are reimbursed by the assigned DRG as determined by geographic location. All procedures performed 72 hours before the stay and 72 hours after discharge are lumped into the DRG. Medicare is broken up into part A, which covers inpatient hospitalization, and part B, which covers physician services, outpatient clinical laboratory, and x-ray (5).

Phases of Immunologic Testing

Preanalytic Phase

How do we take all of this responsibility and incorporate it into being an effective clinical laboratory immunologist? We divide our responsibility into medical and administrative and then further divide medical into the preanalytic, analytic, and postanalytic phases (1). The *preanalytic phase* is being available to communicate with the physician regarding a diagnosis or suspected diagnosis of a patient. The clinical questions that would be posed to assess the patient's immunologic status would take into consideration the physician's knowledge base, background, and training. It is the CLI's responsibility to listen and draw on the physician's clinical experience, respond with his or her own experience, be current in the literature, and form a network of CLI colleagues for his/her own counsel in order to assist the physician with good counsel to pursue a direction of thought that will be productive in a clinical history and examination. It is the further responsibility of the CLI to facilitate the physician with education if needed and guidance if requested. Education can come in many forms, for example, papers in which important statements have been highlighted, 60 to 90 seconds of morsels of concise information, and so forth. Experience would suggest that when a physician calls he or she will most often have a differential in mind, and many times a clinical diagnosis, and is looking for counsel in choosing the correct tests and the sequence in which they should be ordered/performed.

The categories of a physician mentality of testing are: 1) Screen for a particular disease, 2) help confirm a specific diagnosis, 3) evaluate disease activity, 4) assess for target organ involvement, or 5) monitor treatment (7). While listening to the physician discuss the clinical presentation of the patient, the CLI should listen for clinical goals expressed that can be fulfilled by immunologic testing. Tests that could be considered should be explained, and then tests that would be most beneficial to be ordered should be described.

In expressing requested suggestions, one should keep in mind cost-effective testing and ways of maximizing results. Considerations for the clinical value of any test are its sensitivity and specificity as well as positive and negative predictive values. The sensitivity is the percent of patients with disease who have positive results, thus indicating the accuracy of the test to detect disease. The specificity is the percent of patients without disease who have negative results and thus indicates the accuracy for identifying patients without disease. The positive predictive value, which varies with prevalence of the disease in the population, provides the probability that a patient with positive results has the disease, whereas the negative predictive value is the probability of a patient with negative results not having the disease.

An excellent way to assist the physician is to develop manual or computer-driven algorithms. The algorithms provide for another tier of testing, depending on the results of the previous tier. An excellent example is antinuclear antibody (ANA) detection. A significantly positive (=>1:160) ANA with a speckled pattern would move to the next tier of testing for anti-ribonucleoprotein (RNP), anti-Sm, anti-SS-A/Ro, anti-SS-B/La, anti-Scl-70, and so forth (8).

Any test is only as good as the specimen collected. One should make it clear as to whether it is whole blood, plasma, or serum and what are the appropriate volumes required. Any experienced CLI knows that special exceptions must be made available for volumes in newborns and small children. One should learn the assays thoroughly to know specimen requirements, for one does not need the experience more than once of telling a new mother that her baby will need to be restuck because the wrong specimen was collected. Good communication with clinic and hospital staff is quite important in the collection of specimens, especially in the process of implementing new assays, for example, polymerase chain reaction (PCR). *Availability* and the processes that follow are extremely important in specimen requirements and collection.

Specimen processing is another important part of the preanalytic phase, for certain specimens, such as complement specimens, require refrigeration, whereas others, such as CD4 specimens, need room temperature. Some tests require speed of specimen processing whereas others allow the specimen to set. One should take the time to educate hospital and clinic staff as well as one's own processing staff so that each specimen is handled correctly. Experience would suggest that when errors are made the medical staff or processing personnel should be approached and the problem should be corrected in an appropriate manner in the laboratory.

Analytic Phase

In the analytic phase of the process, we do what we have been trained to do and have done very well over the years (1). The clinical immunology laboratory will provide quality results because of the quality assurance and quality control programs that have been in place since the inception of the laboratory. Quality assurance guarantees quality to the best of our ability and the quality controls establish the levels of quality that the laboratory desires to achieve. Any quality laboratory is constantly striving for quality improvement by establishing goals, looking for new reagents to challenge the assay, and adjusting the system to prevent any deficiencies.

Postanalytic Phase

The results that have been so precisely attained must be communicated in a clear and concise manner in the postanalytic phase (1). It is most helpful to the physician, particularly today when many of the gatekeeper physicians do not have the background knowledge in immunology to provide a clear and concise interpretation of the results. If one has the luxury of knowing the physician, knows that immunology is not one of his or her strong points, and is aware that the results could be enhanced by the CLI's involvement, one should call and personally communicate the results to the physician before he or she receives the printed report (9). A good example of such a call would be serology for Epstein-Barr virus (EBV). Interpreting the significance of immunoglobulin M and immunoglobulin G (IgM and IgG) responses to EBV–viral capsid antigens (VCA), total antibody response to the EBV–early antigen (EA), and the antibody response to the EBV–nuclear antigen (EBNA) can be very helpful. A verbal interpretation of how these results support one another can be educational, clinically informative to the CLI and the physician, and time saving for the recipient physician. This builds relationships of trust between the physician and the CLI. Or, the results from an assay may indicate the need for a phone call because of a result that was outside the scope of ordered tests. An excellent example of this is an antimitochondria antibody being observed during an ordered ANA. Many times these calls precipitate further testing or even a discussion of another patient, but they always seem to aid in development of the relationship of trust.

Not only is it the CLI's responsibility to report the results along with a clear and concise interpretation, but he or she must be available to discuss the clinical significance of the results. This is where the CLI has an opportunity to share the knowledge, the literature, the sensitivity and specificity of the test(s), the positive or negative predictive value of the test, and, most of all, the sound orchestration of the training and experience that become good counsel to the physician as to the clinical significance of the results. This is a wonderful opportunity to further educate the physician as well as the CLI, to suggest supportive assays, and, especially, to allow it to be a learning experience for the physician and the CLI such that the knowledge of immunology is expanded. The patient is definitely the beneficiary of such an interaction.

Experience would suggest that a daily log should be kept in order to recall specific conversations that occurred days, weeks, months, and even years earlier. One should organize the log by identifying the physician, patient, and specific pertinent immunologic information. The daily log pays high dividends in subsequent interactions with physicians and their staff and is also helpful in demonstrating usefulness to an administrator.

Last but not least is the billing aspect of the testing effort (5). The correct CPT-4 code(s) must be assigned to the evaluation such that correct billing and thus chances for optimum reimbursement will be initiated.

Clinical laboratory immunologists have opportunities as never before to develop and perform new assays and improve old assays, and also to take an active role in the expansion of the knowledge of clinical laboratory immunology into the field of medicine. CLIs must make that choice, develop a plan unique to their setting, and then implement the plan. That plan must be developed around availability, communication, cooperation, mutual respect, and trust of those they desire to serve.

REFERENCES

1. Peddecord KM, Hofherr LK. Measurement of the effectiveness of immunology testing. In: Rose N, DeMacario E, Fahey J, et al, eds. Manual of clinical laboratory immunology. 4th ed. Washington, DC: American Society of Microbiology, 1992: 52–57.
2. Lantz W, Lantz C. The fifty-one percent principle. Tulsa, OK: Honor Books, 1995:22–43.
3. Sewell DL, Schifman RB. Quality assurance: quality improvement, quality control, and test validation. In: Murray PR, Baron EJ, Pfaller MA, et al, eds. Manual of clinical microbiology. 6th ed. Washington, DC: American Society of Microbiology, 1995:55–66.
4. Morbidity and Mortality. Clinical laboratory performance on proficiency testing samples. United States. Atlanta: Centers for Disease Control, 1996;45:193–196.
5. Jaros ML. Survival of the clinical laboratory in the 1990's. Clin Immunol Newsletter 1996;16:64–67.
6. James K. Impact of managed care on immunology laboratories. Ninth Annual Meeting of the Association of Medical Laboratories, Chicago, 1996.
7. Moder KG. Use and interpretation of rheumatologic tests: a guide for clinicians. Mayo Clin Proc 1996;71:391–396.
8. Homburger HA. Cascade testing for autoantibodies in connective tissue diseases. Mayo Clin Proc 1995;70:183–184.
9. Ringel M. Phone finesse speaks volumes about a reference lab. CAP Today 1995;9:5–10.

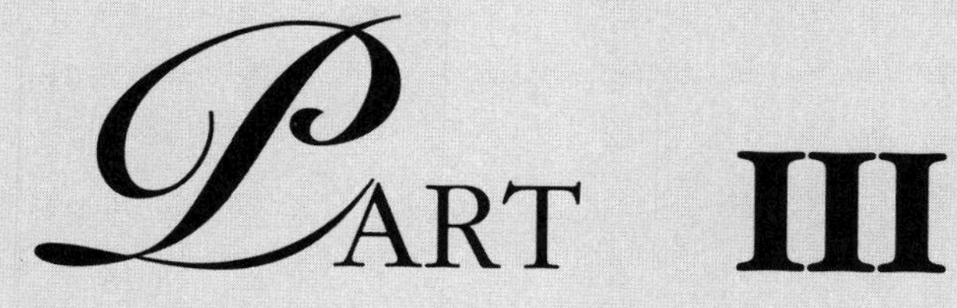

PART III

Recommendations for Quality Assurance, Quality Control, and Standardization of Humoral Analytes

LINDA COOK, EDITOR

CHAPTER 11

Quantitative, Electrophoretic, and Immunochemical Characterization of Immunoglobulins and Serum Proteins

DAVID F. KEREN

Background

Proteins participate in a wide variety of functions, including host defense (immunoglobulins and complement), cell structure (membranes), and movement (contractile proteins), and as regulatory molecules (enzymes, enzyme inhibitors, lymphokines). Characterization of immunoglobulins and serum proteins by electrophoresis and immunochemical methods has become the mainstay for detecting humoral immunodeficiency diseases and some lymphoproliferative conditions such as multiple myeloma and Waldenström's macroglobulinemia, and for evaluating alpha-1 antitrypsin deficiency. Although the detection of a monoclonal component in multiple myeloma is the single most important reason for performing serum protein electrophoresis, a wide variety of other conditions, including acute-phase reaction, cirrhosis, and nephrotic syndrome, can be detected by this technique. In this chapter, the methods, quality control, and quality assurance features for serum protein electrophoresis and the immunochemical characterization of immunoglobulins are reviewed.

Available Assay Procedures

In the 1930s, Tiselius (1) pioneered the use of moving boundary electrophoresis. During electrophoresis, he layered serum on top of buffer in a U-shaped electrophoretic tube. The refraction of light from these proteins as they passed by a sensitive Schlieren band optical system allowed him to define five fractions of human serum protein: albumin, alpha-l, alpha-2, beta, and gamma globulin (1).

Visualization of these fractions was achieved by later workers, who used paper, cellulose acetate, or agarose as a support medium in which proteins could migrate and be stained and quantified. Paper is no longer used as a support medium, however; acetate and agarose in various low- and high-resolution systems are now available commercially. Under conditions of typical electrophoresis with a buffer at pH 8.6, most serum proteins exist as anions, and the acetate or agarose support medium acquires a negative charge relative to the buffer solution. The buffer cations oppose themselves to the negative surface charge of the support medium and flow toward the cathode. This creates an endosmotic flow that pulls neutral or weakly negatively charged proteins toward the cathode. Most immunoglobulins have a weak negative charge, and because of endosmosis migrate toward the cathode instead of toward the anode (2).

Cellulose acetate has been a popular support medium in laboratories because it is easy to use, has a clear background, and gives five reproducible bands. Unfortunately, routine cellulose acetate methods provide an inferior resolution of bands compared to most agarose electrophoresis systems. This inferior resolution makes it difficult to detect alpha-1 antitrypsin deficiency and small monoclonal gammopathies (2). In Europe, the Cellogel high-resolution acetate method has been widely used, but in North America, high-resolution electrophoresis is usually achieved with agarose support media. High-resolution electrophoresis is attained by using highly purified agarose preparations, high voltage, and a cooling method to allow dissipation of excess heat that is generated during electrophoresis (3).

Following electrophoresis on a support medium, the gels are stained with one of several common protein stains (amido black, Coomassie Blue, Ponceau S), washed, and examined visually. In many laboratories, densitometry is used as an adjunct to provide objective information about the quantity of protein that is present in each fraction. It is not recommended that densitometry be used as the sole basis for interpretation of the gels since direct visualization of the gels provides superior information. Densitometry, however, is a useful adjunct to direct visualization.

Recently, capillary zone electrophoresis has been approved by the Food and Drug Administration (FDA) for use in clinical serum samples. This method resembles moving boundary electrophoresis in that the serum passes through thin columns of fused silica to facilitate differential absorption and elution of protein fractions (4). The pattern of separation resembles densitometric scan information, but at a much better level of resolution of the protein fractions. Because each sample takes only a few minutes to complete and can be run consecutively, the capillary zone electrophoresis has the potential advantage of efficiency and minimal technologist time compared to the laborious agarose zone technique. Although still early in its development, this technique has great promise for larger laboratories, where efficiency of processing may be best achieved. Whether this technique will be as sensitive as high-resolution electrophoresis to detect beta migrating monoclonal components and subtle alpha-1 antitrypsin deficiencies needs to be established in peer-reviewed publications.

A newer electrophoresis technique, immunofixation, has recently gained popularity because of its increased sensitivity and short performance time as compared to immunoelectrophoresis. In this method, the sample is electrophoresed in a high-resolution agarose gel in multiple lanes and then each lane is overlaid with immunoglobulin G (IgG)-, IgA-, IgM-, IgD-, kappa-, or lambda-specific antiserum. Antigen-antibody complexes are allowed to form during a short incubation time; then the agarose gel is washed to remove noncomplexed proteins, and finally the gel is stained to detect the presence of the complexed protein. This technique allows the visualization of a band that corresponds to the heavy and light chain type in the gel.

Quantification of Immunoglobulins by Precipitin-Based Assays

Combination of soluble antigen with antibody to form a visible precipitate is termed the *precipitin reaction*. The precipitate is the result of the formation of a relatively large insoluble lattice when the antibody and antigen combine in approximately equivalent molar ratios. In the presence of excess antigen or antibody, soluble complexes are formed. This is why attention to the concentrations of each analyte used is of great importance to avoid false-negative reactions. Indeed, part of our internal quality assurance program requires correlation of all available data, including serum protein electrophoresis, immunoglobulin quantification (usually by nephelometry), and immunofixation (when needed), to be sure that a false-negative nephelometric or immunofixation has not occurred (see below).

Precipitin reactions form the basis for both nephelometry and radial immunodiffusion (RID), the two most commonly used methods to quantify immunoglobulins. Although these methods of analysis are considerably less sensitive than assays that use enzyme, chemiluminescent, or isotopic probes, they are rapid, accurate, and inexpensive for measuring analytes such as IgG, IgA, and IgM, which are present in relatively high concentrations in normal serum. RID and nephelometry are useful in measuring quantities down to 0.5 mg/dL. Nephelometers that use latex particle methods can measure quantities down to μg/dL levels.

For RID, antibody specific for the serum protein to be measured is mixed into the agarose when the agarose is about 50°C. At this temperature, the agarose is liquid enough to allow an even distribution of the antibody in the matrix, but not too hot to affect antibody stability. The agarose that contains the specific antibody is poured onto a slide and allowed to cool, and then holes are punched in the agarose at regular intervals. Standard solutions containing the specific antigen of interest and unknown serum samples are placed in the holes to construct the standard curve. Sera with unknown concentrations of the immunoglobulin are placed in other wells. The immunoglobulin then diffuses radially until the concentration of the analyte in the serum is roughly equivalent to the concentration of the specific antibody in the agarose where a precipitin ring forms. The standard solution to determine the curve and unknown sera must be read at the same time. The concentration of the immunoglobulin in the unknown sera correlates with the size of the precipitin ring (5–7). A precise measurement is determined by comparing the diameter of each unknown serum to that of the standard solution curve (**Fig. 11-1**). Although RID is quite simple, requiring virtually no expensive special equipment, it is slow and not as precise as nephelometry.

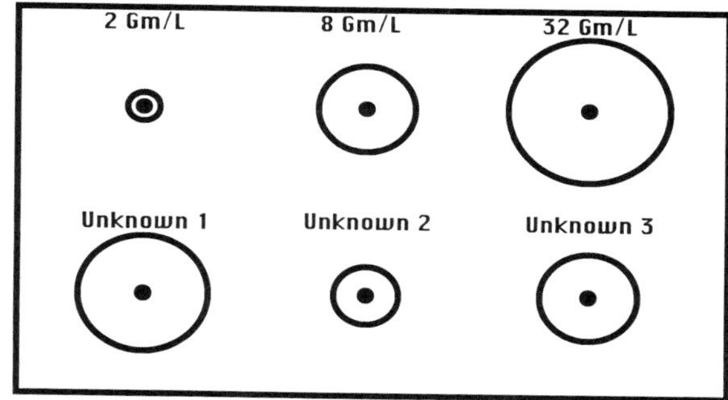

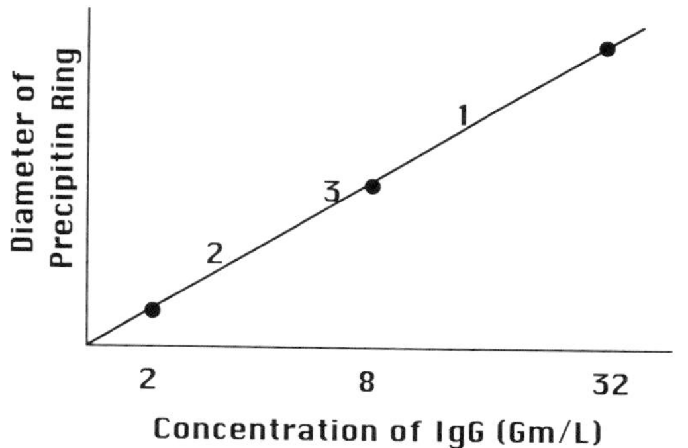

FIGURE **11-1**

Schematic representation of radial immunodiffusion. *Upper panel.* Six wells are represented. The three wells at the top had standard IgG solutions of 2, 8, and 32 g/liter placed in them. The three wells at the bottom of the gel had three unknown samples placed in them as indicated. *Lower panel.* Standard curve is constructed based on the diameter of the three standard samples above (*filled circles*). Then, the concentration of IgG in the three unknown samples is estimated by determining where they fall on this curve.

Nephelometry involves the mixture of the serum and known standards with specific antibody in solution. The immune complexes formed by this procedure will scatter light that is shone through an appropriate reaction cell. Some nephelometers can also use either antigen- or antibody-coated latex particles. The degree of light scatter measured by a standard photomultiplier tube is proportional to the concentration of the antigen being measured (8).

Nephelometry has a great advantage over RID in that it can be performed in a matter of minutes while RID takes 2 or 3 days. Originally, only a single reading of the light scatter would be taken; however, when multiple readings of each sample are taken over time, the rate of the development of light-scattering ability (immune complexes) can be determined. This rate nephelometry is quicker and more precise than the older single point determinations. In order to avoid antigen excess effect that would dramatically underestimate the concentration of a particular immunoglobulin (potentially a great problem if looking at patients with multiple myeloma, who may have a 10-fold increase in the concentration of a particular isotype of immunoglobulin), rate nephelometers run a check for antigen excess by adding additional antigen. Even with this check, however, cases with a falsely low value have been seen that could have resulted in a misdiagnosis if appropriate internal quality assurance programs were not in place (see below).

Falsely low immunoglobulin measurements can be obtained in either monoclonal or polyclonal increases in immunoglobulins. This problem is seen more often in situations in which there is a large increase of a relatively uncommon analyte. It is also frequently seen when urine immunoglobulin quantitations are performed. For instance, an increase in IgG4 (the least common subtype of IgG) may be difficult for a nephelometer to detect with anti-IgG4 reagent, because that assay is standardized to detect small quantities of IgG4. When an IgG4 subclass quantification is requested, the clinician is usually trying to rule out an IgG4 subclass deficiency. Therefore, the assay that is standardized to detect relatively low quantities under normal circumstances will be useful in detecting a deficiency. A patient with an IgG4 myeloma may have a falsely low value in such an assay. Patients may have striking polyclonal increases in IgG4 in several situations: allergy, systemic lupus erythematosus, diabetes mellitus, and Wegener's granulomatosis (9–11).

In a case of Wegener's granulomatosis seen in my laboratory, an unusually broad and dense beta-gamma region band was observed on serum protein electrophoresis. Because of the location, broad nature of the band, and known association with some cases of Wegener's granulomatosis, an attempt was made to quantify the IgG4 subclass using our standard nephelometric procedure. However, when the serum was added directly to the nephelometer, the instrument reading showed IgG4 to be undetectable (**Table 11-1**). Only when the sample was prediluted at 1:216 were we able to correctly measure the 1408 mg/dL of the IgG4 subclass present in the patient's serum. Clearly, antigen excess is a problem even in modern nephelometers and appropriate quality assurance requires comparison of all of the immunologic data available on the patient and demands that the results be consistent. If they are not, the patient's serum should be prediluted and the nephelometric results repeated. In the example shown in Table 11-1, the predilution (shown in parentheses) of the patient's sample made a dramatic difference in the amount of IgG4 that was detected. It should be noted that little effect was seen on the concentrations of IgG1, IgG2, or IgG3 at the two different predilutions run on each of these analytes.

TABLE **11-1**

Dilution and IgG Subclass (total IgG = 3070 mg/dL)

IgG Subclass	First Result (dilution)	Final Result (dilution)
IgG1	741* (1:216)	888 (1:1296)
IgG2	517 (1:216)	597 (1:1296)
IgG3	96 (1:6)	111 (1:36)
IgG4	0 (1:6)	1408 (1:216)
Total	1354	3004

*Results expressed as mg/dL.

Specimen Requirements

For serum protein electrophoresis or immunoglobulin quantification, a blood specimen should be drawn from a fasting individual. Serum should be separated and stored at 2°C to 8°C for up to 72 hours. After 72 hours, however, the sample will deteriorate with loss of the C3 (beta-2 region) band. Freezing the sample at −20°C will preserve the complement for future study.

Internal Controls

For serum protein electrophoresis at least one quality control serum should be included on each electrophoretic strip and each daily run should contain two quality control sera. The migration and concentrations expected for these control samples should be noted visually and recorded by densitometer to compare day-to-day values. These data can be recorded on Levy-Jennings charts for easy daily reference to see if the system is performing consistently (**Fig. 11-2**).

FIGURE **11-2**

Levy-Jennings chart for one month of the albumin concentration in the control assayed each day with the patient electrophoresis samples. Quantity of albumin determined by densitometric scan of the albumin peak. Similar charts are created for each of the five serum fractions.

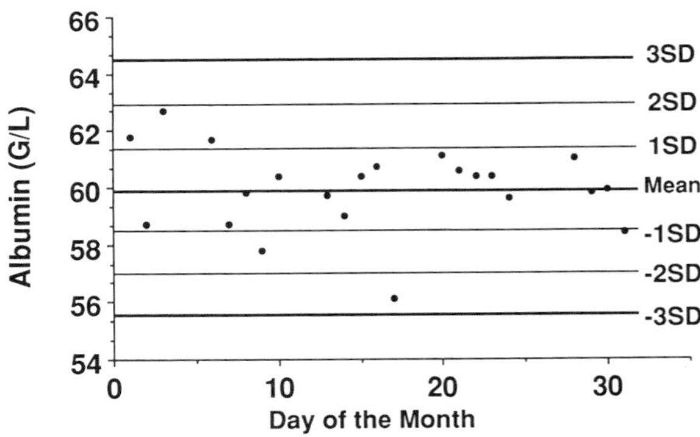

Standards

Most commercial assays are standardized to the International Federation of Clinical Chemistry International Reference Preparation for Plasma Proteins. This material is certified by the Bureau of Reference of the European Community and can be obtained as a Reference Preparation for Proteins in Human Serum from the College of American Pathologists (CAP).

Pitfalls and Troubleshooting

Because nephelometry and RID will only give optimal results in the near equivalence range, it is important that the assays be standardized for the usual range of the analyte in serum. It is important that the technologist who is performing the assay be thoroughly versed in basic immunochemistry. Despite manufacturers' claims that their nephelometric systems will not give problems with falsely low values due to antigen excess effect phenomenon, my experience has been to the contrary (see Table 11-1). Although the case described previously dealt with an increase in the most obscure subclass of IgG (IgG4), unusual nephelometric results may be found even with common components. This is why immunoglobulin quantifications should be interpreted together with serum protein electrophoresis. Occasionally, cases with massive amounts of an IgA lambda monoclonal protein have mistakenly been called alpha heavy chain disease because the nephelometric quantification of kappa and lambda were normal due to antigen excess.

For the initial evaluation of a patient for possible monoclonal gammopathy, immunoglobulin quantification alone is inadequate. Some monoclonal components may be in the normal range; further, patients with biclonal gammopathies may have a normal kappa-lambda ratio.

False positives can occur if abnormalities seen on protein electrophoresis are not further characterized by immunofixation. Protein electrophoresis may demonstrate bands that are not related to immunoglobulins such as fibrinogen, C-reactive protein, and transferrin variants. These must be distinguished by immunofixation to rule out a monoclonal component. The specificity of the antisera used in immunofixation must be determined. False positives due to cross-reactivity of some commercial reagent antisera with other proteins also have been reported (12). This cross-reactivity should be detected by reacting each new lot of commercial antisera with appropriate controls. The controls should include normal serum and plasma (because some patient samples may have fibrinogen–inadequate clotting, those receiving anticoagulants).

When a band on protein electrophoresis does not correlate with the level of immunoglobulin, the immunoglobulin quantification should be repeated with a predilution of the patient's serum. The amount of predilution can be determined after estimating the protein concentration from the densitometric scan of the monoclonal component (13). After the amount of protein in the monoclonal component is estimated, the serum should be diluted to place the quantity of the probable monoclonal component in the middle of the standard curve.

Interpretation

Serum protein electrophoresis and immunoglobulin quantification are the most appropriate screening tests for detection of a monoclonal component. Immunofixation is used to characterize the monoclonal protein. No one electrophoretic pattern is always associated with monoclonal components because of the great diversity of immunoglobulin production. Indeed, even the quantity of monoclonal component that needs to be detected is not established. Newer high-resolution electrophoresis techniques are able to detect monoclonal components as small as 50 mg/dL. It is not clear that such tiny monoclonal components have clinical significance if one wishes to detect solely neoplastic lymphoproliferative conditions. Quantities of monoclonal components much greater than this have been described in patients with infectious and autoimmune diseases, as well as in those with monoclonal gammopathy of undetermined significance (MGUS) (14). Therefore, interpretation of serum protein electrophoresis must give the clinician perspective to judge what the significance of the monoclonal component may be in light of the specific patient's clinical picture.

Tiny monoclonal components that may require immunofixation for detection may be critical to understanding some patients with monoclonal gammopathies in the presence of peripheral neuropathies (15). The older five-band pattern electrophoretic techniques are too insensitive to detect the small monoclonal components that are seen as part of the monoclonal gammopathy with neuropathy syndrome. Therefore, immunofixation is recommended in all patients in whom a monoclonal protein associated with a neuropathy is part of the differential diagnosis.

In addition, patients with some forms of myeloma, including light chain disease, IgE myeloma, and IgD myeloma, may have relatively small or no monoclonal component detectable in the serum protein electrophoresis. Immunoglobulin light chains are small molecules that pass through the glomerular basement membrane. Since tubules can reabsorb up to 1g protein per 24 hours by the time monoclonal free light chains (Bence Jones proteins) appear in the urine, they may have great clinical significance. Serum protein electrophoresis in patients with light chain disease usually contains low-normal gamma globulins, but may have a small restriction, often in the beta region. It is recommended that a urine immunofixation be performed in any case in which the serum gamma globulin is low. Further, even with a small serum monoclonal component, a urine immunofixation should be performed to rule out a Bence Jones protein. Cases with small serum monoclonal components and massive urine Bence Jones proteins are well known (16).

Clinical Rationale and Relevance

Serum protein electrophoresis and immunoglobulin quantifications are indicated in any patient with signs and symptoms of myeloma, Waldenström's macroglobulinemia, or evidence of a lymphoproliferative disorder (**Table 11-2**). The test is useful in detecting a monoclonal process as the etiology of the symptoms and signs listed in Table 11-2. As mentioned previously, however, use of immunoglobulin quantification without protein electrophoresis can lead to false negatives and false positives. There is no way to be certain of the absence of an antigen excess effect without serum protein electrophoresis. False positives for a monoclonal component can occur when the patient has a massive increase in polyclonal immunoglobulins. Usually, the gamma globulin region of serum protein electrophoresis in patients with a polyclonal pattern is very broad. However, occasionally, there are oligoclonal bands and regional restrictions that can mimic a monoclonal component.

Polyclonal and oligoclonal increases in immunoglobulins can be seen under a wide variety of circumstances, many of which overlap with symptoms and signs of lymphoproliferative processes (**Table 11-3**). Typically, antibodies that respond to antigenic stimulation are the basis for the increase in gamma globulins. On occasion the increase is due to inappropriate T-cell stimulation such as in angioimmunoblastic lymphadenopathy (see below). Microorganisms, vaccines, autoimmune diseases, and chronic inflammatory diseases (especially gastrointestinal and inflammatory lung diseases) often are associated with polyclonal and

TABLE **11-2**

Clinical Features that Lead to Serum Protein Electrophoresis and Immunoglobulin Quantification

Disease	Signs or Symptoms
Myeloma	Back pain, osteolytic lesions, pathologic fractures, fatigue, anemia, elevated sedimentation rate, renal failure (amyloid, Bence Jones protein), infections, hypercalcemia, cryoglobulinemia
Waldenström's macroglobulinemia	Fatigue, elevated sedimentation rate, anemia, splenomegaly, lymphadenopathy, lymphocytosis
B-cell lymphoproliferative disease	Weight loss, infection, splenomegaly, lymphadenopathy, anemia, lymphocytosis

TABLE **11-3**

Conditions Associated with Polyclonal Increase in Gamma Globulins

Infections
- Viral
- Bacterial

Autoimmune disease
Vaccines
Lymphoproliferative disease
- T cell—angioimmunoblastic lymphadenopathy
- B cell—rare cases of B-cell lymphoma

oligoclonal increases in gamma globulins. The electrophoretic counterpart of the polyclonal increase in gamma globulins is the broad increase in the gamma globulin area. When IgA is also increased (often part of a cirrhotic pattern, or in mucosal infections), there is often a beta-gamma bridging because IgA preferentially migrates in the beta globulin region. When the increase in polyclonal immunoglobulins is sufficiently high, the serum viscosity may increase to levels that are usually associated with Waldenström's macroglobulinemia.

Expansion of a few clones, recognizable by a few small bands superimposed on the otherwise diffusely staining gamma globulin region, is typically seen in the serum from patients with infections and circulating immune complexes (17–19). Because a particular sample from such a patient may show a large peak that could be mistaken for a monoclonal component, follow-up specimens are important to avoid overinterpreting the significance of these findings (20).

Massive polyclonal and oligoclonal increases in gamma globulins have been reported in patients with the acquired immunodeficiency syndrome (AIDS). Some of the oligoclonal bands described in patients with AIDS have specificity for human immunodeficiency virus (HIV) antigens; 43% of patients who were HIV antibody positive had oligoclonal bands by electrophoresis (21–24).

Polyclonal increases in gamma globulins correlate with interleukin-6 production. Although gamma globulins are usually decreased in the serum of patients with B-cell lymphoproliferative disorders, some cases have small monoclonal or oligoclonal bands (25).

Lymphoproliferative processes develop with increased frequency in patients who are immunosuppressed following a transplantation. It is important to detect these cases of post-transplant lymphoproliferative disorders (PTLD) early because they can regress if the immunosuppressive therapy can be decreased or discontinued (26,27). PTLD has been reported in as many as 20% of patients with heart transplants. In one study, a third of 76 heart transplant patients had oligoclonal bands and 15% of them had monoclonal components (28).

Although most polyclonal increases in immunoglobulins produce a diffuse increase of gamma globulins, occasionally the increase will occur preferentially in one subtype of IgG (29). This will produce a restriction that can resemble a monoclonal component. To distinguish this from a monoclonal component, an immunofixation needs to be performed.

Quality Assurance for Evaluation of a Monoclonal Component

In our laboratory, internal quality assurance for evaluating serum protein electrophoresis and immunoglobulin quantifications for the presence of a monoclonal gammopathy consists of three major components beyond the usual preanalytic concerns about specimen processing, analytic concerns about technique (discussed above), and postanalytic procedures to ensure correct delivery of information.

First, all immunologic information on the patient must be correlated. As stated previously, we do not recommend performing immunoglobulin measurements in the absence of serum protein electrophoresis. In an adult, the indications for immunoglobulin quantification are evaluating a patient for a monoclonal gammopathy and ruling out an immunodeficiency. Since a monoclonal gammopathy is in the differential diagnosis for an adult with a potential immunodeficiency, a serum protein electrophoresis is an important component of this evaluation. Cases with obvious (large) monoclonal components will usually have the correct diagnosis made after immunoglobulin quantification with protein electrophoresis is performed. Smaller monoclonal components will require the additional performance of immunofixation (30). Immunoelectrophoresis is an acceptable technique that is less sensitive than immunofixation, but is acceptable to detect most of the monoclonal components of clinical significance. When correlating the serum protein electrophoresis, immunoglobulin quantifications, and immunofixation (if available), one must demand that all of the information be consistent. If the protein electrophoresis has an unexplained large restriction and none of the immunoglobulin fractions are increased, repeat analysis of the immunoglobulins using predilution of the sample may be warranted. Alternatively, or in addition, an immunofixation should be performed to determine if this is a monoclonal component, or if it represents another protein component such as fibrinogen. Inconsistent findings should not be ignored and should be reported as conflicting, unexplained bits of individual information to the clinician.

Second, comparison between the present sample and all previous samples on that patient should be made. This allows the laboratorian to be sure that the same monoclonal component is present in the current sample that was described previously, and the extent to which it has changed over time. Kyle notes that in about 20% of patients monoclonal gammopathy of undetermined significance evolves into a malignant lymphoproliferative process within 10 years of its detection (31). Comparing previous results and including information on this in the final report to the clinician bring continuity to the care of the patient and allow the clinician to learn of any significant alteration in the monoclonal component or in the normal polyclonal immunoglobulins in that patient that may be of clinical interest. For instance, the development of a hypogammaglobulinemia background in a patient with a previously described monoclonal component may cause the clinician to consider using gamma globulin replacement therapy to combat a pyogenic infection in that patient. The issue of comparing the current to previous samples is becoming even more important as patients begin to undergo more aggressive therapy including bone marrow transplantation for treatment of myeloma. In those patients, the monoclonal band may disappear completely. Reappearance of that band should be distinguished from oligoclonal bands that may occur in these patients.

Third, internal quality assurance should always include direct communication with the clinician when unusual features appear in a case, or when discrepancies are found between the immunoglobulin quantification and electrophoresis information that cannot be resolved by further protein studies. The presence of unexplained bands, the continued presence of large bands, or the demonstration of a pattern consistent with an unusual condition such as heavy chain disease should generate a conversation with the clinician to see how the findings in the laboratory compare to the clinical signs and symptoms. For instance if the laboratory finds what appears to be alpha heavy chain disease, the clinician should be called. In one such case that was recently reviewed in my laboratory, the history was consistent with IgA myeloma, not alpha heavy chain disease. A review of laboratory findings with repeat immunofixation using a new anti–light chain reagent indicated that the original antilambda antisera had been unable to react with the light chain in that case. Direct contact with the clinician is one of the most overlooked techniques available to the immunology laboratory to assure the utility of information that we generate (32,33), and for our friends in managed care it is quite cost effective as well.

External quality assurance consists of proficiency testing. Comparison of the laboratory with other facilities across the country is a great benefit of subscribing to programs such as the CAP. By comparing our results to those of peer institutions, we can be confident that the answers we provide are reproducible by other laboratories. Immunology still has some of the most subjective tests, including electrophoresis, found in laboratories today. Therefore, the participation in an external proficiency testing service is crucial for providing quality results for our patients.

REFERENCES

1. Tiselius A. A new apparatus for electrophoretic analysis of colloidal mixtures. Trans Faraday Soc 1932;33:524–531.
2. Keren DF. High-resolution electrophoresis and immunofixation. In: Methods and rationale for high-resolution electrophoresis. 2nd ed. Boston and London: Butterworth-Heinemann, 1994.
3. Elevitch FR, Aronson SB, Feichtmeir TV, Enterline ML. Thin gel electrophoresis in agarose. Am J Clin Pathol 1966;46:692–697.
4. Kim JW, Park HJ, Park JW, et al. Quantitative analysis of serum proteins separated by capillary electrophoresis. Clin Chem 1993;39:689–692.
5. Fahey JL, McKelvey EM. Quantitative determination of serum immunoglobulins in antibody-agar plates. J Immunol 1965;94:84–92.
6. Finely PR. Nephelometry: principles and clinical laboratory applications. Lab Management 1982; 20:34–41.
7. Mancini G, Carbonara AO, Hereman JF. Immunochemical quantitation of antigens by singly radial immunodiffusion. Immunochemistry 1965;2: 235–342.
8. Nakamura RM. Nephelometric immunoassay. In: Boguslaski RC, Maggio ET, Nakamura RM, eds. Clinical immunochemistry: principles of methods and applications. Boston: Little, Brown, 1984:199.
9. Nagpal S, Namboodiri MS, Rao BS, Rao PV. IgG4 autoantibodies to DNA in systemic lupus

erythematosus patients. Int Arch Allergy Appl Immunol 1991;95:1–6.

10. Bidet B, Beauvais F, Timsit J, et al. Presence of anti-insulin reaginic auto-antibodies of the IgG4 class in insulin-dependent (type 1) diabetic patients before insulin therapy. Int Arch Allergy Immunol 1993;102:27–132.
11. Brouwer E, Cohen Tervaret JW, Horst G, et al. Predominance of IgG1 and IgG4 subclasses of anti-neutrophil cytoplasmic autoantibodies (ANCA) in patients with Wegener's granulomatosis and clinically related disorders. Clin Exp Immunol 1991;83:379–386.
12. Register LJ, Keren DF. Hazard of commercial antiserum cross-reactivity in monoclonal gammopathy evaluation. Clin Chem 1989;35:2016–2017.
13. Keren DF, DiSante AC, Bordine SL. Densitometric scanning of high resolution electrophoresis of serum: methodology and clinical applications. Am J Clin Pathol 1986;85:348–352.
14. Keren DF, Morrison N, Gulbranson R. Evolution of a monoclonal gammopathy (MG) documented by high-resolution electrophoresis (HRE) and immunofixation (IFE). Lab Med 1994; 25;313–317.
15. Freddo L, Yu RK, Latov N, Gangliosides GMI and GDIb are antigens for IgM m-protein in a patient with motor neuron disease. Neurology 1986;36: 454–458.
16. Keren DF. High-resolution electrophoresis and immunofixation. Approaches to pattern interpretation in cerebrospinal fluid and urine. 2nd ed. Boston and London: Butterworth-Heinemann, 1994.
17. Kelly RH, Scholl MA, Harvey S, Devenyi AG. Qualitative testing for circulating immune complexes by use of zone electrophoresis on agarose. Clin Chem 1980;26:396–402.
18. Kelly RH, Hardy TJ, Shah PM. Benign monoclonal gammopathy: a reassessment of the problem. Immunol Invest 1985;14:183–189.
19. Levinson SS, Keren DF. Immunoglobulins from the sera of immunologically activated persons with pairs of electrophoretic restricted bands show a greater tendency to aggregate than normal. Clin Chem Acta 1989;182:21–30.
20. Keshgegian AA. Oligoclonal banding in sera of hospitalized patients. Clin Chem 1992;38:169–170.
21. Keshgegian AA. Prevalence of small monoclonal proteins in the serum of hospitalized patients. Am J Clin Pathol 1982;77:436–442.
22. Papadopoulos NM, Costello R, Ceroni M, Moutsopoulos HM. Identification of HIV-specific oligoclonal immunoglobulins in serum of carriers of HIV antibody. Clin Chem 1988;34:973–975.
23. Taichman DB, Bayer K, Senior M, et al. Oligoclonal immunoglobulins in HIV-antibody-positive serum. Clin Chem 1988;34:2377–2378.
24. Ohsaka A, Saito K, Sakai T, et al. Clinicopathologic and therapeutic aspects of angioimmunoblastic lymphadenopathy–related lesions. Cancer 1992;69:1259–1267.
25. Tienhaara A, Irjala K, Rajamaki A, Pulkki K. Four monoclonal immunoglobulins in a patient with chronic lymphocytic leukemia. Clin Chem 1986; 32:703–705.
26. Craig FE, Gulley ML, Banks PM. Posttransplant lymphoproliferative disorders. Am J Clin Pathol 1993;99:265–276.
27. Godyn JJ, Hicks DG, Hsu SH, et al. Demonstration of passenger leukocytes in a case of Epstein-Barr virus posttransplant lymphoproliferative disorder using restriction fragment length polymorphism analysis. Arch Pathol Lab Med 1992;116:249–252.
28. Myara I, Quenum G, Storogenko M, et al. Monoclonal and oligoclonal gammopathies in heart-transplant recipients. Clin Chem 1991;37:1334–1337.
29. Alberse RC, van der Gaag R, van Leeuwen J. Serologic aspects of IgG4 antibodies. I. Prolonged immunization results in an IgG4-restricted response. J Immunol 1983;130:722–731.
30. Keren DF, Warren JS, Lowe JB. Strategy to diagnose monoclonal gammopathies in serum: high-resolution electrophoresis, immunofixation, and quantification. Clin Chem 1988;34:2196–2201.
31. Kyle RA. Monoclonal gammopathy of undetermined significance (MGUS): a review. Clin Haematol 1982;11:123–150.
32. Keren DF. Proactive pathology. ASCP News August 1995:2.
33. Rao KMK, Bordine SL, Keren DF. Decision making by pathologists: a strategy for curtailing inappropriate tests. Arch Pathol Lab Med 1982; 106:55–56.

CHAPTER 12

Quality Control in the Complement Laboratory

PATRICIA C. GICLAS

Background

The complement system comprises a complex group of circulating proteins and cellular receptors that play important roles in host defense and inflammatory processes. It is beyond the scope of this chapter to describe in detail the activation pathways and control mechanisms of the complement system, but there are a number of review articles and books on the subject to which the reader can refer for further information (1–3).

Patients with congenital or acquired complement deficiencies are at greater risk for infections, as well as increased susceptibility to autoimmune and connective tissue diseases, than are individuals with intact complement systems. Although genetic deficiencies of complement cannot yet be corrected, understanding the complement system's involvement in the patient's disease history can help the physician make intelligent choices for prevention and treatment when symptoms do occur. In acquired deficiencies, analysis of complement activation pathways and determination of the extent of activation, or other factors such as the presence of autoantibodies against complement components, can help to identify the cause of the deficiency so that appropriate treatment can be started. The acceptance of complement as a marker of pathology is becoming increasingly useful to the physician.

The role of the complement laboratory is to provide reliable data from which such decisions can be made. While our understanding of the biochemistry and molecular biology of complement has grown exponentially since the system was first described at the end of the nineteenth century, it is only recently that clinical laboratories have begun adapting more modern techniques to replace many of the assays that were developed years ago. This has been brought about, in large part, by the increased availability of high-quality commercial reagents, including monoclonal antibodies that are specific not only for the native complement proteins, but also for the individual split products and neoepitopes that are created as a result of complement activation. The careful laboratory must still pay close attention to the particular problems presented by complement analysis, particularly in the area of preanalytical concerns, which may not always be under the laboratory's direct control, but which can greatly affect the quality of the results.

Assays Available for Complement Analysis

Complement tests can be based either on the function or on the concentration of the complement proteins that are present in the test specimen. Advantages and disadvantages of each type of test will be discussed.

Hemolytic Assays

Because human serum complement efficiently lyses antibody-sensitized erythrocytes, hemolytic assays have been utilized to analyze complement function (2,3). The CH50 (*c*omplement, *h*emolytic, *50*% lysis) evaluates total classic pathway function: C1, C4, C2, C3, C5, C6, C7, C8, and C9, which act in that sequence, and the AH50 [*a*lternative, *h*emolytic, *50*% lysis; sometimes written APH50 (AP represents *a*lternative *p*athway)] evaluates total alternative pathway function: C3b or C3·H_2O, factor B, factor D, properdin, C3, C5, C6, C7, C8, and C9, acting in that order. Functional hemolytic assays for individual components are modifications of CH50 or AH50 methods in which every component except the one being measured is provided in excess, so that only the component in question is limiting in the test (4).

The major advantage of the functional hemolytic assays such as the CH50 and AH50 is the ability to quickly screen the entire classic or alternative pathway with one test. By performing both CH50 and AH50 on a specimen, a defect can be localized to the classic, alternative, or terminal pathway (shared: C3–C9), thus limiting the number of subsequent tests that are necessary (5). The tests are relatively simple and take only 1 to 2 hours to perform. Advantages of the functional assays for individual components are the exquisite sensitivity of these tests and the ability to detect small changes (5%) in a component's function over time.

The disadvantages of the CH50 and AH50 include 1) the insensitivity of these two tests to relatively large changes (up to 50%) in an individual component's concentration or function, 2) the requirement for dealing with relatively unstable reagents (the erythrocytes) that should be prepared fresh for each test, and 3) the inherent lability of complement, which makes specimen collection and storage methods critical to the test. Disadvantages of the hemolytic assays for individual components include the complexity of the test procedures and the instability of the reagents used. Since most of these reagents are not commercially available, inhouse preparations must be used. There is also a high degree of skill involved in running and interpreting these tests. As with the CH50 and AH50, a major problem for most laboratories is the inherent instability of the analytes themselves. Many of the complement components are heat labile and lose their ability to participate in hemolytic assays if they are not handled and stored correctly. A further complication can occur if the patient has circulating immune complexes, cryoglobulinemia, or C1 inhibitor deficiency, since serum that contains complement activators or lacks inhibitors will often undergo in vitro activation if it is not collected and handled properly.

Immunochemical Assays

Individual complement component concentrations can be measured in serum, plasma, and other body fluids, by standard immunochemical techniques: radial immunodiffusion (RID), rocket electrophoresis, nephelometry, enzyme immunoassays, radioimmunoassays (RIA), and fluorescence immunoassays. Enzyme-linked immunosorbent assay (ELISA) kits are now available for measurement of many complement split products, and while none of these has yet been approved by the Food and Drug Administration (FDA) for diagnostic use, many laboratories are using them as aids in understanding disease processes in a wide variety of clinical settings.

Advantages of these immunochemical methods include their familiarity to most laboratory personnel. Nephelometric methods are widely used and are considered highly reliable by most laboratories. Nephelometric reagents are available for many, but not all, of the circulating complement components. Antisera and monoclonal antibodies for most of the complement components are available commercially, and some tests such as radial immunodiffusion plates are available in kit form, making set-up easier for the laboratory.

Disadvantages include lack of suitably characterized standards and controls for some of the less commonly ordered components. This can be overcome by inhouse development of controls and standards, and with interlaboratory cooperation and sharing of established reagents that are not commercially available. As with the hemolytic assays, the instability of complement components can also be a problem when immunochemical methods are used. Changes in the antigenicity of some of the complement proteins occur after complement activation takes place, because of enzymatic cleavage and conformational changes in the proteins.

Recommended Assay Methods

Hemolytic Assays

The CH50 is still the most commonly accepted test used to determine the functional integrity of the total classic pathway of complement. It represents the reciprocal of the dilution of serum at which 50% of the erythrocytes in the test are lysed. Thus, a CH50 of 125 units/mL means that 1 mL serum dilution of 1:125 would lyse 50% of the red cells under the test conditions. Likewise, the AH50 measures the function of the total alternative pathway and also represents the reciprocal of the dilution of serum at which 50% of the erythrocytes are lysed. As mentioned above, these pathways share the terminal components, and therefore their combined use can pinpoint the location of a complement deficiency to the pathway involved.

Immunochemical Methods

Nephelometry, immunodiffusion methods, enzyme immunoassays, and radioimmunoassays can all be used to quantitate complement components.

Principle

In *hemolytic assays*, initiation of complement activation by either pathway triggers an enzyme cascade in which the individual components are sequentially cleaved or bound in macromolecular complexes, and the end result is the formation of a complex that can insert into a cell membrane, destabilizing it and causing osmotic lysis of the cell. The step that initiates the reaction is a function of the activating substance: The CH50 depends on the activation of the classic pathway of complement by immune complexes formed by antibodies bound to surface antigens of sheep erythrocytes, while the AH50 relies on the direct activation of the human alternative pathway by the surface properties of rabbit erythrocytes (E_{rab}).

The percentage of cells lysed by a given amount of serum is determined by measuring the optical density (OD) of the released hemoglobin in the supernatant, and comparing it with that of a totally lysed aliquot of cells. Regression analysis or plotting of the data can then be used to calculate the dilution that causes 50% lysis for each specimen tested.

There are variations of the CH50 that use only one dilution or volume of serum per specimen, making the assumption that the slope and intercept of the line formed by plotting percent lysis versus the amount of serum will be constant for any specimen used (Diamedix, Miami, FL). Another variation is the CH100 assay, in which sensitized sheep erythrocytes are mixed with low melting temperature agarose and poured into plates similar to those used for radial immunodiffusion. In this test, serum is placed into a well cut in the agarose and the cells lyse as the serum diffuses into the gel. The complement activity is reported as a function of the diameter of the circle of lysed cells surrounding the serum well compared with that of a standard serum.

Two other types of CH50 assay have recently been made available commercially. One of these assays substitutes liposomes for the erythrocytes and can be performed on a Hitachi analyzer (WAKO Diagnostics, Richmond, VA). This assay is very rapid and gives qualitative results that can be further analyzed by other techniques if an abnormal serum is detected. The other type of assay is an ELISA method that depends on activation of the classic pathway by a substance bound to an ELISA plate, and then later detection of activation products by standard ELISA methods (INCSTAR, Stillwater, MN, and Quidel, San Diego, CA). As with all the other CH50 methods, abnormal sera should always be further analyzed to verify the results and identify the defect.

Functional assays for the individual components of the classic and alternative pathways are done by making serial dilutions of the test sera and incubating these with a constant amount of serum that is deficient in, or depleted of, the component being tested. This supplies an excess of all of the components except the one being measured. Care must be taken that these assays are linear in the dilution range used.

Immunochemical assays are based on standard immunochemical methods and are, like other immunoassays, as good as the antisera used. The nephelometric- and immunodiffusion-based assays require a high titer that precipitates antisera specific for the component being measured, and while the enzyme immunoassay methods can be done with polyclonal sera, it is more common these days to find monoclonal antibodies or a sandwich assay using both monoclonal and polyclonal antibodies. Indeed, the assays for some of the components, including the SC5b-9 and C1–esterase inhibitor (C1–INH) ELISAs, are sandwich assays that use an antibody against one component of the complex as a capture antibody, and an enzyme-conjugated antibody specific for another part of the complex as the detector antibody.

Sample Requirements and Specimen Collecting, Handling, and Storage

Hemolytic assays require very little sample (<0.5 mL serum), but the reliability of the results depends greatly on the way the specimen is collected, handled, and stored.

1. Serum is preferred for hemolytic assays because most of the anticoagulants used to prevent clotting also inhibit complement activation. Ethylenediaminetetra-acetic acid (EDTA) chelates calcium and magnesium, required for both pathways, and EGTA, citrate, and oxalate chelate calcium, needed for classic pathway activation; heparin interferes with C1 function and also binds to other components.

2. Many of the complement components are heat labile, and are extremely susceptible to repeated freeze-thaw cycles. For example, 20 to 30 minutes at 50°C is enough to destroy the activity of C2 and factor B, and decrease the activity of C1. Both C1 and C8 are destroyed by heating at 56°C for 30 minutes, and other components are destroyed if the sample is heated longer. These same components are damaged by repeated freeze-thaw cycles, even if the specimen does not get warmed during the process. The practice of leaving specimens for complement analysis at room temperature or even partially thawing a frozen tube in order to relabel it, and then refreezing it, can seriously compromise the results obtained with that specimen.

3. Because of the inherent instability of the thioester bonds in C3 and C4, continuous spontaneous activation occurs at a low level, and the process is greatly speeded up as the temperature increases. Blood, plasma, or serum left sitting at room temperature or in the refrigerator for any length of time will have markedly elevated C3 and C4 split products (iC3b, C3a, C3c, iC4b, C4a, C4d).

4. The usual way of processing blood to obtain serum also contributes to this process: Many of the coagulation pathway enzymes (e.g., kallikrein, factor XIIa, plasmin, thrombin) can cleave complement components and contribute to the loss of complement activity and the generation of complement split products as the blood clots. Tubes that contain clot activators or serum separators enhance this effect.

In the practical setting of most laboratories, the best sample is obtained by drawing blood into a plain glass tube (red-top vacutainer tube with no serum separator or clot activator), removing the cell-free serum rapidly after the clot has formed, and freezing it at −70°C (or on dry ice) if the sample is to be stored for any length of time (more than overnight) before being tested. Short-term storage (up to 6 hr) can be accomplished best by putting the tube into a slushy ice bath, or freezing it quickly and keeping it in a non–frost-free freezer for up to 24 hours. Any time that specimens are to be shipped to another location for analysis, they must be packed in an insulated container with enough dry ice (2–5 lb) to ensure that they will not thaw out en route. It is a good idea for critical samples to be aliquotted into multiple tubes before they are frozen the first time, so that repeated freeze-thaw cycles can be avoided by the testing laboratory.

Immunochemical measurements of complement components, including split products, should be performed on plasma samples that have been collected as quickly as possible after the blood is drawn. Ideally, the blood should be collected in tubes that contain K_3EDTA and centrifuged within a few minutes to separate the plasma from the cells. The cell-free plasma should then be transferred to a clean tube, labeled, and kept frozen at −70°C until the assay is performed. This collection method ensures that little or no complement activation occurs in vitro. For the anaphylatoxins (C3a, C4a, and C5a) an additional protease inhibitor, Futhan, can be obtained from Amersham (Life Science, Little Chalfont, Buckingham-Shire, England), to prevent activation if the specimen must be kept at ambient temperature. Although other anticoagulants can be used for the RID and ELISA methods, the Amersham RIA procedure cannot be performed on samples that contain heparin since this compound interferes with the initial precipitation step. RID and ELISA methods require less than 0.05 mL specimen, while the RIA methods need about 0.5 mL plasma.

All specimens, standards, and controls to be used for all complement assays should be stored at − 70°C. It has been the author's experience that sera and plasmas stored in one-use aliquots and never refrozen and thawed retain their complement activity at −70°C for many years (>20), although some purified components may lose their activity slowly even at −70°C.

Controls, Standards, Available Reference Preparations, and Quality Control Guidelines

Controls run for functional and immunochemical complement tests should include sera with normal and low values established from previous runs. High controls for hemolytic and immunochemical measurements of individual components are often difficult to obtain, although acute-phase plasma will usually have elevated C3, C4, B, C1-INH, and C9. Since the clinically relevant complement defects (except for split products) involve reduced or absent activity or levels, it is more important to have good controls for the low end of the reference range. High controls for split products can be obtained by using serum instead of plasma (intermediate high levels), or by adding activators of complement (zymosan, heat-aggregated gamma globulin) to serum (very high levels). Specimens that fall outside the assay range on the high side should be diluted and retested so that the results are within the control range for the test.

Appropriate controls for hemolytic assays and component measurements include pooled sera from healthy individuals for the normal control, and the same or another pool of serum diluted (1:2 to 1:10) for the low control. Serum should not be diluted more than 1:4 for the alternative pathway hemolytic assays. Sera from patients may contain immune complexes, altered concentrations of complement control proteins (e.g., C1-INH), or other substances that may alter the complement activity with prolonged storage or repeated freeze-thaws, and thus these sera do not make good stable controls. Sera depleted in specific individual components can be purchased (Quidel, San Diego, CA; Sigma Chemical Co, St. Louis, MO), and used as negative controls. For RID or ELISA methods, a series of plasma dilutions can be used to establish the standard curve.

Standard sera and *reference preparations* for some of the components can be obtained commercially. For functional assays, a few good standard sera are available commercially. One source of pooled serum that can be used for this purpose can be purchased from Quidel (San Diego, CA), and the suggested CH50 and AH50 units/mL in this serum are given in the product insert. Diamedix and the other commercially available CH50 methods mentioned previously come with standard sera to be used with the kits. For individual component assays, purified components can be purchased, and calibrated standard sera are available for some of the components (Quidel, San Diego, CA; Calibrator 4, Calibrator 1, and Calibrator 7, INCSTAR, Stillwater, MN). Another way to obtain standards is through exchange between laboratories that employ the same or similar methods. Indeed, this sort of exchange should be encouraged as it would help standardize the complement assays presently in use by the laboratory community, and would make interpretation and comparisons of results done in different laboratories much easier.

For nephelometric and radial immunodiffusion assays, calibrated standards are available from the manufacturer of the instrument's reagents or kit for C3, C4, B, C1-INH, and other commonly measured components. These can be used for other immunochemical methods as well, but should not be utilized for the functional assays because they are not prepared and stored in a way that preserves complement activity. Care should be taken to determine what the preparation has been calibrated against (i.e., another calibrated serum or purified component protein). Purified preparations of many of the individual complement components can be purchased from several sources, including Quidel, San Diego, CA; CalBiochem, San Diego, CA; and Sigma Chemical Co, St. Louis, MO. These can be used to calibrate a plasma or serum pool for inhouse use as a standard.

If a standard serum or reference preparation cannot be found for a given component, a pool of 20 or more normal sera can be arbitrarily defined, for example, as 100% or 100 units. The reference range can then be established by assaying 30 or more normal sera or plasmas using an arbitrarily defined standard and the results can be reported as percent of the standard or the arbitrary assay units. This allows the laboratory to report the results without needing to know the absolute concentration of the component in question.

Most of the available polyclonal antisera against complement components cross-react with the major split products formed when complement activation occurs, and therefore results often include these fragments in estimates of the protein mass in the specimen. For example, some of the commercial nephelometric antibodies and standards for C3 and C4 are prepared using aged sera that contain predominantly C3c and C4c, the end products of complement conversion. Since they do not accurately reflect the amount of native C3 and C4 that are present in the original specimen, a normal C3 or C4 reading can be obtained on a serum that has little or no functional C3 or C4 protein. In order to be more accurate, the results can be verified by a functional C3 or C4 assay or split product measurement. Some laboratories offer C4:C4d ratio determinations to verify the amount of activation occurring in a patient's circulation. The same sort of ratio can be done with C3:C3a (or iC3b), and factor B:Bb levels.

As with other complement reagents, standard and reference sera and plasma should be stored in small aliquots and not subjected to repeated freeze-thaw cycles. Once a standard is adopted for a given method, changing to a new lot should be done in the same way that is employed for other methods: the old standard and the new run in parallel until the value of the new is established relative to the old.

Quality control (QC) is especially important in the complement laboratory because so few laboratories perform the more esoteric tests that comparison and proficiency testing are difficult to obtain. C3 and C4 proficiency tests are available from the College of American Pathologists (CAP), but the other components and the hemolytic assays are not part of this established routine. One of the reasons for this is the lack of standardization of methods and the variability of the reagents used (different sources for antibodies, standards, and controls). The introduction of commercial kits for some of the assays gives the laboratories a common methodology, but even with the same method performed in different laboratories, the results can vary because of differences in sample processing or technicians' skills.

Inhouse proficiency controls can be prepared or voluntarily shared between laboratories that are doing similar tests. Good proficiency controls can be prepared in reasonable amounts from sera treated in various ways to alter the complement levels or functions: Heat inactivation, zymosan (or heat-aggregated gamma globulin) activation, dilution, and concentration are some of the methods that can be used to prepare a series of varied high and low controls that can then be run in a blinded fashion on a regular (2–3 times per year) basis. As with all other complement specimens, these should be stored in single-use aliquots at −70°C.

Quality control parameters that should be monitored for each test run include the values obtained for inhouse and kit controls. These must fall within limits defined either by the kit method insert or by inhouse established limits. For many of the methods, a standard curve is used to calculate the results of the unknowns in the test, and the slope and intercept of the standard curve can be used as QC parameters. Westgard or other accepted statistical rules should be employed for decisions regarding the acceptability of a given run. Specimens that fall ±3 SD outside the normal range should be tested by repeat assay to confirm the results. If possible, ranges should be established for infants as well as adults, since at birth most of the complement values are about half those of the adult values. By the age of 2 to 3 years, the values of complement components and function in children are the same as those in adults.

Practicability: Speed, Level of Operator Skill, Safety, Cost, and Dependability

The *functional assays* for complement are not practical for the small laboratory that receives infrequent requests for the tests. The reagents are unstable for long-term storage and the assays require a great deal of hands-on labor to perform, which drives up the cost per test when small batches must be run. The introduction of the newer tests mentioned above (WAKO's liposome assay and the ELISAs from INCSTAR and Quidel) should make this form of the CH50 more readily available to laboratories that have access to the appropriate equipment, but the more esoteric assays should continue to be performed by reference laboratories that have expertise in complement testing. CH50 and AH50 assays provide relatively rapid screens of complement activity, with results available within 1 to 2 hours. The functional component assays generally take 3 to 4 hours to set up and run. Not included in this time estimate is the amount of time required for preparing reagents and cells for the assays. A high level of skill is involved in performing and interpreting the individual component functional assays. All of these factors increase the cost of the individual component assays over the CH50 and AH50 methods. There are no hazards associated with the functional assays other than those associated with dealing with human blood products. The laboratory that is performing routine complement functions is able to provide reliable results if the quality control and preanalytical concerns are met (i.e., sample integrity).

The *immunochemical methods* are more practical and require less operator skill and time. Most laboratories now have the capacity to perform ELISA or RIA tests, and most of the complement split products (C3a, C4a, C5a, C4d, Bb, iC3b, and SC5b-9) can be performed using commercial kits. The RIA methods involve the use of ^{125}I-labeled proteins, and thus include hazards associated with radioactive reagents and waste materials. RID methods are the easiest to set up, but usually take 24 to 72 hours for the results to be available, while the other immunoassay methods are quicker to perform (10–30 min for the nephelometry, 1–3 hr for the ELISAs, 2–6 hr for the RIAs). Costs of these methods vary, but are usually reagent dependent rather than time dependent. The kits for the RIA and ELISA methods tend to be relatively expensive when used for small runs, and a balance must be drawn by the laboratory management between the cost effectiveness of batching samples against the ordering physician's need for the results. The same number of controls and standards must be run regardless of the number of patient specimens to evaluate. Again, the principal hazard is that associated with handling human blood products.

Pitfalls and Troubleshooting

Many of the problems encountered with complement testing can be avoided by careful attention to specimen collection, handling, and storage procedures. The most common problem is that of the low (but not absent) CH50. The specimen history should be obtained as completely as possible, with times and dates of collection, temperatures of storage and transport, and condition on arrival in the test laboratory. Any deviation from the optimal conditions for assuring sample integrity should be reason for rejecting the result and requesting a repeat specimen on the patient. Sometimes it is not possible to obtain a repeat specimen under the same conditions that the first one was drawn, and in this case the results should be accompanied by a clear explanation to the physician of the problem with the specimen's integrity. One way to control for this is to have a control serum from a healthy individual drawn at the same time as that of the patient and have it sent along with the patient's sample.

The cells used for the hemolytic assays should not have background lysis greater than 5% of total lysis. Cells with high backgrounds can often be restored by washing several times with fresh buffer, followed by resuspension at the desired concentration. No fewer than 2×10^8 cells per milliliter should be used in an assay, as the results tend to be nonlinear. Serum that is badly hemolysed can be used if a series of dilutions run in parallel with those utilized in the assay but with no cells added to them are subtracted from the readings obtained for the same dilutions incubated with the erythrocytes. Another method for dealing with badly hemolysed sera is to perform the assay as normal, centrifuge to pellet the unlysed cells, remove the supernatants, and add an equal volume of distilled water to each cell pellet. This will lyse the remaining cells, and the assay can be calculated by determining the OD of these supernatants and subtracting it from the OD of the 100% lysed control.

Complement-depleted sera used for individual component assays should not give greater than 5% background lysis of the assay cells when incubated at the dilution used for the assay. Traces of the depleted protein could lead to high background lysis. If lysis of greater than 10% occurs, it may be necessary to use a higher dilution, and the degree of depletion should be verified.

The immunochemical methods are usually straightforward and reliable, but problems can occur when the inappropriate specimen is tested. If serum is used instead of plasma for the split products, for instance, falsely high levels will be obtained. Likewise, if plasma is used for C1 function, values will be falsely low. Individual components have peculiarities that require attention to the assay used; since C9 is not absolutely required for red cell lysis, sera with little or no C9 may have normal CH50 or AH50 values. The C9 concentration should be confirmed by immunochemical measurement. Conversely, C8 consists of several gene products (alpha, beta, and gamma chains) that are all required for hemolytic activity. If one chain is missing due to a genetic defect, the C8 produced will not be functional even though normal or near-normal levels are obtained by immunochemical methods. Thus, C8 deficiency should always be confirmed by hemolytic assay, and CH50 and AH50 should both be absent. C4 is the product of two gene pairs and is present in two forms: C4A and C4B. These forms are identifiable by haplotyping methods and they have slightly different properties in terms of immune complex clearance and hemolytic activity (6). It is not uncommon (1 in 100) to have one of the four alleles missing or duplicated, and therefore C4 is the most variable of the complement components in terms of its quantity and function.

Interpretation

Sensitivity and Specificity

The CH50 and AH50 are relatively insensitive tests that are primarily useful as screens for total complement activity. The CH50 depends on the intact classic pathway (C1, C4, C2, C3, C5, C6, C7, C8, and C9). C2 is the limiting component in the CH50, whereas C9 is the least limiting component. The AH50 requires the entire alternative pathway (C3b or C3·$H_2$0, factor D, factor B, properdin, C3, C5, C6, C7, C8, and C9). As above, C9 is the least limiting component, but the entire early pathway must be present for good AH50 activity to occur. In contrast to the CH50 and AH50, the individual component hemolytic assays are exquisitely sensitive tests. The depleted sera used to provide the excess of all components except the one being measured provide high specificity for the methods as well. The best depleted sera are those obtained from patients or animals that are genetically deficient in one component, but sera depleted of a single component by affinity chromatography are also available.

Immunochemical quantitation methods are similar in sensitivity and specificity to those used to measure other analytes. The RIA methods used for C3a, C4a, and C5a are good in the ng range, while the ELISA methods for C4d, iC3b, SC5b-9, and Bb are good in the μg range. These methods have very low cross-reactivity with other components. RID methods are good down to a few mg/mL, and are sensitive enough for most of the circulating components. Factor D is best measured by ELISA, since it is present in very low concentrations.

Handling and Interpretation of Data

Most complement assays, with the exception of the nephelometric methods and the WAKO CH50 method, are not automated, and thus must be dealt with hands on. The data obtained from the hemolytic assays and most other methods based on standard curves can be calculated by plotting or linear regression, with several cautions. Complement-dependent hemolysis follows Poisson distribution, and can be plotted best using probability paper with a log scale for the dilutions and the percentage scale for the lysis (7). Because the curves obtained are not linear except in the center region, points that fall below 15% to 20% or above 80% to 85% lysis should not be used. In the event of a deficient serum in which little or no lysis occurs, the 50% lysis value can be estimated from the lysis obtained in the tube with the lowest dilution and using the slope (but not the intercept) of the line obtained from the control or standard serum. The assay should be repeated using even lower dilutions if possible.

Clinical Rationale and Relevance: When Is the Test Useful?

Complement analyses are useful when a patient has recurrent infections, immune complex disease, autoimmune disease, or angioedema. A family history of similar problems is indicative of a genetic basis for complement deficiency, but often complement-deficient family members are asymptomatic. C1-INH deficiency usually manifests itself in patients by the time they are in their teens or early 20s. Tests for C1-INH deficiency should include CH50, C1-INH level and function, and C4 level. If the acquired form of the disease is suspected, C1q should also be measured. Patients with infections involving *Neisseria* should be tested for complement activity (CH50) and those with low or absent CH50s should be followed up with late-component screens, including C3, C5, C6, C7, and C8. If C3 is low, tests should be done for factors H, I, and properdin (the latter only in males, since the properdin gene is on the X chromosome). C3-nephritic factor, an autoantibody that causes uncontrolled C3 depletion, can also lead to low C3–C9 and set the patient up for neisserial infection (7).

Internal Quality Assurance

Preanalytical concerns have been discussed previously, and primarily involve the handling of the specimen for complement testing. Again, it cannot be stressed too much that proper sample handling is critical to accurate complement analysis. Analytical and postanalytical concerns include assurance that the reagents and antibodies used are of the best obtainable quality, and that the personnel who perform the tests are adequately trained in complement methods including sample handling. Turnaround times must meet the requirements of the ordering physician, and even though cost effectiveness encourages waiting for the accumulation of enough specimens to make a bigger batch, the welfare of the patient is the most important consideration, and a balance should be reached in consultation between the physician/patient (customer) and the laboratory (supplier). Interpretation of the more esoteric tests should accompany the results, and the complement laboratory personnel should be available to answer questions regarding results, the appropriateness of the tests ordered, and the requirements for the specimen.

Comments and Recommendations for Future Improvement

The complement laboratory faces many of the same problems shared by other laboratories, but because of the esoteric nature of many of the complement tests it constitutes a unique branch of immunologic testing. Many of the problems encountered by the physician or other laboratory personnel who deal with complement tests center around inadequate information, improper specimen collection, handling and storage, and ignorance of the many tests that are now available to completely evaluate a complement-related disease state. Complement nomenclature has changed over the years, making it difficult for an "outsider" to know what tests to order or which components are which. This is gradually changing as more publications deal with complement in the clinical setting, and more people become aware of the possibilities that are now available. The biggest improvement in diagnostic complement testing will come through standardization of test methods and the availability of accurately calibrated standards and controls that can be shared by many laboratories. Shared proficiency controls for more components and for some, if not all, of the hemolytic assays will bring different laboratories closer together and provide more reliable data by all involved.

REFERENCES

1. Law SKA, Reid KBM. Complement. 2nd ed. In: Male D, ed. Focus series. Oxford, New York, Tokyo: IRL Press, 1995.
2. Kabat EA, Mayer MM. Experimental immunochemistry. Springfield, IL: Charles C Thomas, 1961:133–239.
3. Platts-Mills TAE, Ishizaka K. Activation of the alternative pathway of human complement by rabbit cells. J Immunol 1971;113:348–358.
4. Harbeck RJ, Giclas PC. Diagnostic immunology laboratory manual. New York: Raven Press, 1991:21–67.
5. Giclas PC. Evaluation of total complement activity and individual complement components. In: Rose NR, DeMacario EC, Folds JD, et al, eds. Manual of clinical laboratory immunology. 5th ed. Washington, DC: ASM Press, 1997.
6. Densen P. Human complement deficiency states and infection. In: Whaley K, Loos M, Weiler JM, eds. Complement in health and disease. 2nd ed. Boston: Kluwer Academic, 1993.
7. Giclas PC, Wisnieski JJ. Autoantibodies to complement components. In: Rose NR, DeMacario EC, Folds JC, et al, eds. Manual of clinical laboratory immunology. 5th ed. Washington, DC: ASM Press, 1997.

CHAPTER 13

Cryoglobulins and Immune Complexes

LINDA COOK

A variety of tests have been described over the last 30 years that detect the presence of complexes of immunoglobulins in the serum. Two commonly used laboratory tests for the detection of immunoglobulin complexes are the cryoglobulin test and the immune complex tests.

Cryoglobulins are immunoglobulins that precipitate out of serum when it is placed in the cold. Cryoglobulins have been classified into three major categories based on the protein content of the cryoglobulin complexes (1). Type I cryoglobulins contain a single monoclonal immunoglobulin and are found in patients with monoclonal B-cell proliferations, including multiple myeloma, Waldenström's macroglobulinemia, lymphoma, and, more rarely, Sjögren's syndrome. The immunoglobulin that is present can be IgG, IgA, IgM, or very rarely IgE and can have either kappa or lambda light chains. Type I cryoglobulins precipitate when cooled down because of insolubility of the protein at elevated concentrations.

Type II cryoglobulins contain a mixture of a monoclonal IgM kappa immunogloblin and polyclonal IgG kappa and IgG lambda immunoglobulin. The complexes form in the cold because the monoclonal IgM kappa has rheumatoid factor activity that causes binding of the IgM to the Fc portion of polyclonal IgG. The IgM-IgG complexes are very insoluble and precipitate in the cold. In the complexes of some patients, complement is also activated, and therefore complement components may also be found in the precipitate. Type II cryoglobulins are found in patients with chronic hepatitis caused by hepatitis C or hepatitis B and in patients with essential mixed cryoglobulinemia. Type III cryoglobulins contain a mixture of polyclonal IgG, IgM, and IgA immunoglobulins and some complement components. Type III cryoglobulins are precipitates formed as large antigen-antibody complexes that are insoluble in the cold. These complexes may also contain complement components, and some of the polyclonal immunoglobulins may have rheumatoid factor activity. Type III cryoglobulins are found in a wide variety of autoimmune and infectious diseases, including systemic lupus erythematosus, rheumatoid arthritis, Sjögren's syndrome, vasculitis, glomerulonephritis, chronic autoimmune hepatitis, chronic viral hepatitis, and human immunodeficiency virus (HIV)-1 infection.

A wide variety of assays for the detection of immune complexes containing antigen-antibody complexes have been described (2,3). Circulating antigen-antibody complexes can be seen in a variety of autoimmune and infectious diseases. In some cases, the complexes are of sufficiently high concentration and are insoluble enough to precipitate as a cryoglobulin. In most cases, however, other assays are necessary to detect the presence of the complexes in the serum. Some immune complexes activate the complement pathway and as a result complement components can be found bound to the complexes. Each of the in vitro assays was developed in an effort to correlate the measurement of complexes in serum or plasma with the in vivo pathologic damage caused by the formation and deposition of complexes and the activation of complement components in a wide variety of tissues of the body.

Available Assay Procedures

There is a single simple method used to detect cryoglobulins that consists of placing serum at 4°C and then examining the serum after 2 to 3 days to determine whether any visible precipitate is present. If a precipitate is detected, a variety of methods can be used to determine the types of immunoglobulins and proteins that are present. Any of a variety of protein electrophoresis methods or immunofixation methods can be used to determine the presence of a monoclonal immunoglobulin. Additional characterization of the precipitate can be done by either of the classic agarose precipitation methods, Ouchterlony or counterimmunoelectrophoresis, to detect the presence of a variety of proteins, or the proteins can be detected with the more quantitative method of nephelometry. In most cases, detection of rheumatoid factor, IgG, IgA, IgM, C3, C4, and fibrinogen should be done. The presence of albumin and fibronectin can also be determined for some cryoglobulins.

A tremendous variety of assay methods have been described that detect immune complexes. In 1978, the World Health Organization (WHO) evaluated 18 different methods for detecting immune complexes in rheumatologic and infectious diseases (4). Only four of the assays, the solid-phase C1q, the C1q binding, the monoclonal rheumatoid factor (RF), and the Raji cell assays, were shown to be sensitive and reproducible enough to detect immune complexes in disease states. Because of the differences between results between the four acceptable assays, the WHO group recommended that at least two assays be used to confirm the presence of immune complexes. More recently enzyme immunoassay (EIA) assays have been developed and commercially produced. The capture reagents in the commercially available assays are one of the following:

1. Human or goat C1q
2. Mouse antihuman C1q
3. Mouse antihuman C3d or C3b,C3dg,C3d
4. Human CRII (Raji cell replacement assay)

In each case, the detection reagent is antihuman IgG coupled to a detection enzyme. Capturing with C1q allows the detection of complexes in the serum that are capable of binding to the C1q molecule. The capture reagent of anti-C1q detects complexes that have already bound to C1q. The final two capture reagents detect complexes containing IgG that have already activated complement and created complement fragments that are bound to the other proteins in the complex. Any of these immune complex assays can be used in the diagnostic immunology laboratory but results will vary between methods. It is important to determine the clinical situations in which the test is being ordered to select the best method to be used.

Sample Handling Issues

Proper collection and sample handling are very important for both the immune complex and cryoglobulin assays. For the immune complex assays, the complexes are fragile and easily degraded, and therefore care must be taken to handle and store the samples carefully to ensure the stability of the complexes. Serum should be separated from the clot within 1 to 2 hours of the draw time and rapidly frozen at −20° or −70°C. Samples should not be exposed to high temperatures, frozen and thawed more than once, or stored in small aliquots in large tubes, as this promotes freezer burn–induced protein aggregation.

For the cryoglobulin assays, it is vitally important to ensure proper collection and sample handling. If the samples are not collected correctly, essentially all of them will be negative. The sample should not be allowed to come to room temperature either during the clotting or centrifugation steps and must not be collected in a tube containing separator gel, as this will result in a loss of cryoglobulin. Improper collection by the phlebotomist or failure to keep the sample at 37°C during processing is a common mistake in most modern laboratories, and therefore constant reminders are essential to ensure the proper sample handling necessary for the consistent detection of low quantities of cryoglobulin that are present in some samples. Laboratory personnel should be very strict in the rejection policies of improperly handled samples to ensure that samples are not reported negative because of improper collection. In most laboratories, this requires constant re-education of phlebotomists and specimen processors by the immunology laboratory personnel.

Recommended Testing Method for Cryoglobulin Testing

The detection of cryoglobulins is a very simple test. The blood sample should be collected into a non-SST (serum separator) tube and the clot tube immediately placed in the water bath at 37°C where it is allowed to clot for 30 to 60 minutes. Then it should be rapidly centrifuged and the serum separated from the clot.

Once the sample has been separated from the clot, two Wintrobe tubes should be carefully filled to the top line with serum. The remaining serum should be placed into a 12 × 75mm tube. One of the Wintrobe tubes should be stored at room temperature and the other Wintrobe tube and the 12 × 75mm tube should be stored at 4°C for 48 to 72 hours. At the end of the incubation time, the two tubes are examined for visible precipitation, which can be seen in the 4°C Wintrobe tube but is absent from the one stored at room temperature. To determine the cryocrit, the 4°C Wintrobe tube is spun in a cold centrifuge to pellet the precipitate to the bottom of the tube. The cryocrit is then read by determining the level of visible precipitate and its corresponding percentage from the tube markings.

To determine the protein composition of the cryoglobulin, 2 to 3mL serum should be placed in a 12 × 75mm glass or plastic tube and stored at 4°C for 48 to 72 hours. Any volume of serum can be used for this analysis but the maximum serum available should be utilized in order to maximize the sensitivity of subsequent detection methods. The volume added to the tube should be recorded. When a visible precipitate is present, the sample should be spun down in a cold centrifuge to pellet the precipitate, and then the precipitate should be washed three to four times with cold saline. The precipitate should then be re-solubilized by adding 100 to 250μL cold saline and the tube then incubated at 37°C until the precipitate is dissolved.

The soluble proteins of the cryoglobulin can then be examined with three methods to determine the presence or absence of immunoglobulins, complement components, and contaminating fibrinogen. For the first method, a few microliters of sample should be loaded on a high-resolution electrophoresis plate and subjected to a standard protein electrophoresis (protein electrophoresis kits from Beckman Instruments, Brea, California or Helena, Beaumont, Texas). After the plate is stained for protein, the electrophoresis lane should be examined for the presence of a single monoclonal band in the gamma region. If the band is present but very weak, an immunofixation electrophoresis can be used to determine the class of monoclonal protein present and the light chain type. For the second method, 100mL of sample should be tested for rheumatoid factor by nephelometry if that assay method is available. If not, a latex agglutination tube or slide method can be done to determine the presence of RF activity in the cryoglobulin. For the third method, an Ouchterlony test is performed by punching a six-well flower pattern in the agar, filling the center well with the soluble cryoprecipitate, and then loading the outer wells with anti-IgG, -IgA, -IgM, -C3, -C4, and -fibrinogen–specific antisera. After 72 hours of incubation, the gel is examined to determine the presence of precipitation lines, which indicate the presence of each of the proteins tested for. If desired, a small sample can be used to determine the total protein present in the precipitate. The quantitative value of mg/dL for the total protein or IU/mL of rheumatoid factor can be calculated by correcting the measured value by the amount that the cryoglobulin was concentrated [value × (cryo reconstitution volume/initial serum volume)].

Based on the results from all these tests, the type of cryoglobulin, type I, II, or III, can be determined. The cryocrit, the type of cryoglobulin present, and the components of the cryoglobulin that are present should be contained on the final report.

Recommended Testing Method for Immune Complexes

For immune complex assays, serum is collected into a non-SST tube and allowed to clot at room temperature for 30 to 60 minutes; then the separated serum is removed and frozen at −20 or −70°C until tested. The serum samples are stable for several weeks at −20°C or for 2 to 3 months at −70°C. All available immune complex assays have 96-well microtiter EIA formats in which the capture protein is immobilized on the well surface. The capture proteins are either C1q, anti-C1q, anti-C3, or CRII.

To perform the assay, the frozen serum is rapidly thawed, and then a serum dilution is added to the wells that contain the capture reagent. The wells are then washed and the detection antibody is added. This is an antihuman IgG coupled to either alkaline phosphatase or peroxidase in all commercially available assays. The wells are then washed again and the substrate is added. At the end of a short incubation, the plate is read with a spectrophotometer and the optical density (OD) of each well is determined. The OD that is present in the patient wells is then compared to the ODs of standard curve points to determine the quantity of immune complexes present. Some samples may have very high levels of immune complexes and give OD results above the top standard of the curve. For these patients the manufacturer's directions should be carefully followed to determine if the sample should be retested at higher dilutions. Since essentially all samples are nonlinear when run at higher dilutions, accurate quantitation of very high levels is extremely difficult and the suggested manufacturer's method should be carefully followed.

Standards and Controls for Cryoglobulins

No standards or controls are available for cryoglobulin testing. Positive controls, especially weakly positive samples that can be used to determine the sensitivity of the method at low cryoglobulin concentrations, are difficult if not impossible to obtain. Samples that contain cryoglobulins can be obtained from a few laboratories that perform the testing and in rare instances plasmapheresis samples can be obtained from patients who need therapeutic plasmapheresis. However, these samples are usually strongly positive, and in addition once they are stored they do not have the same properties they did when they were originally collected. They are usually much more easily precipitated and may not contain the same amount of precipitate as in the original collection.

Negative controls for the cryoglobulin tube are easily obtained. A normal can be drawn at the same time as one is being drawn from the patient and should be handled in an identical manner. This strategy is in practice difficult and usually unnecessary, however. As an alternative, duplicate tubes can be set up on patients that are drawn as an internal blind duplicate control. This strategy will usually work but functions as both a negative and a positive control when the sample is occasionally positive. Except for testing in unusually selected patient populations, the positive rate will be less than 5% of patient samples tested. A negative control can also be generated from a single normal serum sample stored in 2- to 3-mL aliquots at −20°C. In addition, the assay has an internal negative control, the control patient serum tube incubated at room temperature that is very useful to prevent the false detection of fibrinogen and fibrin precipitates as cryoglobulins. Fibrinogen precipitates can be seen when the tube of blood is not allowed sufficient time to clot before the separation of the serum. They can also be seen when samples are tested from patients with coagulation deficiencies or when patients are receiving anticoagulation therapy.

A very useful quality assurance activity is the tracking of all positive cryoglobulin patients in a database. Once a positive result is obtained for a patient and the cryoglobulin type is determined, all subsequent samples from that patient should have the same type. A rare exception to that may be the conversion of a patient with hepatitis C infection from a type III to a type II as the patient begins to produce high levels of monoclonal IgM rheumatoid factor. During therapy for either type I cryoglobulins (chemotherapy directed against the B-cell proliferation) or type II cryoglobulins (interferon directed against the hepatitis C virus), the cryoglobulin amount may be decreased or even disappear. Serial monitoring of cryoglobulin quantities can be useful during interferon therapy for type II cryoglobulin-positive patients. Serial monitoring of cryoglobulin quantities can also be done for type I cryoglobulins, but a more accurate way to measure response to chemotherapy is the nephelometric measurement of IgG, IgA, or IgM quantity, depending on the monoclonal type. When a cryoglobulin sample is measured with the nephelometer, care must be taken to draw and process the sample while keeping it warm, and then the sample must be warmed before it is run on the instrument to ensure the complete solubilization of the immunoglobulin. Thus, the routine monitoring of results from type I and II cryoglobulins can be a useful quality assurance activity when correlated with the therapy of the patient. The tracking of type III cryoglobulins is less useful, as the presence and quantity of cryoglobulin are much less reproducible. However, serial samples from patients with type III cryoglobulins will frequently give similar results, and therefore comparison of results may be useful to ensure the correct performance of the test by all personnel. A database containing a list of all positive type I cryoglobulins may also be a useful quality assurance tool for chemistry and hematology laboratories where cryoglobulins may show interference with the methods used for other testing.

Although a good positive control is not readily available for the detection of cryoglobulins, the subsequent testing of positive cryoglobulins can be controlled with the routine controls available for those tests. For protein electrophoresis, the normal serum used in routine electrophoresis can be utilized to validate the electrophoresis and immunofixation tests. For the rheumatoid factor assay, the negative-, low-positive, and high-positive controls used in the routine assay can be employed. For the Ouchterlony or CIE methods, a normal serum sample diluted to a low level can be used as a positive control for reactivity with each of the antisera that are used.

Standards and Controls for Immune Complexes

For the immune complex assays, the commercially available kits contain standards and controls to be used on a routine basis. Since all immune complex assays are not standardized between vendors' kits, a direct comparison of results cannot be done. An immune complex standard is available from the Centers for Disease (CDC) antinuclear antibody (ANA) reference collection. This standard contains a known quantity of IgG that must be aggregated before use according to the standardized protocol included with the reagent. The standard expresses the amount of immune complex in IgG μg equivalents per milliliter (μg Eq/mL). Inhouse positive and negative controls can be produced by aliquotting small volumes of positive patient specimens and storing them at −70°C. The positive samples are not stable for long periods of time (<1 yr) and frequently give values that are significantly lower than the original assayed value, as the complexes may not be stable during freeze-thaw. This is especially true for immune complex assays that measure complement-containing complexes.

Quality Control Issues for Cryoglobulin Assay

It is also important to thoroughly train all technologists to ensure that the appearance of the cryoglobulin is recognized when it is positive. It should be able to be recognized easily whether it is readily visible as precipitate in the bottom of the tube, or as flakes or slight turbidity throughout the sample, and should be easily distinguishable from small fibrin clots that may be present. Technologists must also be carefully trained to ensure that the cold temperature is maintained during the washing procedure to prevent loss of precipitate. Inadequate washing, especially of samples that contain high levels of precipitate, can leave serum albumin and polyclonal IgG present in the pellet. This can result in an overestimate of the amount of cryoglobulin present and can cause the incorrect interpretation of a type I cryoglobulin as a type II cryoglobulin.

For the follow-up tests that are performed to determine the types of proteins that are present in the cryoglobulin, it is important to keep the cryoglobulin solution at 37°C until immediately before the performance of the test. This is important to ensure that the test results are not invalidated by the presence of complexes in these tests. For the electrophoresis and immunofixation assays, if the sample is kept warm until just before it is loaded onto the gel, the sample will usually run correctly. If, however, a large band of precipitate is visible in the gel at the location of the sample application, the cryoglobulin is precipitating as it cools to room temperature. This artifact can usually be prevented by warming the gel to 37°C just prior to the loading of the cryoglobulin. Warming of the gel may cause slightly faster electrophoresis migration but does not usually result in significant problems with the interpretation of the electrophoresis results.

It is also critically important to ensure that the cryoglobulin is entirely soluble if a nephelometer is used for the quantitation of rheumatoid factor or albumin that may be present. The initial turbidity read by the instrument gives an accurate estimation of the presence of insoluble precipitate that may be present. If a significantly high reading is found, the assay may be invalidated or the results may be falsely decreased. High turbidity of the sample can be prevented by keeping the sample at 37°C until just before loading, warming the sample cuvette, and minimizing as much as possible the time the sample is on the instrument prior to the analysis.

Some cryoglobulins have properties that require slight adjustments to the routine protocol. In rare cases, the precipitate does not form rapidly and may not be visible within 48 to 72 hours. All samples should be maintained at 4°C for at least a week and examined again to determine if precipitate has formed more slowly. In some cases, usually seen in samples with high levels of type I or II, the cryoglobulin is insoluble at temperatures only slightly lower than 37°C, and therefore both the room temperature tube and the 4°C tubes will have precipitate. Usually there is less visible precipitate in the room temperature tube but it may be hard to distinguish the difference when the tube is visually examined. For these samples, one of the tubes can be placed in a 37°C water bath or heating block, where the visible precipitate should disappear within 10 to 15 minutes. This procedure can be used to confirm the presence of any cryoglobulin, as it should be soluble at 37°C within a few minutes. Possible cryoglobulins that do not disappear on heating should be carefully examined to exclude the presence of fibrinogen or fibronectin proteins, or both, as the cause of the precipitate.

Clinical Relevance

The detection of immune complexes with any of the test assays that have been described demonstrates the presence of circulating antigen, systemic immune activation, and a specific antibody response. Unfortunately, because the tests are not designed to detect specific antigens they are only nonspecific measures of immune response. In addition, because the available assays vary significantly in their technical aspects, results obtained when serum samples are tested with different assays also vary significantly. Because of these problems, immune complex assays are not specific or reliable enough to be of significant clinical relevance in most clinical conditions. Immune complex assays are currently not widely used either in the diagnosis or the monitoring of disease. The only clinical situation in which an immune complex assay is useful is in a patient with suspected vasculitis or glomerulonephritis in which no other tests are available that can demonstrate the abnormal immune response and the presence of circulation immune complexes.

The detection of cryoglobulins, in contrast to that of immune complexes, is very important in the diagnosis of affected patients. For patients with type I cryoglobulins, discovery of the cryoglobulin may indicate the presence of an occult monoclonal B-cell malignancy or demonstrate the cause of vascular, cardiac, or circulatory abnormalities that are present. Patients with type I and II cryoglobulins usually have symptoms associated with exposure to the cold, including Raynaud's phenomenon, vascular purpura, bleeding tendencies, cold-induced urticaria, and distal arterial thrombosis with gangrene. For type II patients, symptoms of polyarthritis, vasculitis, glomerulonephritis, neurologic manifestations, weakness, lymphadenopathy, and hepatosplenomegaly may be present. All patients with type II cryoglobulins should be tested for infections with hepatitis C and B, as the majority of cases have been shown to be associated with these two diseases (5,6). Cases of essential mixed cryoglobulin, which are not associated with hepatitis infections or other known cause, have been documented but occur infrequently.

The cryoglobulin test can be useful in the monitoring of response to therapy. The effects can be most dramatic with the chemotherapy given to patients with type I cryoglobulin and with the interferon therapy given to patients with type II cryoglobulin who have hepatitis C infections. Serial cryocrit determinations can be a useful way to document significant changes in the levels of cryoglobulins. Cryocrit determinations can be done on a weekly basis for type II cryoglobulin patients who are receiving interferon therapy. They can also be performed every few days for type I cryoglobulin patients if they are undergoing plasmapheresis as part of their therapy. Depending on the response to therapy, the cryocrit can be significantly decreased within a few days for both of these conditions. For patients with autoimmune diseases and type III cryoglobulins, the cryocrit can be significantly decreased or disappear within a few months after a good response to therapy.

Proficiency Testing

Proficiency samples are not available for testing cryoglobulins or immune complexes. Inhouse testing by blind duplicate replicates or the sharing of samples with other laboratories that perform the testing should be done on at least an annual basis to demonstrate the proper performance of the test.

REFERENCES

1. Brouet JC, et al. Biologic and clinical significance of cryoglobulins. A report of 86 cases. Am J Med 1974;57:775–788.
2. Mannik M. Immune complexes. In: Lahita RG, ed. Systemic lupus erythematosus. New York, New York: Churchill Livingstone, 1992:327–341.
3. Cook L, Agnello VA. Detection of immune complexes. In: Rose NR, DeMacario E, Fahey J, et al, eds. Manual of clinical immunology. 4th ed. Washington, DC: American Society for Microbiology, 1992:110–113.
4. Lambert PH, et al. A WHO collaborative study for the evaluation of eighteen methods for detecting immune complexes in serum. J Clin Lab Immunol 1978;1:1–15.
5. Levo Y, et al. Association between hepatitis B and essential mixed cryoglobulin. N Engl J Med 1977; 296:1501–1504.
6. Agnello V, Romain PL. Mixed cryoglobulinemia associated with hepatitis C virus infection. Rheum Dis Clin North Am 1996;22:1–21.

CHAPTER 14

Cytokines, Growth Factors, and Adhesion Molecules

CONSTANCE EMMETT
KIMBERLY FOSTER

Background and Clinical Relevance

Cytokines, growth factors, and adhesion molecules represent two families of regulatory proteins secreted by white blood cells and a variety of other cells. The pleiotropic actions of these proteins include numerous effects on cells of the immune system, modulation of the inflammatory responses, and homeostasis. Members of the cytokine family include growth factors, interleukins, colony-stimulating factors, transforming growth factors, tumor necrosis factors, chemokines, and interferons, and many smaller families of proteins. Adhesion molecules represent a separate family of proteins that include the immunoglobulin superfamily, the integrins, and the selectins.

Cytokines

A concise and general description of the cytokines is that they are signaling molecules that are low-molecular-weight proteins (5–140kD), secreted by diverse cell types. Cytokines are generally undetectable under normal physiologic conditions, but increase significantly during pathologic states. Production is regulated by various inducers, including other cytokines, at the transcriptional or translational level (1). Cytokine expression is influenced by a number of factors, including the state of growth and differentiation, levels of nutrients, presence of pathogens and cell damage, other cytokines, hormones, and neurotransmitters. Early in the study of cytokines, they were classified as lymphokines or monokines, in order to denote whether they were produced by lymphocytes or monocytes (1). Later, the word *cytokine* was proposed as an umbrella term for all of these molecules that were discovered to be the product of cells other than just lymphocytes and monocytes. Cytokines are produced by a wide variety of cells: lymphocytes, monocytes, neutrophils, mast cells, endothelial cells, fibroblasts, glial cells, neurons, and endocrine organ cells such as the anterior pituitary cells and oocytes (2).

Cytokines have been likened to hormones, and indeed they generally can be described as polypeptide hormones (2). Most cytokines, however, are local mediators that affect growth and metabolism (2). This fact distinguishes them from the hormones produced by endocrine organs, which serve as signaling molecules in distant tissues (2). Most cytokines have a highly regulated expression that must be induced (3). Unlike hormones, which are made by specialized cell types (e.g., insulin is produced by the beta islet cells of the pancreas), cytokines are made by multiple cell types. In fact, these cell types can be widely disparate and produce the same cytokine (e.g., interleukin-8 is produced by macrophages, neutrophils, and mast cells). In addition, diverse stimuli, including those of other cytokines, will induce the expression of the same cytokine. By either inducing or suppressing the expression of other cytokines, cytokines form a network (4). Cytokines, like hormones, function to mobilize and activate a wide variety of target cells to grow and to perform their various functions. Unlike hormones, cytokines maintain a differentiation of the self from the nonself in their various roles in the immune system of the host (1).

Most cytokines interact with cells through specific, high-affinity receptors (K_d 10^{-9} to 10^{-12}) on the cell surface. Even though cytokines are of distinct chemical structure from one another, they may share common cell receptors. In addition to cell surface receptors, soluble receptors corresponding to the binding domains of cytokine receptors and polypeptide hormones have been described (5). The cytokine receptors are discussed in detail in Chapter 16.

Even though the cytokines were basically discovered in the last decade, continued knowledge about their roles in the immune system, physiologic metabolism, pathogenesis, and treatment of disease has burgeoned. Because of their complexity in action and reaction, the cytokine field is certain to continue to expand at a rapid pace. The classes of cytokines, as they are currently used, are briefly described below. Some cytokines fall into more than one category because of structural or functional homology (e.g., interleukin-8 is an interleukin and a chemokine).

Interleukins

In an attempt to develop a better system of nomenclature for new cytokines, the Second International Lymphokine Workshop proposed the term *interleukin* in the late 1970s (1). The term implies that the name is reserved for agents that function to communicate signals between leukocytes, but as the field has expanded that reservation has been discarded. While many cytokines are now termed interleukins, others retain the original names.

The interleukins do not have structural homology to one another; all but interleukin-4 (IL-4) and IL-13 of the first 14 so named have distinct structures (6). They are produced, like all cytokines, by diverse cell types, and each can be produced by more than one cell type (e.g., IL-1 is produced by T lymphocytes, B lymphocytes, mast cells, placental cells, platelets, oocytes, endothelial cells, and astrocytes) (7). The interleukins affect more than one area of the immune system: inflammation, T-cell growth, hematopoiesis, B-cell growth, chemotaxis, and suppression (e.g., IL-4 is a T-cell growth factor, a B-cell growth factor, and a suppressor molecule).

The role of the interleukins in the T-cell helper clone subset switch defines their importance in immunoregulation. T-cell helper clones (Th1 and Th2) first were described in the mouse (8) on the basis of the cytokine patterns produced in response to the presentation of different antigens to an uncommitted or precursor T helper cell (Th0). The existence of the Th1 and Th2 CD4+ subsets in humans was later supported by studies that isolated antigen-specific CD4+ clones from patients (9). It was then found that Th1 and Th2 clones could be derived from healthy donors as well, and that the switch from one subset to the other was antigen dependent. The Th1/Th2 CD4+ subset switch is not absolute; gradations such as Th1/Th0, Th2/Th0 subsets exist, as well as the naive Th0, and respond to the challenge of various antigens. The Th1 phenotype generally results from stimulation of naive Th0 cells by antigens such as intracellular bacteria, viruses, endotoxins, and, most importantly, IL-2, interferon (IFN)-g (10), and IL-12. The Th1 response results in activated macrophages and cell-mediated immunity, which includes the activation of the CD8+ cytotoxic T-cell subset, and delayed-type hypersensitivity (10). The switch to a Th2 phenotype generally results from the stimulation of naive Th0 cells by antigens such as exotoxins, extracellular bacteria, helminths, and, most importantly, IL-4, IL-5, and IL-10 (10). The Th2 response results in the stimulation of B cells and the production of antibodies, including immunoglobulin E (IgE), which is a humoral response (10).

Tumor Necrosis Factors

The tumor necrosis factor (TNF) family is essential in the evolution of an inflammatory response and in the tissue damage that accompanies this response (11). As the name suggests, TNF has been shown to have a direct cytotoxic effect on some tumor cells, and was originally defined by its antitumor activity. Members of this group include the products of the same gene family: TNF-α, produced by macrophages and other cells, and TNF-β, produced by activated lymphocytes and other cells (11). These two distinct molecules share only 30% homology, but they have the same receptors, have similar activity, and can induce each other (12). TNF-α has been implicated in the pathogenesis of many diseases (13), but it is the main mediator in triggering septic shock and tissue injury, and a method to successfully neutralize its effects is the subject of intense scrutiny (13). TNF-β plays a unique and critical role in lymphoid organ development (14), but also induces deoxyribonucleic acid (DNA) fragmentation or apoptosis (14). The TNF activate neutrophils, mediate the activation and differentiation of macrophages and monocytes, and have been implicated in the pathogenesis of autoimmune diseases (12). The TNF also have been the most studied cytokines with regard to their potential relevance to human immunodeficiency virus (HIV) infection (15).

Interferons

Interferons (IFN) are glycoproteins produced and released from virally infected cells (12). IFN and their receptors function by having antiviral activity (16). The members of this group include IFN-α, -β, and -γ. There are at least 22 different isoforms of IFN-α and a single form of IFN-β, which all bind to the same type of receptor (type I receptor) (17). Interferon-gamma is unrelated to the type 1 receptor IFN, and binds to a type 2 receptor (12). It has lower antiviral activity but it is a much more important mediator in the immune system than the other IFN (12). It is critical to the immune response because it inhibits the proliferation of Th2 but not Th1 CD4+ subsets, and on B cells it is directly responsible for immunoglobulin isotype switching (12). It activates macrophages and enhances the inflammatory response by inducing TNF production (12). Interferon-gamma also has a major role in regulating major histocompatibility complex (MHC) class I and II protein expression in a variety of immunologically important cell types (18). Due to its important and pleiotropic role in immunoregulation, the therapeutic potential of the IFN has been examined, but as with the few other cytokines tested so far, the toxicity and unexpected effects have yielded basically unsuccessful results.

Growth Factors

More than 20 proteins are currently identified as growth factors (2). Some, such as platelet-derived growth factor (PDGF) and the transforming growth factors, are not viewed as true cytokines in their activities, and are included in discussions about cytokines mostly because of their role in tumorigenesis (19). Their action is basically one of growth enhancement, with some more directly involved in immune responses than others. PDGF, a dimeric protein, is involved in several pathologic states, such as atherosclerosis and tumorigenesis, as well as regulation of cell growth and differentiation during development and, tissue repair (20,21). PDGF has a role in wound healing and angiogenesis, and stimulates fibroblasts to synthesize collagen and collagenase. It is also a potent vasoconstrictor (22).

Epidermal growth factor (EGF) is a small single-chain (6 kD) polypeptide found normally in the salivary glands, saliva, and milk (23). It is a broad-ranging mitogen for epithelial, mesenchymal, and nonmesenchymal cells (24). EGF has pleiotropic actions that include angiogenesis in immature capillaries and tumors (25) and the promotion of cell proliferation.

Transforming Growth Factors

Two families have been discovered, represented by the transforming growth factor (TGF)-α and TGF-β families, which are distinct peptides with very different biologic activities (26). TGF-α is closely related to EGF, a 6-kD polypeptide, structurally and functionally, and binds to the EGF receptor to produce a mitogenic stimulation (19). TGF-α has been shown to be associated with neoplastic transformation in a variety of transformed cells and tumors. It was first detected in the culture medium of retroviral transformed fibroblasts, where it was demonstrated that TGF-α was able to reversibly transform immortalized normal rat kidney fibroblasts (19). Both EGF and TGF-α are reported to stimulate angiogenesis in vivo (27). TGF-α has been shown to be produced by monocytes and macrophages and numerous transformed and tumor cells (19).

The TGF-β superfamily consists of TGF-β_{1-5}, and factors expressed and regulated during development, such as the inhibins, activins, and bone morphogenetic proteins (28). TGF-β, a 25-kD homodimer, has a role in cell growth and neoplasia, inflammation, and immunoregulation as a potent immunosuppressor (15). In fact, TGF-β has profound immunosuppressive effects on virtually every component of the human system (15). While TGF-β suppresses lymphocyte proliferation and function, it activates several functions of the monocytes and macrophages. TGF-β receptors are found on almost all cells, regardless of origin, which bind TGF-β with high affinity (12). Based on what is known about TGF-β's actions in the promotion of wound healing, fibrosis, angiogenesis, the activation of mononuclear cells, and the immunosuppression of numerous functions of T cells (29,30), TGF-β would seem to be a true cytokine. Recombinant HIV *tat* protein, a viral transcription protein, upregulates the production of TGF-β. TGF-α and TGF-β are both upregulated by HIV in vivo (15). TGF-β has been shown to block HIV transcription in in vitro systems, and to prevent HIV production induced by other cytokines, such as IL-1, IL-6, granulocyte-macrophage colony-stimulating factor (GM-CSF), and IFN-γ, but does not block viral induction by TNF-α (15).

Colony-Stimulating Factors

Colony-stimulating factors (CSF) are low-molecular-weight glycoprotein cytokines, and as typical cytokines, they are produced by many different cell types, including T lymphocytes, macrophages, and neutrophils (2). CSF function mainly to regulate proliferation and differentiation of various types of hematopoietic cells, and have been observed to regulate some functions of fully differentiated hematopoietic cells (2). Colony-stimulating factors have been shown to be valuable in stimulating hematopoiesis after chemotherapy or bone transplant (31).

Members of this group include multi-CSF (IL-3), granulocyte-macrophage CSF (GM-CSF), macrophage CSF (M-CSF or CSF-1), and granulocyte-CSF (G-CSF) (32). A number of cytokines, such as the chemokines (see below) and CSF, have been shown to be involved in the activation and recruitment of neutrophils (33,34). The CSF interact with specific receptors on the neutrophil surface and alter a range of neutrophil functions that result in the inflammation response and its resultant tissue damage (33).

Chemokines

The chemokines are a group of small (8–11 kD) proteins that are produced by endothelial cells, leukocytes, fibroblasts, and keratinocytes (34). Chemokines and their receptors appear to be instrumental in fine tuning the responses to tissue injury. The chemokines are divided into two families, alpha and beta, which are based on structure and selectivity for leukocytes (34), but which also are the products of two related gene families (35). Their structures differ only by an amino acid intervening between the first two cysteines of the amino terminus for the alpha family, which the beta does not have (34).

The alpha family is characterized by interleukin-8 (IL-8), which is a neutrophil chemoattractant and activator (34). Interleukin-8 acts on neutrophils and neutrophil migration across the endothelium membrane (34). It can either upregulate or downregulate neutrophil adhesion to the endothelium (33). Endothelial surface–bound IL-8 helps induce neutrophil transmigration in endothelia, with the priming of IL-1 or TNF-α, by creating a chemotactic and haptotactic gradient over the endothelial surface along which the neutrophils can move (34). This property of IL-8 observed in vitro supports its central role in the accumulation of neutrophils at inflammatory sites in vivo (33). Neutrophil contact with cytokine-activated endothelium can lead to endothelium cell damage, and it seems as though IL-8 prevents this from happening, although this controversial concept is at odds with its role as chemoattractant (33,34). It is known that soluble IL-8 causes nonadherent neutrophils to shed L-selectin (described under Adhesion Molecules, below) and decreases neutrophil-endothelium interactions (34). Interleukin-8 therefore either stimulates or inhibits neutrophils from adhering, depending on whether it is bound or soluble IL-8 (34). IL-8 appears in the circulation of patients with septic shock and endotoxemia, and the levels are higher in the bronchioalveolar lavage fluids of patients in whom acute respiratory distress syndrome (ARDS) subsequently develops, as opposed to those in whom it does not (34,36). Interleukin-8, along with complement 5a and platelet activation factor, has been shown to mediate leukocyte activation. These factors have been demonstrated to induce leukocytes to spread across the endothelium as the precursor step to leukocyte transmigration to the site of tissue injury (37).

The beta family is exemplified by monocyte chemoattractant protein 1 (MCP-1), a chemoattractant for monocytes (34). The MIP-1 family (macrophage inflammatory protein 1) attracts activated T cells, with MIP-1α acting preferentially on CD8+ T cells, and MIP-1β attracting the CD4+ subset (34). The MIP subfamily also contains MIP-2α (i.e., GRO-β), GRO-α, and MIP-2β (i.e., GRO-γ) (34). RANTES (regulated on activation, normal T expressed and secreted) acts as a chemoattractant for unstimulated T cells, monocytes, and eosinophils (34). Other members of the chemokines include platelet factor 4 and IP-10 (an IFN-γ inducible protein) (35).

MCP-1, MIP-1, and RANTES are the mononuclear cell chemoattractant equivalents of IL-8 (34). MIP-1α, MIP-1β, and RANTES have been linked to the control or suppression of HIV infection in vivo (38,39). Uninfected subjects with multiple high-risk sexual exposures to HIV-1 were found to have CD8+ cells with greater anti–HIV-1 activity than unexposed controls (38). RANTES, MIP-1α, and MIP-1β were identified as the major anti-HIV factors produced by these anti–HIV-1 CD8+ T cells (39). Recombinant forms of these chemokines induced a dose-dependent inhibition of different strains of HIV-1, HIV-2, and SIV (39). The CD4+ cells in the HIV-resistant subjects were less susceptible to infection than were those of unexposed control subjects as well (38). Although the CD4+ cells were not resistant to all HIV strains, the resistance observed was associated with the activity of RANTES, MIP-1α, and MIP-1β (38). The chemokines, therefore, are playing an important role in the search for successful means of prevention and therapy of acquired immunodeficiency syndrome (AIDS).

A new chemokine has been identified that appears to be specific for lymphocytes (40). Named *lymphotactin*, this would be the first example of a lymphocyte-specific chemokine, which also shows no chemotactic activity for monocytes or neutrophils (40).

Adhesion Molecules

Adhesion molecules are a family of proteins, distinct from the cytokines, that are involved in leukocyte movement into tissues following tissue injury. The interaction of a leukocyte with the endothelium is guided by an adhesion molecule–driven cascade. The cytokines TNF-α and IL-1 act on adhesion molecules to increase the adhesive nature of the endothelium for bloodstream leukocytes (34,41). Further, these cytokines modulate the interaction between adjoining endothelial cells by upregulating the expression of adhesion molecules on the surface of the endothelium (34). The adhesion molecules and their receptors play a central role in the delivery of leukocytes to the endothelium and eventual transmigration into the underlying tissue where injury has occurred (34). The various subfamilies of adhesion molecules each play a distinct role in this cascade, which has a strong association with inflammation, endothelial activity, and tissue injury. Most of the cell adhesion molecules have an equal role in signal transduction as well as adhesion (42). The adhesion molecules are divided into four families based on their specific structural features (34,42).

Immunoglobulin Superfamily

The molecules in the immunoglobulin superfamily (IG-SF) have IgG-like domains that contain a constant and a variable region (42). There are many roles among this family, but the common function is one of controlling cell behavior. This control is exerted during development, especially of the nervous system, and in the regulation of the immune system (42). This control is exerted by molecules that act as signal-transducing receptors or as intercellular adhesion molecules (42,43).

This family is composed of cell adhesion molecules (CAM) such as intercellular (ICAM), vascular (VCAM), neural (NCAM), and platelet endothelial (PECAM) (34,42). These adhesion molecules, working together with the integrins (see below), aid the T cells in binding to the endothelial cells, and facilitate entry of the T cells into the vessels (43,44). The ICAMs appear to be involved in the activation of resting T cells. ICAM-1 is produced by T lymphocytes, thymocytes, dendrite cells, endothelial cells, fibroblasts, keratinocytes, chondrocytes, and epithelial cells (43). ICAM-1 is expressed constitutively, but expression can be enhanced by IL-1, TNF-alpha (34). ICAM-1 and ICAM-2 engage the neutrophil β_2 integrins, resulting in firm adhesion and flattening of neutrophils on the endothelium (34). PECAM is localized at the intercellular junction of endothelial cells and appears to be involved in leukocyte migration to the tissue site (44).

Integrins

The integrins are a family of heterodimeric membrane glycoproteins expressed on a wide variety of different cell types. Endothelial cells express a number of different integrins that function as interendothelial adhesion or endothelial cell membrane receptors (42). The integrins function in numerous biologic processes such as platelet aggregation, wound healing, tumor metastasis, and tissue migration during embryogenesis (45). The major structural feature is the presence of two noncovalently associated subunits, alpha and beta. Integrins are now believed to also be involved in signaling pathways, both into and out of cells (42).

Cadherins

The cadherins, a subfamily of the integrins, are calcium-dependent adhesion molecules found both within and outside the nervous system (42). Cadherins generally mediate homotypic cell-cell adhesion events (42,45). Unlike the other families of adhesion molecules, they act as both ligand and receptor (42). These molecules appear to play a significant role in selective cell-cell adhesion or cell allocation of different cell types during development (42). An example of a protein in this family is T-cadherin, which is located in the neural tissue and appears to function in guiding axon growth and guidance during embryo development (42). There is evidence to show that the cadherins may play a major role in the intercellular and cell-to-matrix interactions associated with the progression and metastasis of colorectal cancer (46).

Selectins

The three selectins are transmembrane glycoproteins that have a sugar-binding lectin domain (47). The selectins mediate the reversible binding of the leukocytes to the endothelium, which is the first phase of the adhesion cascade (37). E- and L-selectin are found on activated endothelial cells, and L-selectin is also seen on circulating lymphocytes, neutrophils, and monocytes (48). P-selectin is associated with platelets (34,42). All the selectins mediate the rolling of leukocytes along stimulated endothelium, which occurs in regions of inflammation (42,49).

Available Assay Procedures for the Measurement of Cytokines

The demand for cytokine measurements by investigators in research and clinical settings has created many commercially available cytokine assay kits. These kits are designed to quantitate cytokines in sera, whole blood, and other body fluids. Many of the available assays have technical and validation problems, and the interpretation of the results obtained must be restrained by the deficiency of the assay design (50). The main restraint on the interpretation of results, however, should be because of the current lack of understanding of how cytokine networks are regulated in normal versus disease states, and the role of individual cytokines in the disease pathogenesis (50). The bioassays, immunoassays, and nucleic acid–based assays represent the available methods for measuring cytokine levels (50). Each variety of assay will answer different questions about the regulation of cytokines, but the basic faults in assay design and our current understanding of cytokine regulation must be emphasized.

Bioassays

The influence of cytokines on biologic systems has best been defined by following the results of the addition of the cytokine to cell or tissue culture systems. Bioassays for evaluating cytokines are biologically most relevant since they will only detect active cytokines (50,51). The bioassay is also more sensitive since the stimulation of a biologic system is followed over time (50). A drawback to performing bioassays is that they can be difficult and labor intensive to perform (50). Further, results are not obtained for several days, and a target cell line must be carefully maintained in a cell culture facility (50). The bioassay often provides the first line of identification of the biologic importance of a cytokine or other marker (52). However, since this information is obtained in a cell culture environment, it cannot be directly correlated to actual in vivo conditions. The results can be less specific than those derived from immunoassays and results can be ambiguous, since they consist of the observed response of a cell line to a stimulus (50,51). The response is usually cytotoxic or proliferative, which can be difficult to assign to one stimulus in a cell culture environment. Neutralizing antibodies to the specific cytokines are therefore essential to confirming the identity of the cytokine and its role in the observed response in the bioassay (50). Finally, the data analysis of bioassay results is not a trivial task (50).

Immunoassays

The immunoassay represents a positive alternative to bioassays. The assays are usually simple to perform, and results can often be obtained in a matter of hours versus the days required for bioassays (50,51). One drawback inherent to the immunoassay is that the active as well as inactive forms of cytokines are detected, thus lowering the specificity of the assay (50,51). Some of these complications can be overcome by the use of competitive receptor assay formats, which depend on the interactions between an active cytokine and its receptor, and measure both free and receptor-bound cytokines (see Chap. 16 for more details on competitive receptor assays) (50). A wide variety of immunoassay formats are available, including antibody sandwich formats, in which the target antigen is sandwiched in between two specific antibodies, one that captures the target and one that is enzyme labeled to initiate a reaction that can be detected (53). The capture and the detector antibody can be either monoclonal or polyclonal antibodies, and the format in which they interact is an enzyme-linked immunosorbent assay (ELISA) (53). A variation on the standard ELISA uses a nucleic acid to capture the analyte of interest and detector made of nucleic acid rather than antibodies (54). The analyte of interest in this case is a polymerase chain reaction (PCR) product, which is a faithful copy of the unique sequence contained within a cytokine messenger ribonucleic acid (mRNA), copied in large enough numbers to be detected in the ELISA format (53,54). Different levels of elevated cytokine mRNA expression can be detected and quantitated, using internal standards in an ELISA format (50,53–56). This procedure is called reverse transcription PCR (RT-PCR), since the retroviral enzyme reverse transciptase is used to synthesize cDNA from the mRNA (50,54). The cDNA is then copied in the PCR reaction with labeled PCR primers so that enough labeled copies accrue to be detectable (50,53,54). With the use of the internal standard, the resultant number of copies can be quantified and related back to the original number of mRNAs for a particular cytokine (54,55) .

The immunoassay sheds more light on the role of the cytokine in the actual normal or disease state than does the bioassay, since the immunoassay can be performed in biologic fluids, such as serum, and is not limited to cell culture (50). This makes the direct analysis of the cytokine during various disease events or normal states possible. The immunoassay is limited by the sensitivity of the detection method (53) and can be hampered by lack of access to a sequestered cytokine (50). These are some of the issues that should concern the assay developer, as well as the assay user. Both must be aware that if low levels of the cytokine cannot be detected, or if only soluble cytokines in the serum are found, erroneous conclusions may be drawn about the actual in vivo conditions (50,51). This could affect a clinical situation, in which detection of variations in cytokine expression could aid in relevant clinical decisions. New methods in obtaining access to cytokines in cells and tissue, as well as more sensitive detection methods, can help avoid these problems. In addition, new methods that involve the use of nucleic acid–based assays may improve both the sensitivity and specificity of cytokine assays, since cytokine mRNA expression and production are highly regulated (50).

Recommended Assay Methods

As discussed above, the ELISA has superior specificity, ease of use, quickness, ease of analysis, access to total cytokine expression, and relevance to in vivo conditions (50). It also is superior in terms of versatility, since the analyte can be protein, nucleic acid, peptide, or carbohydrate (53). The specificity of the immunoassay is enhanced by the use of a monoclonal antibody as the capture antibody, because it will bind to only one epitope of the analyte (53). The sensitivity of the immunoassay is dependent on the affinity of the antibodies but can be increased by the use of the various detection methods that make the detection of relevantly low concentrations of cytokines possible (53,57) Other factors, such as capture antibody orientation on the solid phase, incubation conditions, and sample size, contribute to the sensitivity of an assay system (53). The limits of assay sensitivity are determined during the validation of the assay. A common method employed to determine the sensitivity, or minimum detectable concentration (MDC), is to assay multiple replicates of the zero standard. The mean optical density (OD), derived from the absorbances of the multiple replicates, plus two standard deviations, is determined to be the minimum detectable concentration attainable for a sample in the assay, as compared to the standard curve.

The sandwich ELISA is so called because it makes use of two antibodies that can be monoclonal or polyclonal in nature. The primary or capture antibody binds the analyte of interest and is immobilized on a solid support, which is most often a microtiter plate, but can also consist of a tube or the various modules used for this purpose in automated systems. The secondary or detector antibody, which is specific for a different epitope on the analyte than the capture antibody, completes the sandwich (53). This detector antibody can be directly labeled with an enzyme label, such as horseradish peroxidase (HRP), alkaline phosphatase, or beta-galactosidase (58). Detection of the target analyte also can be accomplished by labeling the secondary antibody with a small molecule, such as fluorescein isothiocyanate (FITC) (53). This FITC-labeled antibody is bound by a third antibody in the system, an anti-FITC antibody that has an enzyme, such as HRP, conjugated to it. The anti-FITC enzyme-conjugated antibody can be universal in use, since it can complete the sandwich of any two antibodies, or capture and detect nucleic acids, as long as the secondary one is FITC labeled (53). The small size of the FITC molecule (MW 389) on the secondary antibody prevents the steric hindrance problems that are sometimes observed when antibodies are labeled with large enzymes such as HRP (MW 40,000), which interfere with the binding of the antibody to the analyte (53,58). In the case of HRP, the detection is actually accomplished by the addition of an HRP-specific colorimetric substrate solution, such as 3,3′5,5′-tetramethyl benzidine (TMB) (58). The colorimetric reaction that results from this is allowed to develop, then stopped with acid (53,58). The absorbance of the color developed is read at a predetermined wavelength in a plate reader (53). Most plate readers are equipped with computer software so that a standard curve is generated and the sample values are determined from sample absorbances backfit onto that standard curve (53).

Specimen Collection and Treatment

The ELISA system can be used with a wide variety of different sample types, as stated previously. Depending on the sample, the assay may require dilution of the sample into a sample diluent, to prevent nonspecific binding. Traditionally, ELISAs have been used for measuring analytes in serum, plasma, or urine (50). However, new methods have made it possible to evaluate analytes in tissue or lymph biopsies and whole blood (59). Proper and complete solubilization of cellular material must be ensured in order to release cell-associated cytokines and thus reliably measure the cytokines that are present in these samples. The detection and measurement of cytokines bound to their receptors present a unique challenge, which is discussed in Chapter 16.

Cytokines can be detected in a variety of different biologic fluids. All biologic samples should be considered hazardous and handled using good, microbiologic practices of protection from, and disposal of, biohazards. As the detection of cytokines and their receptors has become increasingly important in the clinical arena, so has concern grown over the accuracy of their measurement in serum and other fluids (50). The stability of these analytes has been discussed elsewhere (60,61). Generally, samples can be stored for the short term at 4°C, but long-term storage must be at −80°C. Short-term storage is defined differently for different cytokines; for example, IL-8 is stable for long periods at 4°C, while IL-12 will degrade in a matter of hours at 4°C (personal observations). Processing of samples must occur directly after collection in order to prevent potential degradation problems. The clotting factors in plasma can cause the degradation of some cytokines, thus making serum the preferred sample. When collecting serum, care should be taken to remove the clotted blood cell components from the serum immediately. The processed serum should be placed in the cold immediately to prevent degradation (50).

A relatively new application of an old method consists of the solublization of the cellular membrane with maintenance of the integrity of the analyte. This method has been commercialized by T Cell Sciences, Inc, in its proprietary TRAx technology, for use with whole blood (59). This technology uses a combination of buffered detergents to completely solubilize the cell membrane. However, the treatment is mild enough to allow retention of the integrity of the analyte. This method consists of a simple pre-treatment of whole blood followed by analysis in a standard sandwich ELISA system. The whole blood samples can be lysed, frozen, and analyzed at a later date without deleterious effects on the analyte stability. Once the cells have been solublized, however, they are mixed with the plasma fraction that contains soluble cytokines and receptors. When this mixing occurs, the contribution of soluble versus the cell-associated cytokines to the total measured cannot be determined. In order to be able to gather information about the partitioning of the cytokines, the whole blood can be fractionated into the soluble (serum) portion and a washed cell pellet. Once fractionated, each can be evaluated in the same ELISA assay (59,62).

Assay Development: Validation, Standardization, and Preclinical Evaluation

A major part of assay development is the extensive validation of the robustness, reliability, sensitivity, and specificity of the assay for the detection of the analyte of interest. As part of an assay's performance validation, the specificity of the reagents used is rigorously tested to ensure that they perform within the expected tolerances of the assay system. An immunoassay should contain a standard curve that consists of approximately six standards prepared from well-characterized material (the World Health Organization collects and makes available cytokine standard and reference materials, as do the National Institute for Biological Standards in the United Kingdom and the National Institutes of Health in Washington, DC) (51). The assay should contain three control levels that must represent the dynamics of the standard curve. The standard curve and control performances are then tested by precision analysis or a single assay (representing intra-assay precision), and among multiple assays and operators (interassay precision). An extensive panel of studies, including tests for cross reactivity with markers of similar structure, is always performed. Additionally, antibodies to specific markers are compared with preexisting antibodies in the field. The Human Leukocyte Differentiation Antigen (HLDA) workshop was established to ensure that all new antibodies are subjected to similar analysis. The HLDA is best known for its efforts to type cluster of differentiation (CD) markers. The CD4 antibody classification is a well-known example of this organization's effort to standardize antibody typing on a worldwide level. The use of HLDA antibodies and World Health Organization cytokines in assay development helps ensure that assays accurately measure the cytokine of interest regardless of the matrix. As part of assay development, these materials are used to test the assay's accuracy under all possible conditions (50,51,53,62).

For all the ease of use and simplicity that an ELISA has, the ELISA assay developer faces many problems, which must be anticipated and corrected. Some relevant inhibitors of assay specificity and sensitivity that may be encountered in specimens include antibody purity, cross-reactivity, and the presence of nonspecific binders such as rheumatoid factors or C1q complement complexes (53,57). In addition, some of the factors that bind nonspecifically are actually enhanced by additives common to specimen collection, such as disodium ethylenediaminetetraacetate (EDTA). EDTA releases or activates a variety of blood components, most notably the C1q complement factor, which tends to bind to the Fc portion of antibodies. Removal of the Fc portion of the detector antibody can dramatically reduce or eliminate this problem (53). Antibodies that are digested with pepsin to remove the Fc portion become F(ab)′2 fragments (53). The addition of nonspecific IgG and the use of antibody fragments have been employed with a high level of success to overcome these issues. The use of mouse IgG included in diluents can help to reduce another common interferent, anti-idiotype antibodies (63). These antibodies are found among patients receiving antibody-based therapies, such as OKT3 for immune suppression after organ transplantation (64). All of the possible substances that may be encountered in the matrix of the specimen must be tested during the assay development and validation period. Recovery of a known quantity of the cytokine is attempted in biologic fluids in the presence of elevated levels of bilirubin, cytokines that are structurally related, EDTA, heparin, triglycerides, relevant drugs, and other substances encountered in the specimen environment. Accurate recovery of the cytokine from different sample collection methods is also tested (e.g., serum, plasma, or whole blood collected in EDTA, citrate, or heparin).

Unlike hormone expression, cytokine expression can be regulated by multiple receptors (2). These receptors can be cell bound, but soluble forms are also found in the serum and plasma (50). Cytokines that are bound by their receptors may have the crucial epitope hidden from the antibodies used in the assay, which makes measurement of the cytokines impossible and the assay unreliable. Many nonspecific proteins in the environment, such as β_2-macroglobulin, C1q, rheumatoid factor, and other serum proteins, also can mask the relevant cytokine from detection in the assay (50,53). Performance of dilution linearity, and spike and recovery studies during the assay validation, can help determine whether cytokine-receptor complexes or nonspecific cytokine complexes are creating erroneous assay results. Some investigators have begun to investigate the significance of the free versus bound ratio in the evaluation of cytokine expression and disease monitoring (50,65). These assays make use of competitive assay formats, or multiple capture and/or detection antibody systems. This issue is more thoroughly addressed in Chapter 16.

The question of the significance of the soluble versus cell-associated forms of these analytes is gaining interest. As with other cytokines, red blood cells can specifically bind IL-8 and other chemokines via the Duffy antigen (65). In fact, cell-associated levels of IL-8 have been observed to be as much as 10-fold higher than the soluble levels in stimulated samples (65, personal observation). Investigations of the expression and partitioning of cytokines, that is, soluble, cell associated, and cell bound, may lead to better understanding of their regulation. Once the assay validation is completed, the analyte levels should be determined in 100 to 200 healthy donors in order to establish an expected range for normal samples. Expected levels of the analyte in the patient population of interest are determined as part of a preclinical evaluation, and must be compared to those already determined for the normal population. Normal and patient sample levels of the analyte, as determined by the new assay, must be compared to those determined by an established method, if one is available.

Commercially produced products that are used in the clinical environment are manufactured under defined conditions and must adhere to current good manufacturing practices (GMP). These products must conform to strict requirements in terms of the way that they are produced and the manner in which they perform. A quality assurance program is designed to monitor the manufacturing of products in a manner that will prevent mistakes, provide a record of each step, and ensure the assay's consistent performance.

Once a kit has completed the development phase and entered the manufacturing phase, quality control guidelines and specifications are implemented to ensure consistency and reliability of product performance. The use of standards, as described previously, is that which confers a consistent, quantitative nature upon an immunoassay (66). Assay controls, preferably in a matrix equivalent to patient samples, are routinely run by quality control in order to detect performance trends and ensure consistency. Standards and controls are then included in the assay and used alongside the samples during each assay to create the standard curve and ensure that the kit is performing properly. An internal laboratory control, which is calibrated against a reference standard, should be used in each assay to determine interassay variability and to ensure assay consistency. This control may be a cell line supernatant, serum, whole blood, or other material in which the analyte expression level is known. The assay is only viewed as acceptable as long as these patient sample controls remain within the established ranges. The key question to ask is, "Does the product meet the performance claims stated in the package insert?"

Postanalytical Concern

After successful manufacture and commercialization of a cytokine assay, continued validation is required to ensure consistency of performance over time. The College of American Pathologists (CAP) assists clinical laboratories in maintaining quality by providing programs for quality control assurance, including postanalytical factors. Clinical laboratories are subject to regulation under the Clinical Laboratory Improvement Amendments (CLIA) of 1988. Under subpart K, section 493.1213(b)(1) guidelines, CLIA requirements for quality control mandate that each clinical laboratory obtain the performance specification for accuracy, precision, and reportable range of patient test results established by the manufacturer. The laboratory must also verify that the manufacturer's reference range is appropriate for the laboratory's patient population. The manufacturer's reference range is obtained through the accumulation of patient sample ranges established from initial research and development data, confirmed by quality control data, and continuously updated and verified by the quality control and assurance divisions. After successful manufacture and commercialization of a product, continued validation is required to ensure consistency of performance over time. This is done through the accumulation of patient sample ranges established from initial research and development data, confirmed by quality control data, and continuously updated and verified by data gathered on a routine basis by the quality control/quality assurance divisions. The assay is viewed as acceptable as long as these patient sample controls remain within the established ranges.

Generally, part of the postanalytical concern is ongoing external clinical evaluation of the kit. Results from these external sites are analyzed separately and added to the internal pool of results for subsequent analysis.

External Quality Assurance: Proficiency Surveys and Precision Studies, Clinical Trials

External clinical trials validate the performance of the assay in the population for which the test was developed. These studies stress the robustness, specificity, and sensitivity of the assay. External proficiency studies generally include assaying and evaluating the kit standard curve, kit controls, and a series of unknown patient samples. These studies are performed at multiple sites, usually a minimum of three, and are performed by multiple operators over multiple days.

Following the proficiency studies, the assay is validated with a clinical evaluation among the relevant patient population. These external studies ensure that the kit meets the levels of performance demonstrated by the manufacturer. The Food and Drug Administration (FDA) requirements for in vitro diagnostics kit performance may vary slightly from one analyte to another, but several conditions are generally necessary for FDA clearance: 1) demonstration that the kit meets the established parameters listed by the manufacturer; 2) demonstration of precision at each external site, and between the external sites performing the study; and 3) methods comparison studies between the assay and an FDA-cleared method. These studies require that multiple clinical sites be used to perform the assay and the alternative, FDA-cleared method. Each site must generate more than 100 data points from the same set of samples.

The above studies are necessary for the filing of a 510K with the FDA. In the absence of an existing, FDA-cleared method with which to compare the new assay, an extensive clinical study, or premarket approval (PMA) process, requiring multiple clinical sites and up to several thousand total data points, would be required to validate the new assay.

Comments and Recommendations

The next step in defining the role of cytokines in disease is to better understand their biology. Until the cytokine network's expression and regulation in health and disease are better understood, the clinical relevance and potential therapeutic use of cytokines cannot be properly judged. Crucial to this research is the accurate measurement of their protein levels and gene expression in disease (50). The melding of two relatively new technologies can help provide accurate data on both the true cytokine protein levels and gene expression in health and disease states.

Cytokine mRNA expression is tightly regulated and, as previously described, can be investigated using RT-PCR (50). In recent years, many commercially available products have been released that make the processes involved in RT-PCR less labor intensive and difficult. Many companies offer products that will allow the researcher to easily extract intact mRNA, convert the mRNA faithfully to cDNA, amplify the cDNA by PCR, and quantitate the mRNA expression level, using an internal control. The detection of the PCR product representing the cytokine mRNA can be accomplished easily in an ELISA format.

As previously mentioned, the TRAx technology (59) enables the measurement of soluble and cell-associated cytokine protein levels. This technology couples access to cell-associated cytokines and their detection in an ELISA. It also allows detection of soluble cytokines from the same sample. If the sample is properly prepared, the partitioning of the cytokine, between that which is soluble and that which is cell associated, can be accurately measured.

Any technology used must, however, be utilized as part of an assay that has gone through the rigorous development, validation, and standardization that have been described in this chapter. Any form of the analyte will be misinterpreted if the assay used for detection and quantitation is not specific, sensitive, or reliable.

REFERENCES

1. Oppenheim JJ. Foreword to: Thomson AW, ed. The cytokine handbook. 2nd ed. London: Academic Press, 1994:xvii–xx.
2. Aggarwal BB, Puri RK. Common and uncommon features of cytokines and cytokine receptors: an overview. In: Aggarwal BB, Puri RK, eds. Human cytokines: their role in disease and therapy. Cambridge, MA: Blackwell Science, 1995:3–24.
3. Roberts AB, Sporn MB. The transforming growth factor-βs. In: Sporn MB, Roberts AB, eds. Peptide growth factors and their receptors. I. New York: Springer-Verlag, 1990:419–472.
4. Elias JA, Zitnik RJ. Cytokine-cytokine interactions in the context of cytokine networking. Am J Respir Cell Mol Biol 1992;7:365–367.
5. Fernandez-Botran R. Soluble cytokine receptors: their role in immunoregulation. FASEB J 1991;5: 2567–2574.
6. Zurawski G, deVries JE. Interleukin-13, an interleukin-4–like cytokine that acts on monocytes and B cells, but not T cells. Immunol Today 1994;15:19–26.
7. Mizel SB. The interleukins. FASEB J 1989;3:2379–2388.
8. Mosmann TR, Cherwinski H, Bond MW, et al. Two types of murine helper T-cell clone. I. Definition according to profiles of lymphokine activities and secreted proteins. J Immunol 1986; 136:2348–2357.
9. Moodycliffe AM, Ullrich SE. Role of cytokines in the regulation of hypersensitivity responses. In: Aggarwal BB, Puri RK, eds. Human cytokines: their role in disease and therapy. Cambridge, MA: Blackwell Science, 1995:131–152.
10. Romagnani S. Th1 and Th2 subsets of CD4+ T lymphocytes. Science and Medicine. Sci Am 1994;1:68–77.
11. Vassalli P. The pathophysiology of tumor necrosis factors. Ann Rev Immunol 1992;10:411–452.
12. Hillman GG, Haas GP. Role of cytokines in lymphocyte functions. In: Aggarwal BB, Puri RK, eds. Human cytokines: their role in disease and therapy. Cambridge, MA: Blackwell Science, 1995:37–54.
13. Tracey KJ. Tumour necrosis factor-alpha. In: Thomson AW, ed. The cytokine handbook. 2nd ed. London: Academic Press, 1994:289–304.
14. Ruddle NH. Tumour necrosis factor-beta: lymphotoxin-alpha. In: Thomson AW, ed. The cytokine handbook. 2nd ed. London: Academic Press, 1994:305–318.
15. Poli G, Fauci AS. Role of cytokines in the pathogenesis of human immunodeficiency virus infection. In: Aggarwal BB, Puri RK, eds. Human cytokines: their role in disease and therapy. Cambridge, MA: Blackwell Science, 1995:421–449.
16. Pestka S, Langer JA, Zoon KC, Samuel CE. Interferons and their actions. Ann Rev Biochem 1987;56:727–777.
17. Zoon KC, Miller D, Bekisz J, et al. Purification and characterization of multiple components of human lymphoblastoid interferon-α. J Biol Chem 1992;267:15210–15216.
18. Farrar MA, Schreiber RD. The molecular cell biology of interferon-α and its receptor. Ann Rev Immunol 1993;11:571–611.
19. Suematsu S, Kishimoto T. Autocrine and paracrine role of cytokines as growth factors for tumorigenesis. In: Aggarwal BB, Puri RK, eds. Human cytokines: their role in disease and therapy. Cambridge, MA: Blackwell Science, 1995:525–537.
20. Leibovich SJ, Wiseman DM. Macrophages, angiogenesis and wound repair. In: Barbul A, Pines E, Caldwell M, Hunt TK, eds. Growth factors and other aspects of wound healing: biological and clinical implications. New York: Alan R. Liss. 1988:131–148.
21. Pierce GF, Tarpley JE, Yanagihara D, et al. Platelet-derived growth factor (BB homodimer), transforming growth factor-β, and basic fibroblast growth factor in dermal wound healing. Neovessel and matrix formation and cessation of repair. Am J Pathol 1992;140:1375–1388.
22. Buckley A, Davidson JM, Kamrath CD, et al. Sustained release of epidermal growth factor accelerates wound repair. PNAS USA 1985;82:7340–7344.
23. Carpenter G, Cohen S. Epidermal growth factor. Ann Rev Biochem 1979;48:193–216.
24. Das M, Pengarajo M, Samanta A. Epidermal growth factor. In: Aggarwal BB, Gutterman JU, eds. Human cytokines: handbook for basic and clinical research. Cambridge: Blackwell Science, 1992:365–382.
25. Risau W, Drexler H, Mironov, V, et al. Platelet-derived growth factor is angiogenic in vivo. Growth Factors 1992;7:261–266.

26. Derynck R. Transforming growth factor-β. In: Thomson AW, ed. The cytokine handbook. 2nd ed. London: Academic Press, 1994:317–342.

27. Leibovich SJ. Role of cytokines in the process of tumor angiogenesis. In: Aggarwal BB, Puri RK, eds. Human cytokines: their role in disease and therapy. Cambridge, MA: Blackwell Science, 1995:539–564.

28. Matzuk MM. Gene deletion models to understand cytokine functions. In: Aggarwal BB, Puri RK, eds. Human cytokines: their role in disease and therapy. Cambridge, MA: Blackwell Science, 1995:651–662.

29. Frater-Schroder M, Muller G, Birchmeier W, Bohler P. Transforming growth factor-beta inhibits endothelial cell proliferation. Biochem Biophys Res Commun 1986;137:295–302.

30. Wiseman DM, Polverini PJ, Kamp DW, Leibovich SJ. Transforming growth factor-beta (TGFβ) is chemotactic for human monocytes and induces their expression of angiogenic activity. Biochem Biophys Res Commun 1988;157:793–800.

31. Metcalf D. Colony stimulating factors and hemopoiesis. Ann Acad Med 1988;17:166–170.

32. Lang CH. Role of cytokines in glucose metabolism. In: Aggarwal BB, Puri RK, eds. Human cytokines: their role in disease and therapy. Cambridge, MA: Blackwell Science, 1995:271–284.

33. Liu JH, Djeu JY. Role of cytokines in neutrophil functions. In: Aggarwal BB, Puri RK, eds. Human cytokines: their role in disease and therapy. Cambridge, MA: Blackwell Science, 1995:71–86.

34. Litwin MS, Gamble JR, Vadas MA. Role of cytokines in endothelial cell functions. In: Aggarwal BB, Puri RK, eds. Human cytokines: their role in disease and therapy. Cambridge, MA: Blackwell Science, 1995:102–129.

35. Beneviste EN. Role of cytokines in multiple sclerosis, autoimmune encephalitis, and other neurological disorders. In: Aggarwal BB, Puri RK, eds. Human cytokines: their role in disease and therapy. Cambridge, MA: Blackwell Science, 1995:196–215.

36. Donnelly SC, Strieter RM, Kunkel SL, et al. Interleukin-8 and development of adult respiratory distress syndrome in at-risk patient groups. Lancet 1993;341:643–647.

37. Hogg N, Berlin C. Structure and function of adhesion receptors in leukocyte trafficking. Immunol Today 1995;15:327–330.

38. Paxton WA, Martin SR, Tse D, et al. Relative resistance to HIV-1 infection of CD4 lymphocytes from persons who remain uninfected despite multiple high-risk sexual exposure. Nature Med 1996;2:412–417.

39. Cocchi F, DeVico AL, Garzino-Demo A, et al. Identification of RANTES, MIP-1 alpha, and MIP-1 beta as the major HIV-suppressive factors produced by CD8+ T cells. Science 1995;270:1811–1815.

40. Kelner GS, Kennedy J, Bacon KB, et al. Lymphotactin: a cytokine that represents a new class of chemokine. Science 1994;266:1395–1399.

41. Gamble JR, Harlan JM, Klebanoff SJ, Vadas MA. Stimulation of the adherence of neutrophils to umbilical vein endothelium by human recombinant tumor necrosis factor. PNAS USA 1985;82: 8667–8671.

42. Pigott R, Power C. The adhesion molecule facts book. London: Academic Press, 1993:2–20.

43. Bevilacqua MP. Endothelial leukocyte adhesion molecules. Ann Rev Immunol 1993;11:767–804.

44. Muller WA, Weigl SA, Deng X, Phillips DM. PECAM-1 is required for transendothelial migration of leukocytes. J Exp Med 1993;178:449–460.

45. Hynes RO. Integrins: versatility, modulation, and signalling in cell adhesion. Cell 1992;69:11.

46. Dorudi S, Sheffield JP, Poulson R, et al. E-cadherin expression in colorectal cancer. Am J Pathol 1993;142:981–986.

47. Johnston GI, Cook RG, McEver RP. Cloning of GMP-140, a granule membrane protein of platelets and endothelium: sequence similarity to proteins involved in cell adhesion and inflammation. Cell 1989;56:1033.

48. Mayadas TN, Johnson RC, Rayburn H, et al. Leukocyte rolling and extravasation are severely compromised in P-selectin deficient mice. Cell 1993;74:541–554.

49. Kishimoto TK, Warnock RA, Jutila MA, et al. Antibodies against human neutrophil LECAM-1 (LAM-1/leu-8/dreg-56 antigen) and endothelial cell ELAM-1 inhibit a common CD18-independent adhesion pathway in vitro. Blood 1991;78:805–811.

50. Whiteside TL. Cytokine measurements and interpretation of cytokine assays in human disease. J Clin Immunol 1994;14:327–339.

51. Gearing JH, Cartwright JE, Wadhwa M. Biological and immunological assays for cytokines. In: Thomson AW, ed. The cytokine handbook. 2nd ed. London: Academic Press, 1994:507–524.

52. Feldman M, Brennan FM, Chantry D, et al. Cytokine assays: role in evaluation of the pathogenesis of autoimmunity. Immunol Rev 1991; 119:105–123.

53. Foster K. Microtiter plate–based enzyme immunoassay: the universal format system. In: Immunoassay automation: an updated guide to systems. Academic Press, 1996:277–309.

54. Persing DH. In vitro nucleic acid amplification techniques. In: Persing DH, Smith TF, Tenover FC, White TJ, eds. Diagnostic molecular microbiology: principles and applications. Washington, DC: American Society for Microbiology, 1993: 51–87.

55. Guiffre A, Atkinson K, Kearney P. A quantitative polymerase chain reaction assay for interleukin 5 messenger RNA. Anal Biochem 1993;212:50–57.

56. Platzer C, Ode-Hakim S, Reinke P, et al. Quantitative PCR analysis of cytokine transcription patterns in peripheral mononuclear cells after anti-CD3 rejection therapy using two novel multispecific competitor fragments. Transplantation 1994;582:264–268.

57. Elkins R. Enzyme immunoassay. In: Maggio ET, ed. Boca Raton, FL: CRC Press, 1988:20–52.

58. Technical section. Enzymatic labelling and detection. The Pierce catalog 1994–95:T209–T211.

59. Nicholson JKA, Velleca WM, Jubert S, et al. Evaluation of alternative CD4 technologies for the enumeration of CD4 lymphocytes. Submitted for publication, 1995.

60. Thavasu PW, Loghurst S, Joel SP, et al. Measuring cytokine levels in blood: the importance of anticoagulants, processing, and storage conditions. J Immunol Meth 1992;153:115–124.

61. Fletcher MA, Baron GC, Ashman MR, et al. Use of whole blood methods in assessment of immune parameters in immunodeficiency states. Diag Clin Immunol 1987;5:69–81.

62. Emmett C, Turner M, Millett B, et al. An ELISA for the detection of human interleukin-12 in multiple matrices. Assoc Anal Clin Chem 1996: 356. Abstract.

63. Hunter WM, Budd P. Circulating antibodies to ovine and bovine immunoglobulins: a hazard for immunoassay. Lancet 1980;2:1136.

64. Schroeder TJ, First MR, Mansour ME. Antimurine antibody formation following OKT3 therapy. Transplantation 1990;49:48–51.

65. Marie C, Pitton C, Fitting C, et al. High levels of leukocyte-associated interleukin-8 upon cell activation and in patients with sepsis syndrome. Submitted for publication, 1996.

66. Hamilton RG, Adkinson NF Jr. Quantitative aspects of solid phase immunoassays. In: Kemeny DM, Challacombe SJ, eds. ELISA and other solid phase immunoassays: theoretical and practical aspects. New York: Wiley, 1988:57–84.

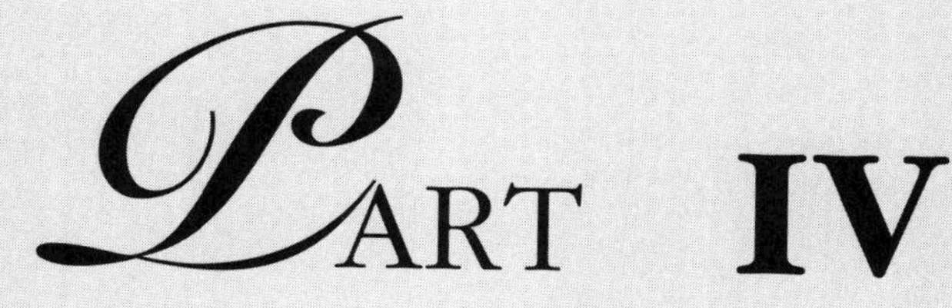

PART IV

Quality Assurance, Quality Control, and Standardization in Cellular and Tissue Assays

C. LYNNE BUREK, ROBERT M. NAKAMURA, EDITORS

CHAPTER 15

Cellular Immune Function Tests

MAURICE R.G. O'GORMAN
ALICE GILMAN-SACHS
LINDA L. BAUM
MARY ANN FLETCHER

In this chapter three broad areas of cellular immune function are reviewed. First and probably the most significant test of the cellular immune system is lymphocyte proliferation; a review of this aspect of cellular immune function is followed by a discussion of natural killer cell function, and lastly granulocyte function, specifically measurement of the oxidative burst reaction. Our goal is not to review the extensive literature that exists in each of these areas but rather to focus on how one performs these functional assays in a clinical setting, using the appropriate methods and controls.

Lymphocyte Proliferation Responses to Antigens and Mitogens by Measurement of Tritiated Thymidine Incorporation: the Whole Blood Assay

The lymphocyte proliferation assay (LPA) has been widely used to help describe the abnormalities associated with diverse congenital immunodeficiencies as well as those considered to be secondary to infectious diseases, cancer, aging, malnutrition, substance abuse, stress, surgery, shock, and autoimmune diseases. Because lymphocytes proliferate only in response to certain specific signals and since this is basic to their immunologic function, measuring their proliferation (or blastogenesis) has found wide application in clinical immunology (1–3). In a sense, such techniques are the in vitro correlate of skin testing for delayed-type hypersensitivity to recall antigens, but with some clear advantages, including easier quantitation (4).

The most widely used system to measure lymphocyte proliferation relies on the incorporation of a radioactive nucleoside ([^{3}H]-thymidine) into cellular deoxyribonucleic acid (DNA). This system makes use of the fact that activated lymphocytes are inclined to divide and that cellular division requires DNA synthesis. If provided with an exogenous source of nucleosides, lymphocytes will transport these molecules into the cell, charge them with triphosphates, and subsequently incorporate them into DNA during chromosomal replication. At the biochemical level it is the conversion of soluble nucleosides into insoluble DNA polymers on which the assay is based. Following incubation with labeled nucleoside, lymphocytes are harvested onto glass fiber filters. Nonincorporated nucleoside is washed away, whereas the label incorporated into DNA remains attached to the solid support. The amount of radionuclide present is then determined by liquid scintillation counting.

Multisite studies, including the AIDS Clinical Trial Group (ACTG) and the Transfusion Safety Study, have instituted standard protocols that use this methodology, in both whole blood (WB) and peripheral blood mononuclear cell (PBMC) approaches. The whole blood approach provides an appropriate and practical means of assessing lymphocyte response in that it requires relatively small amounts of peripheral blood. This attribute is of particular value for studies that involve children or when mul-

TABLE **15-1**

Comparison of Whole Blood and Separated Mononuclear Cell Assays [net CPM (±SD)/10^5 lymphocytes]

Stimulant (μg/ml)	PBMC	WB	[a]	p[b]
C. albicans, 100	13,766 (20,825)[c]	13,574 (5,370)	192	NS
20	12,454 (11,079)	15,962 (5,476)	3508–	NS
10	9926 (8,426)	14,190 (7,491)	4268–	NS
Tetanus toxoid, 10	11,640 (10,362)	11,345 (9,395)	295	NS
5	10,806 (9,558)	7851 (5,546)	2954	NS
2.5	11,252 (8,767)	8600 (9,114)	2652	NS
PPD, 20	7587 (9,199)	22,495 (29,634)	14,908–	NS
10	10,366 (12,497)	25,734 (33,539)	15,367–	NS
0.2	10,378 (12,835)	24,756 (13,092)	14,378–	NS
PHA, 10	31,883 (11,065)	103,861 (51,641)	71,998–	<0.05
PWM, 20	5434 (3,344)	36,865 (5,776)	31,431–	<0.05

NS, not significant.

[a] PBMC net cpm–WB net cpm.

[b] p = 2-tailed p values from Mann-Whitney test; NS = $p < 0.05$.

[c] Standard deviation.

tiple blood samples are to be collected within a short period of time. The WB assay is preferred in situations in which it is best to determine the proliferation of the blood cells without removing or washing away the soluble substances in the whole blood that may influence function of the cells (i.e., hormones, cytokines, neuropeptides). With some stimulants, there is no significant difference between the two methods when results are expressed as net counts per minute (cpm)/10^5 lymphocytes. This is demonstrated in **Table 15-1**, which presents the data from a study of three human immunodeficiency virus (HIV)-infected adults. A single blood draw was obtained. Half of the sample was assayed by the WB method; mononuclear cells were prepared from the rest of the sample and the separated cells were assayed. The net cpm were significantly higher in the whole blood assay when either phytohemagglutinin (PHA) or pokeweed mitogen (PWM) was used as the stimulant. However, no significant difference was noted for the three recall antigens tested. Results using *Candida* are shown in **Figure 15-1**. The variability of the assays was higher when PBMC were used and a larger sample size would likely have shown significantly higher net cpm for purified protein derivative (PPD) using WB.

We recently examined whether there were differences in lymphocyte function as determined by the WB LPA as a function of gender and ethnicity. Gender and ethnic differences in LPA to PHA following a resting period in the seated position were examined in healthy HIV-seronegative individuals. Eighty-five subjects participated (47 men and 38 women). Of the men, 19 were non-Hispanic white, 14 were Hispanic, and 14 were African-American. Of the women, 14 were non-Hispanic white, 13 were Hispanic, and 11 were African-American. Measures were obtained from two blood samples taken at the end of a 30-minute baseline resting period following venipuncture. Subject characteristics for age (18–45 yr), height, weight, and body mass index were assessed. As expected, significant gender differences were found in height and weight; men weighed more and were taller. There were significant ethnic differences in age and height. Hispanics were younger than both blacks and whites and blacks were significantly taller than Hispanics. No ethnicity differences were seen in weight. In addition, there were no differences across ethnicity or gender groups for income and education levels. Analyses of lymphocyte proliferation in response to PHA revealed no significant differences of gender or ethnicity and no interactive effects of these factors. A table of these measures is included (**Tables 15-2** and **15-3**).

Where differences in age, weight, or height were present, the effects of these variables on the immunologic variables were covaried in an additional set of analyses without any difference in the above findings observed. Therefore, together with the limited data available in the

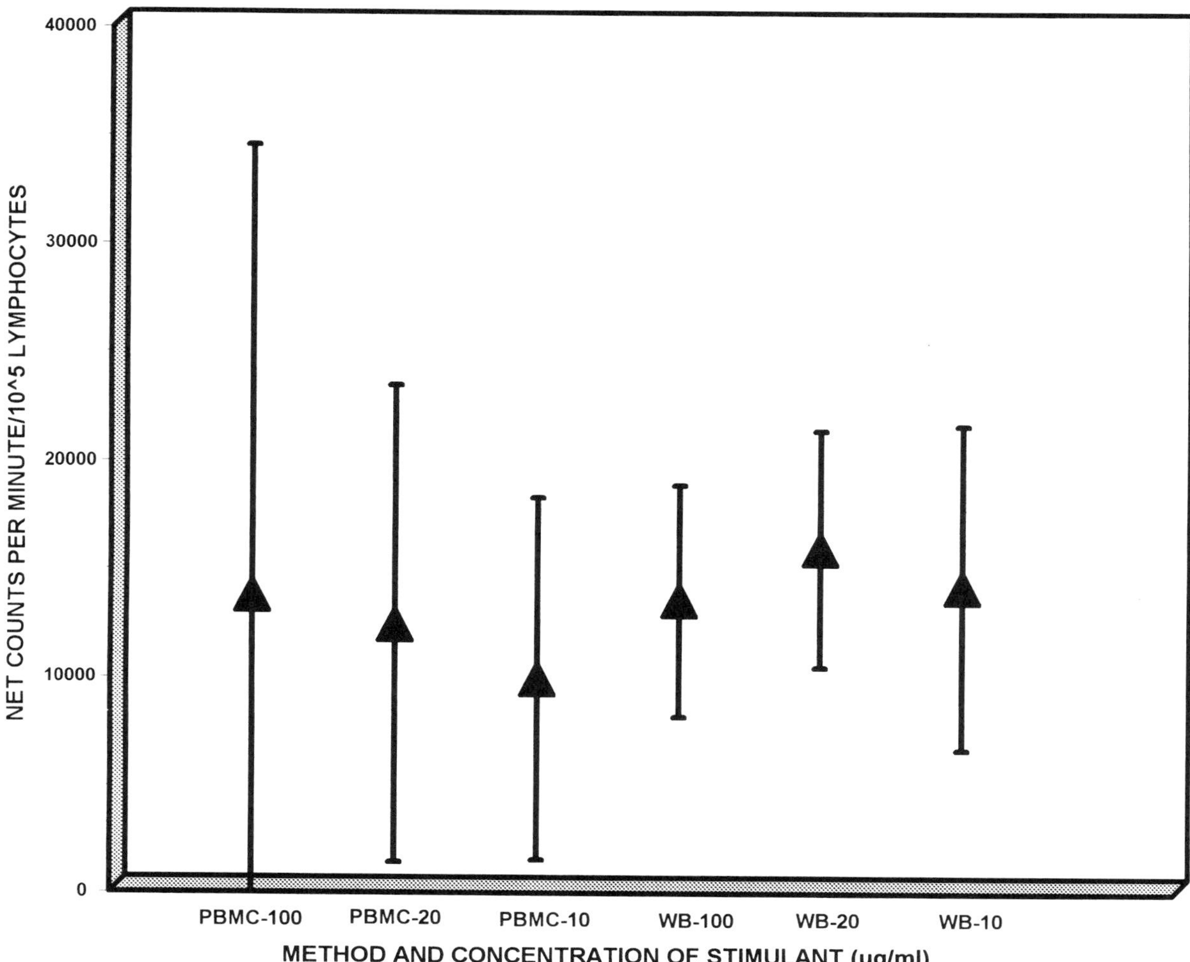

FIGURE **15-1**

Lymphocyte response to *Candida* in HIV-infected adults. Comparison of whole blood (WB) to separated mononuclear cell (PBMC) methods.

TABLE **15-2**

Effects of Ethnicity on Lymphocyte Proliferation (mean +/− standard deviation; NS = $p > 0.05$)

	Whites	**Hispanics**	**Blacks**	p^*
logPHA (net cpm)	5.1 ± 0.2	5.0 ± 0.3	4.9 ± 0.3	NS

*p = 2-tailed p value from Mann-Whitney U test.

TABLE **15-3**

Effects of Gender on Lymphocyte Proliferation (mean +/− standard deviation; NS = $p > 0.05$)

	Males	**Females**	p^*
logPHA (net cpm)	5.0 ± 0.3	501 ± 0.2	NS

*p = 2-tailed p value from Mann-Whitney U test.

literature these data appear to indicate that little or no substantial resting differences exist in lymphocyte response to PHA as a function of gender or ethnicity.

Percent coefficient of variation (%CV) of the WB response to PHA was determined on blood samples from healthy adult laboratory control subjects and the results are presented in **Table 15-4**. The variability (precision) of proliferation assays and the difficulty that this presents in reliably determining a person's "true" lymphocyte function in response to a given stimulus have

TABLE 15-4

Precision Analysis of Whole Blood Response to PHA: Three Subjects Each Assayed 12 Times in 1 Day*

Subject	Stimulant	Mean (cpm)	SD	CV%	Minimum	Maximum
1	None	80	24	30	55	139
	PHA	26,791	6690	25	15,848	40,844
2	None	65	37	57	29	161
	PHA	41,251	12,906	31	22,773	58,216
3	None	85	22	25	65	135
	PHA	22,855	5594	24	16,501	37,997

*Raw cpm are shown uncorrected for lymphocyte count.

been a source of concern for clinical immunologists, particularly in assays that are separated in time but done on the same subject. However, we find that the actual extent of such variability is not so large as to render the data uninterpretable. Reference (3) gives data collected in a longitudinal field study of intravenous drug users. Even in this difficult population, the results of proliferation assays done on HIV-seronegative subjects at three time points over an 18-month period show an acceptable level of variability. We have applied generalizability analyses, as described by Llabre and colleagues (5), to proliferation responses of normal subjects in a whole blood assay of lymphocyte responses to PHA. The design used assessed the generalizability of the proliferation response across days and replications within a day. The results showed that for PHA measurements to be highly reliable across days, determinations are needed either on a single day with three replications, or across 2 days with a single replication on each day (**Table 15-5**). A generalizable estimate should have a dependability coefficient (G*) of ≥0.75. The results indicated that systematic variation due either to visit or to replications was small. The variability associated with individual subjects constituted the largest portion of the overall variation.

An important factor that will influence results is the duration of time from blood draw to assay. We have carried out a study in which blood samples were assayed within 8 hours of blood draw and again at 18 to 24 hours. Between assays the samples were left on the laboratory bench at ambient temperature. Phytohemagglutinin responses expressed as stimulation index (SI) for each of 66 individuals are shown in **Figure 15-2** and as net cpm in **Figure 15-3**. The mean proliferation in response to

TABLE 15-5

Generalizability Study for Lymphocyte Proliferation in Response to PHA

Number of Replications	G* (n = 15) 1 Day	2 Days
1	0.735	0.848
2	0.743	0.853
3	0.746	0.854

*G, coefficients obtained in two separate studies. Data were from HIV-positive gay men aged 24 to 38 years (mean = 31); day 2 sample obtained 10 to 14 days after day 1 sample.

PHA, PWM, and anti-CD3 for day 1 and day 2 is shown in **Table 15-6**. For each stimulant a significant drop in proliferation was seen in the second-day assay. For the two T-cell mitogens, PHA and anti-CD3, the decrease was 25% to 28%. Pokeweed mitogen responses declined only 14% after 24 hours. It should be noted that in all of these assays the lymphocyte counts used to normalize the data to 10^5 lymphocytes were obtained on day 1. Different hematology analyzers differ in the extent of variation observed between fresh and stored samples. Also, shipped samples are likely to be exposed to a much wider variation in temperatures than those stored on the laboratory bench.

Procedural Considerations

Specimen Required, Collection Method, Anticoagulant, Special Restrictions

Heparin (green top) is the required anticoagulant for LPA. Tripotassium ethylenediaminetetraacetic acid (EDTA; lavender top) is the required

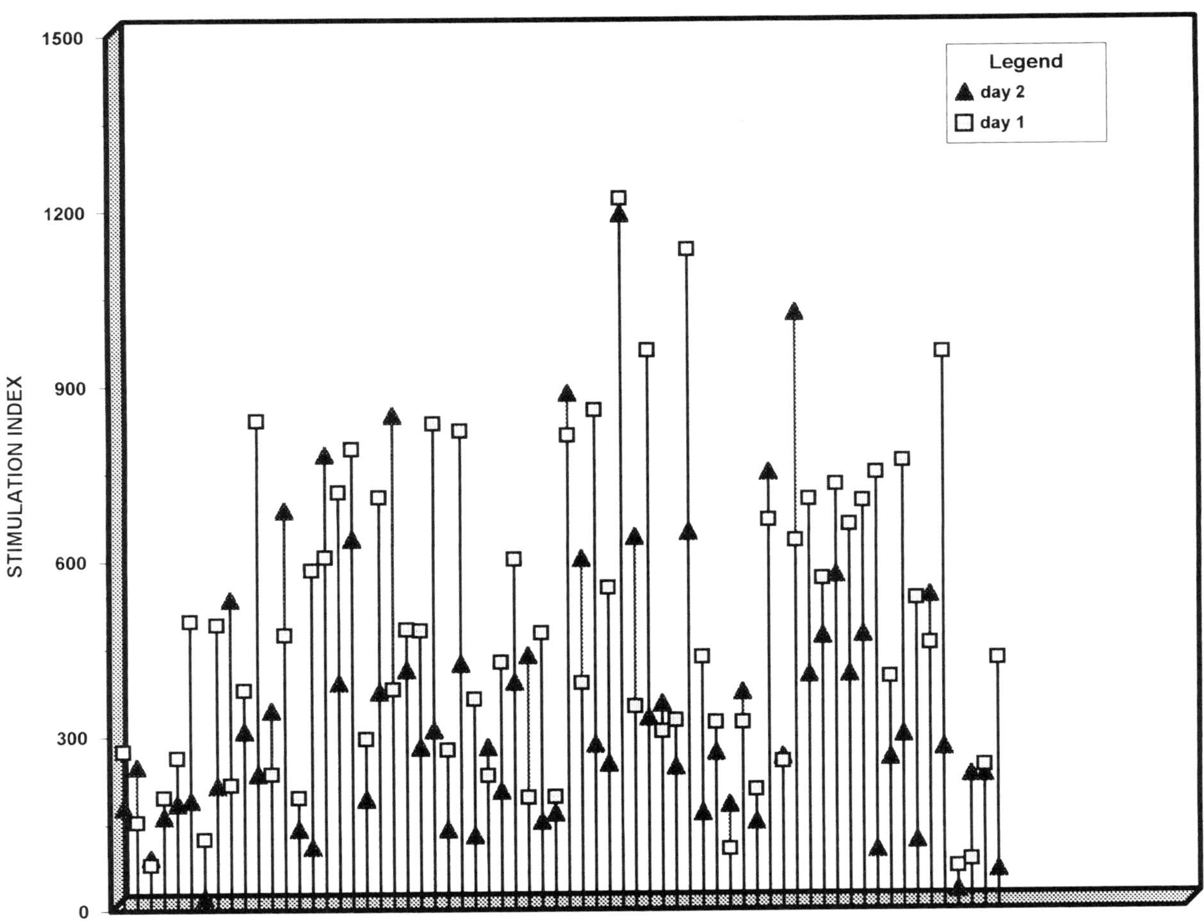

FIGURE 15-2

Whole blood proliferative response to PHA expressed as stimulation index. Comparison of fresh versus 24-hour samples.

TABLE 15-6

Comparison of Fresh Versus Day-Old Blood Sample in Whole Blood LPA

Stimulant	n	Day 1 [mean cpm (±SD)]	Day 2 [mean cpm (±SD)]	Delta cpm (day 1–day 2)	*p**
PHA	66	134,775 (44,914)	101,711 (38,759)	33,063	<0.00001
PWM	66	13,540 (601)	11,969 (642)	1571	<0.05
Anti-CD3	57	42,814 (34,860)	30,793 (35,787)	12,021	<0.02

*p = 2-tailed p value from Mann-Whitney U test.

anticoagulant for leukocyte count and differential analysis, which is needed for analysis of the results of this assay. Blood samples should be held at ambient temperature. If specimens are assayed after 8 hours, the results should be compared to a normal control range obtained on samples also held for more than 8 hours. Sample should be rejected if the blood is lysed or clotted, or if it has been refrigerated.

Reagents, standards, controls, and media used include RPMI 1640 with L-glutamine (Gibco BRL, Gaithersburg, MD); penicillin and streptomycin (P/S); tritiated thymidine ($[^3H]$-TdR; NEN Products, Dupont Wilmington, DE);

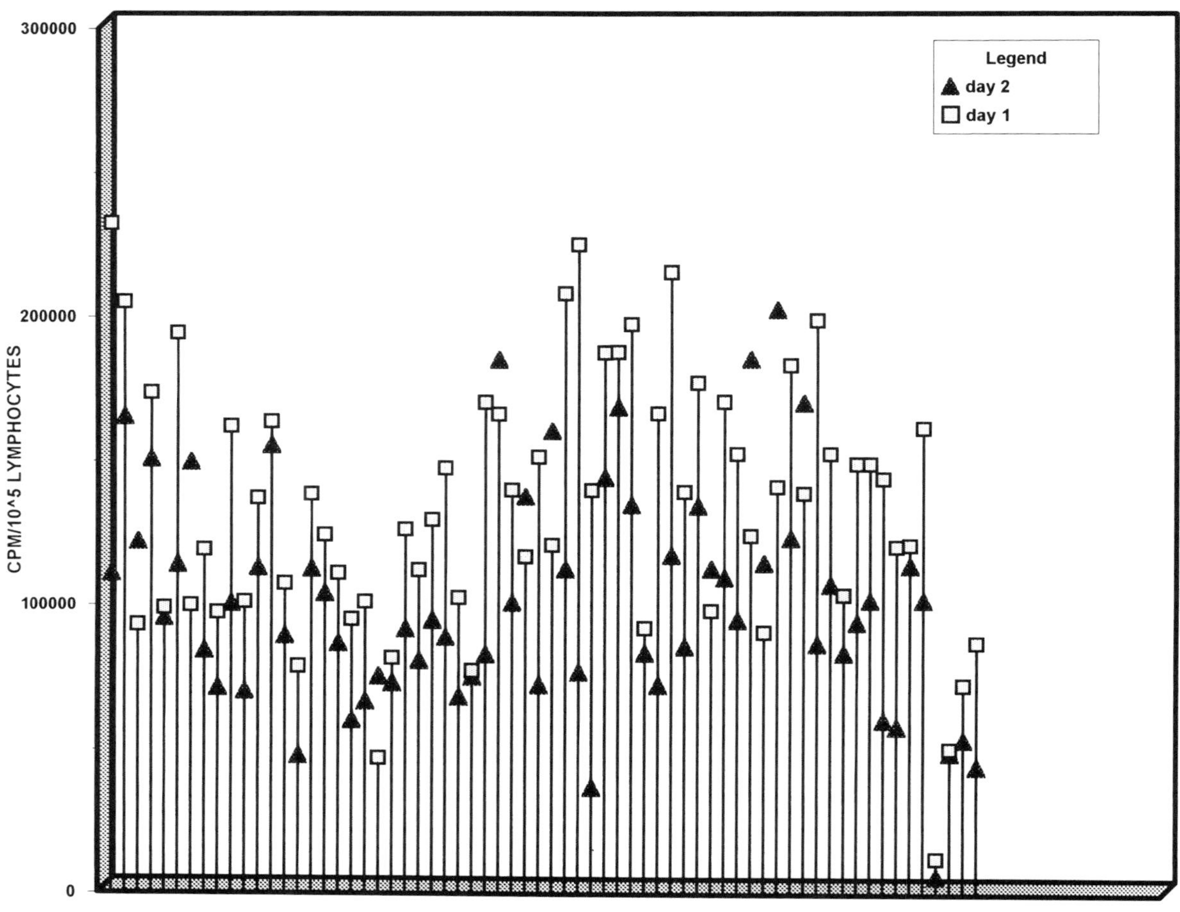

FIGURE 15-3

Whole blood proliferative response to PHA shown as net cpm. Comparison of fresh versus 24-hour samples.

tissue culture grade, sterile, round-bottom 96-well plates with tight-fitting lids (Corning Costar, Cambridge, MA); biodegradable, nontoxic scintillation fluid (Cytoscint, ICN, Costa Mesa, CA); and sterile, disposable pipet tips.

Stimulants

Recall antigens that could find use in clinical studies are numerous, and selection should be dictated by the clinical or research problem at hand. For example, proliferation assays with proteins and glycoproteins associated with HIV-1 may be useful in detecting cellular immune responses to this virus in infected individuals. If response to an antigen to which most people are exposed is to be measured as a marker of general cellular immune competency, *Candida albicans* or tetanus toxoid, or both, are two that are frequently selected. Plant mitogens that have proved useful in studies with human subjects include PHA, PWM, and concanavalin A (Con A). All three can be obtained from the Sigma Chemical Company, St. Louis, MO. A T-lymphocyte–specific stimulant is monoclonal antibody to the CD3 receptor (anti-CD3). This can be obtained from Coulter, Hialeah, FL, or from Becton Dickinson, San Jose, CA. Recall antigens are also useful. *Candida albicans* antigen is obtained from Greer Laboratories, Lendir, NC. Tetanus toxoid is supplied by Connaught Laboratories, Swift Water, PA. HIV-1 peptides can be obtained from NIAID Reagent Program, Rockville, MD. Antigen/mitogen solutions are prepared in RPMI-0 (no exogenous serum) for the whole blood assay or in RPMI-10% fetal calf serum for the PBMC assay.

For each antigen/mitogen in the assay, a solution should be prepared at twice (2×) the intended final concentration in the assay wells. Sufficient volume should be prepared in order to fill the requisite number of assay wells (no. assay wells × 100 μL/well = minimum volume to prepare). Usual 2× working concentrations are as follows:

Candida albicans	20 μg/mL
Tetanus toxoid	2.5 μg/mL
PHA	20 μg/mL
PWM	10 μg/mL
Anti-CD3	1 μg/mL

It is suggested, however, that each laboratory determine optimum antigen or mitogen concentrations. In longitudinal studies, it is wise to obtain a sufficient amount of a single lot of each stimulant. Stock solutions can be prepared in sterile RPMI 1640. These stocks should be dispensed into sterile vials, in suitable volume for one assay, and stored frozen at −20°C.

Assay

One should dispense 100 μL per well of each mitogen concentration being tested. For control wells in whole blood assays, 100 μL RPMI should be dispensed. All test concentrations and control wells are to be done in triplicate. Heparinized blood (1:5) should be diluted with RPMI. Diluted blood, 100 μL per well, should be dispensed to all the wells that contain mitogens/antigens or culture medium (unstimulated control). Plates should be wrapped in aluminum foil, plastic wrap, or plastic bags, and incubated at 37°C in a 95% humidified atmosphere that contains 5% carbon dioxide. This occurs on day 1. Cultures with T-cell stimulants such as PHA or anti-CD3 are generally incubated for 3 days. The B- and T-cell mitogens can be incubated for 3 days or 6 days. Recall antigens are incubated for 6 days. On the morning of the last day of incubation, a working solution of 20 μCi/mL tritiated thymidine in RPMI should be prepared. Sufficient volume should be prepared to dispense 25 μL per well (no. assay wells ×25 μL/well = minimum volume to prepare). Plates should be pulsed with 25 μL (0.5 μCi) of [^{3}H]-TdR. One should then incubate with cells for 6 hours. After 6 hours, one should harvest onto glass fiber filters using a cell harvester. If harvesting cannot be done immediately after the 6-hour pulse, plates can be stored at 4°C until harvested. After harvesting, filters are dried overnight at room temperature and the filter sheets are processed for counting in a beta counter. The appropriate quantity of scintillation fluid should be added and filters left for at least 3 hours in scintillation fluid before counting. Counting should be done on a beta scintillation counter.

Calculations

Data can be expressed in two different ways following determination of mean values of the triplicates: 1) net cpm = (cpm experimental − cpm background unstimulated). For whole blood assays, the mean of the net cpm is transformed to mean cpm/100,000 lymphocytes. The number of lymphocytes present in the culture is determined from total leukocyte count times percent lymphocytes. Both of these values are obtained from the complete blood count with differential. 2) SI = (cpm experimental/cpm background unstimulated).

Quality Control/Quality Assurance

Parallel cultures with samples obtained from normal controls are set up each time patients are assessed. If the results for the control fall out of the normal range the assay should be repeated on fresh samples. The range for the proliferation response of normal humans to a given stimulant is large, as would be expected for this type of functional assay. Appropriately matched controls are essential in clinical research studies in which LPAs are being used to estimate the influence of exogenous or endogenous factors or of experimental therapies on lymphocyte function.

The efficiency of the beta counter and the cell harvester used should be determined and regular preventive maintenance for both instruments should be performed. All of the reagents and mitogens/antigens must be tested for satisfactory performance. This testing is to be documented with source, catalogue number, lot number, date of expiration, date of receipt, date tested, date test reported, and technician responsible for the testing. The list of control variables that must be considered in the analysis of proliferation data includes smoking, alcohol, drug abuse, and medications as well as pyschosocial stressors, including bereavement, anxiety, impending examinations, or anticipation of potentially bad news, such as receiving the results of an anti–HIV-1 test (6,7).

Natural Killer Cell Assays in a Clinical Setting

Natural killer (NK) cells are a heterogeneous population of large granular lymphocytes that have largely been studied because of their participation in host defense against viral infections and the development of cancer (8,9). Natural killer cells in the peripheral blood have been well characterized with respect to both phenotype and function. They can be identified by flow cytometry as large granular lymphocytes (by light scatter) expressing the cell surface markers CD16 or CD56, or both, and not expressing the pan T-cell marker CD3. They are able to spontaneously kill cells that have become malignant or infected with virus. They also produce a repertoire of cytokines that regulate the adaptive immune response and may be important in host defense even if as NK effector cells they are not lytic. Although considerable effort has been directed toward identification of the NK cell surface markers that are responsible for recognition of malignant and virus-infected cells, no single receptor that mediates recognition and leads to lysis of the target cell has yet been identified. Receptors that prevent lysis of normal healthy cells have been described. They are called killer inhibitory receptors (KIR); they protect cells that express normal class I major histocompatibility complex (MHC) molecules from lysis (10).

Natural killer cells may also be important in pregnancy. While the number of NK cells in the blood is usually around 10%, over 50% of the lymphocytes in the decidua (the maternal tissue that is closest to the fetal tissue of the placenta) are CD56+ (11,12). Unlike peripheral blood NK cells, over 80% of these CD56+ lymphocytes lack CD16. Like NK cells from blood, they lack classic B and T cell surface markers. The role of these cells in the decidua is not known. There have been several suggestions that include secretion of cytokines necessary for the growth of fetal tissue, modeling of arteries to allow maternal-fetal exchange, or attraction to the placenta due to the lack of the classic human leukocyte antigen (HLA) expression on this tissue. It is not clear whether the CD56+ cells in the decidua in human pregnancy have lytic activity. During normal pregnancy, the numbers of NK cells in peripheral blood decrease (13); in women with recurrent spontaneous abortions the number may increase (14).

Although NK cell activity is only measured in very specialized clinical laboratories, information about it may be useful in some situations (15). Natural killer cell activity may influence the treatment of patients with cancer or of pregnant women who have had a history of recurrent spontaneous abortions (14). Cancer centers and reproductive immunology clinics may evaluate either the number of NK cells or their function. Natural killer cell activity is often measured in clinical trials, for example, to investigate the contribution of NK cells to host defense against a particular pathogen or to evaluate the effect of a drug or treatment on baseline NK activity. It has been hypothesized that increased NK cell activity may be inversely correlated with the rate of clinical progression in HIV-infected persons (16). Alternatively, it may be informative to determine whether or not certain treatments will affect NK cell activity, for example, in elderly somatotropin-deficient men treated with recombinant human growth hormone (17). There are several other clinical situations in which measurement of NK cell function may be informative; however, a review of these applications is beyond the scope of this chapter. In this section two different procedures that have been developed to monitor NK cell function in a clinical laboratory are reviewed and some of the advantages and disadvantages of each are presented.

A Comparison of Natural Killer Assays

The percentage of peripheral blood NK cells can be measured using the standard flow cytometry immunophenotyping techniques. Monoclonal antibodies against CD56 and CD16 are commercially available and the percentage of CD56+CD16+ or CD56+CD16− lymphocytes in whole blood can be easily determined. However, if information about NK functional activity is required, other assays must be used. Two assays currently in use that measure functional lytic activity are the standard ^{51}Cr-release assay and a flow cytometry–based NK assay. The ^{51}Cr-release assay involves the measurement of radiolabeled chromium released into the supernatant from preloaded tumor cells exposed to a standard number of NK cells. The flow cytometric assay measures the percentage of dead target cells using a viability stain following exposure to a standard number of NK cells (18,19). A few laboratories have adapted the ^{51}Cr-release NK assay for use with whole blood (20,21); however, most laboratories use purified peripheral blood mononuclear cells (PBMC) in this assay.

Both the flow cytometry–based assay and the ^{51}Cr-release assay described herein use separated PBMC as effectors and the human tumor cell line, K562, as the targets. The flow cytometric assay takes less time and measures uptake of propidium iodide (PI) by dead target cells rather than the amount of radioactive chromium that is released. The ^{51}Cr-release assay can be regarded as the "gold standard" and has been used for decades to measure in vitro lysis of target cells (22). The standard ^{51}Cr-release assay takes longer to complete than the flow cytometric NK assay. However, it should be noted that samples processed for NK measurement by flow cytometry must be analyzed immediately whereas once the ^{51}Cr assay is harvested, it can be counted at any time.

In the ^{51}Cr-release assay, K562 target cells in the log phase of growth are washed and incubated for an hour with 100 μCi ^{51}Cr. They are then washed vigorously to remove free ^{51}Cr and resuspended in RPMI that contains 10% fetal calf serum (FCS). Effector cells are either PBMC or lymphocytes purified from PBMC. One hundred microliters of labeled target cells at a concentration of 2×10^4 cells per milliliter are incubated in microtiter trays with an equal volume of effector cells at effector to target cell ratios (E:T) ratios of 50:1, 25:1, or 12.5:1. This range of effector cells should be modified to include a dilution at either end of this range if the patient or trial participants are suspected of having NK activity outside of the normal range. Microtiter trays are centrifuged at low speed to ensure contact of effector and target cells and then placed in the incubator for 3.5 hours at 37°C. After this incubation, the supernatants are harvested and the amount of ^{51}Cr contained in the supernatants is determined using standard gamma counting techniques.

The flow cytometric assay is a modification of the assay described by Hatam et al (18). Briefly, K562 tumor cells in the log phase of growth are washed to remove the FCS which interferes with the membrane intercalating dye PKH-2 used to identify the target cells. The targets are then incubated at room temperature for 2 minutes with 4 μm PKH-2 (Sigma St. Louis, MO) which excites at 488 nm and fluoresces green (530 nm emission, FL1). PKH-2 stably intercalates into the cell membrane and does not significantly affect viability. Fetal calf serum, 1 milliliter, is then added to stop the reaction. After being washed three more times in RPMI that contains 10% FCS, 100 microliters of target cells at a concentration of 5×10^5 cells per milliliter are incubated with 100 microliters of PBMC in 12×75 mm polystyrene tubes. The following E:T are normally used: 50:1, 25:1, and 12.5:1. Included in each incubation mixture is 25 microliters of propidium iodide (PI, FL3) at a concentration of 100 μg/mL, which is used as a viability marker since it will only label cells that have lost their membrane integrity. The tubes are centrifuged at low speed to ensure close contact of effector and target cells and then they are incubated for 2 hours at 37°C.

After this time, each test tube is analyzed on the flow cytometer. Target cells are identified as the green (FL1) positive events and dead targets are identified as green and red (FL1 and FL3) positive events. Background cytotoxicity is defined as the percentage of PKH-2–labeled K562 cells that takes up PI after a 2-hour incubation in the absence of effector cells. The NK cell cytotoxicity (i.e., NK activity) is measured as the percentage of FL1-positive cells that are dual labeled (in the tubes with effectors) minus the background cytotoxicity (dual-labeled cells in the tubes without effectors). The NK flow cytometric assay can be measured using any flow cytometer with an argon laser that will excite PKH-2 and PI at a wavelength of 488 nm. The protocol to analyze the dead targets is a standard two-parameter histogram of green (PKH-2) versus red (PI) (see Fig. 15-4). PKH-26, a stable membrane dye that emits at 570 nm (orange), can also be used to label targets in this assay; however, the spectral overlap with PI is significantly greater than the overlap with PKH-2.

Procedural Considerations

Either PBMC or Lymphocytes Can be Used as the Effector Cells in These Assays

PBMC are usually employed because of the additional time required to remove monocytes

Effector to Target Ratio

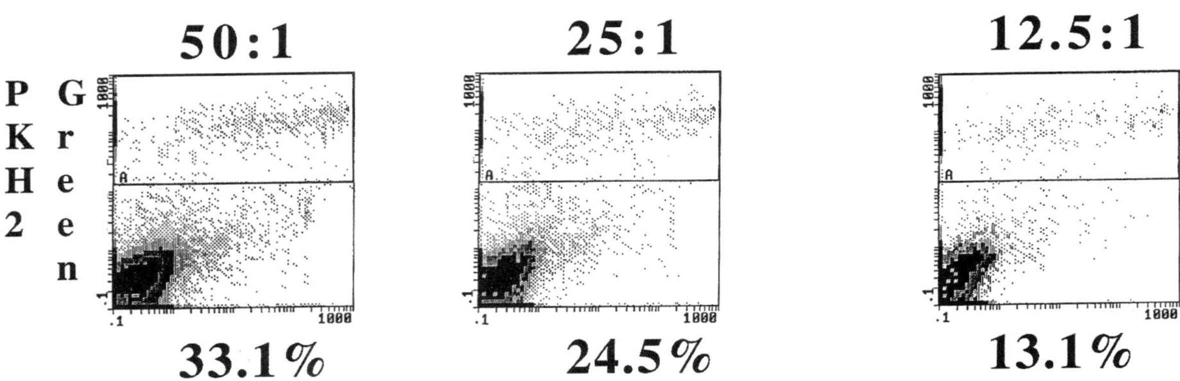

Propidium Iodide (red)
% Cytotoxicity

FIGURE **15-4**

Flow cytometric assay for NK cytotoxicity using PKH-2–labeled K562 target cells. Normal lymphocytes and PKH-2–labeled K562 were incubated for 2 hours at 37°C at E:T ratios of 50:1 (*left*), 25:1 (*center*), and 12.5:1 (*right*) in the presence of propidium iodide (10 μg/mL). Two parameter histograms relate propidium iodide uptake (x-axis) to the number of K562 (y-axis) at each E:T ratio. The percentage of dead target cells for each E:T ratio is shown below the respective histogram. The background of dead target cells in the absence of lymphocytes has been subtracted from percentage shown.

and obtain a suspension of purified lymphocytes. Using the short incubation times described previously, killing by monocytes is assumed to be negligible. Due to the latter and also for practical reasons, PBMC are usually employed when patient samples are being assayed. Removal of monocytes ensures that the NK activity is mediated by lymphocyte NK cells and not by monocytes or macrophages, which can also have NK-like activity. As long as a 2- to 4-hour incubation of effector to target cells is employed, this is not a major concern since monocyte NK-like activity requires approximately 18 hours. Standardizing the number of NK cells added by analyzing the proportion of specific NK cells in the preparation provides information on NK function within specific phenotypically identified NK subpopulations. In fact the whole blood assays express the ^{51}Cr results based on the number of lymphocytes that are phenotypically NK cells present in the blood sample as determined by 2 or 3 color flow cytometry (20,21).

Target Cells for the NK Assay

The standard target cell for the NK assay is the human cell line, K562, which is grown in RPMI with 10% FCS and should be passaged three times each week. These cells are very easy to grow and in fact will remain nearly 100% viable even when in a plateau phase of growth. In order to maintain low background cell death levels for either the flow cytometry or the ^{51}Cr-release assay, target cells must be in the log phase of growth on the day that they are to be used. In order to assure the latter, K562 should be passaged and maintained at a cell concentration of less than 1.2×10^6 cells per milliliter. The day before the assay they should be brought to a concentration of approximately 2.5×10^5 cells per milliliter in fresh culture media and returned to the incubator for use the next day.

A Positive Control Should be Included in Each Assay

It is important to assay the NK activity of a healthy individual with established NK activity each time the flow cytometry or the ^{51}Cr-release assay is performed. Although the results obtained with this individual should not be used to normalize the results, they will alert the investigator if there is a problem with the assay. In our experience, an individual with an average specific release of 55% at a 40:1 E:T ratio in the ^{51}Cr-release assay (with an n of 15) will have activity in the 40% to 70% range on any given day (unpublished results). If, for example, this person is used as a positive control and his or her activity in a particular assay is 20%, the results of that assay would be considered invalid. Establishing expected values on a pool of normal healthy laboratory personnel provides a practical mechanism of ensuring the availability of a positive control. These controls are especially valuable when the patient being evaluated has little or no NK activity. In addition to the "known controls," each individual laboratory should establish its own "normal" reference range on a group of healthy individuals.

The Use of Lytic Units to Evaluate Data

When % specific release values are obtained for at least three E:T ratios, this information can be used to convert the data into lytic units (LU). The LU is a value that is generated by extrapolating a straight line from all of the % specific release values. Lytic units are defined as the inverse of the number of effector cells necessary to kill a defined number of target cells (23). For example, the LU_{20} would be the inverse of the number of effector cells that will kill 20% of the targets. It is easier to compare the information obtained from patient samples because a single number can be used to define the activity of each individual. As an alternative to calculating LU values, some laboratories assay activity at a single E:T ratio. While this provides less complex data, it is risky because if the E:T ratio is not in the log phase of the killing curve, the values obtained may be erroneous. Lytic unit values are frequently used to describe the data obtained in the ^{51}Cr-release assay, but are rarely utilized to present data from the flow cytometry NK assay. There is no reason, however, that LU could not be used for either assay.

The Microcytotoxicity Assay

The ^{51}Cr-release assay that our laboratory has adopted is a modification of the assay described to measure the activity of NK clones (24). This assay requires only 2000 target cells per microtiter well and a correspondingly low number of PBMC from the patient. This "micro" version of the NK assay is useful for pediatric patients, if a particular population is known to have a low lymphocyte count, or if only a minimal amount of blood is obtained. Blood, 10 mL, from patients with normal lymphocyte counts is sufficient for either of the assays described in this chapter even if the microcytotoxicity version of the standard ^{51}Cr-release assay is not employed.

The Effects of Storage and Transport of Blood on NK Cell Assays

The isolation of lymphocytes, the incubation with target cells, and the time necessary to measure the uptake of PI or release of ^{51}Cr can take 6 to 8 hours. Clinical specimens may arrive late in the afternoon necessitating overnight storage. We studied the effect of overnight storage on NK functional activity (flow cytometry assay) in heparinized blood. Specimens were assayed immediately, at 24 hours, and at 48 hours of storage at room temperature or at 4°C. The results indicate that if specimens could not be run immediately it was best to store the blood at room temperature rather than at 4°C. After 48 hours at room temperature, the results were highly variable; the activity in some specimens increased while in others it decreased or remained at the same level as that of fresh samples. In most cases, however, the individuals with extremely high or low activity remained either high or low (Sachs, unpublished observation, 1997). Others have reported that storage of whole blood at 37°C overnight abrogates NK activity (17). When possible, it is best to assay blood samples on the day that the blood is collected; however, since this cannot always be done, the best alternative is to store the blood at room temperature and assay it the following day. Son et al (25) suggested that if PBMC are isolated from blood before storage, it is best to store them at 4°C in RPMI, which contains 10% AB serum before measuring NK activity.

If functional NK assays are performed immediately after the blood is obtained, it does not matter which anticoagulant is used provided that lymphocytes or PBMC are separated from the whole blood. However, if samples are to be stored for any length of time, lymphocytes collected in heparin will maintain their activity better than those collected in EDTA or acid citrate dextrose (ACD) solution. The latter two anticoagulants should not be used in functional whole blood NK assays.

Advantages and Disadvantages of the Standard ^{51}Cr-Release Assay as Compared to the Flow Cytometric NK Assay

The gold standard assay for NK function is the ^{51}Cr-release assay. However, in recent years, it has been recognized that in clinical immunology laboratories, this assay may present some difficulties. One major problem is the use of radioactivity, the disposal of which has become difficult and expensive. Also, handling of radioisotopes requires special training and since the half-life of radioactive chromium is approximately 28 days, a monthly order of this reagent could be expensive.

The lipophilic dyes used to label target cells in the flow cytometric NK assay, PKH-2 or PKH-26, are reasonably priced and fairly stable. Indeed, K562 cells labeled with PKH-2 can be cultured overnight and used as target cells for the next two days (Sachs, unpublished observation, 1997). The cost of a flow cytometer is not trivial; however, many clinical immunology laboratories already have them. Considerable skill is also necessary for performing the flow cytometry–based NK cell assay.

The flow cytometry assay has several advantages. It is possible to determine cytotoxicity on a single target cell basis; this is impossible with the ^{51}Cr-release assay. A third fluorochrome could be used to determine the number of NK cells in the effector cell populations, and the live and dead targets can be distinguished before lysis of the target cell occurs (18). On the other hand, the ^{51}Cr-release assay with PBMC or lymphocytes is easier to perform initially and it provides reliable information about the number of target cells lysed. It does not by itself indicate if the lack of target cell killing is due to a paucity of NK cells or if the NK cells are present but inefficient killers. Due to the nature of the assay, it is not possible to determine whether or not the effector cells were viable at the time of the assay. However, since the ^{51}Cr-release assay is done in microtiter trays, it is easier to set up replicate cultures, thus enabling standard statistical analyses of within run precision. The ^{51}Cr-release assay performed in our laboratory requires five times fewer lymphocytes than the flow cytometry assay, and therefore if the individuals in the particular clinical population are likely to have reduced numbers of lymphocytes, the ^{51}Cr-release assay would be a better choice. When the volume of blood available is very limited (e.g., <2 mL), the whole blood ^{51}Cr-release assay paired with flow cytometric determination of the numbers and viability of NK cells in the sample should be considered (21). Finally, the % specific release values observed when the two assays were run side by side were usually higher in the ^{51}Cr-release assay than in the flow cytometry NK assay (unpublished observation, 1997).

In conclusion, both assays provide a viable way to measure the amount of NK activity in the clinical laboratory. The choice is primarily one of expertise and expense.

Neutrophil Function

Polymorphonuclear (PMN) cell functions are critical to the integrity of host defense against invading microorganisms. Their functions in tissues can be divided into stages: adherence to endothelium, diapedesis through the walls of the blood vessels, and migration toward the offending agent (chemotaxis). The PMN then recognize, adhere to, and phagocytose the invading organism, whereupon the PMN discharge a series of granules into the phagocytic vacuole (degranulate), while generating reactive oxygen intermediates (from the oxidative burst), which kills the pathogen. Clinically the most commonly measured PMN function is the oxidative burst and the products generated from it. The absence of the latter in appropriately stimulated cells is consistent with a diagnosis of chronic granulomatous disease (CGD). We will briefly review CGD and a flow cytometric assay used for the assessment of a normal/abnormal oxidative burst.

Chronic granulomatous disease is a heterogeneous group of inherited disorders and usually manifests itself within the first 2 years of life. Clinically the disease is characterized by repeated and prolonged bacterial and fungal infections of lungs, skin, bones, and liver, often with organisms considered to have low pathogenicity. These patients have a defect in the ability to kill microorganisms because of severely diminished or absent nicotinamide adenine dinucleotide phosphate (NADPH) oxidase activity. Mutations that occur in gp91-phox, p22-phox, p47-phox, or p61-phox have each been shown to produce an abnormal NADPH oxidase, resulting in an inability to generate the oxidative burst product, superoxide. The latter is essential as the precursor of all microbicidal oxidants produced in phagocytic cells. The gene coding for gp91-phox is located on the X chromosome. This form of CGD accounts for approximately 55% of all cases (26). Women with a mutation in this gene would be carriers with a 50% chance of having a male child with CGD. Abnormalities in the expression of the p22-phox membrane component account for approximately 5% of all cases of CGD (27). Defects in the cytosolic component p47-phox account for approximately 33% of all CGD patients, whereas defects in the cytosolic p66-phox are detected much less frequently (approximately 5%) (26). The latter three proteins are not coded for on the X chromosome and appear to be transmitted to offspring in an autosomally recessive pattern. Mutation in these genes leads to either the presence of an abnormal protein or to their complete absence, which results in the abolishment or significant diminishment of superoxide production by intact PMN.

For many years the nitroblue tetrazolium (NBT) dye reduction assay was the gold standard for the laboratory diagnosis of CGD. This test was time consuming, required approximately 10 mL whole blood, and was relatively difficult to interpret, particularly if the patient was a carrier for the mutation. The NBT assay has to a large extent been replaced by flow cytometry–based procedures. We will review a whole blood flow cytometry assay developed in our laboratory for the diagnosis of patients and carriers with CGD (28).

Procedural Considerations

The first flow cytometry–based assay for the diagnosis of CGD was reported by Bass et al in 1983 (29). This procedure was easy to interpret, objective and relatively simple to perform; however, it could not be performed directly in whole blood. Phagocytic cells had to be isolated, washed, and counted before loading with dichlorofluorescein diacetate (DCFH-DA). Many laboratories that perform a flow cytometry–based CGD diagnostic assay use this procedure or a slight modification of it. Unfortunately in whole blood the background fluorescence generated precludes the sensitive and reliable detection of activated versus nonactivated PMN. To establish a procedure that could be performed directly in whole blood we switched to dihydrorhodamine 123 (DHR-123) as the reactive oxygen sensitive indicator.

The use of the uncharged nonfluorescent derivative of the laser dye DHR-123 to measure intracellular reactive oxygen metabolites was first reported by Rothe et al (30). The dye readily permeates most membranes. In the presence of reactive oxygen intermediates (ROI) generated during the respiratory burst, the dye is rapidly oxidized to produce the brightly fluorescent cationic compound rhodamine 123, which localizes in the mitochondria (26). Dihydrorhodamine 123 is a more sensitive indicator of granulocyte respiratory burst activity than DCFH-DA (31). Emmendörffer and colleagues had developed a clinical test utilizing DHR-123 (31–33); however, the test as reported involved sedimentation, erythrocyte lysis, washing, and counting before dye loading and stimulation. Since our goal was to develop a sensitive procedure for the detection of ROI that could be performed rapidly and in a manner similar to that of whole blood procedures for lymphocyte immunophenotyping and other granulocyte function assays, we modified the procedure reported by Emmendörffer (31–33) to allow for dye loading and granulocyte stimulation directly in whole blood. Following the prerequisite incubation periods (with dye and stimulus), erythrocytes are lysed, the leukocytes are fixed, and the fluorescence in individual cells is measured by gating on the appropriate cell populations. This procedure is very sensitive, and easy to perform. In the remaining portion of the chapter, the optimization of this procedure, appropriate controls, specimen requirements, and other quality control issues are reviewed.

Basic Method

Whole blood, 100 μl, is added to the appropriate tubes, diluted 1:10 with calcium and magnesium-free phosphate buffered saline (PBS; Northwestern University Cancer Center, Chicago, IL), and incubated in a shaking water bath at 37°C with 25 μL DHR-123 (Molecular Probes, Eugene, OR) at a final concentration of 2.5 μg/mL. Dihydrorhodamine 123 is stored at a stock concentration of 5 mg/mL in N,N-dimethyl formamide (DMF; Sigma, St. Louis, MO) at −70°C. (*Note*: DMF will dissolve some plastics, and therefore it is essential to pretest the tubes in which the diluted dye will be stored.) The optimal concentration of dye used to load the granulocytes before stimulation with phorbol 12-myristate 13-acetate (PMA) was between 2.5 and 5 μg/mL. The concentration of dye that gives optimal results should be confirmed with each new lot number of DHR-123.

After a 15-minute incubation period with the dye, various stimuli can be added (see below) and the blood is incubated an additional 15 minutes at 37°C in a shaking water bath. Following the last incubation the samples are centrifuged at 400 × *g* for 5 minutes and the supernatant is discarded. The pellet is resuspended in 2 mL erythrocyte lysing solution (Ortho-mune lysing reagent, Ortho Diagnostic Systems, Raritan, NJ) and allowed to stand at room temperature for 10 minutes. The cells are then washed [washing solution, 2.5% sodium azide (Sigma), 10% mL fetal bovine serum (GIBCO, Grand Island, NY), in PBS], resuspended in 0.7 mL of a 1% paraformaldehyde solution (Electron Microscopy Sciences, Washington, PA), and held at 4°C until they are analyzed.

Flow Cytometric Analysis

Following fixation the samples are acquired on the flow cytometer. Both forward-angle and right-angle light scatter signals are optimized for detection of the three major leukocyte populations, that is, lymphocytes, monocytes, and granulocytes. The forward-scatter threshold signal is adjusted to exclude debris and unlysed erythrocytes. It is important to note the following: First, PMA will change the light scatter characteristics of the granulocyte population so that the analysis gate that is set around granulocytes in the unstimulated sample may have to be changed when the granulocytes in the stimulated sample are analyzed. Secondly, in some samples that are held overnight or longer there may be more than one population of granulocytes based on light scatter. It must be recognized that this is due to degranulation and cell death and that the analysis gate must only include undamaged granulocytes. In general the undamaged cells will comprise the population of events with higher forward light scatter signals; however, this is not always straightforward and may require some advanced flow cytometry analysis techniques. Normal PMN and the affected PMN in the blood of a CGD carrier do not differ with respect to light scatter properties; therefore, it is essential that the granulocytes being analyzed comprise a homogeneous light scatter population. All fluorescence parameters are optimized on unstimulated lysed whole blood that has not been preloaded with DHR-123. Fluorescence of this sample is acquired on the photomultiplier tube (PMT), which is used routinely to collect fluorescein isothiocyanate emissions (a band pass filter of approximately 525 ± 10 nm). Logarithmically amplified signals are adjusted such that the peak fluorescence is in the first decade and a clear rise and fall of this negative fluorescence peak are observed. Using these settings, the fluorescence emitted by the cells that were loaded with dye but not stimulated is then measured (background oxidative state), followed by the analysis of the sample that was loaded with dye and stimulated (stimulated). The results are then expressed as a ratio referred to as the neutrophil oxidative index (NOI), which is calculated as the mean fluorescent channel of the dye-loaded nonstimulated cells divided by mean fluorescent channel generated by the dye-loaded and stimulated cells. This formula was first described by Epling et al (34). In cases in which two clear fluorescent populations are observed (i.e., X-linked carriers), the mean fluorescence of both populations is obtained and the NOI for each population is calculated.

Response Curves to PMA, Opsonized Zymosan, and fMLP

Phorbol 12-myristate 13-acetate (PMA), opsonized zymosan, and F-*met-leu-phe* (fMLP) have been assessed for their ability to generate reactive oxygen species as detected in the above flow cytometry–based assay. PMA (Sigma, St. Louis, MO) is diluted in dimethyl sulfoxide (DMSO) and can be stored at a concentration of 5 mg/mL for up to 6 months at −70°C. Working dilutions are made in PBS. We have tested concentrations of 15 to 400 ng/mL PMA.

The zymosan (Sigma) is made up to 0.1g in 10mL sterile PBS, boiled for 10 minutes, washed twice, and resuspended in 10mL PBS. It is opsonized by incubation of 0.1g in 1mL pooled normal human sera in a shaking water bath at 37°C for one hour immediately before use. Following the opsonization procedure, the zymosan is washed and resuspended to 10mg/mL in PBS. Concentrations of 0.1 to 1.0mg/mL have been tested. A 10^{-2}M solution of fMLP (Sigma) is prepared in DMSO and stored as the stock solution at −70°C. Tenfold serial dilutions were made in PBS and concentrations of 10^{-4} to 10^{-9}M have been tested.

The most potent stimulus was PMA at an optimal concentration (maximal fluorescence generated) of 240ng/mL. However, this level was toxic to the cells and resulted in the decreased recovery of granulocytes (as determined by decreased cell counts and a degenerating light scatter pattern). PMA at a concentration of 60ng/mL induced a consistent increase in fluorescence while maintaining the characteristic light scatter pattern of the granulocyte cluster (**Fig. 15-5**). For practical reasons dilutions of 100ng/mL are used for the clinical assay. Zymosan was an effective mediator for the generation of the oxidative burst, with optimal results occurring at a concentration of 0.5mg/mL. Higher levels of the opsonized zymosan in the samples interfered with the light scatter signals. Due to the complexities of preparing opsonized zymosan, it is not used routinely for the clinical procedures. The fMLP generated a very weak response in this assay, resulting in a slight increase in fluorescence at the concentrations used.

Sample Storage Conditions

EDTA- and heparin-anticoagulated whole blood generate comparable results if the samples are assayed in less than 24 hours. Using a slight modification of our assay, Prince and Lapé-Nixon (35) observed that EDTA-, heparin-, or ACD-anticoagulated blood gave reliable results when tested after the blood had been held at room temperature for 4 hours. At 24 hours after the blood draw, only ACD and heparin gave reliable results. At time points greater than 24 hours and up to 72 hours, only heparin-anticoagulated blood was reliable for the assessment of the granulocyte oxidative burst generation. Holding samples overnight after they have been prepared and processed for flow cytometry is not recommended as fluorescence is significantly decreased.

Assay for ROS in Normal Controls, CGD Patients, and X-Linked Carriers

The lower limit of normal for ROI production (calculated as the neutrophil oxidative index, NOI) was established in 33 donors over a 6-month period. With a stimulus of 100ng/mL PMA and a DHR-123 loading concentration of 2.5μg/mL, the mean fluorescence channel in the stimulated granulocytes ranged from 503 to 2248 (mean ± SD = 1400 ± 568 relative linear channel number on a 4-decade log scale on a Becton Dickinson FACScan BDIS, Mountain-View, CA). The mean background fluorescence in this population (i.e., preincubated with DHR-123 but not PMA stimulated) was 13 ± 7 channels. The NOI indices in this population of adult individuals ranged from 32 to greater than 300 with an average NOI of 149. An NOI of greater than 30 is considered to be normal, that is, "not consistent with a diagnosis of CGD" in our laboratory. The average NOI from five patients with CGD was 1.0 ± 0.1. In the X-linked CGD carriers, the average NOI for the population of normal granulocytes was 192 and the average NOI in the abnormal population of granulocytes (i.e., expressing the X chromosome with the CGD mutation) was 2.4.

Figure 15-6 illustrates the results obtained from a CGD family with the X-linked form of the disease. The patient's PMN failed to generate ROS as indicated by the absence of an increase in fluorescence following stimulation with PMA, that is, an NOI of 0.9. His mother's results indicate the presence of both a normal (NOI = 57) and an abnormal population of PMN; that is, cells with the affected X chromosome do not elaborate ROI (NOI = 3). The healthy control's NOI was 125. Finally the father's stimulated PMN were all brightly fluorescent with an NOI consistent with normal ROI production (NOI = 61; data not shown in figure). **Table 15-7** is a summary of the results obtained from four families with at least one child with CGD. Our laboratory has routinely used the nitroblue tetrazolium dye reduction slide test for the diagnosis of CGD and for the

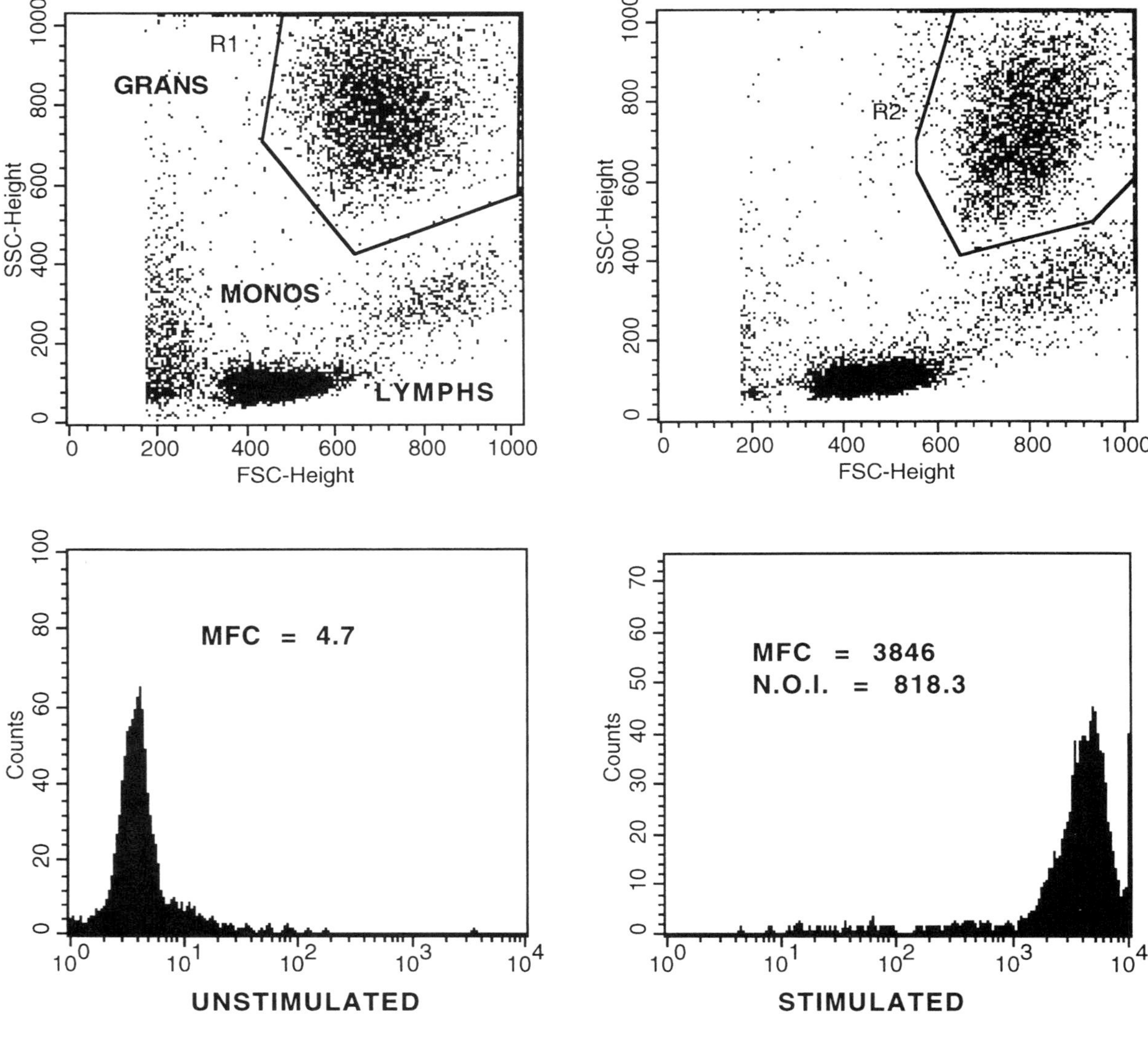

FIGURE **15-5**

Illustrated are the forward- versus right-angle light scatter patterns of whole blood, unstimulated (*left*) and following stimulation with 100 ng/mL PMA (*right*). Below are the levels of fluorescence emitted by the DHR-123 prelabeled granulocytes in unstimulated whole blood (*left*) and DHR-123 prelabeled granulocytes in PMA-stimulated whole blood (*right*). Note the change in light scatter of the granulocyte cluster following stimulation with PMA (100 ng/mL final concentration). Indicated are the mean fluorescent channels (MFC) of granulocytes in both the unstimulated and the stimulated samples, as well as the normal oxidative index (NOI) on this healthy control subject.

identification of X-linked carriers (36). In general the results of the NBT assay correlated very well with the results obtained using the whole blood assay. One of our patient's mother's flow results clearly identified her as a carrier in the flow cytometry–based assay (the affected population was less than 15%). Interestingly, this woman's carrier status may not have been detected in the NBT slide assay, where the normal range is 85% or greater of the cells positive for dye reduction. In a subjective assay, this mother may have been misinterpreted as normal.

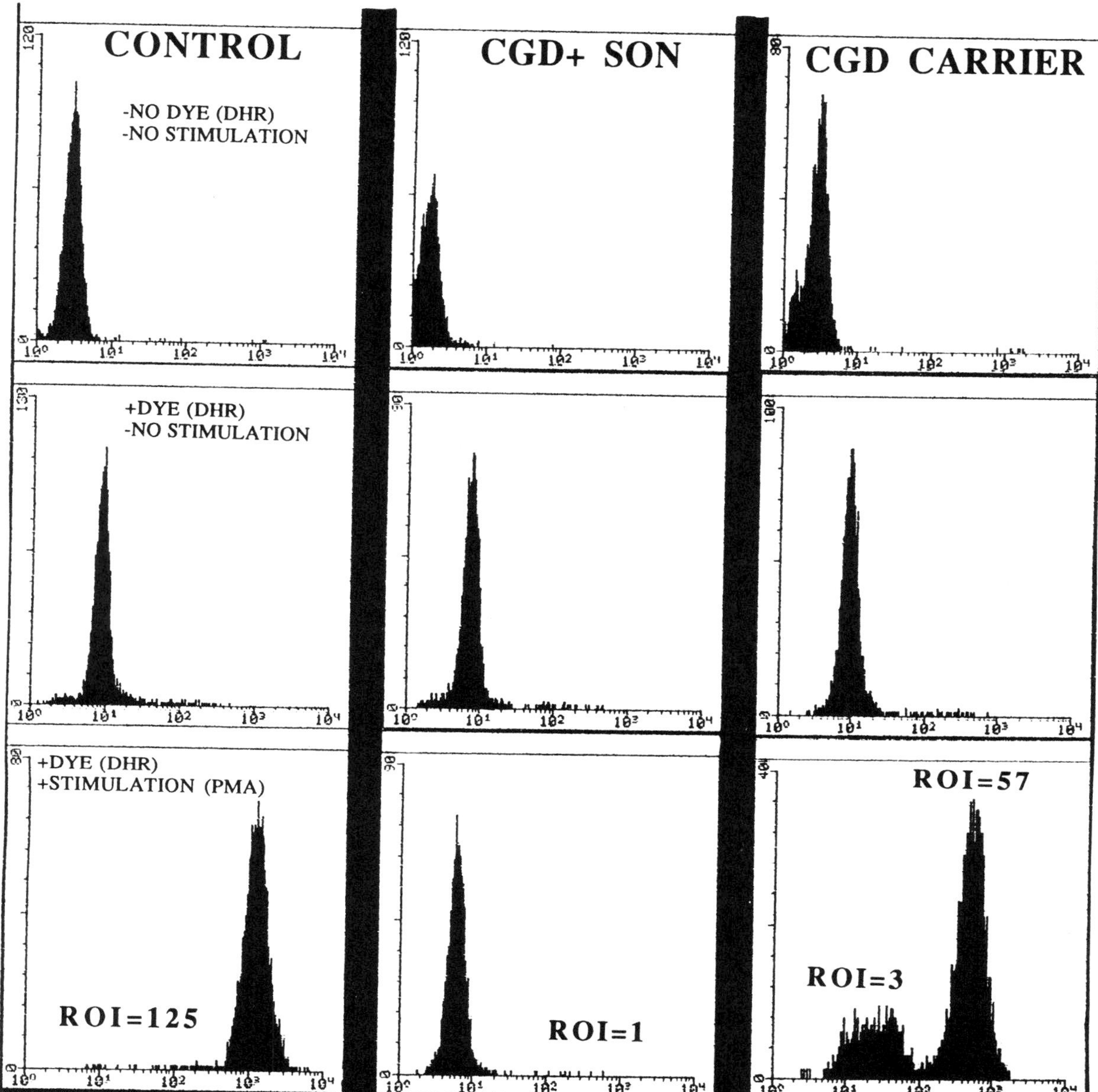

FIGURE **15-6**

The flow cytometric results obtained using the standard assay in a CGD family. The first column is the positive control (father), the second column is the affected son, and the third column is the affected mother. The first row corresponds to the autofluorescent signal generated by untreated cells, the second row is the background fluorescence in cells incubated with dye but not stimulated, and the third row shows the results of the PMA-stimulated samples that have been preincubated with the dye. All results represent the fluorescence in the electronically gated granulocyte population. (Reprinted by permission from ASM publishers, Copyright 1995, [28])

TABLE 15-7

Summary of the Results Obtained with the Standard CGD Flow Cytometric Assay in Four Different CGD Families

	Population 1 (CGD-affected PMN)			Population 2 (normal PMN)			
Family	% of Total PMN	Mean Fluorescence Channel[a] (1–10,000)	NOI[b]	% of Total PMN	Mean Fluorescence Channel (1–10,000)	NOI	NBT % Normal
1. Healthy control[c]	0	NA	NA	100	568	45	96
Mother XXJ[c]	17	38.5	2.9	83	484	36.4	67
CGD son AlXJ#1[c]	100	15.4	1.2	0	NA	NA	0
CGD son AnXJ#2[c]	100	13.7	1.1	0	NA	NA	0
2. Healthy control	0	NA	NA	100	1457	217	98
Mother XXN	82	12.6	1.8	18	1355	199.3	40
Brother EZXN	0	NA	NA	100	1665	146	90
CGD son ELXN #1	100	5.7	0.9	0	NA	NA	3
CGD son RXN #2	100	9.5	1.0	0	NA	NA	0
3. Healthy control	0	NA	NA	100	1296	125.2	95
Father MXH	0	NA	NA	100	626.4	60.8	94
Mother TXM	24	31.6	3.2	76	550.3	56.7	90
CGD son RXM	100	5.6	0.9	0	NA	NA	0
4. Healthy control	0	NA	NA	100	2536	329	NA
Father SXD	0	NA	NA	100	2763	368	NA
Mother SXD	0	NA	NA	73	2640	325.9	NA
CGD daughter AXD	100	12.2	1.4	0	NA	NA	NA
CGD daughter MXD	100	13.9	2.0	0	NA	NA	NA

[a] Mean fluorescence channel from PMA-stimulated cells.

[b] NOI (neutrophil oxidative index) = mean fluorescence channel of PMA-stimulated cells/mean fluorescence channel of nonstimulated cells.

[c] Samples were held overnight before processing and analysis.

Nitroblue tetrazolium (NBT) dye reduction slide assay performed according to standard techniques [see (15)]. Normal = 85% positive or greater for dye reduction. Note mother TXM would have been considered positive by NBT slide assay.

SOURCE: Reprinted by permission from ASM Publishers (28).

Summary

For samples that are going to be processed within 8 hours, the results are equitable whether heparin, EDTA, or ACD is used (35). For routine clinical testing three tubes are processed for each specimen: "no dye, no stimulus" (the nonfluorescent background control), "dye-loaded and no stimulus" (the baseline reactive oxygen state-control) and "dye-loaded and PMA-stimulated" (the positive control). We have previously shown that fMLP generates a rapid increase in the level of expression of β_2-leukocyte integrins on the surface of granulocytes (37). Interestingly, although fMLP stimulated a rapid increase in the surface expression of adhesion molecules, only minimal reactive oxygen intermediates were generated as witnessed by low-level increases in the DHR-123 fluorescence. Some laboratories may opt to use fMLP as a low-level positive control.

The assay allows for the objective determination of carrier status. Interestingly, random X inactivation was observed to be not so "random" (28). None of the CGD "carrier mothers" that we have tested to date have had an equal proportion of normal and abnormal circulating peripheral blood PMN. It is unlikely that the nonrandom X chromosome inactivation observed was due to a selective advantage in those cells with the "normal" X chromosome since one of the mothers had fewer than 20% "normal PMN." Additionally, in the CGD carrier mothers, the abnormal or CGD granulocytes expressed higher fluorescence than the granulocytes from their "CGD" sons. This has been observed by others (33). In a CGD carrier mother with fewer than 20% normal granulocytes, the increased fluorescence in the abnormal granulocytes did not occur. It is our opinion that the observed increase in fluorescence in the affected lymphocytes of carriers may be the result of diffusion of oxidized dye from the normal granulocytes into the abnormal granulocytes and not the result of genetic complementation (28,38). Formal complementation studies may have to be performed to resolve this issue.

In summary, with the appropriate controls this flow cytometry–based, whole blood procedure allows for the objective, rapid, and relatively simple determination of CGD or CGD carrier status with relatively small volumes of whole blood.

REFERENCES

1. Fletcher MA, Baron GA, Ashman M, Klimas NG. Use of whole blood methods in assessment of immune parameters in immunodeficiency syndromes. Clin Diag Immunol 1987;5:69–81.
2. Fletcher MA, Morgan R, Klimas NG, Gjerset G. Lymphocyte proliferation. In: Rose NR, DeMacario EC, Fahey JL, et al, eds. Manual of clinical laboratory immunology. Washington, DC: ASM Press, 1992:213–219.
3. Fletcher MA, Urban R, Asthana D, et al. Lymphocyte proliferation. In: Rose NR, DeMacario EC, Folds J, et al, eds. Manual of clinical laboratory immunology. Washington, DC: ASM Press, 1997:313–319.
4. Klimas NG. Delayed hypersensitivity skin testing. In: Rose NR, DeMacario EC, Folds J, et al, eds. Manual of clinical laboratory immunology. Washington, DC: ASM Press, 1997:276–280.
5. Llbre MM, Ironson G, Spitzer S, et al. How many blood pressure measurements are enough? An application of generalizability theory to blood pressure measurements. Psychophysiology 1988; 25:97–106.
6. Ironson G, Laperriere A, Antoni M, et al. Changes in immune and psychological factors as a function of anticipation and reaction to news of HIV-1 antibody status. Psychosomatic Med 1990;52: 247–270.
7. Goodkin K, Feaster D, Tuttle R, et al. Bereavement is associated with time-dependent decrements in cellular immune function in asymptomatic human immunodeficiency virus type 1–seropositive homosexual men. J Clin Diag Lab Immunol 1996;3:109–118.
8. Robertson MJ, Ritz J. Biology and clinical relevance of human natural killer cells. Blood 1990; 76:2421–2438.
9. Trinchieri G. Biology of natural killer cells. Adv Immunol 1989;47:187–376.
10. D'Andrea AC, Chang C, Bacon K, et al. Molecular cloning on NKB1: A natural killer cell receptor for HLA-B allotypes. J Immunol 1995;155: 2306–2310.
11. King A, Loke YW. On the nature and function of human uterine granular lymphoctes. Immunol Today 1991;12:432–435.
12. Starkey PM, Sargent IL, Redman CW. Cell populations in human early pregnant decidua: characterization and isolation of large granular lymphocytes by flow cytometry. Immunology 1988;65:129–135.
13. Gregory CD, Shaw LP, Lee H, et al. Cytotoxic reactivity of human natural killer (NK) cells during normal pregnancy: a longitudinal study. J Clin Lab Immunol 1985;18:175–181.
14. Kwak JYH, Beaman KD, Gilman-Sachs A, et al. Up-regulated expression of CD56+, CD56+/16+ and CD19+ cells in peripheral blood lymphocytes in pregnant women with recurrent pregnancy losses. Am J Rep Immunol 1995;34:93–99.
15. Whiteside TL, Bryant J, Day R, Herberman RB. Natural killer cytotoxicity in the diagnosis of immune dysfunction: criteria for a reproducible assay. J Clin Lab Analysis 1990;4:102–114.
16. Kaslow R, Ostrow D, Detels R, et al. The multicenter AIDS cohort study: rationale, organization and selected characteristics of the participants. Am J Epidemiol 1987;126:310–318.
17. Rudman D, Shetty KR. Unanswered questions concerning the treatment of hyposomatotropism and hypogonadism in elderly men. J Am Geriatr Soc 1994;42:522–527.
18. Hatam L, Schuval S, Bonagura VR. Flow cytometric analysis of natural killer cell function as a clinical assay. Cytometry 1994;16:59–68.

19. Lane KL, Ashton FA, Schmitz JL, Folds JD. Determination of natural killer cell function by flow cytometry. Clin Diag Lab Immunol 1996;3:295–300.

20. Baron G, Klimas N, Fischl M, Fletcher MA. Decreased natural cell mediated cytotoxicity per effector cell in acquired immunodeficiency syndrome. Diagn Clin Immunol 1985;3:197–204.

21. Patarca R, Fletcher MA, Podack E. Cytolytic cell functions. In: Rose NR, DeMacario EC, Folds J, et al, eds. Manual of clinical laboratory immunology. Washington, DC: ASM Press, 1997:296–303.

22. Brunner KT, Mauel J, Cerottini J-C, Chapius B. Quantitative assay of the lytic action of immune lymphoid cells on ^{51}Cr-labeled allogeneic target cells in vitro: inhibition by isoantibody and by drugs. Immunology 1968;14:181–196.

23. Pross H, Maines M, Rubin P, et al. Spontaneous human lymphocyte-mediated cytotoxicity against tumor target cells. IX. The quantitation of natural killer cell activity. J Clin Immunol 1981;1:51–63.

24. Van de Griend RJ, Bolhuis RLH. In vitro expansion and analysis of cloned cytotoxic T cells derived from patients with chronic T_γ lymphoproliferative disorders. Blood 1985;65:1002–1009.

25. Son BK, Roberts RL, Ank BJ, Stiehm ER. Effects of anticoagulant, serum, and temperature on the natural killer activity of human peripheral blood mononuclear cells stored overnight. J Clin Diag Lab Immunol 1996;3:260–264.

26. Haugland RP. Probes for following endocytosis. In: Larison KD, ed. Molecular probes; handbook of fluorescent probes and research chemicals. Eugene, OR: Molecular Probes, Inc, 1992:99–110.

27. Robesandratana H, Fournier A-M, Chateau M-T, et al. Increased oxidative metabolism in PMA-activated lymphocytes: a flow cytometric study. Int J Immunopharmacol 1992;14:895–902.

28. O'Gorman MRG, Corrochano V. Rapid whole-blood flow cytometry assay for diagnosis of chronic granulomatous disease. Clin Diag Lab Immunol 1995;2:227–232.

29. Bass DA, Wallace P, Dechatelet LR, et al. Flow cytometric studies of oxidative product formation by neutrophils: a grade response to membrane stimulation. J Immunol 1983;130:1910–1917.

30. Rothe G, Oser A, Valet G. Dihydrorhodamine 123: a new flow cytometric indicator for respiratory burst activity in neutrophil granulocytes. Naturwissen 1988;75:354–355.

31. Roesler JM, Hecht J, Greihorst M-L, et al. Diagnosis of chronic granulomatous disease and of its mode of inheritance by dihydrorhodamine 123 and flow microcytofluorometry. Eur J Pediatr 1991;150:161–165.

32. Emmendörffer A, Hecht M, Lohmann-Matthes ML, Roesler J. A fast and easy method to determine the production of reactive oxygen intermediates by human and murine phagocytes using dihydrorhodamine 123. J Immunol Methods 1990;131:269–275.

33. Emmendörffer A, Nakamura M, Rothe G. Evaluation of flow cytometric methods for the diagnosis of chronic granulomatous disease variants under routine laboratory conditions. Cytometry (Communications in Clinical Cytometry) 1994; 18:147–155.

34. Epling CL, Stites DP, McHugh TM, et al. Neutrophil function screening in patients with chronic granulomatous disease by a flow cytometric method. Cytometry 1992;13:615–620.

35. Prince HE, Lapé-Nixon M. Influence of specimen age and anticoagulant on flow cytometric evaluation of granulocyte oxidative burst generation. J Immunol Methods 1995;188:129–138.

36. Windhorst DB, Holmes B, Good RA. Newly defined X-linked trait in man with demonstration of Lyon effect in carrier females. Lancet 1967;1:737–739.

37. O'Gorman MRG, McNally AC, Anderson DC, Myones BL. A rapid whole blood lysis technique for the diagnosis of moderate or severe leukocyte adhesion deficiency (LAD). Ann NYAS 1993;677:427–430.

38. Rabesandratan H, Dornand J. Flow cytometric analysis of oxygen species formation in activated leukocytes. Cytometry 1993;14:695–696. Letter.

CHAPTER 16

Cytokine Receptors

BRYAN MILLETT
KIMBERLY FOSTER
CONSTANCE EMMETT

Background

Cytokines mediate their activity through a large family of structurally and functionally similar receptors, evolved from a common progenitor. The cytokine-receptor complexes form a network of signal mediators that can act synergistically or in a counterregulatory manner.

The pleiotropic actions of cytokines on different target cells can be mediated by the coupling of these high-affinity receptors to different signal-transducing molecules within each type of target cell (1). The selective responses of cells to different cytokines are believed to be, in part, dictated by this repertoire of different receptors expressed on the cell surface. The type of receptor that is expressed by each cell is a function of the type of target cell as well as the cell's stage of differentiation (1). Cytokines and other signaling molecules are believed to transmit signals to cells through receptors that are present at very low concentrations (10–1000 molecules per cell). Since cytokine receptors are present at these low concentrations, the assays to monitor cytokine receptor expression must be equal to the sensitivity required to detect them.

Cytokine receptors have been classified in a number of different ways. Reported here are two classification schemes (2–4). The first classification scheme is historical, and divides the cytokine receptors into three families.

Cytokine Receptor Superfamily

The members of this, the largest receptor family, have in common a 200 amino acid extracellular domain that encodes the ligand-binding domain, with four conserved cysteine residues in the amino terminus (2). Members of this family can be composed of many subunits, and a few can function as monomers (5). Some of the members of this family even share a receptor subunit. Receptors that contain a common beta subunit, which binds the target, combine with a specific alpha subunit to allow signal transduction. The same beta subunit is often shared by different cytokine-receptor complexes: The interleukin-3 receptor (IL-3R) shares its beta subunit with IL-5R and granulocyte-macrophage colony-stimulating factor receptor (GM-CSFR) (6). The IL-2Rγ subunit is shared with the IL-4R, IL-7R, and IL-9R (7).

Immunoglobulin Family

Immunoglobulin family receptors are characterized by extracellular immunoglobulin-like domains, a short transmembrane domain, and cytoplasmic domains of variable lengths. Like the receptors in the cytokine receptor superfamily, these receptors have no intrinsic catalytic activity. Members of this family include IL-1 receptors, interferon (IFN) receptors, granulocyte colony-stimulating factor (G-CSF) receptors, and tumor necrosis factor (TNF) receptors.

Members of the cytokine superfamily and the immunoglobulin receptor family do not have intrinsic tyrosine kinase activity, which means that for signal transduction to occur, they must interact with another protein. For the members of these classes, the binding of the cytokine or ligand to its receptor triggers an association with a novel class of cytoplasmic tyrosine kinase proteins, termed *Janus kinases* (JAK). The JAK allow coupling of the receptor to proteins in the signal transduction pathway. Once this coupling occurs, the cell surface receptors are activated to invoke rapid tyrosine phosphorylation of intracellular proteins, including other receptors. Several articles have recently been published that discuss this new area in detail (8–11).

Tyrosine Kinase Receptor Family

Like the immunoglobulin family, the members of the tyrosine kinase receptor family are characterized by a large, glycosylated, extracellular, ligand-binding domain, and a single transmembrane domain. This family, however, also has an intrinsic intracellular tyrosine kinase catalytic domain. This added activity aids in intracellular signal transduction mechanisms. The family is divided into three subclasses: 1) receptors that are monomers, possessing two extracellular, cysteine-rich repeat sequences, such as the epidermal growth factor receptor (EGFR); 2) receptors that have disulfide-linked structures with cysteine-rich sequences, as exemplified by the receptor for insulin growth factor (IGF-1); and 3) receptors with three to five extracellular immunoglobulin-like domains, such as the receptor for platelet-derived growth factor (PDGF) and colony-stimulating factor (CSF-1) (12).

A second classification scheme, which is similar to that used for the cytokines themselves, is described below. This scheme encompasses the earlier scheme, but further subdivides the receptors into more distinct families.

Hematopoietic Cytokine Receptor Family

The hematopoietic cytokine receptor family has characteristics that are similar to those of the cytokine receptor superfamily. This vast family is involved in the inflammatory response, T-cell growth, chemotaxis, and immunosuppression. This family includes IL-2Rβ and γ subunits, IL-5Rα, gp130, IL-3R, IL-4R, IL-7R, IL-9R, G-CSFR, and GM-CSFRβ subunit. A major feature of this group, which is also found in the cytokine receptor superfamily, is the high level of shared subunits between its members.

Interferon Receptor (IFN-R) Family

Interferon receptors have a single transmembrane glycoprotein, with one or two homologous 200 amino acid extracellular regions. As was previously discussed, the interferons have an extracellular domain that is structurally like immunoglobulin G (IgG) in nature. Signal transduction occurs through interaction with JAK or tyrosine kinase (TYK) protein kinases. The interferons and their receptors have a major role in the modulation response to viral infection. There is evidence to suggest that the interferons have a role in the clearance of poxviruses from infected animals (13). This family includes the interferon receptors, IFN-α-/β-R and IFN-γ-R. The IFN-α-/β- receptor is a common receptor shared by both IFN-α and β. Interferon-gamma binds to a separate receptor (14).

Tumor Necrosis Factor and Nerve Growth Factor Family

The tumor necrosis factor (TNF) and nerve growth factor (NGF) family is characterized by the presence of three to four cysteine-rich repeat sequences that extend about 40 amino acids in their extracellular portion. Members of this family include tumor necrosis and nerve growth factor receptors such as TNF-R1 and -R2, and NGF-R. One of the major functions of the TNF is to mediate activation and differentiation of monocytes and macrophages, which is accomplished through their receptor interactions (15,16). Soluble receptors in this family are produced for the most part as a result of proteolysis from the cell surface.

Transforming Growth Factor-Beta (TGF-β) Receptor Family

The TGF-β receptors are found on almost all cell types. Through interactions with their receptors, TGF-β is a potent inhibitor of cell proliferation, and is involved in inflammatory response, embryogenesis, and carcinogenesis (17). Three distinct types of cell surface TGF-β receptors have been identified, all of which bind the cytokine with high affinity. Receptors

I and III are believed to capture TGF-β and present it to receptor II, which has a transmembrane serine/threonine kinase activity, and therefore imparts the ability to transduce signals to the cytokine-receptor complex (18). A number of soluble TGF-β receptors have also been identified.

Chemokine Receptor Family

The chemokine receptor family is characterized by having a short, acidic extracellular sequence, followed by seven transmembrane domains, with three extracellular and three intercellular loops. Within this family are the alpha- and beta-chemokine receptors. The two IL-8 receptors are representative of the leukocyte alpha-chemokine receptors and are important in neutrophil migration and activation. Leukocyte beta-chemokine receptors are characterized by the receptors for MIP-1α and -1β (monocyte-chemoattractant proteins) and RANTES (regulated on activation, normal T expressed and secreted), and appear to be primarily associated with monocyte activity. These receptors transduce signal by first coupling with GTP-binding proteins, which then allows coupling to signal transduction pathways (19).

Growth Factor Receptor Family

The growth factor receptor family is composed of the epidermal growth factor (EGF) receptors and transforming growth factor–alpha (TGF-α) receptors. Epidermal growth factor receptors are expressed on most known cell types and play a role in stimulating angiogenesis. EGF and TGF-α appear to have similar roles, and may act in concert under a variety of conditions. Soluble receptors are produced by proteolytic cleavage and also by alternative splicing, in which a receptor gene lacks a transmembrane domain. Several growth factor receptors, and cell surface adhesion molecules, including the selectins, contain multiple region homology to EGF, with their extracellular, multidomain structure (20,21).

Adhesion Molecule Receptor Family

The adhesion molecule receptors are employed in the homing and inflammation response of leukocytes. The selectins bind to receptors that contain sialylated and highly glycosylated structural domains, exemplified by the sLe^x and sialylated sLe^a carbohydrate structures (22). The P-selectin glycoprotein ligand I (PSGLI) appears to act as a ligand or receptor for both P- and E-selectin (23). The receptors for ICAM-1(LFA-1), VCAM-1 (CD49d/CD29), the integrins, and the cadherin receptors are also part of this classification scheme. The fundamental molecular mechanisms of the inflammatory response may be a cascade of events brought about by the successive action of the adhesion receptors. Although the adhesion receptors used by neutrophils appear to have been identified, studies with monocytes and T cells indicate that more study is necessary in the structure and function of adhesion receptors in leukocyte trafficking (23).

As evidenced by the diversity of these classification schemes, many of the functions and structures overlap. In a manner consistent with the cytokines, the receptors demonstrate a high degree of redundancy and often act synergistically, which makes it difficult to classify the cytokine receptors in a simple and unambiguous manner.

Soluble Receptors

Cytokine receptors are found in both a cell membrane–associated and soluble form. The roles of both of these forms of the cytokine receptors are important to the regulation of the immune response. Soluble receptors are found to increase in response to various disease states, pointing to their role in disease modulation or regulation. Soluble receptors are generally found in low concentrations in the serum, synovial fluid, and urine (24–28). Soluble interleukin-2 receptor (sIL-2R) is found to increase in disease conditions such as adult T-cell leukemia (ATL), in which extremely elevated levels of sIL-2R have been observed, and the monitoring of which is used to follow the progression of the disease. The expression of soluble receptors appears to be tightly regulated. Soluble receptors can confer on cells and tissues the ability to respond to ligands for which they do not normally express cytokine receptor. Soluble receptors can act as transport proteins to carry cytokines to sites where they are required for biologic activity (29). A good review of soluble cytokine receptors is given by Heaney and Golde (30).

As was mentioned briefly above, soluble receptors are formed by one of two processes:

proteolytic cleavage from the cell surface, or as an alternatively spliced gene product. The exact enzymatic mechanism by which membrane-bound receptors are cleaved is unclear. The process appears to be highly regulated and it is speculated that it occurs through phosphatase or kinase activity, or both (31). This phenomenon is exemplified by the tyrosine phosphorylation that appears to be involved in the activation of the IL-6 receptor of B cells (32). Soluble receptors produced by an alternatively spliced messenger ribonucleic acid (mRNA) transcript lack a transmembrane domain. For that domain, however, the soluble receptor is translated from a dedicated transcript encoding a specific form of receptor, such as the IL-4 receptor (33).

The downmodulation of cytokines and cytokine receptors can be controlled by the shedding of the cell membrane–bound receptor. This solublized receptor then acts as an inhibitor for the membrane-bound version binding the cytokine. In these instances, the extracellular portion of the membrane-bound receptor is shed. The TNF receptors are an excellent example of this phenomenon. Soluble TNF receptors were found to inhibit TNF activity and to limit the severity of TNF-α–induced inflammatory responses in patients with a variety of malignancies and autoimmune diseases (25,34).

Available Assay Procedures for the Measurement of Cytokine Receptors

Defining clinical utility for cytokine receptors has proved difficult due to their complexity, soluble and cell membrane–associated forms, and their ability to modulate the activity of multiple cytokines. Anticytokine receptor strategies in therapeutic design point to a strong involvement of cytokines and their receptors in the pathogenesis of diseases. Their involvement necessitates the creation of detection assays to monitor their levels during normal and disease states. In fact, it is necessary to carefully monitor selected immunologic parameters, including the fluctuations in the levels of multiple cytokines, and both soluble and cell membrane–associated receptors in response to therapeutic intervention. Bioassays, immunocytochemistry, flow cytometry, and immunoassays are some of the currently available methods for measuring receptor levels.

Bioassays

The influence of cytokine receptors on biologic systems is best defined by following the result of addition of cytokine or soluble cytokine receptor to cell culture systems. With the bioassay, the biologic system's response can be followed over time. Drawbacks to the bioassay include the fact that it can be difficult and labor intensive to perform. The bioassay often provides the first identification of the marker and its biologic function and importance. However, this information is obtained in a controlled cell culture environment and cannot be directly correlated with actual disease conditions. Bioassays may require overnight incubations, and provide poor reliability (35,36). Additionally, maintenance of cell lines can lead to decreased sensitivity after several passages of the cells (35). The above limitations of bioassays have led to the implementation of several immunoassay systems.

Immunocytochemistry

Since cytokines act primarily as local mediators, immunocytochemistry can be used to localize cytokines and receptors within a tissue-specific area by combining histologic techniques with the use of available antibodies. Immunocytochemistry can also be used to detect cytokine and receptor genes and mRNA, using nucleic acid probes. This technique is in situ hybridization. Immunocytochemstry therefore can be used to examine the in vivo production of cytokines and their receptors, since it can be used at the site where the physiologic effect occurs. The actual site of inflammation, tumorogenesis, organ injury, and repair might be more biologically relevant to the detection of cytokine-receptor complexes than is peripheral blood (37). These studies, which can be conducted using immunocytochemistry, have merit for the early evaluation of the immunomodulation event, including the specific site where the event occurs.

Flow Cytometry

The most accurate means of measuring cytokine-specific receptors is through the binding of the labeled cytokine. Initial binding studies used radiolabeled cytokines for the detection of the bound receptor. Later, fluorescence labeling replaced radiolabeling for tagging cytokines. With this technology, fluorescence-labeled cytokines, combined with flow cytometry, could be used to follow the binding to cell membrane–bound receptors. Zola (38) reported that through these binding studies the receptor densities ranged from 10 to 1000 molecules per cell on unstimulated cells, and to 100 to 10,000 molecules per cell on stimulated cells. That cells can respond to such low concentrations of receptors emphasizes the importance of cytokines and their receptors in immunomodulation events.

Until recently, flow cytometry offered the only reliable means of measuring cell surface–bound molecules. The other available methods resulted in the destruction of the integrity of the analyte, and thus the loss of reliable signal detection. Cell membrane–associated cytokines and receptors have traditionally been analyzed by flow cytometry. Flow cytometry uses intact cells as the sample to be analyzed. The method detects labeled cytokine or antibody bound at the surface of the cell membrane to its specific receptor (39). The label on the bound cytokine or antibody is then detected by a laser omission within the flow cytometer. The quantitation of CD4+ T-cell levels in human immunodeficiency virus (HIV)-positive individuals is probably the best-known utility of flow cytometry for evaluating cell surface markers. In this example, fluorescent-labeled anti-CD4 antibodies are used to detect CD4 molecules that are present on the surface of T lymphocytes (40).

Although flow cytometry represents an excellent means of examining cell membrane–associated receptors, it requires expensive instrumentation and highly trained personnel. Further, flow cytometry can only be used to examine cell membrane–associated receptors, and not soluble receptor levels.

Immunoassays

With the advent of excellent immunologic tools, immunoassays have allowed the development of rapid, accurate, and simple means of quantitating the levels of analytes in a wide variety of different biologic fluids. The enzyme-linked immunosorbent assay (ELISA) has traditionally been useful for measuring analytes in serum, plasma, synovial fluid, or urine. However, new methods have made it possible to quantitate analytes in tissue, lymph biopsies, and whole blood. Complete solublization of tissue or cellular material must be accomplished to assure accuracy and reproducibility of the analyte detected in these types of samples. This makes direct analysis of the receptor during various disease events possible and demonstrates that the immunoassay is the most versatile method for measuring cytokine receptor levels.

The immunoassay represents a cost-effective, user-friendly alternative to bioassays and flow cytometry. The assays are usually simple to perform and results can often be obtained in a matter of hours instead of the days required for some bioassays. Methods can be used to separate soluble and cell membrane–associated fractions to allow quantitation of both in a single assay. A wide variety of immunoassay formats are available and will be discussed here. [For an extensive discussion of the various microtiter plate formats, see Foster (41).] Assays continue to be developed to detect the cytokine receptor in the soluble fraction. These studies are complicated by the fact that highly specific antibodies are required that cannot bind to epitopes that are in close proximity to the site of binding between the cytokine and the receptor. Still other assays are being developed that detect the cytokine-receptor complex. Each of these assays can provide valuable information regarding the detectable levels of components. In measuring the levels of all these complexes, the presence of the soluble receptor must be kept in mind, as well as the specific analyte that the assay was designed to detect. For example, if an assay has been designed to detect free IL-8, the presence of the soluble IL-8 receptor in the sample and the effect it will have on the overall sample recovery must be considered. Moreover, that same assay will not detect the cell-associated IL-8, for example, in red blood cells, if it was designed to detect only the soluble form.

Immunoassay Development

Several points should be considered when developing an assay. Prior consideration of these facts can resolve potential questions regarding the integrity and utility of the assay.

- Do the antibodies detect only the free receptor?
- Are the antibodies used in the assay directed against epitopes on the receptor that may be

blocked by the binding of the cytokine, thus leading to falsely lowered results?

- Is the free receptor or a complex being measured?
- Which is the biologically significant form? Free or complexed?
- How can the functions of cell membrane–associated and soluble receptors be separated?

Sandwich ELISA

The most common ELISA format makes use of two antibodies, with one antibody immobilized on a solid support, commonly a 96-well microtiter plate. The solid supports also include polystyrene beads and magnetic particles, and other forms commonly used in the automation of assays (41,42). The antibody on the solid support captures the analyte of interest and is usually selected due to its high affinity for the analyte. The second antibody is specific for a different epitope on the analyte and forms the sandwich. This second antibody, referred to as the detector antibody, can be directly labeled with an enzyme, such as horseradish peroxidase (HRP) or alkaline phosphatase. Other detection methods include labeling the second antibody with a small molecule such as FITC (fluorescence thiocyanate), and then detecting the complex with a third anti-FITC antibody, which is labeled with an enzyme such as HRP. The latter example can sometimes be preferable depending on the requirements of the assay system (41). A third anti-FITC antibody, labeled with HRP, is a universal assay reagent since it can be used in many assays, where the specific antibodies are directed against various analytes. The small size of the FITC (MW 389) prevents the steric hindrance problems that are sometimes observed when the detector antibodies are labeled with large molecules such as HRP (MW 40,000). The reaction is detected by reacting with an HRP-specific colorimetric substrate solution, such as 3,3′5,5′-tetra-methyl benzidine (TMB), followed by stopping the reaction with a solution of sulfuric acid. The absorbance is then read at the appropriate wavelength on a plate reader (41,42).

Assay sensitivity is achieved by variations in sample volume, incubation time, and temperature, and experimenting with different buffers and pH. The major limiting factor to sensitivity is the affinity of the capture antibody for the analyte of interest. As part of the assay validation, the lower limit of detection is determined. A common method employed to determine the minimum detectable concentration (MDC), or sensitivity, is to assay multiple replicates of the zero standard. The mean optical density of these replicates, plus two standard deviations, is determined to be the MDC for a sample in the assay, as compared to the standard curve. The biologic MDC is determined by assaying low or artificially depleted samples down to a level that can be consistently discriminated from the zero standard (43,44).

If high sensitivity is not necessary, multiple assays can be designed in which the universal capture antibody is a polyclonal antibody, and detection is accomplished using various monoclonal antibodies, which bind to different, specific epitopes. These assays may also be useful in evaluating the interactions of a single receptor with multiple cytokine targets.

Detection of Cytokine-Receptor Complexes

Complexes of soluble receptors and cytokines can be measured by using a primary antibody directed against the receptor, and a second antibody directed against the exposed epitope of the cytokine. This combination forms a double-antibody sandwich that relies on the presence of both the cytokine and the receptor for detection. This type of assay can be useful for following the expression of complexes in serum.

Competitive Assays

Cytokine assays that are designed in a competitive format are gaining appeal for their ability to detect cytokine receptor levels in the presence of soluble cytokine-receptor complexes. These assays utilize high-affinity polyclonal antibodies that recognize epitopes that are not blocked by interfering proteins. It is now believed that cytokines are present, in the form of cytokine-receptor complexes, at much higher concentrations than were previously thought. Soluble receptors for TNF-α are inducible during inflammation and circulate at levels sufficient to block the in vitro cytotoxicity associated with the TNF-α levels observed in nonlethal infection (45). Many assays that use a standard antibody sandwich format are unable to detect all of the cytokines present because of their inability to detect analyte once it is complexed with its receptor.

Competitive assay formats are designed for the quantitation of total cytokine levels, while the antibody sandwich assays are designed to quantitate the free cytokine levels. Total cytokine levels give a better view of the entire microenvironment. The majority of studies to date have concentrated on the levels of free cytokine, and not on the levels of circulating soluble cytokine receptors, which play a role in immune regulation. These levels can lead to the incorrect assessment of the true level of the cytokine that is present in a sample (46,47).

Sampling and Sample Handling

Immunoassay technologies have made possible the detection of cytokines in a wide variety of different biologic fluids. The immunoassay has been successfully used with urine, synovial fluid, and serum. All samples should be considered potentially hazardous and handled following the Centers for Disease Control guidelines for the handling and disposal of blood samples (48). Serum and plasma represent the biologic fluid most commonly tested. As part of the assay validation, the recovery of the analyte in the various collection methods (e.g., EDTA, citrate, and heparin-treated serum, plasma, or whole blood) must be evaluated, to determine the presence of any variations in recoveries.

Since cytokines and receptors are now used clinically, concern has grown over their accurate measurement in serum and other fluids. The stability of these analytes has been discussed elsewhere (49,50). Generally, samples can be stored for a short time at 4°C, but long-term storage must be at −80°C. The processing (rapid separation and storage in the cold) of samples must occur directly after collection to prevent enzymatic degradation and inactivation of the cytokine proteins. Clotting factors in plasma may act to cause activation of some cytokines/receptors, thus making serum the preferred collection sample. When collecting serum, care should be taken to remove the clotted blood cell components from the serum immediately, and then to put them in cold storage, to prevent any adverse effects. Whatever the sample type, a study must be done to ensure the stability of the sample during collection and storage. This usually involves a time course study to determine the time that the sample can remain at room temperature after collection and before assay analysis. Samples are routinely aliquotted and stored at −80°C, in order to avoid the problems of activation, degradation, and freeze-thaw effects. Storage at −80°C must be evaluated to verify that no adverse effects occur because of extended time in storage or freeze-thaw.

A relatively new application of an old method makes possible the solubilization of the cell membrane with retention of the integrity of the cell-bound analyte. This method has been commercialized by T Cell Sciences, Inc, in its TRAx technology for use with whole blood (51). The method consists of a simple pretreatment of whole blood, which can be immediately analyzed by ELISA, or the samples can be frozen and analyzed at a later date without deleterious effects. Whole blood can also be fractionated into the soluble portion and a washed cell pellet. Once fractionated, each can be evaluated in the same ELISA assay, and the contribution of soluble and cell-bound receptors can be known.

Assay Development and Preanalytical Evaluation

Part of assay development is the extensive validation of the robustness, reliability, sensitivity, and specificity of the assay for detection of the analyte of interest. This performance validation includes rigorous testing of the specificity of the reagents used in the kits to ensure that they perform within the expected tolerances of the assay system. An immunoassay should contain a standard curve made up of approximately six standards and three controls prepared from well-characterized material. Three control levels must be included to represent the dynamic range of the standard curve. The assay is validated over a series of days by multiple operators under conditions within the range of tolerance. The standard curve and the three controls are run by each operator. The reproducibility of the control values and the signals within each assay and between operators are determined. The precision of the standards and controls in a single assay (intra-assay precision) and among many assays and many operators (interassay precision) must also be shown to be acceptable, generally less than 10%.

Component and whole kit stability must be determined as part of the assay validation. The component shelf life is assigned through accelerated studies in which the components are stored at 25 to 27°C and compared to those stored at 4°C. The kit shelf life is determined through real-time and temperature studies. For a shelf life dating of one year, the kit must show no variance in performance for 13 months. The shelf life of the kit is always defined by the least stable component.

An extensive panel of studies including tests for cross reactivity with markers of similar structure is also performed. Common blood components are tested at elevated levels to determine their level of interference in the assay. These studies are done to help predict how an elevated blood component may affect the value obtained for a specific analyte. Generally, the following substances are the minimal blood components tested: serum human albumin, triglycerides, bilirubin, and hemoglobin. A drug panel can be evaluated, depending on the target patient population and the clinical application of the assay. Structurally similar compounds, such as other receptors from the same family, are tested with antibodies employed in the assay system. The specific cytokine to which the receptor will complex is tested to determine the level of interference it will present in the assay. These studies are of particular importance in the evaluation of disease states in which multiple immunomodulation markers may be elevated.

ELISA formats are susceptible to a high-dose hook or prozone effect. Increasing levels of analyte are added to the sample to determine the concentration at which the dose response will begin to decrease. The concentration at which an elevated level gives a signal equivalent to that of the highest standard is the point at which a prozone effect is observed. This effect has relevance in disease conditions in which the analyte of interest can be greatly elevated.

Antibody purity, cross reactivity, and the presence of rheumatoid factors or C1q complement factor are contributing factors to assay specificity (42). Dilution linearity and spike and recovery studies are performed to evalute assay specificity and also the assay kinetics. Accurate results from diluted samples are derived and evaluated by the dilution of naturally elevated samples, or titering of analyte into the sample. The samples are diluted over the range of the standard curve to demonstrate the ability to assign values to samples with levels that are above the highest standard. Spiked samples are prepared by adding analyte to all appropriate sample types. This study is performed to ensure that the analyte can be accurately recovered in sample matrices. Inability to recover the total amount of analyte may indicate the presence of interfering substances, or problems due to matrix differences between the sample and the assay standards.

Once the assay performance has been validated, a patient reference interval must be determined for the analyte in the assay. This is done by measuring the analyte level in approximately 100 to 200 healthy blood donors, exhibiting normal chemistry, to establish an expected range for normal samples. Expected levels of the analyte in the patient population of interest are determined as part of a preclinical evaluation to compare against the normal healthy population. Comparison to an established, accepted methodology is required when available.

Pitfalls and Troubleshooting

Some problems may be encountered in assay development, despite their simplicity and convenience. These problems include nonspecific binding, temperature effects, cross reactivity, and interfering substances (52). Manufacturers of commercial assay kits attempt to anticipate these problems during the development process. Antibodies are thoroughly validated; the addition of proteins, detergents, and other additives is evaluated for the ability to reduce the above problems. Addition of nonspecific IgG and the use of antibody fragments [$F(ab')_2$] have been employed with a high level of success to overcome many of these issues. The use of mouse IgG in diluents can help to reduce another common interfering substance, anti-idiotype antibodies. These antibodies are found among patients receiving antibody-based therapies, such as OKT3 for organ transplant patients (53).

Controls and Standardization of Assays

Whether an assay is designed to be fully or semi-quantitative, all values derived from the assay are based on reference material. Reference or standard material is that which is established by an authority in the field, against which sample materials can be quantified (54). It is important to calibrate the assay to a recognized source of material, such as the World Health Organization (WHO) International Laboratory for Biological Standards, when this is available. Reference materials for the cytokines and their receptors also are available from NIBSC, Blanche Lane South, Mimms Potters Bar, Herts, UK, or, in the United States, from BRMP, National Cancer Institute, Frederick, MD 21701. Unfortunately, the cytokine field is still relatively new and many markers do not have international standard sources available. This has led to great confusion in the field as far as standardization between different testing methods is concerned.

Correlation to existing methodologies such as flow cytometry has proved useful in adding to standardization in this field. This assumes that the existing method is accurately measuring the marker of interest. This can be problematic when the new methodology provides greater sensitivity and accuracy. ELISA, due to its simplicity and convenience, is replacing more labor-intensive and technique-oriented technologies, such as bioassays and flow cytometry. Many times a new unit of measurement must be created or better defined for a correlation to a traditional method.

Internal Quality Assurance

Commercially produced products that are used in the clinical environment are manufactured under defined conditions and must adhere to current good manufacturing practices (GMP). These products conform to strict requirements in terms of the way they are produced and how they perform. A quality assurance program is designed to monitor the manufacturing of products in a manner that will prevent mix-ups, provide a history record, and ensure consistent performance.

Once a kit has completed the development phase and entered the manufacturing level, quality control guidelines and specifications are implemented to allow for consistency and reliability of product performance. The standard material in the kit, used for the standard curve, is the component that confers a quantitative nature on an immunoassay (55). Assay controls, preferably in a matrix equivalent to patient samples, are routinely run calibrated against a reference standard, to monitor assay performance trends and ensure consistency. This control may be a cell line supernatant, peripheral blood mononucleocytes (PBMC), or another material of known analyte expression level.

Clinical Rationale and Relevance

When is the test useful? Research data continue to suggest the importance of cytokines and their receptors in disease modulation, and point to the importance of these markers in therapeutic and diagnostic disease management. Assays to measure individual cytokine-receptor expression, and the interaction between these markers relative to disease state, have made it possible to begin characterizing other factors that contribute to disease and immune regulation in a wide variety of disease conditions. More information will lead to better and more specific assays with regard to the importance of cytokine-receptor networks in disease staging and management. No single cytokine has been demonstrated to successfully diagnose a clinical condition. Panels of cytokines, and other markers such as blood/gas chemistry markers, combined may give a better indication of patient status (56,57).

Postanalytical Concern

After successful manufacture and commercialization of a product, continued validation is required to ensure consistency of performance over time. The College of American Pathologists (CAP) assists clinical laboratories in maintaining quality by providing programs for quality control assurance, including postanalytical factors. Clinical laboratories are subject to regulation under the Clinical Laboratory Improvement Amendments (CLIA) of 1988. Under subpart K, section 493.1213(b)(1) guidelines, CLIA requirements for quality control are that a laboratory must demonstrate that, before reporting patient test results, it can obtain the performance specification for accuracy, precision, and reportable range of patient test results comparable to those established by the manufacturer. The laboratory must also verify that the manufacturer's reference range is appropriate for the laboratory's patient population. This is done through the accumulation of patient sample ranges established from initial research and development data, confirmed by quality control data and continuously updated and verified by data gathered on a routine basis by the quality control and quality assurance divisions. The assay is viewed as acceptable as long as these patient sample controls remain within the established ranges. The key question to ask is, "Does the product meet the performance claims stated in the package insert?" Generally, throughout this period, external clinical evaluation of the kit is ongoing. Results from these external sites are analyzed separately and added to the internal pool of results for subsequent analysis.

External Quality Assurance: Proficiency Surveys

External clinical trials validate the performance of the assay in the test population for which the test was developed. These studies stress the robustness, specificity, and sensitivity of the assay. External proficiency studies generally include running the kit standard curve, kit controls, and a series of unknown patient samples. These studies are performed at multiple clinical sites, usually a minimum of three, and are run by multiple operators over multiple days.

Following the proficiency studies, the assay is validated with a clinical evaluation among the relevant patient population. These external studies ensure that the kit meets the levels of performance demonstrated by the manufacturer. Requirements by the Food and Drug Administration (FDA) for in vitro diagnostics kit performance can be slightly varied from one analyte to another, but several conditions are generally necessary for FDA clearance.

1. Demonstration that the kit meets the established performance parameters defined by the manufacturer
2. Demonstration of acceptable assay precision and control recovery at each clinical site and between the clinical sites
3. Methods comparison with an alternative, FDA-cleared (if possible) method, at multiple clinical sites with greater than 100 data points from each site
4. In the absence of an existing FDA-cleared method, an extensive clinical study would fall under the premarket approval (PMA) process, requiring multiple clinical sites and up to several thousand total data points to validate the method.

Comments and Recommendations

Continued improvements of the competitive and ELISA assays for cytokine receptors with new and better immunologic tools are essential. Deoxyribonucleic acid (DNA) probes to the cytokine-receptor family provide new tools with which to assay. Nucleic acid–based assay techniques offer the advantage of added sensitivity and selectivity. Because of the flexibility of the immunoassay microtiter plate formats, a nucleic acid probe–based format, coupled to ELISA and polymerase chain reaction (PCR) methods, can be readily created.

REFERENCES

1. Arai K, Lee F, Miyajima A, et al. Cytokines: coordinates of immune and inflammatory responses. Ann Rev Biochem 1990;59:783–836.
2. Callard R, Gearing A. Cytokine receptor superfamilies. In: The cytokine facts book. London: Academic Press, 1994:18–26.
3. Pugh-Humphreys RGP, Thomson AW. Cytokines and their receptors as potential therapeutic targets. In: Thomson AW, ed. The cytokine handbook. London: Academic Press, 1994:530–534.
4. Aggarwal BB, Puri RK. Common and uncommon features of cytokines and cytokine receptors: an overview. In: Aggarwal BB, Puri RK, eds. Human cytokines: their role in disease and therapy. Cambridge, MA: Blackwell Science, 1995:3–24.
5. Patthy L. Homology of a domain of the growth hormone/prolactin receptor family with type III modules of fibronectin. Cell 1990;61:13–14.
6. Miyajima A, Kitamura T, Horada N, et al. Cytokine receptors and signal transduction. Ann Rev Immunol 1992;10:295–331.
7. Giri JG, Ahdieh M, Eiseniman J, et al. Utilization of the β and γ chains of the IL-2 receptor by the novel cytokine IL-15. EMBO J 1994;13:2822–2830.
8. Amzel LM, Poljak RJ. Three-dimensional structure of immunoglobulins. Ann Rev Biochem 1979;48:961–967.
9. Ihle JN. Cytokine receptor signaling. Nature (England) 1995;377:591–594.
10. Ihle JN, Witthuhn BA, Quelle FW, et al. Protein tyrosine phosphorylation in the regulation of hematopoiesis by receptors of the cytokine-receptor superfamily. Blood Cells 1994;20:65–82.
11. Taniguchi T. Cytokine signaling through nonreceptor-protein tyrosine kinase. Science 1995;268:251–255.

12. Ullrich A, Schlessinger J. Review: signal transduction by receptors with tyrosine kinase activity. Cell 1990;61:203–212.

13. Ramsay AJ, Ruby J, Ramshaw IA. A case for cytokines as effector molecules in the resolution of virus infection. Immunol Today 1993;14:155–157.

14. Lange JA, Pestika S. Interferon receptors. Immunol Today 1988;9:393–400.

15. Smith CA, Farrah T, Goodwin RG. Mini review: the TNF receptor superfamily of cellular and viral proteins: activation, costimulation and death. Cell 1994;76:959–962.

16. Remaniol A-C, Boussir F, Herbelin A, et al. Induction of soluble tumor necrosis factor receptor (sTNF-R75) release by HIV absorption on cultured human monocytes. Eur J Immunol 1994;24:2055–2060.

17. Sporn MB, Roberts AB. Transforming growth factor β: multiple actions and potential clinical applications. JAMA 1989;262:938–941.

18. Lin HY, Lodish HF. Receptors for the TGF-β superfamily: multiple polypeptides and serine/threonine kinases. Trends Cell Biol 1993;3:14–19.

19. Ahuja SK, Gao J-L, Murphy PM. Chemokine receptors and molecular mimicry. Immunol Today 1994;15:281–287.

20. Murphy PM. The molecular biology of leukocytes chemoattractant receptors. Ann Rev Immunol 1994;12:593–633.

21. Derynck R. Transforming growth factor α. Cell 1988;54:593–595.

22. Magnani J. AS_3 adhesion structures subpanel 3, selectin ligands/carbohydrates $CD15_s$ and $_sLe^a$. In: Schlossman SF, ed. Leukocyte typing: white cell differentiation antigens. London: Oxford University Press, 1995:1524–1528.

23. Hogg N, Berlin C. Structure and function of adhesion receptors in leukocyte trafficking. Immunol Today 1995;15:327–330.

24. Baumheter S, Singer MS, Henzel W, et al. Binding of L-selectin to the vascular sialomucin CD34. Science 1993;262:436–438.

25. Fernandez-Botran R. Soluble cytokine receptors: their role in immunoregulation. FASEB J 1991;5:2567–2574.

26. Fernandez-Botran R, Vitetta ES. A soluble, high-affinity, interleukin-4 binding protein is present in the biological fluids of mice. PNAS 1990;87:4202–4206.

27. Gunther N, Betzel C, Weber W. The secreted form of the epidermal growth factor receptor. J Biol Chem 1990;265:22082–22085.

28. Symons JA, Eastgate JA, Duff GW. Purification and characterization of a novel soluble receptor for interleukin-1. J Exp Med 1991;174:1251–1254.

29. Barlow PN, Baron M, Norman DG, et al. Secondary structure of a complement control protein molecule by two-dimensional ^{1}H NMR. Biochemistry 1991;30:997–1004.

30. Heaney ML, Golde DW. Soluble cytokine receptors. Blood 1996;87:847–857.

31. Mui A-F, Kay RJ, Humphries RK, Krystal G. Ligand-induced phosphorylation of the murine interleukin-3 receptor signals its cleavage. PNAS 1992;89:10812–10816.

32. Nakajima K, Wall R. Interleukin-6 signals activating junB and TISII gene transcription in a B-cell hybridoma. Mol Cell Biol 1991;11:1409–1418.

33. Sempowski GD, Bechmann MP, Derdak S, Phipps RP. Subsets of murine lung fibroblasts express membrane-bound and soluble IL-4 receptors: role of IL-4 in enhancing fibroblast proliferation and collagen synthesis. J Immunol 1994;152:3606–3614.

34. Kalinkovich A, Engelmann H, Harpaz N, et al. Elevated serum levels of soluble tumor necrosis factor receptors (sTNF-R) in patients with HIV infection. Clin Exp Immunol 1992;89:351–355.

35. Eskandari MK, Nguyen D, Kunkelm S, Remick D. WEHI 164 subclone 13 assay for TNF: sensitivity, specificity and reliability. Immunol Invest 1992;19:69–79.

36. Abe Y, Miyake M, Miyazaki T, et al. Nonspecific reaction in the sandwich immunoassay for human tumor necrosis factor α (hTNF-α). Clin Chim Acta 1989;181:223–230.

37. Vitolo D, Zerbe T, Kanbour A, et al. Expression of mRNA for cytokines in tumor-infiltrating mononuclear cells in ovarian adenocarcinoma and invasive breast cancer. Int J Cancer 1992;51:573–580.

38. Zola H. Detection of receptors for cytokines and growth factors. The Immunologist 1994;2:47–57.

39. Alderson MR, Armitage RJ, Maraskovsky E, et al. Fas transduces activation signals in normal human T lymphocytes. J Exp Med 1993;178:2231–2235.

40. Koepke JA, Landay A, et al. Precision and accuracy of absolute lymphocyte counts. Clin Immunol Immunopathol 1989;52:19–27.

41. Foster KA. Microtiter plate–based enzyme immunoassay in the universal format system. In: Chan D, ed. Immunoassay automation: an updated guide to systems. New York: Academic Press, 1996:277–309.

42. Elkins R. In: Maggio ET, ed. Enzyme-immunoassay. Boca Raton, FL: CRC Press, 1988: 20–52.

43. Elkins R. Misunderstanding about assay sensitivity and precision. Ligand 1981;4:60–65. Letter.

44. Millett B, Sullivan AM, Morimoto M, Parsons GA. Third generation immunoassay for tumor necrosis factor-alpha. Biotechniques 1994;17:1166–1171.

45. Van Zee KJ, Kohno T, Fischer E, et al. Tumor necrosis factor soluble receptors circulate during experimental and clinical inflammation and can protect against excessive tumor necrosis factor alpha in vitro and in vivo. PNAS USA 1992;89: 4845–4849.

46. Dinarello CA. ELISA kits based on monoclonal antibodies do not measure total IL-1β synthesis. J Immunol Methods 1992;148:255–259.

47. May LT, Viuet H, Kenney JS, et al. High levels of complexed interleukin-6 in human blood. J Bio Chem 1992;267:19698–19704.

48. Birenbaum MS. A guide to OSHA requirements for clinical laboratories. St. Louis: American Association of Bioanalysts and the International Society for Clinical Technologists, 1990.

49. Thavasu PW, Loghurst S, Joel SP, et al. Measuring cytokine levels in blood: importance of anticoagulants, processing, and storage conditions. J Immunol Methods 1992;153:115–124.

50. Fletcher MA, Baron GC, Ashman MR, et al. Use of whole blood methods in assessment of immune parameters in immunodeficiency states. Diag Clin Immunol 1987;5:69–81.

51. Nicholson JKA, Velleca WM, Jubert S, et al. Evaluation of alternative CD4 technologies for the enumeration of CD4 lymphocytes. J Immunol Methods 1994;177:43–54.

52. Kemeny DM, Antler S. An introduction to ELISA. In: Kemeny DM, Challacombe SJ, eds. ELISA and other solid phase immunoassays: theoretical and practical aspects. New York: Wiley, 1988:1–29.

53. Schroeder T, Frist MR, Mansour ME. Antimouse antibody formation following OKT3 therapy. Transplantation 1990;49:48–51.

54. Hamilton RG, Adkinson NF Jr. Quantitiative aspects of solid phase immunoassays. In: Kemeny DM, Challacombe SJ, eds. ELISA and other solid phase immunoassays: theoretical and practical aspects. Wiley, 1988:57–84.

55. Chevret S, Roquin H, Ganne P, Lefrere JJ. Prognostic value of an elevated CD8 lymphocyte count in HIV infection. Results of a prospective study of 152 asymptomatic HIV-positive individuals. AIDS 1992;6:1349–1352.

56. Fierro MT, Lisa F, Novelli M, et al. Soluble interleukin-2 receptor, CD4 and CD8 levels in melanoma: a longitudinal study. Clin Lab Invest 1992;184:182–189.

57. Sullivan AM, Carangelo E, Turner M, et al. Use of a panel of cytokines to evaluate patient outcome in heart transplant samples. Anal Assoc Clin Chem 1996:Abstract No. 634.

CHAPTER 

Flow Cytometry: DNA Ploidy and Cell Cycle Analysis

THOMAS S. ALEXANDER

Many cancers are associated with genetic alterations. These alterations can lead to chromosomal translocations, gene duplications, or gene deletions. The end result of these genetic anomalies is the uncontrolled cellular growth associated with cancer. This unregulated growth also implies that a larger percentage of neoplastic cells will be in the actively dividing phases of the cell cycle (S, G2, or M), as compared to normal cells from the same tissue. Indeed, "number of mitotic figures per high-power field" is a value that is routinely used by pathologists in evaluating and staging malignancies. Many individuals have postulated that the sum total of the genetic anomalies or the number of actively dividing cells in a tumor population, or both, may have prognostic implications. Thus, the clinical determination of "ploidy," that is, the amount of deoxyribonucleic acid (DNA) in a cell, and the percentage of tumor cells in the S and/or G2/M stages of the cell cycle may benefit the patient with cancer.

Flow cytometric DNA ploidy and cell cycle analysis were originally described by Van Dilla et al in 1969 (1). The proliferation of cytometers with air-cooled, 110-voltage lasers during the 1980s fueled a dramatic increase in publications concerning DNA analysis, and, according to one source, from 1983 to 1993, over 2500 studies were published on clinical applications of DNA analysis (2). In a Medline search I found over 400 additional articles published from 1994 through September 1996 concerning clinical flow cytometric DNA studies. In general, tumors with aneuploid cell populations or elevated S-phase fractions, or both, tend to be more aggressive than diploid tumors with low S-phase values. DNA analysis can be performed prospectively on fresh or frozen tissue, as well as retrospectively on tissue that has been formalin fixed and paraffin embedded. Results have not always been consistent, however, and the field has long suffered from a lack of standardized procedures and reagents. A DNA Cytometry Consensus Conference was held in 1992 to address these issues, and the reader is referred to the resulting articles in *Cytometry* that summarize the results of that conference (3–8) for a review of the clinical application of DNA and cell cycle analyses. This chapter concentrates on the laboratory, quality control, and quality assurance aspects of the procedure.

Specimen Selection

The most important aspect of performing DNA analysis is obtaining an appropriate specimen. DNA studies are normally performed on "tumors"; however, a tumor rarely consists of a homogenous cell population. From a quality assurance standpoint, the higher the percentage of neoplastic cells in a specimen, the more accurately the DNA results will reflect the true ploidy and cell cycle distribution of the disease process. Thus, a pathologist should grossly examine fresh tissue and microscopically examine paraffin-embedded tissue to determine the most appropriate areas for sampling. Shankey et al (3) recommend that the sample contain at least 20% tumor cells. For fresh tissue, one should analyze as large a piece of tissue as is practical. We request a piece of the tumor, approximately 0.5 to 1.0 cm^3, for DNA analysis. Due to earlier detection, however, many breast biopsies are much smaller, perhaps 2 to 5 mm^3 in their entirety. That specimen must be used for frozen sections, permanent histologic sections, and estrogen receptor/progesterone receptor (ER/PR) analysis in addition to DNA analysis. Thus, we often receive specimens that are much smaller than the ideal size. The College of American Pathologists' (CAP) *Reference Guide for Diagnostic Molecular Pathology/Flow Cytometry* (9) recommends 0.1 to 0.5 g tissue rather than a specific size. The DNA Consensus Conference suggests that monitoring the number of cells obtained per gram of tissue can be used as a quality control monitor for tissue processing (3). An alternate sampling method for a moderate-sized biopsy is to insert a needle into the tissue, and aspirate cells for analysis. Multiple specimens from a single tumor may improve the ability to detect an abnormal cell population; however, this is also not practical with small biopsies. A laboratory must further consider the cost-benefit ratio of performing multiple analyses, and whether or not multiple billings may be generated. Finally, a cytospin preparation made from the single cell suspension derived from fresh tissue (see below) will help to confirm the presence of malignant cells, although morphologic studies do not always conclusively identify neoplastic cells (3).

Although fresh, unfixed tissue yields a higher-quality analysis, it is often easier to document the presence of tumor in formalin-fixed tissue obtained from a paraffin block. Normally, three to four 50-μ-thick sections are used for DNA analysis on paraffin-embedded tissue. A pathologist should review thin hematoxylin and eosin stained sections taken immediately before and immediately after the flow cytometry sections are cut, to document that tumor is present in that portion of the block.

Finally, as part of the quality assurance for DNA analysis, the CAP flow cytometry inspection check list requires that laboratories specify which tumors are appropriate for DNA analysis in their procedure manual. We state in the Summa Health System procedure manual that we will accept breast, ovarian, lung, prostate, colon, lymphoid neoplasms, and "other tumors following consultation between the physician or surgeon and the Scientific or Medical Director of the Flow Cytometry Laboratory." This meets the CAP guideline, but also allows us to evaluate specific clinical conditions for which the clinician or pathologist examining the tissue thinks DNA analysis may be of some value.

Quality Control Cells

In addition to analyzing a tumor specimen, laboratories should perform DNA analysis on cells of known DNA content for quality control. Control cells serve two purposes in DNA analysis. First, they provide documentation that the staining procedure worked properly, and second, they assist the analyst in determining the channel number in which a diploid population of cells would reside. The cells that are most commonly used as controls in fresh-tissue DNA analysis include chicken red blood cells, trout red blood cells, normal human lymphocytes, and "normal" cells obtained from the same individual as the tumor specimen. The best diploid control, however, is normal, non-neoplastic cells contained within the patient specimen (3). When propidium iodide (PI) is used as a DNA stain, chicken red blood cells have a DNA content of 0.33 times and trout red blood cells have a DNA content of 0.8 times that of normal human fresh or frozen diploid cells (10). Selecting a control cell population for DNA analysis on tissue obtained from paraffin blocks is more problematic, however. The embedding and deparaffinization processes result in less PI being taken up by diploid cells. In our hands, paraffin-embedded tissue often displays a diploid peak at a channel similar to where fresh chicken red blood cells stained with PI tend to fall (i.e., the cells display about one-third the fluorescence found in fresh, unfixed tissue). The control cells of choice for fixed tissue are normal cells that are present in the same paraffin block as the tumor. In this case, any fixation artifacts may be similar for both the normal and neoplastic cells; however, uneven fixation may also produce different staining characteristics on cells within the same block (3). A pathologist who examines the block can identify the presence of normal cells. Often, however, normal cells will not be present in the block, and an alternate diploid control should be sought. The second choice for a paraffin-embedded control would be normal tissue from a different block from the same patient. If this is also unavailable, a similarly prepared block from another patient that contains normal tissue can be used, although minor variations in DNA staining of diploid cells may occur if the fixation and embedding processes were not identical. No commercial control preparations for paraffin-embedded tissue are available.

Specimen Processing

Fresh Tissue

Tissue can be processed immediately or stored in RPMI 1640 tissue culture medium at 4°C for up to 6 hours according to the CAP guide (9). We have found acceptable histograms from tissue stored in RPMI for up to 24 hours. Longer storage should be at −70°C (dry, not in media) or in liquid nitrogen until it is processed. Frozen tissue should be thawed rapidly in a 37°C water bath and immediately processed. The tissue should not be refrozen for later analysis, as this can introduce artifacts. The initial step in tissue processing is to dissociate the tissue into a single cell suspension. We prepare our suspensions in RPMI 1640 tissue culture medium by cutting the tissue into small pieces with a scalpel, teasing the tissue apart as much as possible using a straight and curved forceps, and, using the curved forceps, rubbing the remaining tissue pieces over a fine mesh screen. If the suspension still contains clumps, one can aspirate the suspension through needles with decreasing orifice sizes. For example, one should start with an 18-gauge needle, followed by a 20-gauge needle, going down in size to a 25-gauge needle. The cell suspension is then strained through a 40-μ nylon mesh. An aliquot of the filtered cell suspension is used to prepare a cytospin slide to allow a pathologist to document the presence of tumor cells in the specimen.

Automated Tissue Processing

A semiautomated system has been developed to prepare tissue specimens for DNA analysis. This system includes the Medicons tissue cassette and the Medimachine tissue processor, which are currently being marketed by Phoenix Flow Systems (San Diego, CA). This instrument can reduce a small tissue specimen to individual cells in under 5 minutes. I have not found published, controlled studies using this instrument; however, we have evaluated it in our laboratory and found good correlation between tissue obtained from the Medimachine system and our manual, teasing procedure described above. The Medimachine does have the advantage of processing the tissue within a cassette, reducing the technologist's exposure to potentially infectious materials. This instrument also may be useful in laboratories that analyze a large number of tissues. The lack of published studies using this system suggests that each laboratory considering this instrument should carefully evaluate its applicability to the laboratory's particular needs.

Formalin-Fixed, Paraffin-Embedded Tissue

Hedley (11) has described procedures for performing DNA analysis on formalin-fixed, paraffin-embedded tissue. As with fresh tissue, it is important to document the presence of tumor cells in the specimen. Thus, for quality assurance, a pathologist should choose a tissue block with a high percentage of tumor cells. Three to four 50-μ sections should be cut from this block. Formalin-fixed, paraffin-embedded tissue must be deparaffinized, and the cytoplasm enzymatically digested away before staining. Following deparaffinization with xylene and rehydration with solutions of increasing aqueous content, cells can be stored in distilled water for up to 1 week until staining. We have found a correlation between length of time in distilled water and the amount of debris in the specimen, and recommend staining the cells within 24 hours after rehydration.

Staining Procedures

Following tissue dissociation, the cells must be stained with a fluorescent dye that can stoichiometrically indicate the amount of DNA that is present in the cell. A number of dyes, including Hoechst 33342, DAPI, acridine orange, and PI, have been described that bind to double-stranded nucleic acids, or DNA specifically. Hoechst 33342 and DAPI are highly specific for DNA, but require ultraviolet light for their excitation wavelengths (12). Most clinical laboratories have flow cytometers that have a 488-nm laser, however, and these instruments cannot excite Hoechst or DAPI. Acridine orange and PI will stain single- and double-stranded nucleic acids. Acridine orange will demonstrate different fluorescence characteristics in either DNA or ribonucleic acid (RNA), making this dye useful for discriminating DNA from RNA (12).

Propidium iodide is a dye that intercalates into double-stranded nucleic acids, is excited by 488 nm light, and is the principal dye used for clinical DNA studies.

Two major technical problems must be overcome when PI is used. First, the molecule is too highly charged to cross a viable cell membrane (12) and thus the cell must be killed or the cell membrane and cytoplasm must be digested away before PI staining. Second, PI will intercalate into any true double-stranded nucleic acid, or any nucleic acid that appears double stranded because of intramolecular folding, such as transfer RNA. Thus, cells to be stained with PI must first be treated with RNAse to destroy any RNA that might bind the dye and give erroneous results.

The principal procedure used in clinical laboratories is derived from Vindelov et al (13), and uses three solutions, each prepared in a stock TRIS-based diluent that contains a detergent such as Noniodet P40, along with spermine tetrahydrochloride. Solution A is a trypsin solution designed to permeabilize the cell membrane. Solution B contains a trypsin inhibitor along with ribonuclease A, and is designed to stop the trypsin activity and eliminate any interference by RNA. Solution C contains PI for DNA staining, and should be handled as a toxic solution due to the carcinogenic effects of that reagent.

Many laboratories purchase the chemicals directly and prepare their own solutions. At least two commercial sets of these solutions are also available, along with an additional commercial staining solution. Coulter (Hialeah, FL) markets the DNA prep, which is an instrument designed to automate the staining process. The instrument is modeled after their Q-Prep, and adds Coulter-supplied Vindelov-type solutions to a prepared single cell suspension, with proper incubations and vortexing. New Concept Scientific Company (Burlington, Ontario, Canada) markets DNA-Assay, a single reagent that contains detergent, ribonuclease, and PI, as a single solution for the Vindelov staining method. BioSure (Grass Valley, CA) also markets a PI staining solution, designed to substitute for Vindelov solution C. The commercial solutions do provide an alternative to preparing the carcinogenic PI solution in the laboratory. Chicken or trout red blood cells (RBC) can be added to the tumor cells before staining as an internal control for the staining process (10).

Flow Cytometry

Flow cytometers differ in their specific procedures; however, the following information can be used to ensure optimal results, and will apply to all clinical instruments, such as the Coulter Profile and XL, the Becton Dickinson FACScan, and the Ortho CYTORONABSOLUTE.

1. The instrument should be calibrated to ensure linearity, following the manufacturer's recommendations. Commercial beads or fixed fowl red blood cell nuclei can be used for this purpose.
2. The sample flow rate should be set on low, or 20 to 25 μL/min.
3. The fluorescence should be monitored using a filter that is appropriate to read red fluorescence. The emission maximum of PI occurs at 623 nm.
4. Ten thousand to 20,000 events should be collected in list mode.
5. The PI staining should be monitored using a linear scale. The gains or photo multiplier tube (PMT) voltages, or both, should be set to put the diploid population of normal human peripheral blood leukocytes (PBL) in the range of channel numbers 50 to 60 on a 256-channel scale (10). This will allow the G_2M fraction of a tetraploid population to appear on the high end and the CRBC peak to appear on the low end of the scale.
6. A two-parameter histogram or cytogram plotting integral fluorescence versus peak fluorescence can be used to gate out doublets (2), although most cell cycle software programs, such as Verity's (Topsham, ME) ModFit or Phoenix Flow System's (San Diego, CA) Multicycle, recommend that all events be collected in list mode, and the software modeling will eliminate doublets from analysis.

Quality Control Review of the Flow Cytometry Data

The flow cytometrist must review the DNA histograms to ensure that the data meet quality control (QC) guidelines. Each laboratory should develop acceptable ranges for the coefficient of variance (CV) of the diploid G0/G1 peak, and for a minimum number of cells required for a valid analysis. We initially established an acceptable CV of less than 5% for diploid G0/G1 peaks derived from fresh tissue, as suggested by Dressler (10), and less than 8% for those obtained from paraffin-embedded tissue, in line with the recommendations of the DNA Consensus Conference (3). In practice, these values are normally between 2% and 3% for fresh tissue, and 4% to 7% for paraffin-embedded tissue. The paraffin CVs are higher due to more debris in the specimen. The debris can appear as a shoulder on the diploid peak, increasing the peak's CV and possibly masking the presence of any near diploid peaks. In severe situations, the shoulder may actually mimic a near diploid peak (3). The wider diploid peak also reduces the power of any S-phase calculations (3). We have found that peak CV values are highly technique dependent, and that an individual technologist's CVs do drop as his/her technique improves. We attempt to collect 20,000 events for analysis, with a minimum of 10,000 cells required for a valid ploidy and S-phase analysis, although we will make a ploidy determination on a good-quality histogram (CV < 5%, background debris < 20%) with less than 10,000 events, consistent with the recommendations of the DNA Consensus Conference (3). As a check of stoichiometric staining linearity within the cell population, the ratio of the mean channel of the G2/M peak to the G0/G1 peak should be 2.0 In practice, this value is often between 1.9 and 2.0.

Quality Assurance Review of the Flow Cytometry Data

The flow cytometrist must ensure that the data are put in the proper clinical context. We perform three QA checks during our procedure. First, we have a pathologist select and verify that the tissue we analyze is representative of the neoplastic process. Second, the surgical diagnosis is cross referenced in the flow cytometry report for easy correlation by the clinician. Finally, all reports are signed out by the flow laboratory Scientific Director and the pathologist who signed out the surgical report. This ensures that all available clinical and pathologic data are considered when interpretations are issued. If any discrepancies between clinical, surgical, and flow reports are found, we contact the clinician, and consider additional testing to resolve those discrepancies. The CAP also requires that all flow reports that identify aneuploid peaks contain a definition of aneuploidy as described by Hiddemann et al (14).

Proficiency Testing

The CAP flow cytometry survey (FL) provides three DNA challenges semi-annually. One specimen is always a diploid control, corresponding to normal PBL, and the other two represent unknown tumor specimens. The survey evaluates ploidy, DNA index, and S-phase calculations and represents a check for fresh tissue staining and analysis. The survey does not control for tissue dissociation procedures or paraffin-embedded tissue analysis. Clinical Laboratory Improvement Act (CLIA-88) competency testing must be developed in each individual laboratory in order to document each technologist's ability to perform the assay. Large specimens can be split, and the assay can be performed by different technologists, or a portion can be sent to an outside laboratory for confirmatory testing. It is important to remember that tumor specimens are not uniform throughout, and that differences in ploidy or S-phase results may be due to cellular differences in the regions analyzed by each individual or laboratory, and not due to technical flaws.

Cell Cycle Analysis of the Flow Cytometric Data

A variety of software packages exist for analyzing cell cycle data. The two most commonly used are ModFit, from Verity Software Corporation (Topsham, ME), and Multicycle, available from Phoenix Flow Systems (San Diego, CA). Each of the commercial programs has the ability to automatically analyze the data, or the user can manually determine ploidy and the cell cycle regions. Descriptions of the various models of S-phase determination can be found in the literature (2,15). In this section, interpretative guidelines for cell cycle analysis are discussed.

Ploidy

The number of chromosomes present in a cell is referred to as ploidy. The number of chromosomes found in a normal, nonneoplastic somatic cell vary from diploid during the G0 and G1 stages of the cell cycle to a tetraploid number of chromosomes in cells in the G2 stage, just before mitosis. Cells in S phase contain an amount of DNA between diploid and tetraploid. An example of a normal diploid cell population is shown in **Figure 17-1**. Ninety-six percent of the cells are in the diploid G0/G1 peak. S-phase and G2/M regions contain approximately 2% of the cell each. Tumor cells that have undergone genetic or chromosomal abnormalities may have a DNA content in their G0 or G1 phases, which is different from diploid. This is referred to as aneuploidy. A strict definition of aneuploidy is a nondiploid number of chromosomes. DNA analysis using PI as described in this chapter does not determine the specific number of chromosomes in cells, but rather the total amount of DNA present in the cell. Thus, in clinical practice, the term *aneuploid* refers to a nondiploid amount of DNA in a G0/G1 cell, not a nondiploid number of chromosomes (3).

FIGURE **17-1**

Flow cytometric histogram of normal peripheral blood lymphocytes. Diploid G0/G1 = 96% of events at mean channel 54; G2/M = 2% of events at mean channel 108; S phase = 2% of events; diploid CV = 2.5%; total events = 17,619.

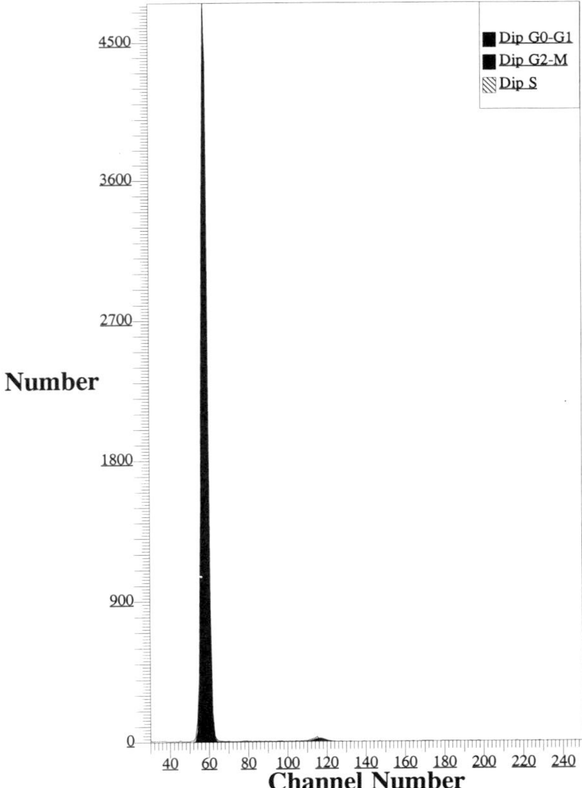

Identifying Aneuploid Populations

Two peaks must be present in the histogram to identify an aneuploid peak. Aneuploid populations are described as populations with a G0/G1 cell DNA content that is different than that of diploid. They present on DNA flow cytometric histograms as G0/G1 peaks in a channel different than that where the diploid content would reside. An identifiable S-phase and G2M component should also be present. Aneuploid peaks are described by their DNA index, which is the ratio of DNA in the aneuploid G0/G1 population to that in a diploid population. This is numerically defined as

$$\frac{\text{Mean channel of G0/G1 aneuploid population}}{\text{Mean channel of G0/G1 diploid population}}$$

Figure 17-2 is a histogram obtained from a well-differentiated, node-negative breast carcinoma. Two cell populations are present; diploid and aneuploid. The aneuploid peak has a DNA index of 1.99, identifying it as a tetraploid population. In Figure 17-2, the tetraploid population represents 75% of the events, and has visible S- and G2/M-phase regions. Identifying tetraploid populations can be difficult when a small fraction of the cells appear in that region. In histograms with a small tetraploid population, it is difficult to determine if one is viewing a separate tetraploid population or the G2/M of the diploid population. The DNA Consensus Conference defines tetraploidy as a DNA index between 1.9 and 2.1, and recommends that the peak contain at least 15% of the total events, or contain a number of events greater than two or three standard deviations above the control G2/M mean value (3). **Figure 17-3** also shows two G0/G1 peaks; however, both are close to the channel where one would expect to find the diploid peak. To determine which was actually the diploid peak, we added normal human PBL to the breast tissue, stained with PI, and reanalyzed the specimen. As seen in **Figure 17-4**, the right-hand peak increased in size compared to the aneuploid peak as a result of the addition of diploid cells. This identified the aneuploid peak as a hypodiploid peak, with a DNA index of 0.83. If normal cells are added to identify a diploid peak, as in this instance, the histogram cannot be used to measure S phase. This hypodiploid tissue represents a special case when adding normal cells to a tumor helps to differentiate near diploid and aneuploid

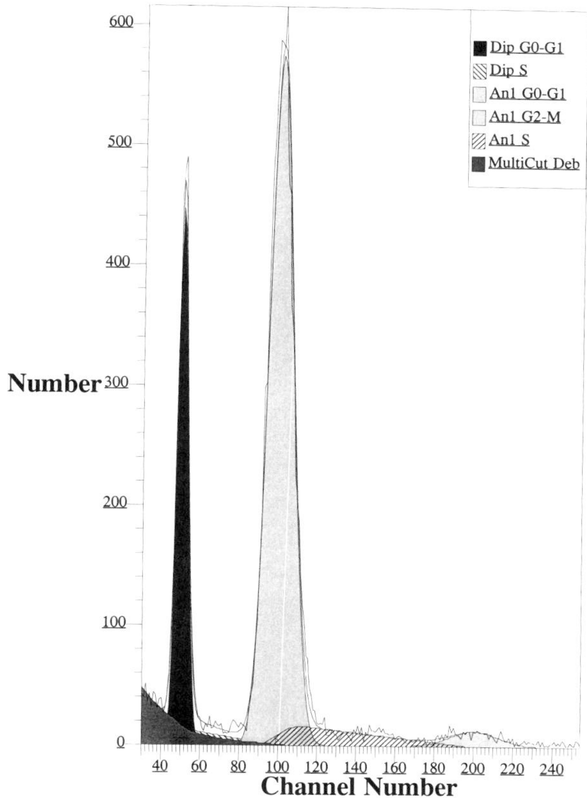

FIGURE 17-2

Flow cytometric histogram of a well-differentiated ductal breast carcinoma showing a diploid and tetraploid population. Diploid cycle = 25% of events; aneuploid cycle = 75% of events; total events = 14,304; aneuploid DNA index = 1.99; aneuploid S phase = 9.0;% background, aggregates, and debris = 2.3%.

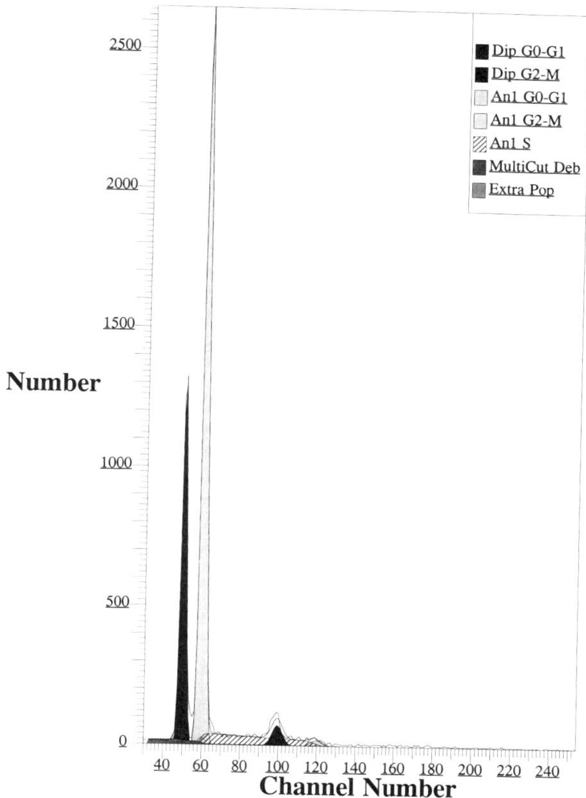

FIGURE 17-3

Flow cytometric histogram of a poorly differentiated ductal breast carcinoma. Note the two distinct populations close to the expected diploid G0/G1 channel. The software program automatically chose the left-hand peak as diploid and the right-hand peak as aneuploid with a DNA index of 1.2.

diploid peaks. Normal cells should not routinely be added to fresh tumor populations, however, and never to paraffin-embedded tissues (3).

S-Phase Analysis

In addition to ploidy, the number of cells in S phase has been shown to be a prognostic indicator, especially in breast carcinoma (5). S-phase calculations become complex because of the presence of debris, overlapping cell populations, and the distribution of DNA content in cells in the other phases of the cell cycle (see Fig. 17-2). Complete descriptions of S-phase calculation methods are available in the literature (2,15), and a detailed review of the analysis methods is beyond the scope of this chapter. Both ModFit (Verity Software Corp) and Multicycle (Phoenix Flow Systems) apply the major methods of S-phase analysis to flow cytometric–generated data, and each contains models that correct for background debris and aggregates. Both programs have autoanalysis routines that determine a best-fit model for the histogram data, and allow the user to manually override and select another model if desired. Separate analysis models are available in the programs for paraffin-embedded tissue that take into account the fact that one will have many sliced nuclei in the specimen.

A major concern regarding S phase is what values should be considered as being within a reference range. There is no universally accepted value of what constitutes elevated S phase (3). The ideal situation is for each laboratory to determine the range in which 95% to 99% of a particular class of tumor's S-phase values fall, and to report the percentile in which

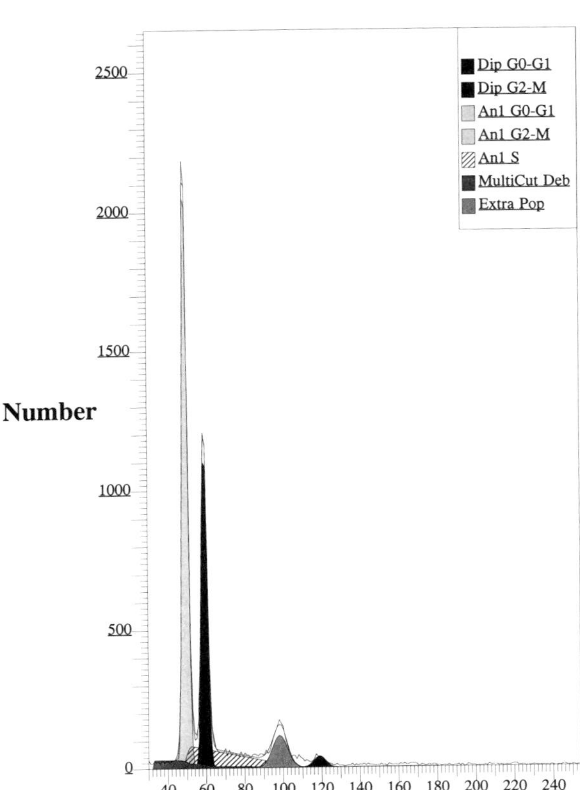

FIGURE 17-4

Flow cytometric histogram of a combination of normal peripheral blood lymphocytes and cells from the poorly differentiated ductal breast carcinoma shown in Figure 17-3. Note the increase in the size of the right-hand peak, identifying it as the diploid peak. Diploid cycle = 59% of events; aneuploid cycle = 41% of events; aneuploid DNA index = 0.83; aneuploid S phase = 26%; % background, aggregates, and debris = <1%.

a particular tumor's S-phase value occurs. This implies different reference ranges for diploid and aneuploid tumors, as well as for each tissue. This approach is not practical for most clinical laboratories due to expense and lack of sufficient material to develop a statistically meaningful range for each tissue or ploidy class. We provide the specific S-phase value on our reports, along with three levels of S-phase interpretations: low (<8% for breast tissue), borderline (8–12% for breast tissue), and high (>12% for breast tissue), in line with the DNA Consensus Conference recommendations (3).

Finally, from a quality assurance standpoint, it is useful to demonstrate that the S-phase results reported represent the malignant process and not the S phase of the normal diploid cells that are present within the tumor. If the specimen contains an aneuploid peak, this is not a problem. One can report the aneuploid S-phase value. If the specimen is diploid, however, one can perform DNA analysis combined with a fluorescence thiocyanate (FITC)-conjugated antibody to a marker for the tumor cells (e.g., cytokeratin for breast tumors), and perform DNA analysis only on the cytokeratin-positive cells. This would ensure that only cells of epithelial origin were included in the S-phase analysis (3). It is possible that normal epithelial cells would be present, but at least any lymphoid or stromal cells would be excluded from analysis.

Summary and Recommendations for Future Improvements

DNA ploidy and cell cycle analysis provide useful information that clinicians can use for prognosis, treatment decision, and monitoring of a patient's disease. Retrospective analysis using archived paraffin-embedded tissue has provided a sound scientific rationale on which to base clinical decisions. Fresh-tissue analysis on current clinical specimens can help a clinician classify a particular patient's disease process. Advancements in tissue processing, staining techniques, instrumentation, and software allowed this field to grow during the past 15 years. Many issues still need to be resolved, however. These include

1. Defining a good, reproducible diploid control for paraffin-embedded tissue
2. Improving sampling techniques for fresh tissue to ensure that a high percentage of tumor cells will be analyzed from smaller specimens
3. Improving the ability of cell surface markers to be used along with DNA staining to identify tumor cells
4. Developing standardized approaches to S-phase analysis so that results from different laboratories and studies can be directly compared
5. Determining clinically useful reference ranges for S-phase values.

REFERENCES

1. Van Dilla MA, Trujillo TT, Mullaney PF, Coulter JR. Cell microfluorometry: a method for rapid

fluorescence measurement. Science 1969;163: 1213–1214.

2. Riley RS, Mahin EJ, Ross W. DNA ploidy and cell cycle analysis. In: Riley RS, Mahin EJ, Ross W, eds. Clinical applications in cytometry. New York: Igaku-Shoin, 1993:251–322.
3. Shankey TV, Rabinovitch PS, Bagwell B, et al. Guidelines for implementation of DNA cytometry. Cytometry 1993;14:472–477.
4. Wheeless LL, Badalament RA, de Vere White RW, et al. Consensus review of the clinical utility of DNA cytometry in bladder cancer. Report of the DNA Cytometry Consensus Conference. Cytometry 1993;14:478–481.
5. Hedley DW, Clark GM, Cornelisse CJ, et al. Consensus review of the clinical utility of DNA cytometry in carcinoma of the breast. Report of the DNA Cytometry Consensus Conference. Cytometry 1993;14:482–485.
6. Bauer KD, Bagwell CB, Giaretti W, et al. Consensus review of the clinical utility of DNA flow cytometry in colorectal cancer. Cytometry 1993; 14:486–491.
7. Duque RE, Andreeff M, Braylan RC, et al. Consensus review of the clinical utility of DNA flow cytometry in neoplastic hematopathology. Cytometry 1993;14:492–496.
8. Shankey TV, Kallioniemi OP, Koslowski JM, et al. Consensus review of the clinical utility of DNA content cytometry in prostate cancer. Cytometry 1993;14:497–500.
9. College of American Pathologists. Reference guide for diagnostic molecular pathology/flow cytometry: fascicle VII. Northfield, IL: College of American Pathologists, 1996.
10. Dressler LG. Controls, standards and histogram interpretation in DNA flow cytometry. In: Darzynkiewicz Z, Crissman HA, eds. Methods in cell biology, flow cytometry. vol. 33. San Diego: Academic Press, 1990:157–172.
11. Hedley DW. Flow cytometry using paraffin embedded tissue: five years on. Cytometry 1989; 10:229–241.
12. Waggoner AS. Fluorescent probes for cytometry. In: Melamed M, Lindmo T, Mendelsohn M, eds. Flow cytometry and sorting. 2nd ed. New York: Wiley-Liss, 1990:209–226.
13. Vindelov LL, Christensen IJ, Nissen NI. A detergent-trypsin method for the preparation of nuclei for flow cytometric DNA analysis. Cytometry 1983;3:323–327.
14. Hiddemann W, Schumann J, Andreeff M. Convention on nomenclature for DNA cytometry. Cytometry 1984;5:445–446.
15. Dean PN. Methods of data analysis in flow cytometry. In: Van Dilla M, ed. Flow cytometry: instrumentation and data analysis. Orlando: Academic Press, 1985:195–220.

CHAPTER 18

Tissue Immunofluorescence Microscopy

VIJAY KUMAR
M. RAJADHYAKSHA

Immunohistochemistry is a simple, yet powerful, tool that is used with ever increasing frequency in clinical immunology and immunopathology laboratories. When applied under well-standardized conditions, this method facilitates confident analysis of specimens and thus aids in making a definitive diagnosis (1–5). There are two primary immunohistochemical detection systems: the immunofluorescence (IF) method and the enzyme immunohistochemical technique (4,6). The methods chosen by a laboratory largely depend on an individual's expertise, preferences, and objectives. In general, both methods will provide precise, and specific information when applied under standardized conditions.

Immunofluorescence is a simple, specific, sensitive, and versatile technique that is the mainstay for detecting antigens and antibodies with exquisite sensitivity in the clinical laboratory. An extremely small number of fluorescein molecules (as few as 50 cuμ) can be detected. Immunofluorescence microscopy has advantages over enzyme immunohistochemical methods in that it can be used over opaque objects. There are certain disadvantages associated with fluorescence microscopy in comparison with enzyme immunohistochemical methods. These include instrument costs and fluorescence fading of the specimen upon excitation. However, with advances in laboratory medicine, some of these limitations have been minimized. The fading of the specimen, for instance, can be minimized by the use of antifading agents in the mounting medium.

In the clinical immunology laboratory, two basic test systems are employed: direct immunofluorescence methods and indirect immunofluorescence techniques. The direct immunofluorescence method is used for in vivo detection of immune deposits in tissues such as skin, kidney, lung, and so forth. The indirect IF method is used for detection of various autoantibodies in patient sera, the most common being antinuclear antibodies (ANA) for systemic lupus erythematosus and other collagen vascular disorders.

Immunofluorescence

Fluorescence microscopy was first described in 1941 by Albert Coons et al (7) and is now routinely used for studying the distribution of substances that are present in small amounts. The fluorochrome has a special property: When irradiated with incident light of a certain wavelength, it absorbs some of the energy, transforming the fluorochrome to a high-energy excited state (excitation). When the electrons drop from the excited state to the ground state, fluorescence is generated (emission). Because of the loss of vibrational energy from excited to ground state, the emission spectrum is shifted to longer wavelengths (Stroke's shift). The greater this shift, the better the fluorochrome, as it becomes easier to separate excitation from the emission light. The various fluorochromes that are primarily used in immunofluorescence microscopy are fluorescein, rhodamine, Texas red, and phycoerythrin. Of these fluorochromes, fluorescein is widely used in IF microscopy. In principle, fluorescence microscopy is similar to the enzyme immunohistochemical method, as described in Chapter 19, except that fluorochrome, instead of an enzyme, is used as the label.

Two basic test systems are used to detect and localize antigens or antibodies, direct immunofluorescence and indirect immunofluorescence (**Fig. 18-1**).

Direct Immunofluorescence

In the direct IF method, fluorochrome is conjugated to the primary antibody, which can then directly react with the antigen in the tissue. Direct IF is used routinely for immunopathologic examination of skin and kidney biopsies for the detection of in vivo bound immune deposits. Briefly, the direct IF method entails the following steps:

1. Place cryostat cut sections of tissue biopsy on microscope slide.
2. Rinse in phosphate-buffered saline (PBS) for 5 to 10 minutes. Remove excess liquid.
3. Place a drop or two of the conjugate appropriately diluted in PBC containing 2% to 4% bovine serum albumin.
4. Rinse the slide in PBS for 2 × 10 minutes.
5. Wipe excess PBS around the sections.
6. Cover the section with a drop of the mounting medium and cover slip.
7. Examine for specific fluorescence under the fluorescence microscope.

Indirect Immunofluorescence

Indirect IF methods are used routinely for the detection of antibodies in the serum of patients with various autoimmune disorders. The steps involved in the indirect IF method include the following:

1. Place cryocut sections of tissue containing the appropriate antigen, the cell smear, or the culture of cells on the microscope slide. Fix the slide with appropriate fixatives.
2. Place patient serum appropriately diluted on the antigen substrate. Incubate for 30 minutes in a humid chamber.
3. Rinse slide in PBS for 2 × 10 minutes.
4. Wipe excess PBS around the substrate. Cover the substrate with one to two drops of the secondary antibody conjugate appropriately diluted. Incubate for 30 minutes in a humid chamber.
5. Rinse the slides in a Coplin jar that contains PBS. Remove excess PBS from the slide. Cover the slide with drops of the mounting medium and cover slip.
6. Examine for specific fluorescence under the fluorescence microscope.

Types of Fluorescence

The type of fluorescence observed on staining can be categorized into one of the following four categories:

1. *Desired or specific staining*: Specific staining is true staining and is a result of antigen-antibody reactions. The intensity of the fluorescence reaction is a function of antigen and antibody concentrations, and the labeling ratio and the conjugate antibody concentration of the conjugate.
2. *Undesired but specific staining*: This type of staining, though specific, is not desired and, hence, is unwanted. This undesired reaction is due to the presence of cross-reactive antibodies in the conjugate to other than the target antigen. This type of staining reaction could be minimized either by using affinity purified conjugates or by absorbing conjugates with cross-reactive antigens.
3. *Nonspecific staining*: The nonspecific staining is primarily a function of the degree of fluorochroming, and of free fluorescein in the conjugate, in addition sometimes to the nature of the antigenic substrate.
4. *Autofluorescence*: Autofluorescence is due to the presence of natural substance in the antigenic substrate that fluoresces on excitation. In tissue sections, collagen and elastic fibers quite often exhibit autofluorescence. Examination of the antigenic substrate without treatment with the conjugate could help in distinguishing autofluorescence from other types of fluorescence.

Standardization

To obtain reproducible and meaningful results in fluorescence microscopy, the following factors are significant and must be controlled.

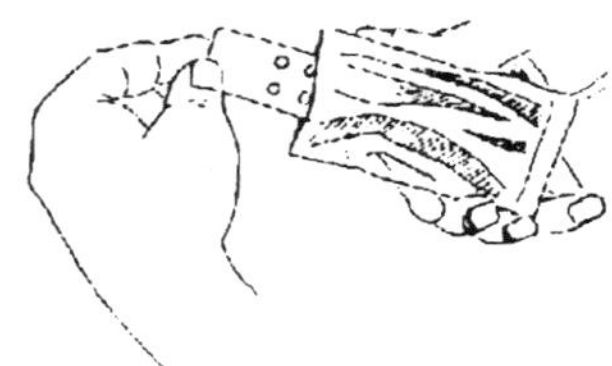

1. Let pouch equilibrate to room temperature, then remove slide(s) from pouch.

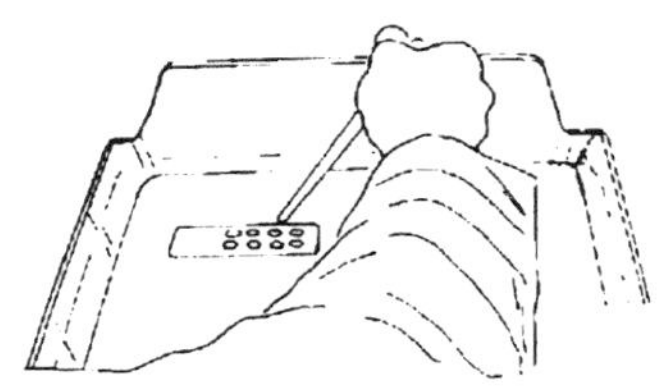

2. Place slide(s) into moisture chamber and add samples and controls. Cover and incubate 30 minutes.

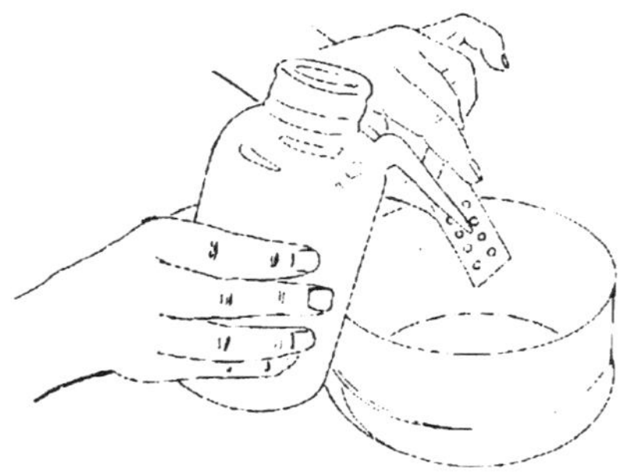

3. Rinse the slide. Avoid hitting substrate with buffer stream.

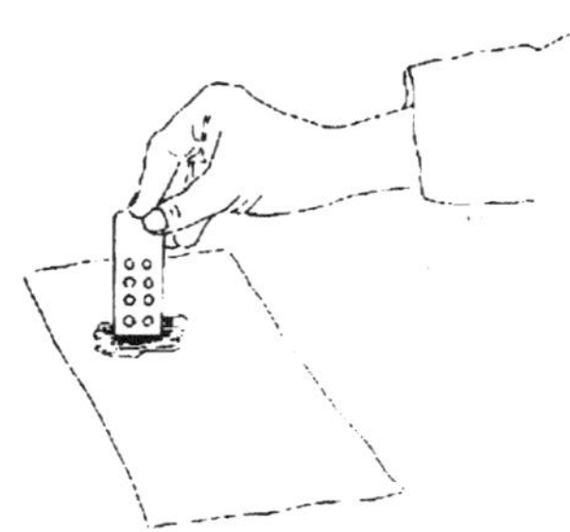

4. Blot edge of slide(s) on absorbent paper. Proceed immediately with next step.

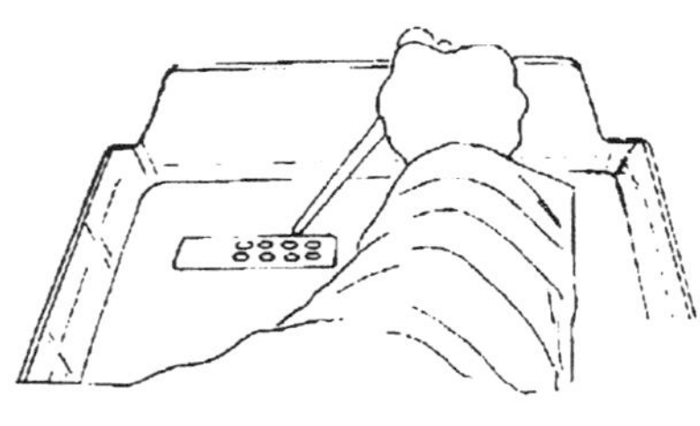

5. Apply conjugate to each well. Cover and incubate 30 minutes.

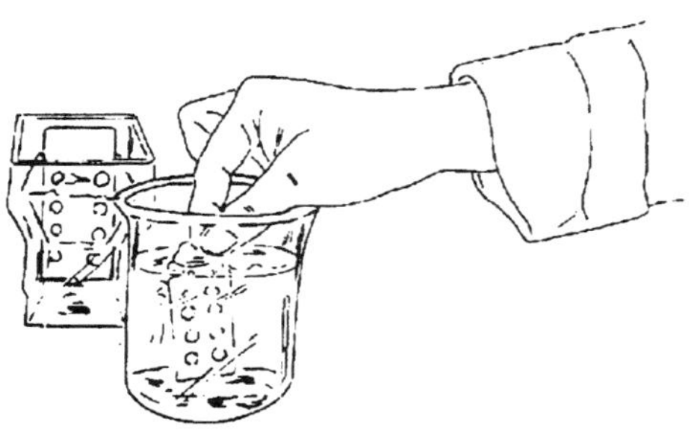

6. Dip slide(s) into beaker with PBS. Wash 10 minutes in staining dish.

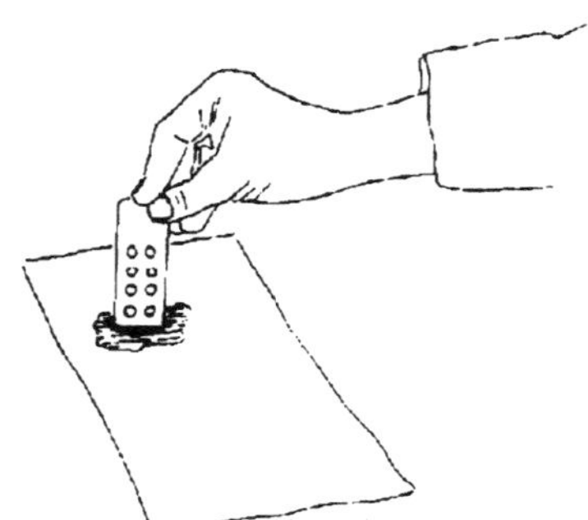

7. Blot edge of slide(s) on absorbent paper. Proceed immediately with next step.

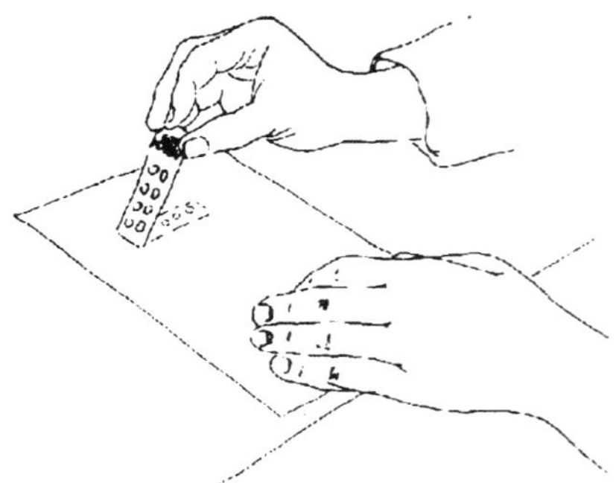

8. Mount cover slip and read under fluorescent microscope.

FIGURE **18-1**

Steps required in performing indirect immunofluorescence (IF). For direct IF, steps 2–4 are not needed. In direct IF, the reactions proceed directly with the addition of the conjugate. PBS, phosphate-buffered saline.

Tissue Preparation

To preserve the tissue and cell morphology and to retain the antigenicity of the substrate, it is essential that tissue obtained is processed appropriately. Quick freezing immediately after collection of the tissue in liquid nitrogen is usually the method of choice for processing the specimen. Alternatively, the tissues can be frozen on dry ice in the cryostat as per the manufacturer's instructions. The frozen tissues must be stored in a low-temperature freezer ($<-70°C$) until use. Sections of the tissue should be cut at 2 to 6μ in thickness and fixed to preserve cell morphology and antigen reactivity, and to increase permeability. For prolonged storage and to preserve the antigenicity and morphology, the slides can be placed in a Mylar bag and sealed in dry nitrogen. The selection of the fixatives is essential; whereas certain fixatives may preserve the morphology, they can alter the antigenicity, rendering the cell impermeable to reactions with antibody or the conjugate, or both, or they can enhance the background reactions. The optimum fixative should be the one that preserves the morphology and maintains the antigenicity with minimal background reactions. The various fixatives that have been employed in fluorescence microscopy include the following.

Acetone

Acetone is an excellent preservative and is routinely employed to fix and permeabilize the tissue sections, cell smear, or cell preparations. Fixation for 5 to 10 minutes in ice-cold acetone is recommended.

Ethanol

Ethanol fixation is useful for antigens that display carbohydrate-containing epitopes, such as surface cell antigens. Both acetone and ethanol fixatives are employed on cryostat sections, cell smears, and cell cultures, and not on tissue blocks.

Formaldehyde

Formaldehyde is the most commonly used fixative for tissues for paraffin sectioning. Formaldehyde fixatives are the fixatives of choice for cell membrane–associated antigens. Intracellular antigens are usually not demonstrable on formaldehyde-fixed substrate. Another disadvantage of formaldehyde fixation is that some of the antigens may not be demonstrable after fixation in formaldehyde. Limited proteolytic digestion of the tissue sections and cell substrates may expose the antigenic determinants and can be employed.

Conjugate

To achieve optimal and reproducible results, in addition to the proper processing of the specimen, the appropriate selection of the conjugate to attain desired specificity and sensitivity is important. The characteristics of the conjugates that affect the performance of the immunofluorescence reaction include the specificity of the antiserum used for conjugation and the degree of labeling of the antibody to the fluorochrome.

Specificity

Specificity is a measure of the degree of cross-reactivity of the conjugate to dissimilar antigens or epitopes. Although conjugates obtained from commercial sources are usually of good quality and in many cases may provide the desired specificity, it is the responsibility of the laboratory that uses them to make certain that the conjugate obtained possesses the desired specificity. In situations in which conjugates of desired specificity are not obtained commercially, they could be manufactured inhouse using well-defined methods (1,3,8,9). The specificity of conjugates can be determined by simple methods such as gel diffusion and immunoelectrophoresis. However, these methods may not be adequate to assess the specificity of the conjugates. The best method, of course, is the method in which these conjugates are to be used. Gel diffusion, also referred to as gel immunoprecipitation, is a simple method that could be used to determine the specificity and the strength of the conjugate. Similarly, immunoelectrophoresis can also be used to assess the specificity of the conjugates. Because of the lack of sensitivity of these methods, these tests should be followed by the immunofluorescence method on a number of substrates using monospecific antibody-positive primary controls. For example, to evaluate anti-human immunoglobulin G (IgG) conjugate, class-restricted antinuclear antibody–positive serum could be employed on mouse kidney section or on Hep-2 cells.

Sensitivity

The sensitivity of the immunofluorescence method is dependent upon the antibody content and the degree of conjugate labeling with the fluorochrome (2,4). Conjugates of higher antibody affinity render greater sensitivity to the method. Similarly, conjugates with higher antibody content are desirable, as the higher the antibody content of the conjugate, the higher the working dilution that could be used to obtain the desired optimum reaction without much nonspecific reaction.

When obtaining conjugates from commercial sources, one should request a copy of the certificate of analysis for the conjugate. The certificate of analysis should provide data on specificity, total protein, antibody content, and fluorescein-protein (F/P) ratio. In general, conjugates must have at least 10% of the total protein to be a specific antibody with a molar F/P ratio of about three. Conjugates with molar F/P ratios higher than five tend to give background reactions. Similarly, conjugates with low F/P content will not be desirable as they will not provide the required sensitivity.

Use Dilution

To obtain a high degree of reproducibility and minimum background reactions and to optimize costs, it is desirable that the conjugates be used at optimum working dilutions. Optimum working dilutions of the conjugate can be determined by a checkerboard titration method of the type shown in **Table 18-1**. This is usually done by making serial twofold dilutions of the conjugate and testing them directly on the antigenic substrate in the direct method and by first incubating the substrate with an antibody-positive serum of known titer at varying dilutions followed by incubation with conjugates of different concentrations in the indirect IF method. Even though the checkerboard titrations of the type shown in Table 18-1 are ideal in determining the use dilution of the conjugate, simpler methods, such as a unitage assay or the antibody content provided by the manufacturer, or both, can provide a reasonable guide in determining the appropriate dilution of the conjugate. The unitage assay is a simple gel precipitation method of titrating conjugates against a fixed (1 mg/mL) concentration of the homologous antigen using a standard template. Dilutions of the conjugate of 1/2 to 1/8 unit/mL have been found to work in the majority of situations.

TABLE **18-1**

Checkerboard Method of Determining Optimum Use Dilution of the Conjugate

		Conjugate					
	Ab Concentrated (μg/mL)	**100**	**50**	**25**	**12.5**	**6.25**	**3.12**
	Units	**1/2**	**1/4**	**1/8**	**1/16**	**1/32**	**1/64**
	Dilution	**1:8**	**1:16**	**1:32**	**1:64**	**1:128**	**1:256**
Direct IF	Specific staining	+++	+++	+++	+++	++	+
	Nonspecific staining	+/w	+/−	−	−	−	−
				Use dilution 1:32			
Indirect IF	PBS	+/−	−	−	−	−	−
	NHS	+/w	+/−	−	−	−	−
	ANA positive control dilution						
	1:40	+++	+++	+++	+++	++	+
	1:80	+++	+++	+++	+++	++	+
	1:160	++	++	++	++	+	+
	1:320	+	+	+	+	+	w
	1:640	+	+	+	+	+	w
	1:1280	w	w	w	w	w	−
	1:2560	−	−	−	−	−	−
				Use dilution 1:32			

IF, immunofluorescence; Ab, antibody; PBS, phosphate-buffered saline; NHS, normal human serum. +++, ++, +, w, +/−, − represent fluorescent staining intensities, +++ being strong positive and − being negative.

When the antibody content of the conjugate is available, approximately 25 to 100 μg/mL of the antibody has been found to work in many situations.

Microscope

Early fluorescence microscopes utilized transmitted light illumination with oil darkfield substage condensers (5,10). Of the various disadvantages of the substage or transmitted light-illuminated microscope, the most important was that the excitation light irradiates much of the specimen outside the field of view being observed, reducing the sensitivity of the method. However, since the advent of vertical illumination, epifluorescence microscopes are the microscopes of choice (**Fig. 18-2**). The epifluorescence microscope has several advantages over the substage illumination: 1) The objective serves as a condenser and image-forming light gatherer, and always is in correct alignment; 2) most of the unwanted or unused excitation light that reaches the specimen travels away from the objective and hence can be used on thick and opaque specimens; 3) the area of illumination is restricted to the area being observed; and 4) full numerical aperture of the objective is utilized, providing bright illumination.

The various aspects of the microscope that affect the specificity and sensitivity are light source, filters, and optics.

Light Source

To attain sufficient excitation light intensity to furnish emission that is capable of detection, powerful light sources are needed in fluorescence microscopy. The most common light sources are 100- and 200-W high-pressure mercury bulbs. Although these are sufficient for routine diagnostic use, other systems such as xenon arc burners and lasers provide high-excitation light and a significant increase in the sensitivity of detection. Xenon arc provides twice the fluorescence of the 200-W mercury bulb; however, it does not have very high spectral intensity peaks, which are characteristics of mercury bulbs. The intensity of light emitted by lasers is 1000-fold higher than that of mercury lamps. Of the types of mercury bulbs available, the 100-W bulb is the brightest, offering a life of 200 hours. Frequent on-off switching reduces lamp life. During changing of the bulb, it should not be handled with bare fingers to avoid etching.

Filters

There are basically three categories of filters: exciter, barrier, and dichroic beam splitter. Proper selection of filters is essential in fluorescence microscopy. Exciter filters allow lights of selected wavelengths to pass through to the specimen. Barrier filters absorb unwanted emission lights and allow lights of only selected wavelengths toward the eye. Dichroic mirrors selectively reflect emission wavelengths and pass emission wavelengths. In epi-illumination microscopes, excitation, barrier, and dichroic mirrors are provided as filter cubes. The function of the cube is to selectively employ a particular excitation and a barrier filter suited for the fluorochrome.

Optics

In fluorescence microscopy, the role of the objective is crucial as it serves to gather light from the specimen. In epifluorescence microscopy, the intensity of light reaching the eye varies proportionately to the fourth power of the numerical aperture (NA) of the objective and inversely to the square of total magnification (intensity = NA/mag). It is thus clear that objectives of high NA are desirable, as they will yield images of higher intensity. As an example, 40 objectives with an NA of 1.0 will provide images that are five times brighter than 40× objectives with an NA of 0.65. Optical sensitivity of the microscope can be determined using optical standard slides.

Calibration

The optical sensitivity of the fluorescence microscope is greatly affected by the optical system alignment, numerical aperture of the objective, type and age of the light source, filter combination, alignment of the light and the instrument, and characteristics of the conjugate used in the IF reactions. These parameters could affect the IF results. Haaijamn and Schaeffer (11) recommended the uranyl glass slide as a stable reference material to achieve standardization and measure the performance of the fluorescence microscope. However, the use of this material was limited because of the radioactivity of the

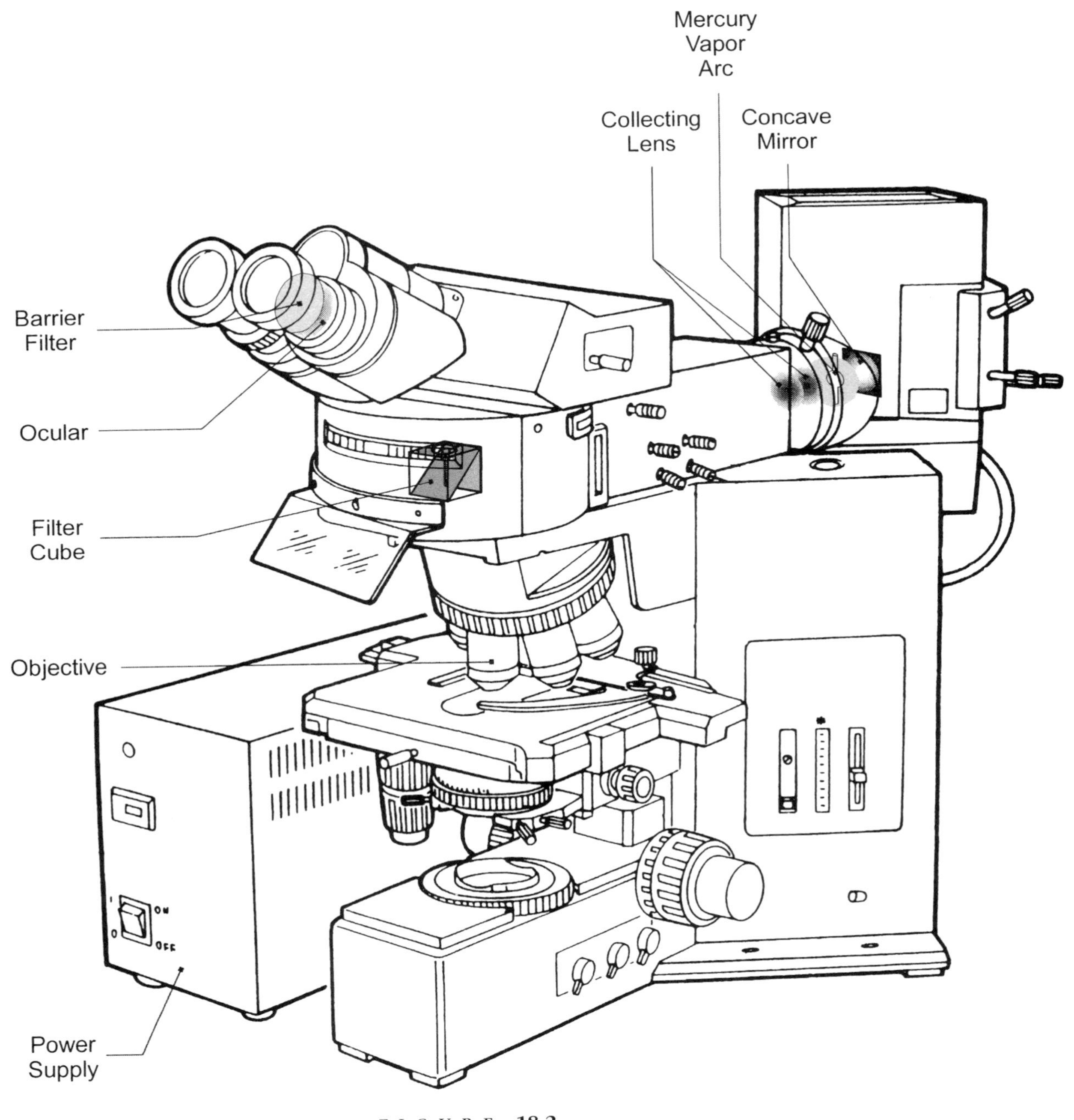

FIGURE **18-2**

Schematic diagram of an epifluorescence microscope.

uranium. The optical standard (OS) slide (IMMCO Diagnostics, Buffalo, NY) offers the fluorescent microscopist a practical approach to standardize the methodology and measure and optimize the performance of the fluorescent microscope (12). The OS slide could be used to 1) monitor the emission of the light bulb, since the readings of the OS slide provide a more reliable criterion than recording the hours of bulb usage; 2) assure optical alignment and correct filter selection; and 3) improve inter- and intralaboratory proficiency. The OS slide is a standard microscope slide with eight wells that contain uniform-sized microspheres of different fluorescent intensities. To monitor microscope performance, the OS slide is placed on the microscope stage and the fluorescence of each well is read visually to determine the end point. An end-point titer that is different than expected indicates inadequate performance of the fluorescence microscope, and remedial actions should be taken. These may include checking for 1) the optical alignment of the microscope as per the manufacturer's instructions; 2) a dirty objective or eyepiece, or both; 3) an inappropriate filter cube; and 4) a spectral emission of the light source that is not optimum, as the bulb may have reached the end of its rated lifetime. Correcting one or more of these should solve the problem. If it persists, the microscope manufacturer should be consulted.

Controls

Controls (positive and negative) are necessary to ascertain the performance of the test method. Without use of the proper controls, the validity of the immunofluorescent reactions, especially when negative, is subject to question. In addition, regulations in certain states mandate that negative, high, and low positive must be run for every qualitative test performed. Serum controls, also referred to as procedural controls, provide a measure of the process of IF staining. In screening or in qualitative IF procedures, the controls could be used at predetermined, fixed dilutions. However, when performing quantitative antibody titers, we recommend titrations of the positive control. In addition to the antibody or serum controls, tissue controls can also be considered in the quality control. Tissue controls are necessary in evaluating the performance of the method and during standardization of the procedure. The tissue controls are of importance in virologic studies during which the positive viral reactions need to be differentiated from the negative reactions.

Mounting Medium

The mounting medium keeps the substrate moist. This is necessary for fluorescence observations. Basically two kinds of mounting medium are employed in fluorescence microscopy. One is buffered glycerin, which is prepared by mixing nine parts of glycerin and one part of the buffer [usually PBS (pH 7.4)]. The disadvantage of this mounting medium is that the fluorescence undergoes rapid photo-bleaching (fading). The fading is a reduction of emission intensity on reradiation of light thereby reducing fluorescent intensity. In addition, the slides mounted in buffered glycerin cannot be stored for prolonged periods.

The other kind of mounting medium used is referred to as semipermanent, polyvinyl alcohol–based medium and is useful in preserving the fluorescent-stained slides for a prolonged period. In addition, the fading is less if slides are mounted in this medium, as compared to buffered glycerin. This medium can be prepared by mixing 20 g polyvinyl alcohol (Gelvatol 20–30, Monsanto) with 80 mL PBS or TRIS buffer for 16 to 24 hours at room temperature. Once in solution, 40 mL glycerol is added and the mixture is stirred for another 16 hours. The preparation is centrifuged at about 10,000 rpm for 15 minutes to remove undissolved materials and the pH is adjusted to 7.2.

One of the limitations of fluorescent microscopy is that fluorescent preparations fade upon excitation. Even though the exact mechanism of fading is not entirely known, the various mechanisms proposed include irreversible decomposition of the fluorescent molecule by the light intensity in the presence of oxygen. In addition to the excitation intensity, other factors include the polarity and viscosity of the mounting medium. The rate of photo-bleaching varies and is characteristic of the fluorochrome. Some fluorochromes undergo rapid photo-bleaching whereas others may be more stable. Photo-bleaching is dependent upon intensity of light irradiation and increases with the magnification of the objective. The fading can be reduced if the mounting medium contains antioxidants such as dithiothreitol, p-phenylenediamine, n-propyl gallate, or β-mercaptoethanol (13,14). The efficacy of these chemicals in reducing fading varies, depending on the type of fluorochrome. p-Phenylenediamine in buffered glycerin or polyvinyl alcohol mounting medium retards fading of the fluorescein but not that of rhodamine-labeled conjugates. Sodium azide, dithiothreitol, dithioerythritol, sodium hydrosulfite, n-propyl gallate, and ascorbic acid are useful in reducing fading. We have found that 1% n-propyl gallate in polyvinyl alcohol mounting medium, or 0.3 M 1,4-diazobicyclo-(2,2,2)-octane (DABCO) in buffered glycerine serves as an effective antifading agent (1).

Applications of Fluorescence Microscopy in Diagnostic Immunology

Immunofluorescence is a simple and powerful tool used with ever increasing frequency in clinical and research laboratories. Applications in the clinical laboratory include virology, parasitology, bacteriology, and immunology. **Table 18-2** summarizes some of the applications of immunofluorescence in the diagnosis of autoimmune disorders.

Acknowledgment

We sincerely appreciate many colleagues and associates who, during the past many years, helped contribute to standardizing the immunofluorescence methods, transforming them from art to science. Our gratitude to Kevin Lawson of IMMCO Diagnostics for his help in reviewing the manuscript and in the design of figures.

TABLE **18-2**

Diagnostic Significance of Immunofluorescence in Various Autoimmune Disorders

Disease	Direct IF	Indirect IF
Vesiculobullous		
Pemphigus	Intercellular deposits of IgG in the epidermis (>90%)	Intercellular antibodies of IgG > 90%
Pemphigoid (bullous pemphigoid, cicatricial pemphigoid, epidermolysis bullosa acquisita)	IgG and/or complement C3 in BMZ; linear almost 100%	BMZ antibodies; 70% in bullous pemphigoid, 25% in epidermolysis bullosa acquisita, 10% in cicatricial pemphigoid
Herpes gestationis (HG)	Complement C3 100%, IgG 30–50% in BMZ	HG factor ~50%, IgG-BMZ antibodies in ~20%
Linear IgA bullous dermatosis	IgA ~100%, C3 rarely in BMZ	IgA-BMZ antibodies ~10%
Dermatitis herpetiformis	IgA in dermal papillae ~100%	IgA-EMA in ~70%, ARA in ~25%
Collagen vascular		
Lupus erythematosus	IgG, IgM, IgA, C3 at DEJ (lupus band) over 90%	ANA (SLE ~95%, SCLE ~70%, DLE ~5%)
Mixed connective tissue disease (MCTD)	IgG in epidermal cell nuclei	ANA in ~100%
Sjögren's syndrome	Usually negative	ANA ~55%
Scleroderma	IgG in epidermal cell nucleoli	ANA ~85% (speckled, nucleolar, centromere)
Poly-/dermatomyositis	Usually negative	ANA ~80%
Endocrine		
Insulin-dependent diabetes (IDDM)	NA	Islet cell Ab ~50–70%
Thyroid diseases	NA	Thyroglobulin and microsomal
Addison's disease	NA	Adrenal antibodies 38–74%
Gastrointestinal/liver		
Celiac disease	NA	EMA ~100%, ARA ~60%
Pernicious anemia/atrophic gastritis	NA	Parietal cell Ab–pernicious anemia 85–95%, atrophic gastritis 30–60%
Primary biliary cirrhosis	NA	Antimitochondrial ~95%
Autoimmune hepatitis	NA	Smooth muscle, liver-kidney microsomal

BMZ, basement membrane zone; EMA, endomysial antibodies; ARA, reticulin antibodies; NA, not applicable; DEJ, dermal-epidermal junction; SLE, systemic lupus erythematosus; SCLE, subacute cutaneous lupus erythematosus; DLE, discoid lupus erythematosus.

REFERENCES

1. Beutner EH, Kumar V, Krasny SA, Chorzelski TP. Defined immunofluorescence in immunodermatology. In: Beutner EH, Chorzelski TP, Kumar V, eds. Immunopathology of the skin. 3rd ed. New York: Wiley, 1987:3–40.
2. Kasten F. Methods for fluorescence microscopy. In: Clark G, ed. Staining procedures. 4th ed. Baltimore: Williams & Wilkins, 1981:29–103.
3. Beutner EH, Binder WL, Kumar V. State of the art of immunofluorescence techniques in tissues. In: Keitges P, Nakamura RM, eds. Diagnostic immunology: current and future trends. Skokie, IL: College of American Pathologists, 1980:89–99.
4. Kumar V. Immunofluorescence and enzyme immunomicroscopy. In: van Oss CJ, van Regenmortel MH, eds. Immunochemistry. New York: Marcel Dekker, 1994:829–847.
5. Rost FWD. Fluorescence microscopy. vols. 1 and 2. Cambridge, UK: Cambridge University Press, 1992.
6. Nagle RB. Immunohistochemistry. In: Nakamura RM, Folds JD, eds. Clinical diagnostic immunology. Cambridge, MA: Blackwell Science, 1998.
7. Coons AH, Creech HH, Jones RN. Immunological properties of an antibody containing a fluorescent group. Proc Soc Exp Biol 1941;47: 200–202.
8. Beutner EH, Nisengard RJ, Albini B, eds. Defined immunofluorescence and related cytochemical methods. Ann NY Acad Sci 1983;420: 1–432.
9. Beutner EH, Nisengard RJ, Kumar V. Defined immunofluorescence: basic concepts and their application to clinical immunodermatology. In: Beutner EH, Chorzelski TP, Bena SF, eds. Immunopathology of the skin. 2nd ed. New York: Wiley, 1979:29–75.
10. Abramowitz M. Fluorescence microscopy. vol. 4. Olympus America Inc. 1993.
11. Haaijman W, Schaeffer M. Fifth International Conference of Immunofluorescence and Related Staining Techniques. Ann NY Acad Sci 1975;254: 1–627.
12. Rostami R, Beutner EH, Kumar V. Quantitative studies of immunofluorescent staining. Int Arch Immunol 1992;98:200–204.
13. Rodriquez J, Deinhardt F. Preparation of a semipermanent mounting medium for fluorescent antibody studies. Virology 1960;12:316–317.
14. Johnson GD, Davidson RS, McNameeke G, et al. Fading of immunofluorescence during microscopy. A study of the phenomenon and its remedy. J Immunol Methods 1982;55:231–242.

CHAPTER 19

Immunohistochemistry Quality Assurance

KATHERINE M. SCOTT
RAY B. NAGLE

There is a common misconception among surgical pathologists who are unfamiliar with the vagaries of protein chemistry that immunohistochemical staining is comparable to other special staining procedures that use organic dyes. The fact that immunohistochemistry involves the detection of epitopes that may be conformation dependent and the use of antibodies that are susceptible to denaturization raises important new issues in terms of the run-to-run reproducibility of these tests. We attempt to address these issues in this chapter.

Antigenic Characteristics

Native proteins assume three-dimensional configurations that are dictated by their specific amino acid sequences. These configurations may be further stabilized by interchain cross-linking and are additionally altered by assembly with other protein subchains to form complex quaternary structures. An antigenic site or epitope is composed of an exposed sequence of amino acids that may be continuous, that is, a linear sequence of amino acids from one portion of a protein, or discontinuous, that is, amino acids that cluster together but may be from different areas of a sequence in a given protein chain, or may even be from different chains in an oligomeric protein that is composed of more than one subchain. These epitopes usually contain charged amino acid side chains with their antigenicity in part due to their three-dimensional structure. Posttranslational modifications such as glycosylation or phosphorylation can also modify an epitope and can increase or destroy its antigenicity.

For most proteins that have been extensively studied, five to six major epitopes reside in exposed areas of the native protein, one of which is usually at the C-terminal sequence. An important observation to remember is that polyclonal antisera raised against the protein will generally contain clones of antibodies that are specific for all of the epitopes. In contrast, a monoclonal antibody will usually detect a single epitope.

Fixation Issues

Fresh tissue snap-frozen in a manner that prevents ice crystal distortion, that is, at −150°C, is the single most effective way to preserve the three-dimensional structure of protein epitopes. Historically, this has been the preferred method of preservation and is still used for certain applications. Most modern immunohistochemistry laboratories have been forced to adapt their detection systems to use on tissue specimens that are routinely fixed in buffered formalin and embedded in paraffin (1,2).

Formaldehyde exists in solution in equilibrium with its hydrated form, methylene glycol ($CH_2[OH]_2$) (2). The equilibrium favors the glycol so that at any given time very little aldehyde is present. This explains why fixation with buffered formalin solutions is very slow and requires small pieces of tissue for complete and uniform optimal fixation. The aldehyde reacts with a number of amino side chains to create methyl cross-links between adjacent protein chains within the same molecule or between molecules (2,3). In practice one often sees this cross-linked fixation at the periphery of a tissue block where the fixative has penetrated while the central region was fixed by precipitation due to alcohol exposure during graded alcohol dehydration. This phenomenon of heterogenous fixation can lead to confusing patterns of immunoreactivity. With epitopes that are destroyed by cross-linking but preserved by alcohol precipitation, one may see an outer rim of nonreactivity with only the central zone of tissue showing reactivity. With other epitopes in which detection requires adequate cross-linked fixation, one may see a rim of immunoreactivity and a central area in which the antigenicity was destroyed due to autolysis. These fixation problems are the major limitation of this discipline and can only be controlled by ensuring maximal uniformity of fixation during the initial tissue selection.

To control for these variables, tissue fixed in the same formulations that are used in the surgical pathology unit should be utilized for all tissue controls. Control blocks that contain tissue fixed at various time intervals, for example, 2, 4, 8, 24, and 48 hours, and using various routine fixatives can be embedded in the same block. This type of control block can be used to assess the sensitivity of a given antigen to fixation and is a very useful tool for titration of new lot numbers and or new antibodies that are being introduced into the laboratory.

The use of an antibody that detects a ubiquitous antigen is also a useful control. In our laboratory we routinely use antivimentin antibody to detect vimentin, which is expressed by most connective tissue cells and all endothelium. This allows one to generally determine the adequacy of fixation in a given block, and one can restrict interpretation to that portion of the specimen that is adequately fixed.

Tissue Processing

As discussed above in the section on fixation, the preservation and detection of antigen represent the major goal in immunohistochemistry. Each antigen is different in its characteristics. When dealing with monoclonal antibodies we are basically looking at the preservation of a single epitope. Recent developments in this area indicate that, whereas the vast majority of monoclonal antibodies were not usable in formalin-fixed paraffin-embedded tissue, with heat retrieval of antigens many antibodies can now be applied to formalin-fixed material (4–6). This technique depends on heating, usually using a microwave oven. This procedure apparently causes release of methyl cross-linking and retrieval of epitope reactivity. At this time, the exact chemistry of how this works is not clear.

Other techniques involve the clipping of proteins by preincubation with enzymes (7). In these procedures the partial cleavage of the proteins allows unmasking of certain antigens, probably because of the release of cross-linked proteins that are covering up epitopes. Another possibility is that the enzymatic cleavage of a protein allows an epitope that is deformed to resume its three-dimensional antigenic conformation.

Whichever of these techniques is employed for recovery of antigens, it is clear that the reactions must be carefully controlled. Proper pH control by the use of buffers is important. It is also obvious that these antigen retrieval techniques require the use of control tissue that is fixed in a manner similar to that of the test tissue, and the control tissue must be subjected to the same antigen retrieval procedure. We have found that these antigen retrieval procedures often change the sensitivity and specificity of the antibodies, and for these reasons the use of antigen retrieval techniques requires retitration of the primary and secondary antibodies. Heat recovery may cause some undesirable effects such as increased reactivity of intrinsic biotin (8).

Antibody Controls

Each primary antibody used in the laboratory must be titrated with the secondary antibody detection system. This is usually carried out by making serial dilutions of the primary and secondary antibodies and, of course, these titrations must be carried out on the same type of material used in testing. For example, if a laboratory uses 10% formalin, the titrations must be carried out in tissue fixed in 10% formalin over a variety of time periods (as discussed above) and embedded with the procedure that is being used.

The problem of a negative control is an important issue. Theoretically, the best negative control would be a primary antibody made against another epitope but of the same idiotype as the testing antibody. This should be reacted with tissue of a similar nature as that to be tested and should be run each time the antibody is used. In many laboratories this idealized control is impractical and omission of the primary antibody is used as the negative control. For example, phosphate-buffered saline (PBS) is incubated rather than the primary antibody. In general, in most clinical applications multiple antibodies are being tested simultaneously so that each serves as a control for the other.

It is extremely important to ensure that the secondary antibody is species specific. Some automated systems overcome this by using a universal secondary antibody that consists of a mixture of antimouse, antirat, antirabbit, and antigoat antibodies. It is important that the secondary concentration is titrated against the primary antibody concentration to obtain ultimate results.

Detection Systems

The secondary antibodies can be conjugated to a variety of enzymes (1,2,9). Most commonly the secondary antibodies are biotinylated. These labeled antibodies are then developed using avidin conjugated with either a horseradish peroxidase or alkaline phosphatase. These, in turn, are used to reduce uncolored substrates to a color read-out product. Because these oxidative reduction reactions are sensitive to light and degeneration, the most commonly encountered problems of immunohistochemistry often are a result of degeneration of the color reagent. For this reason, it is extremely important that these be stabilized in solution. Many of the commercially available automated systems contain oxygen scavengers and other preservatives that ensure that these reagents do not degenerate with time. If they are being made up by hand, they must be carefully buffered and made fresh for each run. A note of caution is that these preparations should be made under a hood since the 3,3′-diaminobenzidine (DAB) is considered extremely carcinogenic.

Counterstaining

The ideal counterstain should contrast sharply with the selected immunohistochemical chromogen and not interfere with interpretation of weak reactions. Ideally, the counterstain is complementary to the chromogen. For DAB, a brown chromogen, or AEC (3-amino-9-ethyl carbazole), a red chromogen, optimal contrast is achieved with blue or green counterstains (e.g., methylene blue or methyl green). A hematoxylin counterstain for DAB or AEC can actually mask weak immunocytochemical reactions and render interpretation of nuclear stains difficult to impossible.

Tissue Controls

Positive and negative controls should be handled in a manner identical to that used with the patient's own tissue, and run simultaneously with the patient's tissue whenever a specimen is processed for immunohistochemistry. This allows for an overall evaluation of antigen preservation, antibody specificity, and the successful performance of all steps of the immunostaining procedure. When using automated systems the control tissue optimally should be placed on the same slide as the test tissue.

Often patient tissue will have areas of recognizable cells with known antigenicity that serve as an internal control, both positive and negative (mesenchymal tissue, hematologic cells, and normal tissue in the margin of the sample), but this is not always available, and it is best to use separate tissue handled as discussed above. The patient's tissue should always be carefully examined for the immunoreactivity of all cells in reference to the interpretation of the cells being studied.

Nonspecific staining has a diffuse appearance; excessive formalin fixation can destroy (mask) antigenicity, and also cause sporadic staining of connective tissue. Necrotic and degenerating cells often stain nonspecifically (1).

Positive Controls

A positive control is a tissue selected for the purpose of obtaining a definite positive reaction; that is, it has the antigen in question. Fresh surgical biopsy or autopsy material can be used, fixed, and processed in an identical manner to that utilized with patient material. Tissue selected as controls (reactive tonsils, skin, colon, etc.) usually contains a heterogeneous cellular composition that provides individual cells and structures for positive and negative reactions in a single tissue. It may be desirable to include several pieces of tissue in a single paraffin block ("sausage roll") to provide a range of antigenic expression, including both positive and negative controls.

Negative Controls

A negative control is a tissue selected for the purpose of obtaining a definite negative reaction; that is, it lacks the antigen in question. Fresh surgical biopsy or autopsy material can be used, fixed, and processed in an identical manner to that utilized with patient material. The negative control is quite useful for evaluation of specific and nonspecific background staining.

Scoring and Recording

Different laboratories must decide on quantitation of reactivity. Generally, a semiquantitative method is acceptable, and one system uses a range of 0 for no staining to 4+ for intense staining. There is generally good agreement among observers using a semiquantitative method, and this allows a method of following strength of reactivity of the final product, which reflects on all steps from the processing of the material up to the final reading of the glass slides. In this way, any differences in staining pattern are available for review and the reviewer is able to monitor all steps in the immunohistochemical staining process.

A daily record should be kept of the positive control tissue results, and evaluation of discrepancies can be instituted immediately or retrospectively. Some laboratorians prefer to attach the results of the appropriate controls to the patient's report, and others opt to keep a separate log of positive results. Each method has advantages: The first allows persons reading the report to know the interpretation of the controls at the time the report is issued, and the second allows an internal check of reactivity strength on a cumulative basis.

Troubleshooting

There are several aspects to troubleshooting problems encountered in immunohistochemistry, and it is always appropriate to begin with a review of the identification of the sample, the controls, and the handling of the material. Differences in fixation of the patient material from the method usually employed in the laboratory is a common difficulty and may result in problems with tissue adherence to the glass slides, reactivity of the antibodies to the tissue antigen, and altered strength of expression.

All methods must be validated in the laboratory, and if the expected results are not obtained in the patient's tissue, it might be advisable to repeat the staining using the same reagents by a different but equivalent method, that is, by machine if the usual method is manual and vice versa. Various strategies can be developed depending on the problem encountered; that is, if there is no staining of the specimen but the control is stained, the tissue handling might have been too harsh or the antigen may be masked. If the control slide stains well but the specimen tissue stains weakly, the antigen may be partly destroyed or present in too low concentration. Weak staining of all slides may be multifactorial, and review of buffers, substrate mixtures, and incubation times should be performed.

Whenever automated equipment is used, all steps that are routinely evaluated by hand staining should be reviewed for proper working order not only as suggested by the manufacturer, but as determined within the laboratory. A quick review of the hand or mechanical procedure may solve the problem, allowing for a repeat of the staining if necessary.

REFERENCES

1. Taylor CR, Cote RJ. Immunomicroscopy: a diagnostic tool for the surgical pathologist. Philadelphia: Saunders, 1994.
2. Larson L-I. Immunocytochemistry. Theory and practice. Boca Raton, FL: CRC Press, 1988.
3. Mason JT, O'Leary TJ. Effects of formaldehyde fixation on protein secondary structure: a calorimetric and infrared spectroscopic investigation. J Histochem Cytochem 1991;39:225–229.
4. Gown AM, de Wever N, Battifora H. Microwave-based antigenic unmasking: a revolutionary new technique for routine immunohistochemistry. Appl Immunhistochem 1993;1:256–266.

5. Battifora H, Alsabeh R, Jenkins KA, Gown A. Epitope retrieval (unmasking) in immunohistochemistry. Adv Pathol Lab Med 1995;8:101–118.

6. Cattoretta G, Pileri S, Parravicini C, et al. Antigen unmasking on formalin-fixed, paraffin-embedded tissue sections. J Pathol 1993;171:83–98.

7. Ordonez NG, Manning JT, Brooks TE. Effect of trypsinization on the immunostaining of formalin-fixed, paraffin-embedded tissues. Am J Surg Pathol 1988;12:121–129.

8. Fan Z, Clark V, Nagle RB. An evaluation of enzymatic and heat epitope retrieval methods for the immunohistochemical staining of the intermediate filaments. Appl Immunohistochem 1997;5: 49–58.

9. Elias JM, Gown AM, Nakamura RM, et al. Quality control in immunohistochemistry. Report of a workshop sponsored by the Biological Skin Commission. Am J Clin Pathol 1989:92(6) 836–843.

CHAPTER 20

Image Analysis of Tissues

THOMAS GAHM
RAPHAËL MARCELPOIL

The assessment and analysis of tissues are the classic domain of pathology. Although during the last decades methodologic and technologic developments have turned digital image analysis into one of the most efficient tools to assist cytopathologists in their eagerness to interpret images more and more accurately (1), a large gap separates computer-assisted cytopathology from computer-assisted histopathology. If image analysis techniques contribute substantially to provide cytologists with accurate, reproducible, and objective cellular analysis, histologic interpretation techniques still rely heavily on the subjective analysis of specimens, with variable intra- as well as interobserver agreement. The reason for this is obvious: The evaluation of tissue sections using image analysis is far more difficult than the individual cell assessment that is usually required in cytologic analysis.

Initially image analysis of tissues was basically confined to technologies developed for the analysis of cytologic specimens. For this purpose, if possible, the tissue samples were either enzymatically disaggregated (2), with the task of analyzing tissue reduced to the evaluation of a cytologic slide, or the three-dimensional character of the histologic section was roughly taken into account through the introduction of a stereologic correction factor (3).

With the evolution and easy availability of high-performance computers, local and wide area communication, cheap database and storage technology, and affordable high-resolution digital cameras and scanners, the situation is now changing. More sophisticated algorithms, which for lack of central processing unit (CPU) power could never before be applied to tissue sections in a routine environment, can now be used to assess and quantify tissue-specific features related to the tissue architecture. At the same time a far more comprehensive support for a reproducible and more standardized visual assessment of tissue sections has become available based on the initial step in image analysis, the creation and management of digital images. This is especially true in the fields of quality control (QC), quality assurance (QA), and standardization. Digital images of difficult cases can be exchanged with reference pathologists via telepathology to get a second opinion (4). They can be effectively used for proficiency testing. Digital images are the basis of powerful image reference databases, which can be accessed via network, and they play an increasingly important role in the documentation of cases and evaluation results, especially in comprehensive electronic or printed reports.

Slide Preparation

The way a histologic slide is prepared from a piece of tissue has a vast impact on the results that can be expected from a subsequent evaluation by means of image analysis. The preparation can be divided into the three steps of sampling, cell collection, and staining.

The correct sampling obviously is the sole responsibility of the pathologist. He or she has to make sure that the correct part of the tissue under consideration also gets processed.

For cell collection the tissue basically can either be enzymatically disaggregated or cut into sections of a specific thickness (5). With the first procedure a slide with nicely separated whole cells or at least whole cell nuclei is the result. Although this kind of preparation is ideally suited for a subsequent evaluation via image analysis, the information of the tissue architecture is lost completely.

In the second procedure the cells still preserve their original arrangement. The important drawbacks with this kind of preparation are cut cells and cell nuclei, a certain number of overlapping cells depending on the section thickness and the kind of tissue under consideration, and in general the problem of having to deal with a third dimension, for which information is incomplete or totally missing. The quantitative evaluation of these slides is one of the biggest challenges in the field of image analysis.

The staining, often in combination with specific markers, determines what kind of information will be visible under the microscope and hence can be used for the quantitative evaluation via image analysis. It also is the determining factor for the contrast of the cells or cell nuclei within the images, which will be the basis for subsequent processing.

The Basic Steps of Image Analysis

Once a tissue slide is prepared, a pathologist visually examines it under the microscope. If image analysis should be applied to the slide, the microscope must be at least equipped with a camera, which is connected to a computer system via a special interface. The camera samples the optical microscopic image. As a result a digital image is collected in the memory of the computer and displayed on the monitor. The acquisition of these digital images has to be done in such a way that the important details of the optical images are still correctly represented (6).

The creation of a digital representation of a tissue slide alone, even without any further processing, has huge consequences for standardization, QA, and QC. This is discussed below.

The next step for a quantitative assessment of the digitized images is the segmentation, which sometimes includes an additional intermediate step of preprocessing. During the segmentation the cells or cell nuclei are separated from each other and from the image background. Although it looks like an easy task for a human being, this is the most difficult and most error-prone step in image analysis. For slides in which the cells are nicely separated and stained in such a way that good contrasts occur in the digitized image, segmentation can be done very reliably for most of the cases. As soon as one of the above conditions is not fulfilled, however, highly sophisticated and time-consuming segmentation algorithms, using additional a priori knowledge about the cells and their relationship to each other, have to be applied and the results are often not satisfactory. This is especially true for tissue sections, where most of the cells are no longer nicely separated on the slide but are touching and overlapping each other. Once the meaningful areas of an image are determined the feature extraction takes place. For each cell or cell nucleus a set of densitometric, morphometric, and texture features is measured, which characterizes the individual cells as comprehensively as possible.

To evaluate the arrangement of cells within tissue sections, the center of each cell nucleus has to be determined. Connecting these centers according to certain rules creates web-like two-dimensional graphs, from which feature sets can be extracted that characterize the relationship between cells within clusters or even bigger entities. This is described in more detail below.

The last step is the presentation of the raw data and their compilation into meaningful results. Very often the result output of an image analysis system has to match the form of visual and semiquantitative grading systems that are already in use by the pathologist in order to be easily applicable in routine use.

The Pathology Workstation for Tissue Evaluation

The platform for the evaluation of tissue samples via image analysis is shifting more and more from the initial general purpose image analyzer to highly specialized dedicated "pathology workstations" (7). These workstations are designed for routine work. They combine all the tools that are needed to provide the pathologist with the necessary information to derive the best results possible. The major components of such a workstation are outlined in **Figure 20-1**.

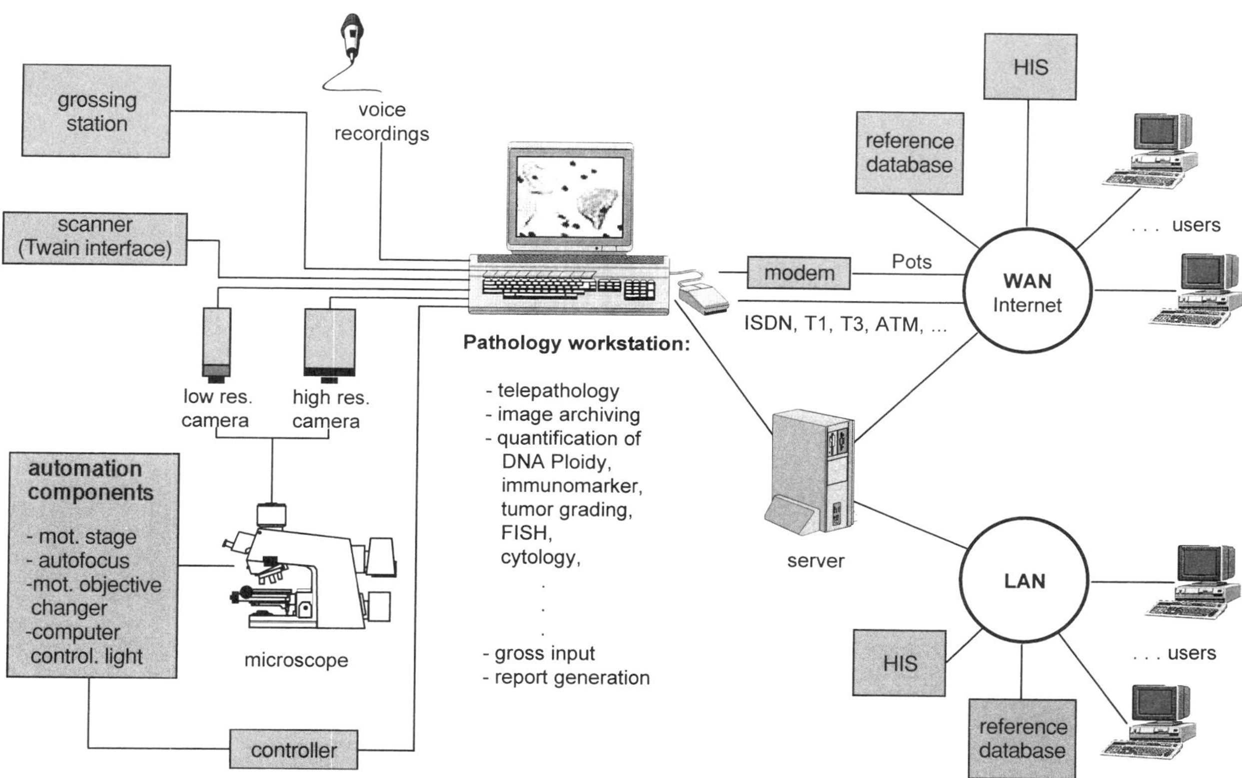

FIGURE **20-1**

Pathology workstation. WAN, wide area network; LAN, local area network; DNA, deoxyribonucleic acid; FISH, fluorescent in situ hybridization; HIS, hospital information systems.

The central part of the workstation is the microscope. It is equipped with robotic parts, including a motorized stage, automatic focus, objective changer, and light-intensity adjustment. Different input devices such as cameras for fast automatic focusing and acquisition of high-resolution images, scanners for printed image and document acquisition, grossing stations, and voice recording devices are linked to the workstation. The workstation can be part of a local area network (LAN). It supports different communication protocols, so that available communication channels, such as the standard telephone line, ISDN, T1, T3, and ATM, can be used to easily connect the workstation with other places in the world (wide area network, WAN).

If the pathology workstation operates in an integrated environment, the LAN or WAN connection, or both, will give it access to existing reference databases (8) and hospital information systems (HIS). In this way new cases can easily be compared with the pictures and accompanying information of reference cases that have been accumulated over time. Images acquired from the slides under review can be complemented with the patient and case history.

The pathology workstation outlined in Figure 20-1 is ideally suited for a very comprehensive tissue evaluation. Starting with information and digital pictures of the initial gross piece, images of the slides prepared from the tissue can be taken. The patient and case information, the images themselves, and quantitative information about the cell components of the tissue sample and its architecture can all be stored in the same database.

If a second expert opinion is needed or if the slide is used for training or proficiency testing (9), the communication capabilities along with the microscope automation enable the workstation to be used as a telepathology system. High-resolution images that characterize the open questions of the slide of interest are sent to the reference expert or to the audited candidate. To get an overview picture of the slide, the motorized microscope can be initialized to scan the whole slide automatically on a field-per-field basis and the corresponding digital images stored in the computer memory. The edges of adjacent fields are precisely matched using correlation algorithms, so that the result is one large overview image of the entire slide.

This overview image helps the reference pathologist to assess the correctness of the information that has been sent. He or she also can use it as a navigational tool for remotely controlling the microscope from his/her own site to acquire the images that he/she considers necessary for a correct assessment of the slide. This is shown in **Figure 20-2**.

To support the visual screening of a slide, the computer tracks the stage movement. As shown in **Figure 20-3**, the screening path is graphically displayed on the monitor (screening map) to give the pathologist a feedback of which parts of the slide he or she has already seen and which parts were missed.

All of the information accumulated by the workstation for one case, such as images, measurement results, graphic presentations of these results, patient data, preparation data, and screening maps, can be selected to be part of a report that can either be printed or signed out electronically via network. This report provides a very comprehensive picture of the case under evaluation and represents a large step in the direction of quality assurance and standardization.

Quantification of Disaggregated Tissues

The need to enzymatically disaggregate tissue samples for quantitative evaluation may arise if features have to be measured that require the entire cell or the whole nucleus to be in one piece. This is especially the case for diagnostic deoxyribonucleic acid (DNA) cytometry (10). Cell nuclei are stained quantitatively according to the Feulgen reaction (11) for their DNA content. Nuclear DNA can be used as an aid in diagnosis, to predict prognosis, and to determine management of certain neoplasms. The measured feature of interest, which is proportional to the stained DNA content of a nucleus, is the summed-up optical density. After calibration it translates into ploidy values.

In tissue sections a large number of nuclei are cut. The number depends upon the thickness of the section and the kind of tissue that has to be evaluated. The cut nuclei introduce severe problems for calibration and for the final interpretation of the ploidy distributions (12).

Quantification of the Cell Arrangement and Assessment of Tumor Heterogeneity

Tissue section analysis using image processing and analysis is far more difficult than individual cell analysis, which is usually required for cytologic analysis. Nevertheless, we can expect for histopathology a similar evolution as cytopathology, for which quantification has helped substantially to improve accuracy and robustness of interpretations. Bringing quantification into the field of tissue section analysis certainly represents one of the best solutions for improving quality control and quality assurance in this field.

As the tools are becoming more powerful, however, they are also often becoming more complex to use. Therefore, a large effort needs to be made to provide the cyto- and histopathologist with reliable internal quality control and quality assurance (13,14).

Quantification and Requirements

Recent developments in image processing techniques provide new tools to bridge the gap between cytology and tissue section analysis. Among these tools, very efficient ones, mainly issued from the mathematics of graphs (15,16), are designed to provide descriptors of tissue architecture as well as objective methods to sample and weigh cytologic results according to contextual information.

Based on the mathematics of graphs (17), sometimes called cellular sociology or syntactic structure analysis, this theory is primarily based on the neighborhood relationships extracted from the Voronoi diagram or its subgraphs such as the minimum spanning tree (18). Such methods, used together with the more "usual" image analysis descriptors (shape, densitometry, texture), provide the finest image processing and mathematical tools to help histopathologists objectively describe tissue organization regarding the functionality of cells considered along with the contextual information. In the near future this should allow pathologists to investigate specific regions of interest within a tissue section and objectively normal-

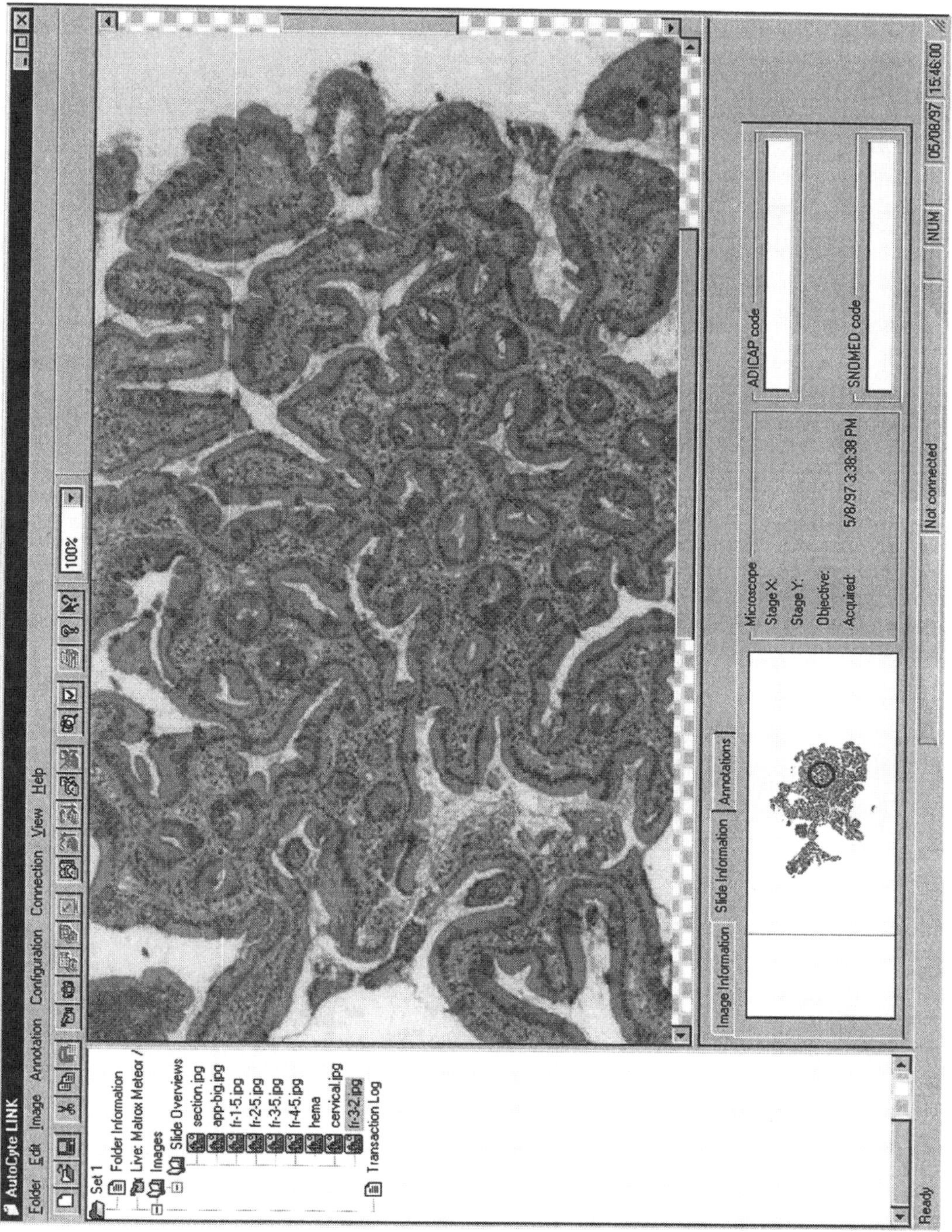

FIGURE 20-2
Slide overview and image folder for remote consultation (AutoCyte, Inc, Elon College, NC).

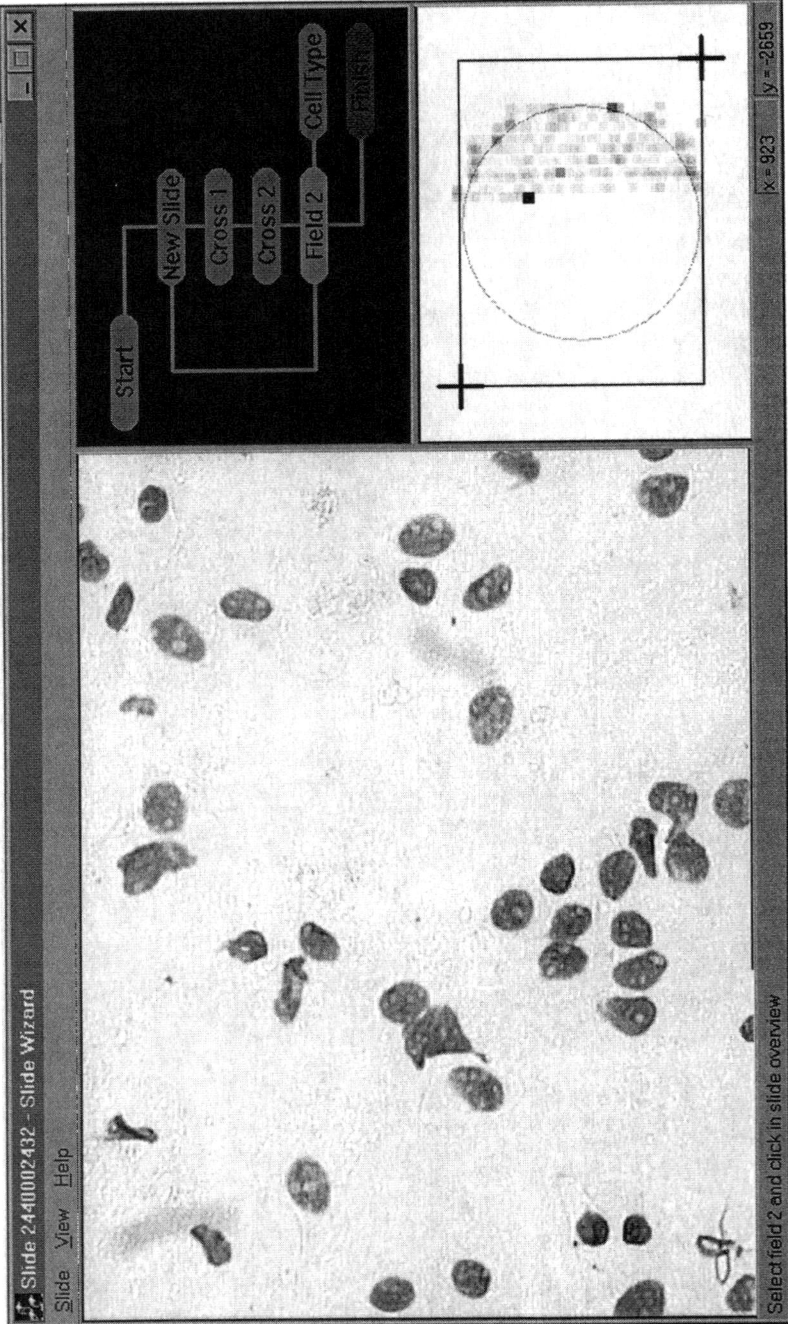

FIGURE 20-3

Screening map (*right bottom corner*) graphically tracing the stage movements (AutoCyte, Inc, Elon College, NC).

ize information according to their cytologic or histologic context, or both.

The main difficulty in tissue section analysis is the "segmentation" procedure, which is designed to extract from the original image a mask of the objects of interest, for example, the cells.

As was mentioned previously, once an image is digitized and stored in an image analyzer or a pathology workstation, the pictorial information offers the possibility of extracting quantitative data and can eventually be improved for qualitative human interpretation as well. Compared to single cell preparations, histopathologic sections present microscopic images of higher complexity, making segmentation a very sensitive issue for subsequent analysis and interpretation.

In the field of image processing, segmentation (i.e., partitioning of the image into identifiable objects) has always been a major problem. Usual segmentation approaches are based on the identification of regions within the image, which adhere to a given set of homogeneity criteria or are well separated from each other by transitional contours (19).

The diagnostic assessment of a histopathologic section is indeed based on the microscopic image, but the process relies to a very large extent on information that is not offered by the microscopic image itself (20). A tissue sections analyzer thus requires more sophisticated methods, with built-in external knowledge or the capability of referring to an external set of a priori laws when facing a specific problem.

The first antagonism encountered when working with light microscopic images is the antagonism of resolution versus space and time. In other terms, the more details that have to be revealed and assessed in a preparation, the larger the magnification needs to be. This results in a very small field of view and a much longer time to process the data. To solve this problem and get a good understanding of the biologic case, pathologists have developed the "muiti-scale analysis" concept. To get a good overall understanding of the region of interest under consideration, pathologists tend to screen parts of the slide at a given resolution, switching the objectives back and forth from low to high magnification. In this way they reveal either structural information or fine cellular details.

This multiscale analysis concept, adopted and in everyday use by histopathologists all over the world, is obviously a very good solution to help with segmentation. In effect, the result of the segmentation performed at a given resolution can be efficiently used as external knowledge to help the segmentation performed at a different resolution. A feedback loop can even be initiated by comparing the results of segmentation performed at different scales on single objects or groups of objects.

If good segmentation is a sine qua non requirement to perform the architectural analysis of tissue sections, the two basic requirements to help histopathologists with the interpretation of a case are as follows.

Present Conventional Data in an Efficient and Normalized Manner

The final report should contain the patient and case information together with a selection of images, presenting the overall region of interest, and some high-resolution images that illustrate the clues on which the final decision was based. If the overall region of interest covers several microscopic fields of view even at low magnification, the system should be able to construct an overview image by matching the related microscopic fields.

Provide Additional Information and Measurements that Are Difficult to Perform by a Human

Numerous studies have been devoted to cellular interactions and to cellular pattern analysis in order to elucidate the way that cell differentiation acts on cell scattering and clustering, or vice versa, to organize the living matter. It appears that there is an increasing importance in both general comprehension of mechanisms that govern cellular interactions and development of therapeutic applications to determine the organization and the kind of relations that cells are able to set up between themselves. A cell is not born in an information-free environment, but in a universe of signals sent out by its fellows. Thus the cell environment has to be considered as an environment organized by elementary exchanges between the population members where communication plays a structural part. Study of the way cells structure their own environment should therefore increase the knowledge of homeostatic tissular controls and of tumor heterogeneity, and allow us to draw information from spatial alterations seen in pathologic slides.

The purpose of tissue section analysis is to explore the relationships between cellular functions and spatial positions. It is possible to reduce cells to points by locating their centers of gravity and to treat such data sets as spatial point patterns. Studies based on statistical analysis or graph constructions have been used to search for parameters that describe order and disorder in tissues. Most of these approaches converge toward the use of graphs based on spatial partitioning such as the Voronoi paving, that is, the Voronoi diagram (21). The Voronoi diagram is a tesselation or subdivision of the two-dimensional space into partitions formed by polygons around the cell nuclei, such that any location of the space within a specific polygon is closer to the nucleus that gave rise to the polygon than to any other polygon. An example of local architecture computation based on the Voronoi diagram is presented in **Figure 20-4**. The basis for this graph is a picture of human prostatic tissue presented in **Figure 20-5**. To draw the overall region of interest, this picture was matched and stitched together out

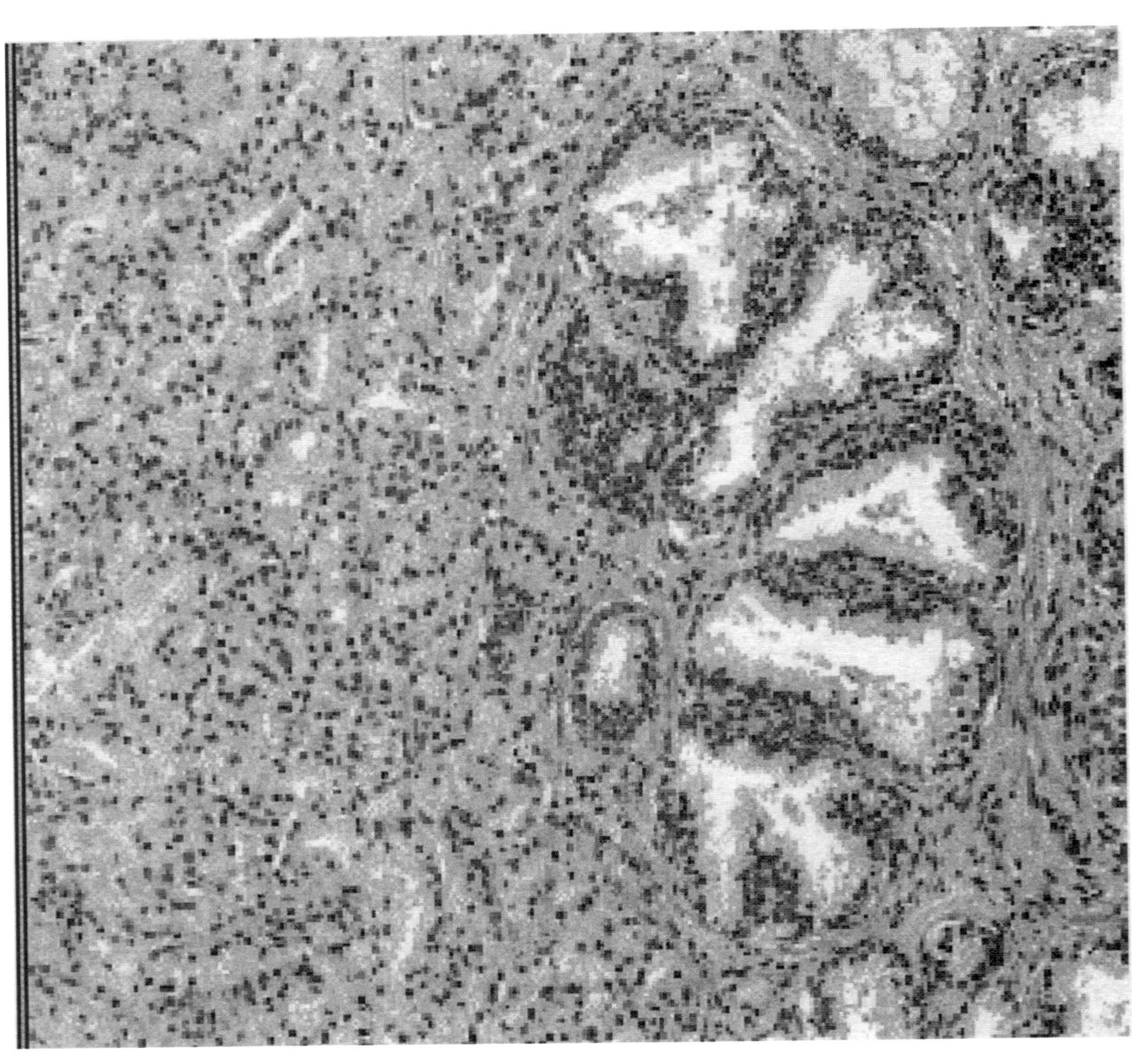

FIGURE 20-4

Local architecture evaluation of the image in Figure 20-5 based on the Voronoi diagram.

of nine adjacent fields, which were acquired with a 40x magnification objective.

This specific region of interest presents on its left side a prostatic cancer and on its right a more "normal-hyperplasia" type of prostatic tissue. The segmentation applied on the high-resolution images allowed a fine separation of the cell nuclei from the rest of the image. From the gravity centers of the nuclei, a Voronoi diagram was built and local configurations around each cell were measured, giving rise to a feature space, which is presented in false color on the synthetic image. The false color look-up table reveals a clear separation of the cancerous region from the normal one based on the computation of local topographic information extracted from the Voronoi diagram.

Three-Dimensional Imaging and Analysis

In the last decade a large improvement has been made to three-dimensional studies, primarily by the use of confocal laser scanning microscopy (CLSM). The CLSM bridges the gap between the traditional light microscope and the scanning electron microscope. It offers particularly high resolution—both lateral and in the direction of the optical axis—and a large signal-noise ratio, so that good signals can be obtained even from weak reflecting/fluorescing surfaces. A confocal aperture (pinhole) is placed in front of the photodetector so that the fluorescent light from points on the specimen that are not in the

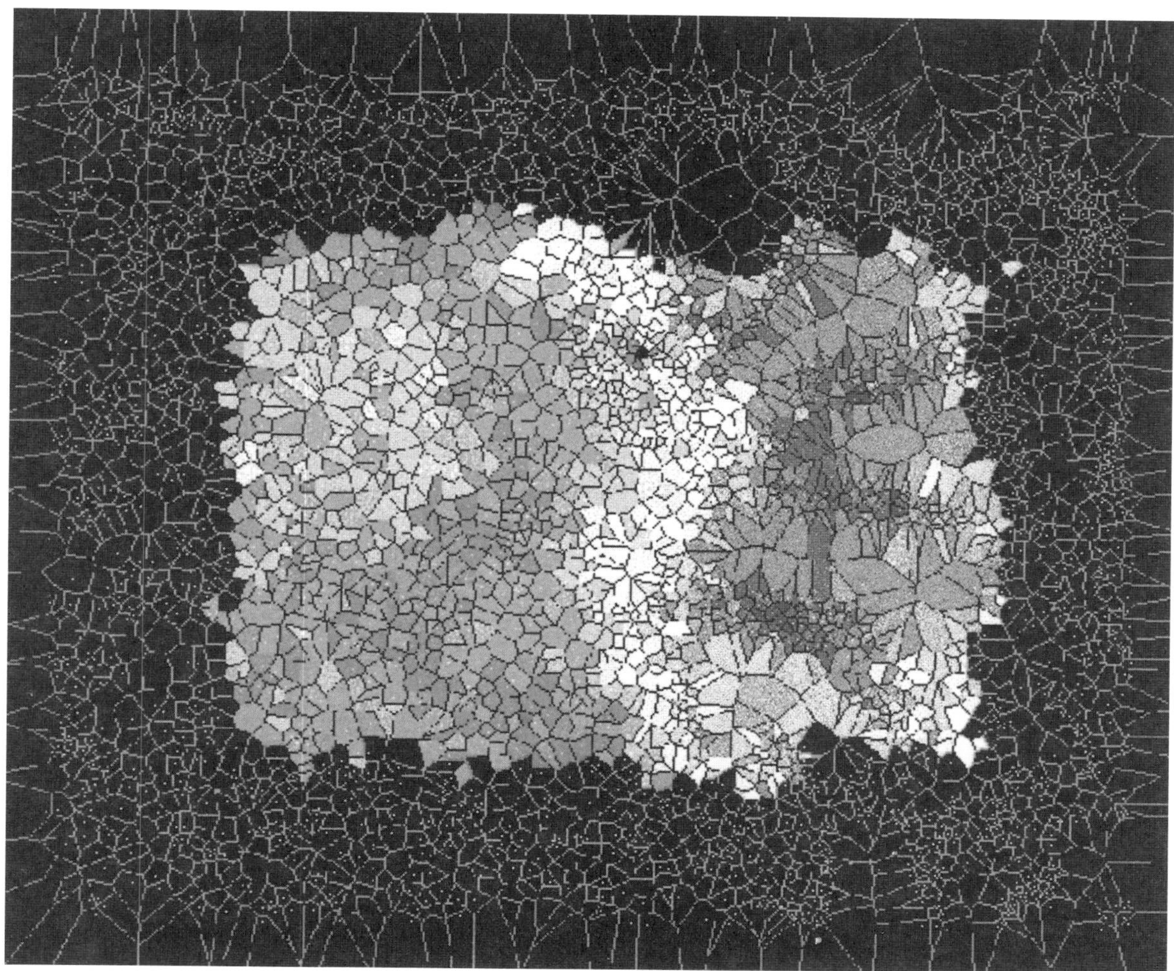

FIGURE **20-5**

A prostate tissue section matched and stitched together out of nine adjacent fields acquired with a 40x objective.

object plane in focus will be strongly de-emphasized by the pinhole. In this way, information from structures outside of the object plane is suppressed by the pinhole and the images produced are always sharp. The out-of-focus information, both above and below the focal plane, is greatly reduced, allowing an optical sectioning of even thick specimens.

Surfaces, tissue, cells, cell compartments, and microstructures within the cell can be imaged precisely in three dimensions and measured. This type of microscopy is therefore useful for investigations in pathology research that require fine three-dimensional analysis of surfaces and structures (22).

To build a three-dimensional data block from the specimen, the data of the object are recorded by moving a laser beam over the object in x and y direction and slightly displacing the object in z when a new plane needs to be acquired. Optical sectioning suppresses the usual distortion artifacts and the difficulty of precisely matching different layers. Typical focus motors can adjust the focal plane in as little as 0.1-μ increments. A three-dimensional reconstruction of a specimen can be generated by stacking two-dimensional optical sections collected in series.

Summary

Within the last decade vast methodologic and technologic improvements in the field of image analysis have changed the concept of the general purpose pathology image analyzer to a dedicated and comprehensive workstation for the routine pathology. These workstations are designed for routine work. Connected to large hospital information systems, they combine all the tools that are needed to provide the pathologist with the necessary information to arrive at the best results possible. These pathology workstations therefore contribute substantially to providing cytopathologists and histopathologists with accurate, reproducible, and objective data derived from cellular and tissue analysis.

Even if the evaluation of tissue sections using image analysis is far more difficult than the individual cell assessment usually required in cytologic analysis, new segmentation algorithms and an extensive use of the mathematics of graphs make it possible to measure both the global topography of a tissue section and the structure of the local environment of the cells. It is now possible to describe a tissue section and quantify specific features related to the tissue architecture and the functional status of the underlying cells. At the same time a far more comprehensive support for a reproducible and more standardized visual assessment of tissue sections has become available based on the creation, enhancement, and management of digital images.

Introducing quantification in the field of tissue section analysis will represent a large step in the direction of quality control, quality assurance, and standardization in the field of histopathology.

REFERENCES

1. Brugal G. Image analysis of microscopic preparations. Meth Achiev Exp Pathol 1984;11:1–33.
2. Hedley DW, Friedlander ML, Taylor IW, et al. Method for analysis of cellular DNA content in paraffin-embedded pathological material using flow cytometry. J Histochem Cytochem 1983;31: 1333–1335.
3. Mairinger T, Gschwendtner A. Comparison of different mathematical algorithms to correct DNA-histograms obtained by measurements on thin liver tissue sections. Anal Cell Pathol 1996; 11:159–171.
4. Krupinski EA, Weinstein RS, Bloom KJ, Rozek LS. Progress in telepathology: system implementation and testing. Adv Pathol Lab Med 1993;6: 63–87.
5. Ross JS. DNA ploidy and cell cycle analysis in pathology. New York, Toyko: Igaku-Shoin, 1996.
6. Gonzalez RC, Woods RE. Digital image processing. Reading, MA: Addison-Wesley, 1992:111–119.
7. AutoCyte, Inc. Product information. 112 Orange Drive, Elon College, NC 27244.
8. Schubert E, Gross W, Siderits RH, et al. A pathologist-designed imaging system for anatomic pathology signout, teaching, and research. Semin Diagn Pathol 1994;11:263–273.
9. Becich MJ, Gross W, Schubert E, Blank G. Building an information training program for pathology. Semin Diagn Pathol 1994;11:237–252.
10. Böcking A, Giroud F, Reith A. Consensus report of the European Society for Analytical Cellular Pathology Task Force on Standardization of

Diagnostic DNA Image Cytometry. Analytical and quantitative cytology and histology. 1995;17.

11. Whitaker BP, Stigliano WW, Carson FL, Lynn JA. Thionin Feulgen stain for DNA (ploidy) quantitation by image analysis. J Histotechnol 1993; 16:113–116.
12. Sapi Z, Hendricks JB, Pharis PG, Wilkinson EJ. Tissue section image analysis of breast neoplasms. Evidence of false aneuploidy. AJCP 1993;99:714–720.
13. Bigras G, Marcelpoil R, Brambilla E, Brugal G. Cellular sociology applied to neuroendocrine tumors of the lung: quantitative model of neoplastic architecture. Cytometry 1996;24:74–81.
14. Van Diest PJ, Baak JPA. Reproducibility and prognostic value of syntactic structure analysis in invasive breast cancer. In: Quantitative cyto- and histoprognosis in breast cancer. Amsterdam: Elsevier Science, 1992:99–107.
15. Bertin E, Parazza F, Chassery JM. Segmentation and measurement based on 3D Voronoi diagram: application to confocal microscopy. Comput Med Imaging Graphics 1993;17:3–4.
16. Toussaint GT. Pattern recognition and geometrical complexity. In Proceedings of the 5th International Conference on Pattern Recognition, Miami Beach, 1980. Catalog no. 80CH1499–3, pp 1324–1347.
17. Preparata FP, Shamos MI. Computational geometry. New York, Springer-Verlag, 1985.
18. Marcelpoil R. Normalization of the minimal spanning tree. Anal Cell Pathol 1993;5:177–186.
19. Chassery JM. Microscopic imaging. In 13th Annual International Conference of the IEEE EMBS, Orlando, FL, 1991;13:1113–1114.
20. Bartels PH, Gahm T, Thompson D. Automated microscopy in diagnostic histopathology: from image processing to automated reasoning. Int J Imaging Systems Technology 1997;8:214–233.
21. Okabe A, Boots B, Sugihara K. Spatial tesselations: concepts and applications of Voronoi diagrams. Chichester, UK: Wiley, 1992.
22. Usson Y, Parazza F, Jouk P-S, Michalowicz G. Method for the study of the three-dimensional orientation of the nuclei of myocardial cells in fetal human heart by means of confocal scanning laser microscopy. J Microsc 1994;174:101–110.

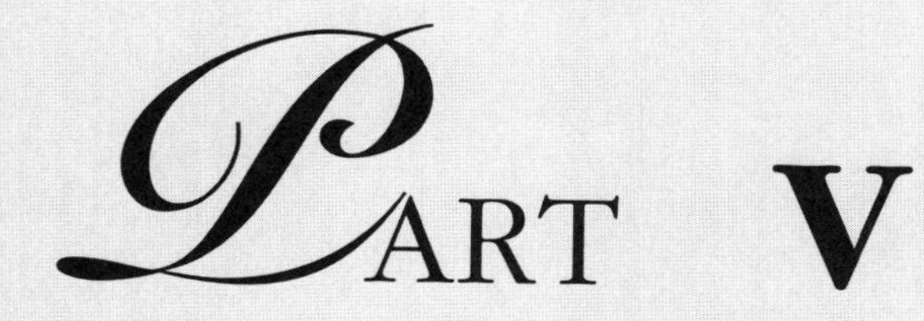

Part V

Recommendations for Quality Assurance and Standardization of Laboratory Procedures for Evaluation of Diseases Mediated by Immune Mechanisms

C. LYNNE BUREK, EDITOR

CHAPTER 21

Assessment of Immunodeficiency Diseases

C. KIRK OSTERLAND
A. FARHOUDI

One of the major challenges in modern immunology practice is the development of procedures that can be used routinely to guide physicians in the diagnosis of dysfunction of discrete elements of the host defense mechanism. The immune defense mechanisms work against foreign microorganisms in a preventive manner, and by aggressively responding to and attacking them. In addition, they provide a surveillance mechanism against malignant cell change and some control of the expression of autoimmune cells. The host defense mechanisms can be assessed by laboratory tests that measure specific cellular and humoral immune systems, and elements of the nonspecific defenses. The latter are often induced by activated immune cells, to amplify the effectiveness of specific immunity.

The host defense mechanisms can be impaired in many ways: as partly congenital defects seen predominantly in the pediatric age group, or as acquired conditions, secondary to infections, other primary diseases, or various forms of drug therapy. In selecting the appropriate diagnostic tests for a patient who exhibits recurrent infections and is suspected of having immunodeficiency, one naturally considers the clues given by the clinical presentation, such as age of the patient; growth and development history; types of infection, for example, pyogenic organisms (humoral), fungal (cellular), *Neisseria* (complement), and skin (macrophages or immunoglobulin E); and the family history.

A useful classification of the immunodeficiency disorders has been issued by the World Health Organization (WHO) (1), and specific descriptions of the clinical pictures of defects in individual components of the host defense system are well reported in a number of publications and are not reproduced here (2–12). Humoral immunodeficiency is the most common, but mild to severe impairment of cellular immunity can accompany many general conditions, including virus infections, nutritional defects, and malignancy. When defects are significant enough to result in repeated infections, the immunodiagnostic tests become most useful in defining the pattern of involvement of components of the immune mechanism. This will direct appropriate corrective steps.

The immune system provides the specificity of the activity of the host defense mechanisms. Receptor molecules on lymphocytes—surface immunoglobulins and T-cell receptors—interact with great precision with key epitopes of infectious organisms. Evidence for a normally operating immune system comes through the identification of clonal and polyclonal proliferation of T- and B-lymphocyte populations, or indirectly through the demonstration of elaborated soluble factors or activities that amplify the defense mechanisms, providing effector activity to the defenses. Examples of such systems are antibody-activated complement components and cytokine release by activated lymphocytes (13).

The clinical problem of immunodeficiency occurs in all age groups, but usually for different reasons. A spectrum of congenital immunodeficiency states have been described in the pediatric age group (2,11,12); some involve discrete elements of the host defense system (13,14), and others have a defective function of many elements. It seems surprising to find redundant and functionally overlapping elements in the host defense system. One element can be completely dysfunctional, yet the normally functioning mechanisms are able to compensate. This is a powerful and multilayered system.

The adult forms of immunodeficiency are more likely to be acquired than congenital. Human immunodeficiency virus (HIV)-related disease has clearly been the most remarkable and devastating example of these in recent years. The immunodeficiency states of acquired immunodeficiency syndrome (AIDS) have been studied intensively in relationship to the patterns of infection that occur, and this has increased the understanding of the components of host defenses that seem to be most critically important for protection against various types of infection. Other important forms of immunodeficiency in the adult are those secondary to primary diseases that affect the immune apparatus (e.g., lymphomas) or the effect of drugs given as part of the treatment protocol in autoimmune disease or transplantation medicine.

The laboratory procedures for assessing the status and the functionality of the host defense mechanisms can be considered in three parts: those that are most useful for humoral immunity, those for cellular immunity, and those that reflect the amplification of the expression of the first two by "nonspecific" effectors such as macrophages and soluble mediators. The focus here is on tests that have achieved standard use and are generally available in the clinical situation. Other tests that fit into a more advanced specialized category are mentioned primarily to point out their potential and the directions of future test development. These latter specialized tests are not available in all routine laboratories; their usage is often not supported by sufficient data showing adequate precision for diagnostic use. Advanced procedures are most often done as part of a research laboratory activity, and they often define the functional integrity of discrete components of the defense mechanisms. Because they have not been standardized, their principal usefulness is gained when the defect in the system being tested is pronounced. When they have achieved a sufficient degree of performance standardization and quality assurance that they can be relied on as a routinely available test, they will enrich the growing repertoire. This is a very dynamic field of diagnostic medicine, as the intricacies of the immune response are well characterized. The exciting part of diagnostic immunology will be seen when new standardized tests ultimately make it possible to measure surrogate markers for the function of all individual components of the immune system, and thus provide a really practical guide to immunotherapy. Therapeutics in immunology is becoming equally sophisticated, making it possible to consider boosting or replacing individual factors that may be defective in an individual.

Laboratory Assessment of the Integrity of Function of the Humoral Immune System

Most of the techniques used for assessing humoral immunity involve the principles of immunochemistry (4,6,15). By and large these tests are sensitive, quite specific, and highly accurate. These factors, along with the knowledge that the immunoglobulin (Ig) levels that are measured in the serum and other body fluids give a fairly true reflection of the functional level of humoral immunity, make this one of the more satisfactory parts of the overall assessment of host defense mechanisms. (In the case of measurements on lymphocytes or cytokines, the elements most critically involved in the defense against the disease process may not be best reflected in the peripheral blood specimens which are usually the ones available for analysis.)

Screening Procedures

Immunoglobulin measurement levels are dependent on a number of factors—age, sex, ethnic origins—so that a system of normal ranges must be established by each institution that reflects these interpopulation differences (4,6). What has happened is that quite broad ranges of normal values are used by most laboratories that undoubtedly reflect some patient heterogeneity. It is likely that the current quantitation technologies could allow the establishment of a more narrow range of normal values for selected age groups. As it stands there must be a considerably reduced value for Ig levels present to be referred to as hypogammaglobulinemia; it is likely that there are patients with impaired function of their humoral mechanisms who exhibit how normal or borderline Ig levels in the wide ranges used.

In routine practice only IgG, A, M, and E are measured to assess the presence of humoral immunodeficiency. Immunoglobulin D can be measured, and is usually absent in agammaglobulinemia, and often raised in hyper IgE syndromes (16). However, it rarely adds much to the clinical assessment. Immunoglobulins M, G, and A are present in highest concentrations in serum, although the IgA of greatest functional significance is that in mucosal surfaces and secretions, where it is present in the form of dimers and tetramers along with a J chain and a secretory component (14). The IgE is also produced largely in mucosal sites and, due to its high affinity for receptors on mast cells and basophil, practically all of it is located as a tissue-bound form.

The methods used most commonly for Ig measurements are zone electrophoresis (for total Ig) and nephelometry (for individual isotypes). Zone electrophoresis is simple and very inexpensive, but it requires an experienced operator to make the judgment on the zone for quantitation in a reproducible fashion, if the technique is to be used serially for following changes in the total Ig value. Some protein stains are differentially taken up by the various proteins so that corrections must be used for this. Electrophoresis alone can establish gamma globulin deficiency, but only when this involves IgG. The quantities of IgA and M in serum are not sufficient by themselves to reduce the total Ig zone below a normal range, even when these are absent.

Nephelometry that uses high-affinity sera specific for each individual Ig isotype has made this an accurate and very practical screening procedure (6). The problems of antiserum specificity, and of accurate quantitation of monoclonal gammopathies, have been largely overcome. Of greater relevance to the assessment of immunodeficiency are the preparation and quality control of special kits that have made measurement of low-level antigen concentrations much more accurate. Immunoglobulin G subclasses can be measured by low-level nephelometric kits, with or without a particle enhancement. Because this latter method increases the background signal and gives a small measuring range of turbidity, IgG subclasses and IgE are still frequently done by enzyme-linked immunosorbent assays (ELISA). The use of automated instrumentation has reduced the error in these that comes from the large dilution step of the samples that is used in performance of these assays.

Table 21-1 outlines some of the many forms of selective humoral immunodeficiency that may exist (15,17,18). Defects in IgG subclasses and individual isotypes are mainly restricted to pediatric practice although some

TABLE **21-1**

Immunoglobulin and Humoral Immunodeficiencies

Deficiency	**Remarks**
Nonselective	
Hypogamma IgG, A, M	Sometimes IgE normal or raised
Selective	
IgA	Most common, respiratory
IgM	
IgE	Sometimes with IgA
IgG1	Involved as opsonins
IgG2	Infections with encapsulated organisms
IgG3	Involved as opsonins
IgG4	Unclear significance; may have complement deficiency (18)
Other patterns	
Hyper IgE	Phagocyte dysfunction (16)
Hyper IgA, hypo IgM	Wiskott-Aldrich syndrome
Hyper IgM with hypogamma	Failure of isotype switch, X-linked, CD40L deficiency
M protein with "agamma"	Plasma cell dyscrasias with low physiologic Ig

forms of common variable immunodeficiencies seen in adults may also have isolated IgG subclass deficiencies. In measuring IgG subclasses it is useful to remember that if the total IgG is reduced, IgG1 almost certainly is involved. The other subclasses can be deficient and predispose to a humoral immunodeficiency state, even though total IgG values appear to be normal.

Measuring Antibodies

When an immunodeficient state appears to exist in the presence of normal Ig levels, it is useful to be able to measure specific antibody activities to assess humoral competence (19). This type of testing is probably best done in a central location, by a laboratory that is performing these tests in a sufficiently high volume to produce reliable results. The quantitative techniques for determination of most of these responses to specific antigenic stimulation are ELISA-type assays. The immunization technique and the specimen processing must be standardized to get the best, interpretable, results. A response to typhoid O antigen is dominantly IgM (as are the presence of ABO isoagglutinins in blood group A, B, or O subjects); responses to typhoid H, diphtheria, and tetanus toxoids are dominantly IgG, with those against pneumococcus being relatively specific for IgM and IgG2 subclass.

Antigen challenge results are particularly meaningful if done in a standard fashion. The antibody response is a reflection of the normal functioning of the phenomena involved in antigen recognition, processing, and cellular cooperation for producing help and cell proliferation signals. This is a highly labor-intensive procedure that is ultimately quite expensive; standardization is essential.

Secretory Humoral Immunity

Immunoglobulin A deficiency is the most common form of selective immunodeficiency, affecting 1/500 of the normal population (14). It may not be attended by symptoms of immunodeficiency, but this is more likely to occur when it is associated with IgG2 or IgG4 deficiencies as well. The latter population usually suffers from a high frequency of respiratory infections.

Most IgA is present in the body as secretory IgA found in almost all mucosal surfaces and secretions. More IgA is synthesized daily than IgG and it exists in two isotopic forms, termed IgA1 and IgA2. The latter is more prominent in secretions. Secretory IgA can be measured directly in properly harvested secretions, and with serum IgA deficiency, it is also usually absent. In medical practice it is not common to do quantitative tests to demonstrate selective secretory IgA deficiency. This may be a more useful procedure than is generally appreciated, and probably requires further studies.

B-Cell Measurements

The specific surface phenotypic markers, such as sIg, CD19, and CD20, make it possible to make quantitative B-cell measurements in peripheral blood (15). However, this has not become a very useful screening measurement for deficient humoral immune function. The B-cell count of peripheral blood has a rather wide and poorly established range, and it is, furthermore, influenced by many factors. Activated B lymphocytes that appear in peripheral blood are really in transit from a central lymphoid organ, and they may home to peripheral lymphoid sites on a single pass through the spleen, lymph nodes, or marrow. At a technical level, measurement of B lymphocytes by virtue of their surface Ig or their Fc receptors can be difficult to quantitate due to nonspecific surface absorption of Ig to the cells and reaction of receptors with the Fc domains of detector antisera. There are ways to correct for these difficulties, such as by staining for kappa and lambda determinants on B cells, which should show distinctive cell populations, and by use of $F(ab)_2^1$ reagents. Nonetheless, the usefulness of flow cytometry as a means to assess humoral immunodeficiency is probably still reserved for more use as an advanced-type procedure and to confirm certain types of B-cell deficiency.

Miscellaneous Procedures

In vitro mitogen responses can be a useful procedure for confirming the defect at the cellular level of an abnormality in the activation and maturation of B cells. It is also a useful method for analyzing B-cell development steps, in the research laboratory, and for determining the responsiveness of the maturing B cells to various growth and differentiation signals. However, these can hardly be used as standard procedures for the assessment of defective humoral immunity. All such tests are highly specialized, labor intensive, and therefore expensive, and they are poorly standardized.

Biopsy of lymphoid tissue can be of considerable value in precisely defining some forms of immunodeficiency, especially in the pediatric population. The availability of labeled antisera against epitopes that are specific for B cells at various stages of development have made this an even more powerful procedure. This aspect of immune testing is dealt with elsewhere in this volume.

Evaluation of the Integrity of the Cell-Mediated Immunity Mechanism

Of the two major adaptive arms of immune function, the cellular system is of prime importance (8,12,15). The T-lymphocyte receptors allow the cells to recognize and respond to peptide epitopes derived from proteins of infectious agents when these are presented in the context of major histocompatibility antigens. The T lymphocytes exist in multiple different forms that are distinguishable by their surface phenotypic markers. These different forms underlie the complex activities of T-lymphocyte cellular immunity, which range from the regulation of the immune response to its expression, as predominantly antibody or cytokine formation or as cytotoxic cellular activity.

It is possible to assess discrete components of T-cell functional activity in cases of apparent clinical immunodeficiency. It is generally accepted that cellular immunodeficiency predisposes to infection with intracellular organisms such as viruses and mycobacteria. However, as a result of the role of T cells in the regulation of the immune response, other types of infections may be seen with cellular immunodeficiency, such as gram-negative bacterial, fungal, protozoal, and so forth. Primary cellular immunodeficiencies are not common, but they are lethal if left untreated. Secondary forms of cellular immunodeficiency are common, often due to immunosuppressive drug therapy, malnutrition, viral infections, and other primary diseases. The methods that can be used to assess the integrity of T-cell function range from the very simple ones to the very complex. The latter are performed in low volume in most institutions, and are, thus, probably best done in a central reference laboratory, which can perform them in large enough volume to obtain the desired level of accuracy and precision, and some cost containment through the economy of scale.

Peripheral Blood Lymphocyte Counts

This is the most simple test for cellular immune competence. A lymphopenia is generally a count of less than 1500 cells/μL. However, marked age-related differences in lymphocyte counts exist and reference to these ranges must be made (4,15). A lymphopenia can represent a true depletion of T lymphocytes or it may also reflect mainly an abnormality in cell recirculation, and tissue redistribution due to a primary disease process or some drug effects. In the latter cases the lymphopenia may not be a constant or sustained finding. Primary immunodeficiencies commonly exhibit lymphopenia (severe combined immunodeficiency, enzyme deficiencies) while in those that are secondary to viral infections, malnutrition, lymphoma, and immunosuppressive therapy are variable. Lymphopenia is a common and useful parameter in assessment of immunodeficiency.

Delayed-type Hypersensitivity (DTH) Skin Testing

This is the most direct way of evaluating the integrity of cell responsiveness for cell-mediated immunity. It is a valuable screening method; normal reactivity confirms the intact functioning of antigen processing and presentation and recognition by specific memory T cells followed by a response with synthesis of lymphokines (at least those that are predominant in the DTH reaction such as interferon-alpha) (20).

Delayed-type hypersensitivity testing is done with a panel of antigens derived from common pathogenic microorganisms. A high proportion of the adult population is expected to show reactivity against at least one or two of these antigens 48 hours after intradermal injection. Unfortunately the standardization of antigens is imperfect and proper screening might require some repeat testing with increasing amounts of antigen. Nonreactivity to the commonly used *Candida* antigen may exist as an isolated specific immune defect in some patients who harbor chronic *Candida* infections.

Positive DTH skin reactions probably exclude significant intrinsic cell-mediated immunodeficiency. However, quantitating the vigor of the cellular immune mechanism by this method is difficult. Attempts have been made to make it more quantitative by preparing a multitest plate that contains reproducible, small standard amounts of antigen on each of several needle projections used for introducing the antigen intradermally. This should be technically a more satisfactory procedure than the traditional tuberculin syringe injection of 0.1 mL antigen intradermally, but, in fact, it is not always easy to apply the antigens in the multitest apparatus equally to all the skin sites. The reactions that occur are very small due to the minimal quantities of antigen used. However, the scoring is a quantitative sum of the diameters of induration given by all of the antigens, and it does give some element of quantitation and a reference score for subsequent testing if needed. For all DTH skin testing procedures, it would be useful (in the case of apparent anergy) to have a test antigen that would always give a positive reaction in normal subjects, and another that would demonstrate the ability to express a local inflammatory response reaction. The mitogen phytohemagglutinin (PHA) has been used by some laboratories as a standard positive DTH skin test reagent. It is not clear why this should give a universal response and it has not achieved widespread use. No commercial supplier has ever marketed a standard preparation for clinical testing. A maneuver that might be a useful future addition in DTH testing is a local cytokine application to a test site in an attempt to bring out or rescue DTH responsiveness in an anergic state and at the same time point to specific deficiencies.

Delayed-type hypersensitivity remains the best, although an imperfect, method for assessing cellular immune integrity. The technique needs even further standardization if it is to remain a gold standard. In its behalf, a large medical literature has pointed to the anergic state as being a highly unfavorable clinical prognostic factor for the progress of surgical and other patient populations. This is practical knowledge that can be applied as improved methods become available for "boosting" the activity of the cellular mechanisms.

Use of In Vitro Lymphocyte Proliferation Assays

These assays include short-term cultures of patient and control lymphocytes, in the presence of specific antigens, mitogens, and/or allogeneic cells (12,15). Mitogens such as PHA give specific stimulation indices of over 50 of nucleotide incorporation by the stimulated cells and true nonreactivity undoubtedly denotes significant cellular immunodeficiency. The mixed lymphocyte culture (MLC) specific stimulation indices are about 10 while those against specific antigen range from 2 to 4. There is a wide range between normality and reduced reactivity that makes this difficult to interpret and use in a medical decision-making situation. In vitro testing is expensive and time consuming, and requires costly equipment, radioisotopes, and so forth. The method is probably very low in precision, except when done by laboratories that regularly and routinely perform such tests. There is considerable day-to-day and person-to-person variation in numbers. This is not really part of a routine assessment; conceivably, proliferation assays could become more routinely useful if it were possible to modify the assay, making it much shorter and less dependent on cell separations. The use of changes of surface markers on cells by flow cytometry as they respond to antigen or mitogen, which can occur much earlier than deoxyribonucleic acid (DNA) synthesis (thymidine incorporation), is the direction for the future. However, considerable effort will be required to determine the optimal markers to assess and then to standardize the methodology and sample preparation before it can become a test that can influence clinical therapeutic decision making.

Flow Cytometry—T-Cell Subset Enumeration

The flow cytometer provides a very powerful tool for enumerating lymphocytes and their subsets (8). This can be extremely useful in helping to define the nature of the immune deficiency, and it can also point to quantitative changes, as in the case of the CD4/CD8 measurements in HIV infections.

Examples of lymphocyte markers that are well defined and that can be useful in assessing T cells are seen in **Table 21-2**. It seems probable that this technique will be used increasingly in the future to quantitate T-cell subsets that underlie discrete functions in cellular immune expression. The greatest obstacles to general use will be in the standardization of the methods. This is an example where the

TABLE **21-2**

Some Useful Phenotypic Markers Used in Evaluation of Cellular Immunodeficiency

Lymphocyte Population	Phenotype Marker	Normal Values (%)
Total	CD45, CD2	95–100
T cells	CD3	75–95
T helper/induced	CD4	40–60
T cytokine/suppressor	CD8	20–35
Natural killer	CD56	5–20
Activated T	HLA-DR	1–5
Interleukin-2 receptor	CD25	15–40

technical details in sampling and processing of the specimen will have extreme importance. The percentage values for various cell subpopulations may have little significance if the peripheral blood lymphocyte population itself is depleted or is being actively influenced by changes in recirculation and homing phenomena as a result of an active disease process or drug therapy (21,22). Flow cytometry is considered in Chapter 17.

Cytokine Measurements

The cytokines (CK) form a complex network of hormone-like proteins that have multiple overlapping activities (23). Functional properties in the immune system include growth stimulation, cell activation and differentiation regulation, and effectors in inflammation-related events.

Measurement of specific lymphokines would seem to be an ideal way to assess lymphocyte function, and it may be so in the future in some instances. Currently, as a means to assess the integrity of the cellular immune function, it probably only has use in procedures that combine in vitro culture with CK assay of the supernatants. Because most secreted cytokines function as autocrine or paracrine hormones, and not endocrine, the measurements on blood do not necessarily point to deficiencies. However, this may change, as immune assays are becoming more specific rather than tests that rely on biologic activities. At this time, the most promising CK measurements are ones used in assessing natural immunity, such as interferon (IFN), tumor necrosis factor (TNF), and interleukin (IL)-1 and -6, all of which do exist in a measurable amount in serum, with sufficient half-life to make assays feasible. Cytokine measurements remain expensive and highly specialized. Testing is still probably best done in a centralized laboratory, performing an adequate volume of assays and better standardizing the results.

It may ultimately be that the best way to use CK assessment will be through molecular techniques. A quantitative assay of messenger ribonucleic acid (mRNA) that specifically encodes cytokines could provide a superior index of immune cell function, and obviate the difficulties of short half-life, diurnal variation and drug and nutrition effects that influence blood CK measurements.

Other Measurements

Enzyme Defects

Evaluation of adenine deaminase (ADA) and purine nucleoside phosphorylase (PNP) enzymes is established and useful in the primary pediatric immunodeficiency population (2,3). Enzyme deficiency causes the accumulation of purine nucleotide metabolites that are toxic to developing T cells. These measurements could conceivably become of greater value in adult immunodeficiency diseases, as some immunosuppressive and cytotoxic drug therapies may influence the same nucleotide metabolite pathways. However, there are no substantial data on this point.

Tissue Biopsies

Lymph node and thymic tissue biopsies are of value primarily in primary pediatric population immunodeficiencies and through evaluation of phenotypic markers, and may yield critical information on the functionality of both T-cell and B-cell populations. This aspect of immunopathology is reviewed elsewhere in this volume.

Molecular Biology

Molecular techniques have contributed considerable new information to the diagnosis and treatment of the primary immunodeficiencies (5) by showing defects in cell receptor rearrangements. The role of molecular techniques in the assessment of the acquired immunodeficiencies may be quite different from this in the future. A quantitative estimate of lymphokine release from lymphocyte subpopulations done indirectly by an reverse-transcriptase–polymerase chain reaction (RT-PCR) method on mRNA extracted from a subject's cells could be quite useful since this will not be influenced by the many factors mentioned previously for serum cytokine measurements.

Tests for Non–Antigen-specific Host Defense Parameters and Amplifying Factors

There are many procedures in use that can test for the functional integrity of non–T- and non–B-cell related host defense functions. Some of these can identify important causes for a clinical immunodeficiency state. Unfortunately, many of the tests are difficult to perform, expensive, or still in a developmental, rather poorly standardized state. As with many procedures used in assessment for immunodeficiency, such low-volume tests are best done at a centralized facility. There is difficulty in assuring standardizing all of the details of sample procurement and processing that greatly influences results, especially for institutions that perform complex procedures only on rare occasions. With time standard procedure for these tests should improve adequate accuracy and precision so that their impact on clinical decision making will be highly possible.

Complement System

Most often the complement system of serum proteins and receptor molecules is assessed to demonstrate immune activation during ongoing disease activity (10). However, a number of genetic deficiencies of individual complement components are associated with a predisposition toward immunologic diseases, either autoimmune or immunodeficiency (18). Because of the latter group, it may be relevant in some cases of suspected immunodeficiency to screen for selected complement factors. Examples of complement deficiencies with defective host defenses are listed in **Table 21-3**.

When a patient with an apparent immunodeficiency state that is not due to a defined Ig or cell mediated immunity (CMI) defect has a decreased (or absent) CH50 level, isolated complement component deficiency is suspected. Commercial kits are available for measuring most of the complement components, or units such as the C6, 7, 8 membrane attack complex utilizing nephelometry or ELISA techniques. Interestingly, the major pattern of infection with complement deficiencies is bacterial and often neisserial, indicating the importance of opsonization and perhaps membrane attack bacteriolysis in the normal host defenses against these organisms.

TABLE **21-3**

Complement Deficiencies with Defective Host Defenses

Complement Activity	Infectious Complications
CH50, AH50	Bacterial infections
Factor H (alternative pathway)	Meningococcal infections
C3	Bacterial infections
Late components C5, 6, 7, 8,9	Neisserial infections
C5aR	Mucosal infections (32)

Cell Surface Adhesion Molecules

The effective immune response requires the cellular interaction between lymphocytes and macrophages. These cells are able to interact as a result of membrane molecules that are present on their surface either constitutively or induced transiently as part of the immune activation process. When these surface molecules are defective, a state of immunodeficiency can result (24).

The analyses for many of these surface molecules on individual cell types are highly specialized and not yet really in general use for screening cases with immunodeficiency. This will likely change over time as the reagents become even better, and when some standardization of methods and ascertainment of normal values are obtained.

The technique used is generally flow cytometry, a rapid and powerful technique when optimal antisera and specimen processing are available. It will remain to be seen if certain phenotypic determinations on cells such as the macrophage CD11, complement receptor molecules, or Fc determinants can ultimately be used as a satisfactory means to routinely estimate the functionality of various cooperating cell types of the immune system. This active area of development is already supported by several bodies interested in the standardization of the methods, a fact that should lead to increasing utilization of such tests in immune status assessment (21,22).

Cytotoxic Lymphocyte Assays

An example of analysis of a component of the host defense system [natural killer (NK) cell activity] has recently been described, using flow cytometry (25,26). The usual cytotoxic assays for NK cells using ^{51}Cr release techniques are time consuming and expensive, and have high variability, making them of questionable value as part of routine screening procedures. Yet measurement of the NK activity could be of considerable use in the assessment of immune function integrity in certain patients. If the phenotyping of peripheral blood leukocytes (PBL) for CD69 or other membrane antigens is specific to the NK population, it will make quantitative testing of this activity much more accessible.

Phagocyte Function—Neutrophil Function Tests

Neutropenias (and monocytopenias) can occur in a number of settings, secondary to primary diseases and due to drug or radiation effects, and this can represent a serious problem in host defenses. A number of specific conditions have been defined in which the defect in host defense is one that involves the phagocytic mechanisms, for example, Chédiak-Higashi chronic granulomatous disease (GGD) leukocyte adhesion molecule (selectins, integrins) defect, and Schwachmann's syndrome. The simple blood count may be deceiving, as when leukocytosis is present in the cases with adhesion molecule defects.

Many assays have been described to assess neutrophil functions such as chemotaxis, bactericidal activity, and superoxide production. Only a few of these have been standardized sufficiently and give enough precision to establish a defect in function in a given patient, unless the defect is extremely marked. When tests on macrophages requires the purification of cells before the assay, frequently a problem of metabolic activation of the cells has occurred during the isolation process. The nitroblue tetrazolium dye reduction reaction and a chemiluminescence assay have been the most extensively used for phagocyte testing (7,27). These procedures detect the functional ability of an individual's polymorphonuclear leukocytes (PMNs) to phagocytose particulate matter and generate either a metabolically induced reducing activity within the cytoplasm or emit a light signal that is amplified by luminescent compounds. The techniques have been used for years and are sufficiently well standardized to give a satisfactory assessment of phagocytic function. This is especially so when marked impairment exists such as in chronic granulomatous disease of children (27,28).

Macrophages are somewhat more difficult to assess individualiy than are PMNs. They can be tested in the same phagocytic and chemiluminescence systems as the PMNs but their activity signals are lower, requiring the isolation of the macrophages from PMNs before testing. This adds considerable labor and expense, and can also result in spurious activation in the cells. This is an area where it would be useful if a flow cytometric phenotype analysis could substitute for the labor-intensive assays that are available. However, to date, surface phenotype cannot be equated with functionality.

Standardization and Quality Assurance

In testing for the integrity of function of the various cellular and humoral components of the immune system, it is critical to attain both a high degree of test precision and standardization of techniques so that there will be good agreement between different laboratories (29,30). There are many difficulties in the standardization of immunologic procedures that are not only due to technical differences in methodology and instrumentation being used, but also to the methods used for specimen acquisition and processing. Factors that involve the timing of the specimen, speed of processing, sample storage, influence of drugs, and other factors may all greatly influence results. This can be a major difficulty in tests that are relevant to the assessment of cellular immunity. Since it will probably remain a fact that peripheral blood will be the main specimen available for testing, standardization and interpretation of results require special consideration. The most disease-relevant lymphocytes might not be what will be measured in such specimens; those are accumulating in pathologic tissue sites or central lymphoid organs. The normal values for various subsets of PBL will have to be determined under rigorously standardized conditions with such factors in mind, plus the possible confounding influence of active antigen exposure and drugs. Expert interpretation is required for accurate diagnostic conclusions to be drawn from tests done cellularly on peripheral blood leukocytes.

What has been very useful has been the establishment, through international workshops, of standardized assay samples for Ig and complement components, available from organizations such as WHO, the College of American Pathologists (CAP), and others. Antisera to leukocyte phenotype antigens have been well standardized through international workshops so that what remain are the rigorous standardization of the techniques of sample handling and measurement and the establishment of a known normal range of values for cellular subtypes under various standard conditions (21–23,31).

Immunochemistry measurements should be possible with good interlaboratory agreement. There are variations in values obtained that are instrument related, but these should be minimized by the use of calibration specimens and external standards (6). Nephelometry has come to be the method most often used, with individual preferences for the rate versus the steady state end-point analysis. The coefficient of variance (CV) of both methods has now achieved a very acceptable level. The difficulties in the assays of individual proteins become progressively greater as one moves into the enzyme immunoassays of low-level proteins, especially where significant background signals reduce the useful measuring range. This is part of the reason why the use of various cytokine-related measurements to assess the immune system integrity is still not at a level of unqualified acceptance.

The intricate details of the steps and sequence of events in immune function and the immune response are being defined in precise detail. It should ultimately be possible to select laboratory markers that will serve as accurate surrogate markers for measuring the integrity of discrete components of host defense mechanisms, as well as immune activation events.

The effective quality assurance program for all tests that assess immune integrity will include routine use of internal laboratory standards and calibrators, use of selected controls in sample runs, and the participation of laboratories in interlaboratory performance surveys. In addition to this, as has been pointed out, the technical problems of sample acquisition and processing will have to be rigidly standardized in order to be able to accurately interpret measured data on what are likely to remain less than ideal clinical specimens.

REFERENCES

1. Rosen FS, Wedgwood RJ, Eibl M, et al. Primary immunodeficiency diseases: report of WHO Scientific Group. Clin Exp Immunol 1995; 1(suppl. 99):1–24.
2. Conley ME, Stiehm ER. In: Stiehm ER, ed. Immunologic disorders in infants and children. 4th ed. Philadelphia: Saunders, 1996:201–252.
3. Markert ML. Purine nucleoside phosphorylase deficiency. Immunodeficiency Rev 1991;3:45–81.
4. Stites DP, Channing Rodger RP. Clinical laboratory methods for detection of antigens and antibodies. In: Stites DP, Wells JD, Wells JV, eds. Basic and clinical immunology. 7th ed. Lange, 1992.
5. Conley ME. Molecular approaches to the analysis of X-linked immune deficiencies. Ann Rev Immunol 1992;10:1063.
6. Zola H, Roberts-Thomsan P, McEvoy R. Diagnostic immunopathology. Cambridge, UK: Cambridge Press, 1995.
7. Farhoudi A, Harvey BA, Soothill JF. Neutrophil mobility defects. Arch Dis Childhood 1978;53: 625–630.
8. Rose N, DeMacario E, Fahey J, et al. Manual of clinical laboratory immunology. 4th ed. Washington, DC: ASM Press, 1992.
9. Sandberg ET. The secondary immunodeficiencies. In: Stiehm ER, ed. Immunologic disorders in infants and children. 4th ed. Philadelphia: Saunders, 1996:553–601.
10. Gaither TA, Frank MM. Complement. In: Henry JB, ed. Clinical diagnosis and management by laboratory methods. 18th ed. Philadelphia: Saunders, 1991:830–847.
11. Ochs HD, Winkelstein J. Disorders of the B-cell system. In: Stiehm ER, ed. Immunologic disorders in infants and children. 4th ed. Philadelphia: Saunders, 1996:296–338.
12. Hong R, Gatti RA. Disorders of the T-cell system. In: Stiehm ER, ed. Immunologic disorders in infants and children. 4th ed. Philadelphia: Saunders, 1996.

13. Buckley RH, et al. Disorders of the IgE system. In: Stiehm ER, ed. Immunologic disorders in infants and children. 4th ed. Philadelphia: Saunders, 1996.

14. Cunningham-Rundles C. Disorders of the IgA system. In: Stiehm ER, ed. Immunologic disorders in infants and children. 4th ed. Philadelphia: Saunders, 1996:423–442.

15. Hong R. Assessment of T and B lymphocytes in primary immune deficiency. In: Rose N, DeMacario E, Fahey J, et al. Manual of clinical laboratory immunology. 4th ed. Washington, DC: ASM Press, 1992:387–399.

16. Leung DY, Geha RS. Clinical and immunologic aspects of hyper IgE syndrome. Hematol Oncol Clin North Am 1988;2:81–100.

17. Ochs HD, Wedgewood RJ. IgG subclass deficiencies. Ann Rev Med 1987;38:325–340.

18. Bird P, Lachmann PJ. The regulation of IgG subclass production in man: low serum IgG with deficiencies in classical pathway of C3 activation. Eur J Immunol 1988;18:1217–1222.

19. Insel R. Interpreting vaccine responses. Pediatr Infect Dis 1990;9:424–433.

20. Gorden EN, Krause A, Kinney JL. Delayed cutaneous hypersensitivity in normals: choice of antigens and comparison to in-vitro assays of cell-mediated immunity. J Allerg Clin Immunol 1983;72:487–494.

21. American Society for Histocompatibility and Immunogenetics. Standards for clinical flow cytometry and cell phenotyping. American Society for Histocompatibility and Immunogenetics, 1986.

22. Calvelli T, Denny T, Paxton H. Guidelines for flow cytometric immunophenotyping. Cytometry 1993;14:702–715.

23. Romagnani G. Lymphokine produced by human T cells in disease states. Ann Rev Immunol 1994; 12:227–257.

24. Mach B, Steimle V, Reith W. MCH class-II deficient combined immunodeficiency. Immunol Rev 1994;138:207–221.

25. Kane KL, Ashton F, Schmitz J, Folds J. Determination of natural killer cell function by flow cytometry. Clin Diagn Lab Immunol 1996;3:295–300.

26. Hatam L, Schuval S, Bonagura V. Flow cytometric analysis of natural killer function as a clinical assay. Cytometry 1994;16:59–68.

27. Quie GP, et al. Disorders of the polymorphonuclear phagocytic system. In: Stiehm ER, ed. Immunologic disorders in infants and children. 4th ed. Philadelphia: Saunders, 1996:443–468.

28. Quie PG, Herron J. Neutrophil assessment. In: Rose N, DeMacario E, Fahey J, et al, eds. Manual of clinical laboratory immunology. 4th ed. Washington, DC: ASM Press 1992:419–420.

29. Hancock JJ, Taylor RN, Johnson C, et al. Quality of laboratory performance in testing for HIV type I antibody. Arch Pathol Lab Med 1993;117: 1148–1155.

30. Roberts-Thompson P, McEvoy R, Gale R, et al. Quality assurance of immunodiagnostic tests on Australia. Pathology 1991;23:125–129.

31. US Department of Health and Human Services. 1979 Quality Control for Immunologic Tests. HHS Publication No. CDC-82-8376.

32. Hopken U, Lu B, Gerard NP, Gerardi C. The C5a chemoattractant receptor mediates mucosal defence. Nature 1996;383:86.

CHAPTER 22

Systemic Rheumatic Diseases

ROBERT M. NAKAMURA
C. KIRK OSTERLAND

The hallmark for laboratory diagnosis of systemic rheumatic diseases is the identification of abnormal *bands* of autoantibodies that are specific for nuclear and cytoplasmic antigens (1–4). Many of these cellular autoantigens are involved in essential cellular functions such as deoxyribonucleic acid (DNA) in replication, proteins that are active in ribonucleic acid (RNA) processing and splicing of precursors to messenger RNA (1–4). Considerable progress has been made in the understanding of the biologic events, pathogenesis, and immune mechanisms of the various systemic rheumatic diseases during the past decade. The role of many of these autoantibodies is not clear; their intracellular location seems to render them inaccessible to potentially noxious autoantibody. However, the close correlation between disease patterns and the specific autoantibodies formed implies a close correlation between the autoimmunity and disease.

Classification of Types of Diseases

The classification of the systemic rheumatic diseases has been difficult, both from the laboratory and clinical aspects, since in many of the diseases, a definite etiology is still unknown (5). A modified classification from JL Decker and the Glossary Subcommittee of the American College of Rheumatology (5) is shown in **Table 22-1**. Many of the systemic rheumatic diseases have a distinctive profile of autoantibodies used in established precise diagnosis (1–4).

Some examples of several of the major autoantibodies and their disease associations are listed in **Table 22-2** (1–4,6). Systemic lupus erythematosus (SLE) is the prototype of the systemic rheumatic autoimmune diseases, and patients exhibit multiple abnormalities of the immune system with evidence of hyperactivity of the B cell–related humoral immune system (6). The tissue injury that occurs in SLE is largely mediated by immune complexes such as DNA–anti-DNA. The patients demonstrate a heterogeneous polyclonal antibody response; the typical case of SLE has an average of *three* different circulating autoantibodies against tissue antigens simultaneously (7). More than 25 different specificities of autoantibodies have been identified in SLE (7). Most of the common autoantibodies of these are listed in **Table 22-3** (6).

Role of the Immunology Laboratory in the Diagnosis, Evaluation, and Management of Diseases

The clinical immunology laboratory may be extremely helpful in establishing a diagnosis or in ruling out a specific diagnosis, confirming a suspected diagnosis, or subclassifying a systemic autoimmune disease. This is essential for optimal treatment and for determining prognosis (8).

The immunology laboratory professional should work closely with physicians to provide education and information concerning the best use, application, and limitations of the various tests that are available for diagnosis and evaluation of the specific disease. These tests are useful for establishing precise diagnosis and classification of a case of systemic

TABLE 22-1

Systemic Rheumatic Diseases and Related Disorders

1. Systemic lupus erythematosus (SLE)
2. Discoid lupus erythematosus (DLE)
3. Lupus-like syndromes
4. Drug-induced lupus erythematosus
5. Sjögren's syndrome
6. Scleroderma/CREST syndrome (calcinosis, Raynaud's, esophageal dysmotility, sclerodactyly, and telangiectasia)
7. Rheumatoid arthritis
8. Dermatomyositis and polymyositis
9. Mixed connective tissue diseases (MCTD)
10. Overlap syndromes
11. Connective tissue disease syndromes that have been poorly defined as to clinical category

autoimmunity; however, they are not the best ones to use for monitoring the course of the disease and impacting on therapeutic management.

The role of the diagnostic immunology laboratory in medical practice has been summarized as follows (8):

1. Provide laboratory evidence of specific immune responses to disease-related antigens (i.e., diagnosis and classification)
2. Assess the status and state of activation of the immune system (disease monitoring)
3. Ascertain the value of various laboratory tests in the diagnosis and evaluation of patients (clinical research procedures, evaluation)

TABLE 22-2

Nuclear and Intracellular Autoantibodies and Disease Associations

Antibody To	Disease Association
Double-stranded (native) DNA	Highly specific for SLE (40–60% incidence) when in moderate to high titer
Single-stranded (denatured) DNA	Present in SLE, in other rheumatic diseases, and in nonrheumatic diseases
Individual histones H1, H2A, H2B, H3, H4	SLE (70%), drug LE (>95%), RA (15%)
Histone complexes H2A-H2B, H3-H4	SLE (70%), drug LE (>95%)
Sm (25K, 16K, 10K, 9K, and other proteins with U-RNAs)	SLE (30%), highly specific
U1-RNP (19K, 70K, and other proteins with U1-RNAs)	MCTD (>95%), SLE (35%)
SS-A/Ro (protein with small RNAs)	SS (70%), SLE (50%), other CTDs
SS-B/La (45K protein with RNA pol III transcripts)	SS (40–50%), SLE (15%)
Proliferating cell nuclear antigen (PCNA)	SLE (3%)
Ku (DNA-binding proteins)	SLE (10%)
K1 (nuclear protein 32 kDa)	SLE (31%)
Scl-70	70% in diffuse scleroderma
Centromere/kinetochore	70–80% in CREST, diffuse scleroderma (10–20%)
RNA—pol I	4–20% in scleroderma
Fibillarin	8% in scleroderma
Jo-1 (histidyl tRNA synthetase)	Polymyositis/dermatomyositis (23–36%)
PL-7 (threonyl tRNA synthetase)	Polymyositis/dermatomyositis (4%)
M_{1-2} (proteins 53 and 61 kDa)	Polymositis/dermatomyositis (5–35%)
PM-Scl (complex of 11 proteins)	Polymyositis/dermatomyositis (8–12%)

TABLE 22-3

Antigens and Autoantibodies in Systemic Lupus Erythematosus

Antigen	Molecular Structure	Autoantibody Frequency (%)
Native DNA	Double-strand DNA	40
Denatured DNA	Single-strand DNA	70
Histones	H1, H2A, H2B, H3, H4	70
Sm	Proteins, 29(B′), 28(B), 16(D), and 13(E) kDa, complexed with U1, U2, and U4–U6 snRNAs; splice some component	30
Nuclear RNP (U1-RNP)	Proteins, 70, 33(A), and 22(C) kDa, complexed with U1-snRNA; splice some component	32
SS-A/Ro	Proteins, 60 and 52 kDa, complexed with Y1–Y5 RNAs	35
SS-B/La	Phosphoproteins, 48 kDa, complexed with Y1 nascent RNA pol III transcripts	15
Ku	Proteins, 86 and 66 kDa, DNA-binding proteins	10
Ki	Nuclear protein, 32 kDa	31
PCNA/cyclin	Protein, 36 kDa; auxiliary protein of DNA polymerase	3
Ribosomal RNP	Phosphoproteins, 38, 16, and 15 kDa associated with ribosomes	10
Hsp 90	Heat-shock protein, 90 kDa	50
S10	Ribosomal small subunit protein, 20 kDa	11
Cardiolipin	Anionic phospholipids	20–40

4. Provide laboratory assistance in clinical decision making (through evaluation of test procedures in the clinical setting).

Laboratory Tests for Diagnosis and Evaluation of Systemic Rheumatic Diseases

In the clinical and laboratory evaluation of systemic rheumatic diseases, screening tests are used to detect the presence of antibodies to nuclear, cytoplasmic, and sometimes membrane antigens. Secondary, more definitive tests are then used to identify the specificity of the antibody detected by screening.

The commonly used methods for autoantibody detection are listed in **Table 22-4** with a notation on their laboratory characteristics. The most commonly used screening test in the clinical laboratory today is immunofluorescence microscopy (IFM), which is quite sensitive in providing evidence for the presence of a large number of tissue antigens. Immunoenzyme analysis, which is very sensitive, can also be used as a screening test if a substrate that contains multiple known tissue antigens is used (9,10).

A second level of more definitive tests is used for specific identification of autoantibody specificities. These include immunodiffusion, counterimmunoelectrophoresis (CIE), particle agglutination, immunoenzyme tests, enzyme-linked immunosorbent assay (ELISA), and a combination of procedures as with "Western" immunoblotting (9–11).

Immunofluorescence Microscopy (IFM) Test

The IFM test, first described by Robbins et al (12) and Friou (13) in 1957, is still a very important means of evaluating patients with systemic rheumatic diseases. The immunofluorescence microscopy test, often called the indirect

TABLE **22-4**

Methods for Detection of Autoantibodies

Method	Antigen Source	Sensitivity and Use
Immunofluorescence microscopy (IFM)	Tissue sections; cell lines	Sensitive assay; used often for screening
Double immunodiffusion (ID)	Tissue and cell extracts (thymus and spleen)	Requires precipitin reaction and high specificity but not very sensitive immunologic procedure
Counterimmunoelectrophoresis (CIE)	Tissues and cell extracts (thymus and spleen)	Increased sensitivity and speed as compared with ID procedure
Particle agglutination	Purified native or recombinant antigens	Sensitivity is greater than immunodiffusion; specificity is dependent on purity of antigens
Immunoblotting (IB)	Cell extracts	Very sensitive; permits detection of antibodies against soluble and insoluble antigens
ELISA	Purified native or recombinant antigens	Very sensitive; quantitative; can determine antibody class

immunofluorescent antinuclear antibody (IF-ANA), or just ANA, has undergone modifications in recent years to bring about better standardization of the tissue substrates used in the screening procedure. The use of a continuously growing culture of human epithelium-derived cells has become an accepted standard substrate. The monolayers of Hep-2 cells must be handled by the same method in washing, fixation, using the same buffers for reaction and washing, to achieve optimal reproducibility and standardization. The patient's antibody binds to the nuclear and/or cellular constituents of the Hep-2 cell and is subsequently visualized using an anti-human immunoglobulin (Ig) that has a standardized amount of fluorescent label. Visualization of the staining pattern is most often done now with incident illumination fluorescence microscopy (14).

The test result is reported as negative or positive if positive fluorescence is seen at a defined screening dilution. The test and its reading are further refined by doing end-point dilution to titer the autoantibody, and by defining specific patterns of nuclear and cytoplasmic staining that relate to antibody specificities.

Standardization of the IFM Test

Standardization of the screening test for ANAs has been difficult. Many factors influence the test, including substrate and fixation variations, microscopic optics, and methods of "quantitating" results. Concerted efforts have been made to establish reference ranges and some uniformity in the interpretation of results. The difficulties associated with standardization of screening (5,14–16) and the quantitative analysis of ANA have been discussed in the report of the College of American Pathologists (CAP) Proficiency Survey and in the Centers for Disease Control's results in diagnostic immunology (15).

A National Committee for Clinical Laboratory Standard Document 1/LAZ-T Guideline, "Quality Assurance for the Indirect Immunofluorescence Test for Autoantibodies to Nuclear Antigens (IF-ANA)," was revised in 1992 (14). The standardization has been improved with the use of reference ANA sera, uniform assay conditions, and standardization of the optical systems (5,14–6).

The following guidelines were recommended in the performance of the IF-ANA test:

1. Each laboratory should establish a range of reference values for 95% of the population with representative patients from age groups younger than 40 and older than 40. Usually the screening procedure that is used should not give a positive result in more than 2.5% to 5.0% of a "normal" test population.
2. In performance of the quantitative tests, one should have a uniform section of substrate that is reacted with a defined amount of serum dilution. The primary immunofluorescent (or immunoenzyme conjugate) should be added in excess to the washed

tissue substrate that has been reacted with test serum or controls, or both.

3. The result of the reaction done at screening conditions can be roughly graded as positive, strongly positive, and negative. More quantitative end-point titrations of the test serum can determine the "amount" of antibody in the patient's serum.
4. An ideal way to report immunofluorescent ANA would be to establish an end-point titer of the specimen and to report the result as positive at a particular dilution in relation to the normal range. The interpretation of normal or abnormal would be the laboratory interpretation of a sufficiently strong reaction rather than a clinical assessment.
5. A low-titer ANA control serum should be included in the assay run, as most difficulty occurs in the identification of weak but significant positive ANAs.
6. Each lot of substrate slides should be checked to see if the test will detect SS-A/Ro antibodies; that is, the culture cell line expresses sufficient amounts of this protein. Reference sera for help in standardization of IFM or IF-ANA tests are available from the World Health Organization and the Arthritis Foundation (9).

Clinical Interpretation of the IFM Screening Test for Nuclear and Intracellular Autoantibodies

The high sensitivity of this test leads to the detection of ANA in patients with a wide variety of conditions and in 5% of non-elderly normal persons (11,17). The IFM test is sensitive but has a low diagnostic specificity for SLE (20–35%) (17). A patient with a negative IFM-ANA test has less than a 0.14% chance of having SLE. Therefore, the IFM-ANA can be primarily used to exclude the diagnosis of SLE (18). It is a relatively easy to perform and useful screening test.

IFM-ANA is a good test for the diagnosis of SLE but not for monitoring its clinical course and therapy. As with most serologic procedures, there is a poor correlation between response to therapy and quantitative titers of IFM-ANA. A 50% reduction of autoantibody might reduce the end-point titer by only one dilution.

The tests that are most useful for monitoring the course of SLE and making decisions from this on therapeutic measures are generally ones that reflect the activation status of the immune system or the intensity of the ongoing inflammatory reaction, or both. These include cell counts, complement component determination, and the measurement of some serum proteins whose levels serve as indices of inflammation or immunologic activity. These are useful but imperfect techniques; a great deal of further clinical research is needed to better evaluate the usefulness of such measurements as flow cytometry for specific activation markers on cells, complement component activation products, and some cytokine products. It is possible that molecular methods may provide a better measure of some of these than do the more traditional immunochemical methodologies. There are tests directly relevant to the expression of the autoimmune process that are still considered useful for the monitoring of SLE (3–5,7):

1. *Double-stranded (ds)-DNA antibodies.* The presence of high titers of these antibodies is an unfavorable prognostic factor and is related to disease activity. The SLE patient with these antibodies is at risk when tissue destruction (i.e., high exposure to ultraviolet sunlight) has occurred, allowing subsequent formation of increased quantities of DNA–anti-DNA immune complexes; both reflect the activity of a major pathogenetic process in this disease.
2. *Serum immune complexes and complement assays.*
3. *Early proteinuria.* This indicates injury to the kidney and can be an indirect indicator of ongoing formation of noxious immune complexes. SLE is often complicated by immune complex glomerulonephritis, resulting in an active urine sediment and proteinuria, and later by decreasing renal function.

The IFM-ANA is positive in 68% of patients with Sjögren's syndrome, 16% of individuals with juvenile rheumatoid arthritis (RA), and 25% to 50% of patients with rheumatoid arthritis. A negative result may be observed in patients with Sjögren's syndrome, polymyositis, rheumatoid arthritis, and scleroderma, yet some such patients may demonstrate nuclear antibodies and cytoplasmic proteins by other specific immunologic tests. When these particular rheumatoid diseases are clinically suspected, one should consider tests that will identify the specific antibody activities that are part of the screen (1–5).

Are There Patients with SLE Who Are Antinuclear Antibody Negative?

In the past, there have been reports that the amount of SLE serum testing ANA negative may be as high as 5% of the total population of SLE patients (19). Today, ANA-negative SLE patients are still recognized, but, with the improved supplementary diagnostic tests, patients rarely have gone undiagnosed and untreated because of a negative IFM-ANA test and these individuals constitute only a small percentage of patients. The IFM-ANA may give negative nuclear staining in some cases of SLE but show antibodies restricted to cytoplasmic constituents (7). The ANA test is sensitive and therefore very useful as a screening procedure. It does not serve as a diagnosis of systemic immunity, but a negative test nonetheless makes this diagnosis highly unlikely.

Recently, it has been brought to the attention of the clinical laboratories that quality assurance programs designed to detect SS-A/Ro antibodies with their screening tests are needed (20). The inability to detect SS-A/Ro antibodies may account for a significant percentage of so-called ANA-negative SLE cases. The tissue substrate must contain sufficient amounts of Ro antigen and it should be remembered that Ro can be present in both nuclear and cytoplasmic compartments.

Autoantibody to SS-A/Ro is present in high frequency in a clinical subset of lupus called subacute cutaneous lupus erythematosus. Many patients with subacute cutaneous lupus erythematosus have been falsely labeled as having ANA-negative lupus. It has now been shown that many of these individuals will demonstrate a positive IFM-ANA test result on substrate of human tumor KB and Hep-2 cells containing increased amounts of the SS-A/Ro antigen (20).

Variations in Methodologies Used for Detection of Autoantibodies to Nuclear Intracellular Antigens

The various tests used for antibody detection vary greatly in specificity and sensitivity. For example, the primary antibody-binding assays, such as enzyme immunoassay and IFM for ANA, may be 1000 times more sensitive in picking up some detectable signal than the immunodiffusion assay. On the other hand, techniques are available to enhance the precipitin band formation in the gel diffusion method. It should be emphasized that though gel diffusion is less sensitive, assays usually demonstrate a higher specificity in the diagnosis and characterization of a specific disease (9,21). For this reason, and because of the difficulty in interpreting weak or borderline optical density (OD) values in the immunoassays, gel diffusion methods remain popular.

The best studies regarding the different methods for the detection of autoantibodies to intracellular antigens were reported by a European Consensus Study Group (22,23). The European Consensus Study Group for the Detection of Autoantibodies to Intracellular Antigens in Rheumatic Diseases was formed in 1988 and has conducted four annual workshops from 1989 to 1992. The 1988 and 1989 consensus workshops were conducted to define interlaboratory concordance in the detection of autoantibody specificities in rheumatic diseases. Twenty-eight laboratories participated in the study using various methodologies (22,23). The objectives of the consensus study initiated in 1989 were 1) define the interlaboratory consensus in detecting autoantibodies and specificities, 2) test whether discrepancies were due to the methodology used, and 3) make recommendations for improved quality of results with improved sensitivity and specificity. Some of the conclusions of the study are summarized below.

IFM Method

The European Consensus Study found that culture cells (Hep-2) were the preferred method for the detection of autoantibodies. The culture cells in mitosis were needed to detect anticentromere antibodies; antibodies against antigens usually found in the cytoplasm, such as Jo-1, Ss-A/Ro, ribosomal-RNP (rib-RNP), and protein P, were easily missed. It is probable that greater experience with the currently available cell lines done in conjunction with specific antibody assays will further improve the sensitivity of this screening method.

Immunodiffusion (ID) Method

Double immunodiffusion analysis has been used to determine specificity of several ANAs. Assay specificity in double immunodiffusion is generally dependent on the quality of other control sera used in the procedure as well as the purity of the antigen preparation. The same is true for enzyme immunoassays, but one deals only with a printed OD value rather than the visual evidence of some lack of monospecificity. Although the ID tests are not very sensitive, their high degree of specificity continues to make them useful as a diagnostic marker in certain rheumatic diseases.

The European Consensus Group Study has reached the following conclusions:

1. The ID method is much less sensitive than the counterimmunoelectrophoretic technique. However, CIE only works well with antigens that are sufficiently negatively charged that they can migrate to encounter the IgG antibodies that are moving in a cathedral direction by endosmosis.
2. The detection rate of SS-A/Ro antibodies was very poor, with an overall detection rate of 42% in the 1991–1992 study. The reasons for this are still not clear and the method for this relatively important autoantibody specificity needs to be better standardized.
3. The CIE method had a 97% detection rate in the European study, while the immunoblotting (IB) method results were very poor, with a 50% detection rate.
4. In the determination of antibodies to Scl-70 by ID with use of rabbit thymus extracts, a concentration of 60 to 80 ng/mL concentrated extract had to be used to obtain satisfactory results. The extracts that contain antigen are very stable to −20°C and can be stored at −70°C.
5. Antibodies to rib-RNP were difficult to detect by ID or CIE.

Counterimmunoelectrophoresis (CIE)

The counterimmunoelectrophoresis method is similar to the ID but approximately 10 times more sensitive if the gel medium and pH conditions are ideal for the antibody and antigen to become concentrated together by the electrophoresis. However, the final test result is again an immunoprecipitin line.

In the European study, the following observations were also made:

1. Most laboratories used rabbit thymus extract (Pel Freez) as antigens.
2. There was good overall performance for antibodies to SS-B/La, Sm, and nuclear ribonucleoprotein (nRNP). When mixed specificities were present in the serum, such as Sm/nRNP, the anti-Sm antibody often appeared to hamper the detection of a weak anti-nRNP activity. Conversely, anti-nRNP can hamper detection of anti-Sm by CIE or ID. This effect can be overcome by using trypsin treatment of the antigen preparation, which eliminates the NRNP epitope but which apparently does not destroy the Sm.
3. The Jo-1 and Scl-70 activities were missed by 33% and 50% of laboratories, respectively, with the use of CIE. When extracted from rabbit thymus, the Jo-1 and Scl-70 antigens are quite unstable when stored at −20°C. The use of fresh concentrated extracts of thymus is recommended for Jo-1 and Scl-70 assays. The extracts should be stored at −70°C to ensure better stability of the antigen.
4. The anti–rib-RNP, when assayed by CIE, was missed by most laboratories. A few laboratories reported an unidentified precipitation line. A reference serum for anti–rib-RNP is recommended to ensure that the antigen extract contains immunochemically reactive rib-RNP.
5. The SS-A/Ro antibody was detected by CIE by most laboratories. An antigen extract of spleen is necessary for this test.

Immunoblotting (IB)

Immunoblotting is sensitive and is an important means for characterization of the specific nature of the antigens and the isotopes of the autoantibodies. However, as suggested by the European study, its rate of detecting antibody is much less than that of the CIE method. An important advantage of the technique is that a specific antibody can be identified with use of crude cell extract antigen preparations such as Hep-2 cell extracts. That is to say, the combination of zone electrophoresis on a gel separating a mixture of proteins by size gives an extra dimension for identifying precipitin bands formed by overlying with test sera. However, the disadvantage of immunoblotting is that, in the procedure, the proteins are denatured by sodium dodecyl sulfate (SDS) before immunoblotting (24) and the immunoblotting procedures are difficult to reproducibly quantitate.

The European Consensus Study observed the following with the immunoblotting procedure (22,23):

1. The antigen preparation is very important in the IB procedure. That is to say, a full spectrum of antigenically intact proteins must be present, most usefully in equimolar concentrations.
2. The detection of antibodies to NRNP, Sm, and Scl-70 was acceptable. This method can be very helpful in the detection of multiple specificities of antibody in the same specimen.
3. The method requires careful controls to monitor molecular weight bands. For example, histone bands can be confused with a centromeric antigen (CENP-A, 19-kDa), and Scl-70 (topoisomerase I) can be confused with other 100-kDa bands.
4. Protein degradation can occur in the antigen cell extract used for IB, especially Scl-70 and centromere antigens.
5. The anti-Sm is distinguished by the presence of anti-D (the D antigen is a 16-kDa protein contained in all major NRNP particles).
6. Anti-SS-B/La is readily detected by IB. Anti–SS-A/Ro is, however, poorly detected by IB and is insensitive. The SS-A/Ro antigen may not demonstrate the proper epitopic structure in the immunoblotted band for recognition.

ELISA

An increasing number of enzyme immunoassays have been developed over the past decade with use of standard purified and recombinant antigens (22,23). This should provide a major improvement in this form of testing. Many of these enzyme immunoassays have proved to be more sensitive than comparable immunodiffusion methods (9,21). Thus, because of the high sensitivity of enzyme immunoassays, *one needs to determine carefully the reference range of normal patients and the proper cutoff values.*

Compared with immunodiffusion tests, the ELISA test results show much greater sensitivity but lower specificity. Further, the ELISA tests were frequently positive in low titers of antibodies in sera of patients with rheumatic diseases other than SLE. It must be carefully re-established, in light of new data with ELISA measurements, just how disease specific various antibody specificities are. For example, the presence of antibodies to Sm as assayed by immunodiffusion is considered to be highly specific for SLE. However, in ELISA tests, the Sm antibody was positive in 23% of 54 RA patients, 25% of 24 patients with systemic sclerosis, 9% of 11 polymyositis patients, and 2% of 59 normal patients (25). Increasing sensitivity and decreasing specificity might result in false-positive test results.

In the European Consensus Studies of 1988 and 1989, it was observed that many false-positive reactions were noted in the clinical laboratories using ELISA tests. Authors of the study believed that the false-positive reactions were due to poor blocking reagents in the procedure and the presence of impure antigen preparations used as substrates. In the 1990 and 1991 cooperative study, the laboratories that used ELISA performed much better, with few false-positive or extraneous negative results. The ELISA assays also performed well in sorting out sera with multiple specificities. The percentage of clinical laboratories that used ELISA increased from 25% to 47% over a 4-year period, from 1989 to 1992.

Profiles of Autoantibodies in Various Systemic Rheumatic Diseases

It has been observed that distinct profiles of ANA are seen in different systemic rheumatic diseases. The important characteristics include the presence or absence of certain antibody specificities and their mean titers (1-5,26).

The following features are noteworthy:

1. Multiple ANA frequently seen in SLE generally included high levels of antibodies to native DNA.
2. Distinctiveness of anti-Sm for SLE.
3. Restriction of ANA in drug-induced SLE to antihistone.
4. Antibodies to U1-RNP or nuclear antibodies to RNP present in several rheumatic diseases with different frequencies.
5. The restriction of ANA in mixed connective tissue disease (MCTD) to U1-RNP or nuclear RNP antibodies.
6. Sjögren's syndrome sera characterized primarily by the presence of antibodies to SS-A/Ro and SS-B/La.
7. Patients with scleroderma showing a profile consisting of antibodies to Scl-70, the centromere/kinetochore antigen, and nucleolar antigens.
8. The frequent presence of RF, AKA, APF, anti-Ra 33, and RANA in rheumatoid arthritis.

9. The appearance of Jo-1, M_{1-2}, PM-Scl, and 56-kDa autoantibodies in polymyositis/dermatomyositis.

Quality Assurance

Several reference preparations are available for nuclear and cytoplasm antibodies. However, there are no currently available reference preparations for specific antibodies that have been validated by ELISA and immunoblotting. Currently, the AMLI Standards Committee is in the process of preparing reference preparations that will be useful for ELISA and immunoblotting procedures.

Clinical laboratory proficiency surveys are available. The College of American Pathologists provides the most comprehensive survey for the various autoantibody tests.

Summary

The recommended procedure for a screening test for intracellular and nuclear antibodies at this time is the indirect IFM test with the use of Hep-2 cell substrate, which can detect most antinuclear antibodies, including SS-A/Ro antibody.

A patient with a negative IFM-ANA has less than a 0.14% chance of having SLE. Therefore, the IFM test can be primarily used to exclude the diagnosis of SLE.

Negative IFM test results may be observed in patients with Sjögren's syndrome, polymyositis, rheumatoid arthritis, and scleroderma, although such patients demonstrate specific nuclear antibodies by other immunologic tests. When these particular rheumatic diseases are clinically suspected, one should consider tests that will identify the immunologic specificity of the ANA.

The secondary definitive tests for specific identification of ANA utilize immunodiffusion, counterimmunoelectrophoresis, particle agglutination, immunoblotting, and immunoenzyme (ELISA).

Immunoprecipitin and double immunodiffusion analysis have been used to determine specificity of several ANAs. Assay specificity in double immunodiffusion is generally dependent upon the quality of the control serum used in the procedure as well as the nature of the antigen preparation. The immunodiffusion tests are not very sensitive. The positive tests by immunodiffusion have a high degree of specificity as a diagnostic marker in certain rheumatic diseases.

Commercial immunodiffusion kits are available for detection of antibodies to RNP, Sm, SS-A/Ro, SS-B/La, and Scl-70 as well as other less prevalent markers.

In the future, reference preparations to specific antibodies will be needed that are useful for evaluation of ELISA and immunoblotting assays.

REFERENCES

1. Tan EM. Antinuclear antibodies: diagnostic markers for diseases and probes for cell biology. Adv Immunol 1989;44:93–151.
2. Tan EM. Autoantibodies to nuclear antigens (ANA): their immunobiology and medicine. Adv Immunol 1982;33:167–240.
3. Nakamura RM, Peebles CL, Rubin RL, Tan EM. Autoantibodies to nuclear antigens. In: Advances in laboratory tests and significance in systemic rheumatic diseases. 2nd ed. Chicago: American Society of Clinical Pathologists, 1985:1–163.
4. Nakamura RM, Tan EM. Update on autoantibodies to intracellular antigens in systemic rheumatic diseases. Clin Lab Med 1992;12:1–23.
5. Decker JL. Glossary Subcommittee of ARA Committee on Rheumatologic Practice. Arthritis Rheum 1986;26:1029–1032.
6. Nakamura RM, Bylund DJ. Contemporary concepts for clinical and laboratory evaluation of systemic lupus erythematosus and "lupus-like" syndromes. J Clin Lab Anal 1994;8:347–359.
7. Reichlin M. Systemic lupus erythematosus. In: Bijazzi PE, Reichlin M, eds. Systemic autoimmunity. New York: Marcel Dekker, 1991:163–199.
8. Osterland CK. Laboratory diagnosis and monitoring in chronic systemic autoimmune diseases. Clin Chem 1994;40:2146–2153.
9. Nakamura RM, Bylund DJ, Tan EM. Current status of available standards for quality improvement of assays for the detection of autoantibodies to nuclear and intracellular antigens. J Clin Lab Anal 1994;8:360–368.
10. van Venrooij WJ, Maini RM. Manual of biological markers. Norwell, MA: Kluwer Academic, 1993–1994.
11. Teodorescu M, Froelich CJ. Laboratory evaluation of systemic lupus erythematosus. In: Lahita

RG, ed. Systemic lupus erythematosus. 2nd ed. New York: Churchill Livingstone, 1992:345–368.

12. Robbins WC, Holman HR, Deicher H, Kunkel HG. Complement fixation with cell nuclei and DNA in lupus erythematosus. Proc Soc Exp Biol Med 1957;96:575–579.
13. Friou G. Clinical application of lupus nucleoprotein reactions using fluorescent antibody technique. J Clin Invest 1957;36:890.
14. Nakamura RM, et al. Area Committee of Immunology and Ligand of NCCLS. Quality assurance for the indirect immunofluorescence test for auto-antibodies to nuclear antigens (17-ANA). NCCLS Document I/LAZ-T, September 1992.
15. Nakamura RM, Rippey JH. Quality assurance and proficiency testing for autoantibodies to nuclear antigens. Arch Pathol Lab Med 1985;109:109–114.
16. Molden DP, Nakamura RM, Tan EM. Standardization of the immunofluorescence test for autoantibody to nuclear antigens (ANA): use of reference sera of defined antibody specificity. Am J Clin Pathol 1984;82:57–66.
17. Schur PH. Clinical features of SLE. In: Kelly WN, Harris ED, Ruddy S, Sledge CB, eds. Textbook of rheumatology. 4th ed., vol. 2. Philadelphia: Saunders, 1993:1017–1042.
18. Griner PF, Mayewski RJ, Mushlin AI, Greenland P. Selection and interpretation of diagnostic tests and procedures. Ann Intern Med 1981;94:453.
19. Maddison PJ, Provost TT, Reichlin M. Serological finding in patients with "ANA-negative" systemic lupus erythematosus. Medicine 1981;60:87.
20. Bylund DJ, Nakamura RM. Importance of detection of SS-A/Ro autoantibody in screening immunofluorescence tests for autoantibodies to nuclear antigens. J Clin Lab Anal 1991;5:212–218.
21. James K, Meek G. Evaluation of commercial enzyme immunoassays compared to immunofluorescence and double diffusion for autoantibodies associated with autoimmune diseases. Am J Clin Pathol 1992;97:559–565.
22. van Venrooij WJ, Charles P, Maini RN. The consensus workshops for the detection of autoantibodies to intracellular antigens in rheumatic diseases. J Immunol Methods 1991;140:507–511.
23. Charles PJ, van Venrooij WJ, Maini RN. The consensus workshops for the detection of autoantibodies to intracellular antigens in rheumatic diseases 1989–1992. Clin Exp Rheumatol 1992; 10:507–511.
24. Dunbar BS. Protein blotting: a practical approach. New York: Oxford University Press, 1994:1–242.
25. Maddison PF, Skinner RP, Vlachoviannopoulos P, et al. Antibodies to nRNP, Sm, Ro(SSA) and La(SSB) detected by ELISA: their specificity and inter-relations in connective tissue disease sera. Clin Exp Immunol 1985;62:337.
26. von Mühlen CA, Tan EM. Auto-antibodies in the diagnosis of systemic rheumatic syndromes. Semin Arthritis Rheum 1995;24:323–358.

CHAPTER 23

Rheumatoid Arthritis and Rheumatoid Factor

LINDA COOK

Rheumatoid arthritis is an inflammatory joint disease in which there is an immune reaction in the synovium that destroys the joint. It usually affects women in young adult or middle age although all ages and both sexes can have the disease. The disease generally begins in the small joints of the hands and feet. In the early stages the main symptoms are pain and swelling in these joints that are especially significant in the early morning or after periods of inactivity. Early in the disease the inflammatory reaction is found in the synovial membrane; later the inflammation causes erosion of the synovial cartilage and the bone. The synovial tissue can be shown to be hypertrophied with finger-like processes and granulation tissue that extends into the cartilage tissue. As the disease progresses, additional joints are affected in a symmetric manner to involve the knees, hips, elbows, shoulders, and spine. Significant damage and joint dislocations result in essentially all affected joints. The damage is clearly immune mediated, as synovial fluid has been shown to contain high levels of inflammatory cells, including macrophages, lymphocytes, immune complexes, rheumatoid factor, and complement breakdown products.

In addition to the joint disease, many patients have systemic manifestations, including fibrosing alveolitis, vasculitis of the skin, granulomas, subcutaneous nodules, atrophy of the skin and muscle, malaise, fever, and weight loss. Some patients with rheumatoid arthritis may develop Felty's syndrome, which is a combination syndrome of rheumatoid arthritis, leukopenia, and lymphoid hyperplasia manifested as either lymphadenitis or hepatosplenomegaly.

Patients with rheumatoid arthritis exhibit classic degenerative joint changes on x-ray. Initially the joint displays soft-tissue swelling and juxta-articular demineralization. Next the articular cartilage destruction causes joint space, which narrows to be visible. Then bony erosions develop at the junction of the synovial membrane and the bone next to the articular cartilage. Finally, destruction of the cartilage and stretching of the ligaments cause maladjustment and subluxation of the joint surfaces. End-stage disease results in loss of joint function.

Early in the disease rheumatoid arthritis can be difficult to distinguish from a wide variety of diseases that present with swollen and painful joints. Diseases that should be considered in patients with hand and foot pain and swelling include systemic lupus erythematosus, Reiter's syndrome, gout, psoriatic arthritis, degenerative osteoarthritis, chronic inflammatory bowel disease, and a variety of infectious diseases that can infect the joints or cause systemic joint pain. Once the classic articular changes are visible on x-ray and a strongly positive rheumatoid factor is present, the diagnosis is easily made.

Rheumatoid factors (RFs) can be detected in a variety of clinical diseases. High titers (>1:160) of RFs can be found in the serum of 75% to 80% of patients with rheumatoid arthritis (1). The remaining patients may have immunoglobulin (Ig) G, IgA, or monomer IgM RFs that are not well measured by the most commonly used RF assay (2). Immunoglobulin E class RFs have also been reported (3). High titers of RFs may also be seen in the majority of patients with Sjögren's syndrome, and essentially all patients with type II cryoglobulinemia. Lower titers of rheumatoid factors are found in systemic lupus erythematosus as well as in a variety of infectious diseases, including rubella, cytomegalovirus (CMV), infectious mononucleosis, influenza, malaria, leprosy, tuberculosis, bacterial endocarditis, syphilis, and human immunodeficiency virus (HIV)-1. Rheumatoid factors can also be seen in sarcoidosis, chronic liver diseases, and pulmonary disease, and can be found in low levels in normal elderly individuals. High levels of rheumatoid factor may be present before the development of clinical symptoms consistent with the disease. High levels of rheumatoid factors can also be detected in the synovial fluid of inflamed joints from patients with rheumatoid arthritis.

Test Selection Rationale

The rheumatoid factor assay is one of the earliest described immunoassays. Rheumatoid factors were originally discovered and described by Waaler in 1940 (4). The original assay described by Waaler characterized the reactivity of some patients with rheumatoid arthritis that caused the agglutination of sheep erythrocytes coated with rabbit IgG. Although rheumatoid factors were initially described in patients with rheumatoid arthritis, subsequent studies found the IgG reactivity in the serum of patients with a variety of other diseases. Further studies determined that rheumatoid factors were immunoglobulins that have autoantibody activity specific for epitopes found in the CH2 and CH3 regions of the Fc portion of IgG. They are usually IgM, but IgG and IgA rheumatoid factors also have been described.

Most currently commercially available assays utilize small latex particles coated with IgG. The source of IgG is a critical factor that determines the reactivity of the assay in a variety of patient conditions. If the IgG used is from a human source, the assay is positive in most patients with rheumatoid arthritis, but in addition it will be positive in patients with a variety of other rheumatic diseases and some infectious diseases. This broad reactivity makes the test useful as a nonspecific marker of inflammation in addition to its use in the diagnosis of rheumatoid arthritis. If the IgG used is from a rabbit source, the nonspecific reactivity is much less and the test is much more specific for rheumatoid arthritis. This is because the rheumatoid factors present in the serum of patients with rheumatoid arthritis have high reactivity to human IgG but also have high cross-reactivity with IgG from a variety of other species including rabbit IgG (5). Rheumatoid factors present in serum from patients with other conditions do not cross-react with other species as well. Thus, the use of rabbit IgG minimizes the positive RF reactivity for patients with diseases other than rheumatoid arthritis. The rabbit IgG test is consequently much more specific for rheumatoid arthritis.

A wide variety of manual agglutination assays that utilize latex or red cell–coated particles in either a slide or tube assay format are commercially available. These assays all perform well if done according to the manufacturer's recommended methods and are simple, fast, and inexpensive to perform. The major disadvantage to the rapid slide and tube assays is the subjective interpretation of the agglutination and the inaccuracy of the endpoint titer, which is variable within a fourfold dilution range.

In the 1980s, a new method was developed to measure RFs (6,7). The assay was automated by developing reagents for use on the nephelometer immunoassay instruments. Currently, the assay is available from two different nephelometry manufacturers, the Beckman ARRAY and QM-300 models (Beckman Instruments, Brea, California), and the Behring nephelometers and turbidimeters (Behring-Dade, San Jose, California), and the Sanofi nephelometer. For the nephelometric method, the amount of light scattered by soluble protein complexes is very sensitively measured. For the Beckman nephelometers soluble aggregated IgG is mixed with a dilution of patient serum. The presence of rheumatoid factors in the patient serum causes increased complexes to be formed that can be sensitively detected by the nephelometer. Some nephelometers can also be used to detect the agglutination of small latex particles that are coated with antigen. For the Behring nephelometer, small latex particles are coated with IgG and mixed with a dilution of patient serum. The presence of rheumatoid factors in the patient serum causes agglutination of the latex beads that can be detected by the nephelometer. For both types of nephelometry assays, the quantity of rheumatoid factor present is determined by comparing the light scatter of the patient to the light scatter values of a standard curve. The standard curve values are reported in units of rheumatoid factor per milliliter of serum (U/mL). The assays available from both of these companies are relatively inexpensive, rapid, and with significantly decreased variation.

The newest RF assays to be developed and used in clinical testing are the enzyme immunoassay (EIA) microtiter assays for the detection of IgM, IgA, and IgG RFs. In the 1990s, these EIA assays have been utilized to more carefully study the quantitative levels of IgG and IgA rheumatoid factors in addition to the more frequently measured IgM rheumatoid factors (8,9). Some studies have demonstrated that the measurement of IgG and IgA rheumatoid factors can increase the sensitivity and specificity of the test for the diagnosis of rheumatoid arthritis. EIA assays have also been developed to more accurately measure IgG rheumatoid factor that exists in vivo as self-associated dimers in which one IgG is bound to another via the antibody combining site. These new EIA assays have been shown to be positive in approximately half of the patients with "seronegative" rheumatoid arthritis in which all other rheumatoid factor assays have been negative. Unfortunately, the EIA assays are more expensive and significantly more labor intensive than the slide agglutination and the nephelometric methods and have not yet been routinely used in a majority of diagnostic laboratories. However, with the rapid development of automated instrumentation for autoimmune and infectious disease serologies, inexpensive and rapid EIA assays should be available on automated instruments.

The RF titer is not directly correlated with the severity of the disease. Some patients with very high titers will be minimally affected while some patients with significant disease will have minimal titers. This is because RFs vary significantly in their avidity and affinity for the rabbit IgG. However, serial titers in many individual patients will be correlated with disease progression or remission. Serial studies can be done that will show increased levels during active disease and decreased levels during inactive disease periods. However, since the levels of RF do not show a very rapid response to therapy or the changing clinical condition of the patient, the test is not useful clinically to monitor the patient. In general, results from different laboratories can only be roughly correlated because of the many different methods that are currently being utilized by immunology laboratories (10). The more accurate and precise nephelometric and EIA assays may enable serial studies of patients to be of more clinical relevance and allow the more direct comparison of results from different laboratories.

A number of other autoantibodies have been described in patients with rheumatoid arthritis, including antihistones, anti–single-stranded deoxyribonucleic acid (ss-DNA), anti-intermediate filaments, anti-RA nuclear antigen, anticollagen, and antielastase. Each of these antibodies can be found in a significant number of patients with the disease but none of them has been found to be superior to the RF assay in the diagnosis of rheumatoid arthritis.

Testing Methods

Rheumatoid factors are usually IgM but can be either IgG, IgA, or IgE. They are autoantibodies that react with the self-antigen IgG. The reaction between the IgG and the rheumatoid factor can be demonstrated by coating the IgG onto a latex particle and mixing the RF with the latex-coated particle. The IgM rheumatoid factor will bind to IgG that is present on at least two coated beads and will cause clumping of the beads.

In the manual slide (or card) method, a 1:20 dilution of the patient serum is made in a phosphate buffered saline (PBS) buffer and placed on one well of the slide. A solution containing IgG-coated beads is then added and the slide is incubated while being rotated gently. At the end of the incubation period, the slide well is examined for evidence of clumping of the latex particles. Any well with visible precipitate is considered positive. The slide test is considered too inaccurate to determine the titer of RF that is present. The most accurate manual method to determine the titer uses the same antigen as the slide method, but the test is done in solution in test tubes. All positive samples are used to make a series of twofold serial dilutions, 1:20, 1:40, 1:80, and so forth. Then the latex antigen is added and the tubes are incubated at 37°C to allow for binding of the RFs to the beads and for clumping to occur. The tubes are then centrifuged and examined for the presence of latex clumps and clearing of the latex from the suspension. The last dilution that shows visible precipitation of the latex beads is determined to be the titer of the sample.

In the nephelometric method the instrument makes a dilution of the patient serum into a buffer and then adds the diluted sample into the reaction cuvette. A volume of the aggregated IgG or the IgG-coated latex beads are then added and the solution in the reaction cuvette is mixed. After an incubation period, the solution in the reaction cuvette is read to determine the amount of light scattered by any soluble complexes (or clumped beads). The light scattered is then compared to the light scatter of RF standard solutions and the amount of RF is determined for each sample. The automated RF assays are standardized to a World Health Organization (WHO) or a Centers for Disease Control (CDC) reference serum with a defined number of RF units.

In the EIA method, IgG is coated onto the surface of the microtiter plate, and then a dilution of the patient sample is added to duplicate wells. After an incubation period, the wells are washed with buffer and then an enzyme-conjugated F(ab) or $F(ab)_2$ antibody specific for IgG, IgA, or IgM is added. After a second incubation period, the wells are again washed with buffer and the substrate specific for the enzyme is added. The plate is incubated and then read with a spectrophotometer to determine the amount of color present (optical density, OD). The OD of each patient sample is compared to that of the ODs of the standard curve to determine the amount of RF that is present in each sample. The IgM RF assays may be standardized with the WHO/CDC preparation but no standard exists for the IgG and IgA RF assays. Great care must be taken in the interpretation of the IgG assays, as in this case the IgG in the patient's serum is both the antigen and antibody. This can lead to problems of self-associating RFs and cause high background binding with this assay. In addition, great care must be taken by the commercial manufacturers to ensure that the enzyme-conjugated antibodies are free of the Fc region of the molecule or the conjugated antibody can become the antigen and be bound by the patient's RF rather than detecting the specific heavy chain determinants desired.

All three methods, manual latex, nephelometric, and the EIA assays, will generate acceptable results that can be used in the diagnosis of rheumatoid arthritis. The manual screening assay and the nephelometric assays are the simplest and least labor intensive. The manual tube dilution assay and the EIA assays are more labor intensive. For large-volume testing the nephelometric assay is simplest. The manual latex method is the easiest method when small-volume testing is needed but has the major drawback of requiring the labor-intensive and least accurate tube dilution method to determine the RF titer. Both the nephelometry and manual latex assays are reasonably inexpensive compared to the EIA method although this ignores the expenses related to the nephelometer and the fact that the EIA assays are not currently used by many laboratories. Expenses of the EIA assays may decrease as more laboratories utilize them. The EIA assays are the only method that can determine the IgA and IgG RF levels and therefore are probably the most sensitive for the detection of rheumatoid arthritis.

Serum samples for RF testing do not require any special handling. Blood can be allowed to clot and then the serum is separated and stored at 4°C for up to 7 days for most assays before testing. If the testing is done on patients with suspected cryoglobulins, the samples should be handled as for the cryoglobulin assay and be clotted and separated at 37°C to ensure that the RF is not lost in a cryoprecipitate. All samples to be tested for RF that have been stored at 4°C should be observed for cryoprecipitation, either type II or type III, which may have occurred during storage. The sample should be carefully examined before testing for the presence of fibrin or fibrinogen clot fibers; this is especially important to eliminate for the nephelometric assays. The RF assay may give false-positive results in patient samples with very high C1q levels and in the EIA assays with samples that have high immune complex levels.

Standards and Controls

Good positive and negative controls are commercially available for all three methods. For all methods, a negative, low positive, and high positive should be run on each assay run. For the manual latex assay, the low positive can be a sample that is positive at the 1:20 end point; as an alternative the titer of the high positive can be determined and that dilution then run on all subsequent runs as the low-positive control. For the nephelometry and EIA assays, a low positive at the bottom of the standard curve near the cutoff should be run. The high-positive sample should give a value in the top third of the standard curve range. In addition, a negative control should be run with each assay for all three methods. This can be a purchased negative control or a patient sample determined to be negative on a previous run. The negative cutoff range should be determined for each assay based on the testing on age- and sex-matched normal samples. In general, a 1:20 dilution has been used for the manual latex assay, but up to 10% to 15% of elderly patients without rheumatic disease will be positive at this level. Each of the nephelometry and EIA assays has established normal cutoff ranges based on studies done by the manufacturers but this should also be verified by inhouse normal testing. Currently accepted ranges of normal are around a cutoff of greater than 30 to 35 U/mL.

For the manual titer methods, screening assays should always have a negative, low-positive, and high-positive control with each run. If both controls are not positive then patient samples should be rerun and accepted only when all three controls have acceptable results. For the tube titration method, a negative and titer control should be run with each assay run. An expected titer range should be established for the positive control, and patient sample results only accepted if the positive control results are within a twofold dilution of the target end-point titer.

For the nephelometry and EIA assays, negative, low-positive, and high-positive controls should be run with each assay. The positive controls should span the standard curve measuring range; one should be in the bottom of the range near the cutoff value and the other should be in the top third of the range to ensure good linearity of the assay throughout the measuring range. When the assay is first used, dilutions of several high positives or linearity standards should be utilized to ensure that the measuring range is linear. Quality control (QC) ranges should be established for both the low and high positives and results for each run of patient samples should not be accepted unless both positive controls are within established ranges and the negative control is negative. QC ranges for the nephelometer should be set at 4% to 5% for the nephelometer, whereas ranges for the EIA method will need to be higher, especially for the low control, in which the variation may be 20% to 30% from run to run. If a patient value is obtained that is above the top of the standard curve range for the nephelometry method, the instrument should be programmed to immediately make a further dilution of the sample and the assay should be rerun to determine the U/mL of the high-positive sample at a higher dilution. For the EIA assays, a result above the top of the standard curve range should be rerun at additional dilutions to determine the U/mL at the higher dilution and then the final result should be calculated. Since many of the samples will show nonlinearity at higher dilutions, the value from the least dilution should be reported for these nonlinear samples.

An international RF standard is available from the WHO (11) and a United States standard can be obtained from the CDC (12). The standards are defined as U/mL for both standards. The standard number of units has roughly the same magnitude as the titer units. For example, a sample with a titer of 1:160 will have approximately 160 U/mL of RF. However, this correlation between titers and units is very loose, as in many samples there will be little correlation of results between methods, and much less than the tighter correlation seen when manual versus automated IgE and antistreptolysin O (ASO) titers are compared. Many samples will give significantly different results even with the same methods when reagents are obtained from different commercial vendors. The correlation between titers and units is very difficult because of the wide variety of antigens used and the variability of the RF populations of antibodies being tested. Comparisons between methods and vendors are especially bad for samples less than 200 U/mL or titers lower than 1:160.

Because of these significant variations with patient samples when different methods are used, it is important to carefully select the RF method used in each clinical laboratory. It is vital to establish good communication between the immunology laboratory and the clinicians who are utilizing the test results to ensure that the assay method selected is producing clinically useful information.

A useful quality assurance monitor is to follow the percent of positive RF results and their distribution of titer or unit value. A good method with stable reagents will generally give a low percentage of positive results. The percent of positive samples will generally stay fairly constant over time and allow the early detection of problems to be seen when the percentage of positive results increases significantly.

Proficiency Testing

Samples are available for interlaboratory comparisons of RF assay results from the College of American Pathologists (CAP) on the general immunology surveys. Results from the manual methods are somewhat variable, as could be expected by the wide variety of manufacturers of reagent kits. Results for the nephelometric determination of RF are less variable when compared within each instrument/method. Results from EIA assays are limited and unavailable at this time for IgA and IgG RFs.

REFERENCES

1. Wolfe F, Cathey MA, Roberts FK. The latex test revisited. Rheumatoid factor testing in 8287 rheumatic disease patients. Arthritis Rheum 1991;34:951–960.
2. Procaccia S, et al. ELISA determined IgM, IgG, and IgA rheumatoid factors in rheumatoid arthritis and in other connective tissue diseases. Clin Exp Rheumatol 1987;5:335–342.
3. Zuraw BL, et al. Immunoglobulin E–rheumatoid factor in the serum of patients with rheumatoid arthritis, asthma, and other diseases. J Clin Invest 1981;68:1610–1613.
4. Waaler E. On the occurrence of a factor in human serum activating the specific agglutination of sheep corpuscles. Acta Pathol Microbiol Scand 1940;1:172–188.
5. Williams RC, Kunkel HG. Separation of rheumatoid factors of different specificities using columns conjugated with gamma globulin. Arthritis Rheum 1963;6:665–675.
6. Blume P, Greenberg LJ. Application of differential light scattering to the latex agglutination assay for rheumatoid factor. Clin Chem 1975;21:1234–1237.
7. Desjarlais F, Daigneault R. Rheumatoid factors measured in serum with a fully automated laser nephelometer and correlation to agglutination tube titers. Clin Chem 1985;31:1077–1078.
8. Johnsson T, Arnason JA, Valdimarsson H. Enzyme linked immunosorbent assay (ELISA) screening test for the detection of rheumatoid factor. Rheumatol Int 1986;6:199–204.
9. Visser H, et al. Diagnostic and prognostic characteristics of the enzyme linked immunosorbent rheumatoid factor assays in rheumatoid arthritis. Ann Rheum Dis 1996;55:157–161.
10. Jaspers JP, et al. Nine rheumatoid factor assays compared. J Clin Chem Clin Biochem 1988;26:863.
11. Anderson SG, et al. International reference preparation of rheumatoid arthritis serum. Bull WHO 1970;42:311–318.
12. Taylor RN, et al. Quality control for immunologic tests. US Department of Health, Education and Welfare Publication No. (CDC)79-8376. Atlanta: Centers for Disease Control.

CHAPTER 24

Autoimmune Endocrine and Gastric Diseases

C. LYNNE BUREK

The stringent definition of an autoimmune disease is a condition in which structural or functional damage, or both, are produced by humoral and/or cell-mediated immune reactions to normal components of the body. Criteria for this designation of an autoimmune disease were proposed by Witebsky et al in 1957 (1). The postulates include the following: The relevant antibodies or cell-mediated immune reactions should be demonstrated; the responsible antigen should be defined, isolated, and used to induce an immunologic response in experimental animals; and the pathologic changes that are similar to those seen in human disease should appear in the corresponding tissue of the immunized animal. However, the more conventional interpretation of autoimmune disease is one in which a strong autoimmune element is associated with the particular disorder, even though no experimental evidence proves that the autoimmunity is actually causing the disease.

These autoimmune conditions are customarily classified "systemic" or as "organ (tissue) specific." The systemic group of diseases, which includes systemic lupus erythematosus, progressive systemic scleroderma, and so forth, is distinguished by an autoimmune response to antigens that are common to various organs and tissues, such as nuclear antigens. Systemic diseases are discussed in Chapter 22. The second group of diseases is characterized by autoimmune responses to tissue- or organ-specific antigens, that is, antigens present in only one particular tissue or organ. This group of diseases includes autoimmune thyroiditis, Graves' disease, insulin-dependent diabetes, atrophic gastritis, and others.

Although the autoimmune responses to tissue-specific antigens frequently may have both humoral and cell-mediated immunity directed to the specific organ or tissue, at present, the detection of humoral responses (autoantibodies) has greater clinical utility. This chapter presents information concerning laboratory methods for the evaluation of autoantibodies found in autoimmune endocrine and gastric diseases. Methods to assess autoantibodies associated with diabetes are evaluated in Chapter 25.

Types of Diseases

The information in this chapter emphasizes laboratory tests to detect autoantibodies to specific autoantigens found in autoimmune endocrine disorders of the thyroid, adrenal, and gastric tissue. Other endocrinopathies are discussed briefly. These diseases usually result in hyporesponsiveness of the particular organ in question. An exception is the hyperthyroidism of Graves' disease, as described below.

Autoimmune Thyroid Disease

Autoimmune thyroiditis is known by many names. It has been referred to as lymphocytic thyroiditis, chronic lymphocytic thyroiditis, Hashimoto's thyroiditis, or, simply, thyroiditis. End-stage disease results in signs and symptoms of hypothyroidism. There are also biochemical signs of disease, for example, low levels of the thyroid hormones such as thyroxine (T4) and high levels of thyroid-stimulating hormone (TSH). Immunologic hallmarks for autoimmune thyroiditis are autoantibodies to two of the major autoantigens of the thyroid gland, thyroglobulin (Tg) and the microsomal antigen of the thyroid epithelial cell, recently identified as thyroperoxidase (TPO). These autoantibodies are accompanied by lymphocytic infiltration of the thyroid gland with inflammation and destruction of the thyroid follicles. The mechanisms by which the immunologic response contributes to the thyroid cell destruction has still not been clarified. Autoimmune thyroiditis is considered to be a multifactorial disease with both genetic and environmental components.

Other thyroid conditions that have an association with the Tg and TPO antibodies include myxedema, certain types of goiter, thyroid cancer, and Graves' disease. Graves' disease is an exception to the concept that the disease causes organ hyporesponsiveness. Graves' disease results in hyperthyroidism because of autoantibody binding to the thyrotropin receptor, mimicking the action of TSH. No feedback loop is in operation, and therefore signs and symptoms of hyperthyroidism result. The biochemical signs of Graves' disease are elevated T4 and reduced TSH levels. The immunologic marker and cause of the condition are autoantibodies to the thyrotropin receptor, called thyroid-stimulating antibody (TSAb). Additional details about these clinical conditions are covered in detail elsewhere (2).

Other Autoimmune Endocrinopathies

Autoimmunity also develops against other endocrine organs, such as the adrenals, pancreas islet cells, parathyroid, pituitary, ovary, and testes (sperm). The autoantibodies are much less prevalent than with thyroid disease but, if present, help in diagnosis.

Autoimmune Gastric Disease

Autoantibodies to antigens of gastric parietal cells (parietal cell antibodies) occur with high frequency in patients with pernicious anemia and atrophic gastritis. Autoantibodies to gastric parietal cells frequently are found simultaneously with thyroid antibodies, although these cells are not usually considered as part of the endocrine system.

Role of the Immunology Laboratory in the Diagnosis, Evaluation, and Management of the Autoimmune Diseases

Autoantibodies are antibodies that have the capacity to bind to antigens of one's own tissue. In some cases autoantibodies may actually cause disease, such as the thyroid-stimulating antibody found in Graves' disease. However, more frequently they are used as markers in a variety of ways. Autoantibodies are evaluated for a number of reasons:

1. Autoantibodies can be used as an aid in diagnosis of disease, either by inclusion or exclusion. For example, virtually all patients with autoimmune thyroiditis have autoantibodies to one or both of the commonly detected antigens of the thyroid, Tg or TPO. In this instance the diagnosis is confirmed by the laboratory. If results are negative, autoimmune thyroiditis can almost be excluded. On the other hand, antibodies to the gastric parietal cell (PCA) do not occur in all patients with atrophic gastritis. If PCA antibodies are found, a diagnosis can be confirmed taken with other signs and symptoms of disease, but their absence does not necessarily rule out disease, as all patients with atrophic gastritis do not present with PCA antibodies. The total picture of the patient must always be considered. In addition, autoantibodies can also be found in normal individuals.

2. Autoantibodies may help distinguish between different forms of a condition, which may result in using different therapeutic strategies. For example, in cases of adrenal insufficiency, it is important to differentiate the disorder due to an infectious cause compared to disease associated with autoimmunity.

3. A change in antibody quantity may be a monitor of successful therapy or be a predictor of disease exacerbation. For disease of endocrine origin, however, changes in titer have less relevance in the management of the disorder; for these diseases a change in titer is frequently unrelated to clinical status. Often the symptoms are treated without "curing" the disease. Replacement therapy for the hyporesponsiveness is initiated to normalize signs and symptoms of disease without treating the underlying immunologic cause. In many cases the immunologic mechanism of the disease has not yet been clarified and is the topic of considerable research. Until the etiology and immunopathogenesis have been determined, immunologic interventions are unlikely to succeed.

Autoantibodies can be used as indicators of individuals at risk for future diseases, such as in endocrinopathies that are familial. Another case where this may be important is in postpartum thyroiditis (PPT), in which the existence of thyroid autoantibodies before pregnancy or their development during pregnancy imparts a much higher risk of PPT after delivery (3).

Autoantibody tests should never be used by themselves for diagnosis of disease, as they are also found in normal individuals. Autoantibodies in normal individuals range in frequency according to age and sex. Generally, the lowest frequency is in young males, the highest in elderly women.

Rationale of Test Selection for the Diagnosis, Evaluation, and Monitoring of Autoimmune Endocrine and Gastric Diseases

Techniques for demonstrating autoantibodies are prescribed by the location and properties of the antigen and the required level of sensitivity. Early assays, some of which are still used today, included agglutination and precipitation techniques. Precipitation in fluid or gelified media (e.g., immunodiffusion) is less sensitive than most assays and is not used as a routine clinical test for endocrine or gastrointestinal autoantibodies. However, it is still appropriate for the demonstration of antibodies to complex-mixture soluble antigens, such as certain nuclear antigens that have not yet been purified.

Indirect immunofluorescence (IIF) is the most commonly used test for detection of tissue-specific autoantibodies because of its versatility. It can detect multiple antibodies on a single tissue or on a multiple tissue block, and thus has considerable value as a screening test. Autoantibody isotype can be determined by using heavy chain–specific anti-immunoglobulin conjugates. IIF is particularly valuable in testing for autoantibodies for which the antigen has not yet been characterized or for unexpected antibodies. Autoantibodies may be missed by an assay that uses a single purified antigen. With IIF, the reaction site can be seen. Thus, the location of the cellular antigen can be determined and, in addition, other antibodies to the tissue can be detected. IIF can be considered as semiquantitative, as a serum titer can be established for a particular sample. A titer is considered to be the reciprocal of the last serum dilution to give a positive response.

In a few cases, however, the major autoantigen associated with a particular autoimmune disorder has been isolated. Subsequently, more sensitive semiquantitative tests, such as hemagglutination (HA), enzyme-linked immunosorbent assay (ELISA), or radioimmunoassay (RIA), have been developed using the isolated antigen fraction and have replaced or supplemented IIF. Autoantibody isotype that is detected in these indirect tests can also be evaluated by using heavy chain–specific or subclass-specific anti-immunoglobulin conjugated to a detection marker (fluorochrome or enzyme). The results of these tests can be expressed as a titer if serial dilutions are performed. The titer is the reciprocal of the last dilution to give a positive response. An alternative is to develop ranges of reactivity (e.g., nonreactive, low medium, high) that can be compared to control values that have previously been determined. Many of the commercial ELISA or RIA kits evaluate sera in this fashion. Another way is to express the results based on international units. Few autoantibody tests are set up this way, as an international standard of antibody preparation is essential. Expression of results as international units has the one advantage of being able to compare one laboratory result to another and should be considered as a goal for the future. A further method of expressing results that is truly quantitative is expressing in actual amounts of μg/mL. For this method of expression, an affinity-purified antibody that has been assayed for total immunoglobulin G (IgG) and IgG subclass quantity is necessary.

Laboratory Methods for the Detection of Thyroid Autoantibodies

As was previously discussed, the most commonly detected thyroid autoantibodies are those to the antigens Tg and TPO (microsomal antigen). Detection of autoantibodies to the TSH receptor is not a routine test; it is very specialized and is only available in special centers. The tests are complex, require a high level of technical skill, and use very specialized reagents (4,5).

The College of American Pathologists (CAP) conducts a proficiency survey for detection of autoantibodies to thyroidal Tg and microsomal (TPO) antigens. It is part of the Diagnostic Immunology Series 2 Survey. The address of the CAP is: CAP, 325 Waukegan Road, Northfield, IL 60093-2750; telephone: 800-323-4040.

Thyroid Antigens

Thyroglobulin

Thyroglobulin is the main component of the colloid in the thyroid follicle. It plays an essential role in the storage of iodine and the synthesis of iodinated thyroid hormones, T4 and tri-iodothyronine (T3). It is a 660-kDa protein that consists of two identical 330-kDa polypeptide chains; it also has a high carbohydrate content. Thyroglobulin autoantibodies can be demonstrated by several procedures, such as precipitation in agar, IIF, indirect hemagglutination of cells coated with Tg, RIA, and ELISA. At present, hemagglutination is the most commonly employed technique for the detection of antibodies against Tg. The ELISA is being used increasingly often for the measurement of antibodies to Tg, and will also detect antibodies that are nonagglutinating. IIF is rarely used. At least one laboratory has reported a quantitative ELISA assay for Tg antibodies (6). This assay uses an affinity-purified anti-Tg antibody that was well characterized for immunoglobulin quantity.

An international biologic standard for anti-thyroglobulin antibodies is available through the National Institute for Biological Standards and Control. Information about receiving a sample can be obtained by contacting the organization at: NIBSC, PO Box 1193, Potters Bar, EN6 3QH, United Kingdom; e-mail address: standards@nibsc.ac.uk.

Assay Methods

The assay methods for discussion here include only the most commonly used techniques of detection of autoantibodies: HA, IIF, and ELISA. Most of the methodologies described here are similar for the individual autoantibodies with differences in tissue substrates or antigens.

Hemagglutination

Hemagglutination is a technique that employs stable suspensions of erythrocytes coated with the appropriate soluble antigen. Autoantibodies crosslink the coated particles, forming the complex lattice structure of agglutination. Group 0 red cells are used routinely in this procedure to prevent agglutination due to blood group antibodies.

Passive hemagglutination tests with the use of tanned erythrocytes [tanned-cell hemagglutination (TCH)] or chromic chloride-treated erythrocytes [chromic chloride hemagglutination (CCH)] are very sensitive. Experimental details are described elsewhere (5). Thus, these techniques detect antibodies to Tg in a variety of conditions other than thyroiditis, a possible disadvantage from the diagnostic point of view.

Erythrocytes treated with tannic acid are capable of adsorbing protein antigens on their surface. When added to serial dilutions of the patient's serum, these erythrocytes will react with the appropriate antibody, if present, with a visible agglutination reaction. Tanned erythrocytes coated with thyroid extract or purified Tg are employed to detect antibodies to Tg. This method is highly sensitive, but requires fresh erythrocytes and reagents for best results. It can be replaced by the CCH method for adsorption of antigen to the red cells. Chromic chloride can be used to couple Tg to erythrocytes, providing a simpler alternative to the tannic acid method (5).

There are several commercially available kits that are widely used. They vary in sensitivity, and no standardized assessment of the different kits has been performed. However, the availability of these kits has allowed many laboratories to perform evaluation of Tg antibodies without the onus of reagent preparation of Tg or of preparing preparations of antigen-coated red cells.

ELISA

The technique of ELISA is an indirect method of antibody assessment. It is performed in specialized microtiter plates, which are coated by individual antigens. Antibody dilutions are incubated in the wells; antibody, if present will bind. Excess proteins are washed away. The second antibody, antihuman immunoglobulin, is conjugated to an enzyme. This reagent is incubated in the wells and, again, excess proteins are washed away. An enzyme substrate is added to the wells that is hydrolyzed by the enzyme that causes a color change of the substrate. The change in color is dose dependent on the initial antibody that is bound. This can be read in a spectrophotometer and expressed as a particular optical density (OD). The results are expressed in comparison to known positives and negatives. It is also essential to have a conjugate-only control to determine nonspecific reactivity of the conjugate itself. Details of the ELISA procedure have been described previously (5,7) Factors to consider when preparing an ELISA are 1) antigen coating the plate (concentration, volume, etc), 2) whether the blocking step is necessary, 3) incubation times for the individual steps, 4) anti-immunoglobulin concentration, 5) time of substrate incubation, 6) expression of results, and 7) interpretation of findings.

Requirements for an ELISA to Tg have been described previously (8,9). Commercially available ELISA is also available. It is essential to follow the manufacturer's instructions rigorously. The method is especially useful for large-scale studies. An advantage of the ELISA is that it can detect thyroid autoantibodies that are not hemagglutinating antibodies. Another advantage of the ELISA is that specific isotypes of the Tg antibody can be determined (10,11). Although this may be a controversial issue now, and should be regarded as a research tool at the moment, additional investigation of isotypes may provide insight into the subsets of the disease. A quantitative ELISA has been developed (6).

While ELISA readily detects antibody to thyroglobulin in those sera that have medium to titers of autoantibodies determined by HA, it may not readily discriminate between negatives and those samples with low titers (8). The reason for this lack is not clear, especially since ELISA has proved to be as sensitive as the isotopic assay in other antibody detection systems. Possibly the ELISA is less sensitive to particular subclasses of antibody to Tg.

Recent evidence shows that there is a difference in the antigenic specificity of autoantibodies to Tg in patients with thyroiditis compared to those with antibody but no disease. The naturally occurring antibodies from normal individuals are directed primarily to sites on the molecule that are shared among species (i.e., conserved), whereas those found primarily in patients are directed to human-specific regions (12).

Indirect immunofluorescence is rarely used for detection of Tg autoantibodies. Details of this procedure are described fully below. If IIF is used, special handling of the thyroid tissue is necessary because Tg is water soluble and will leach off the slide. Therefore, the tissue is fixed in methanol at 56° for 3 minutes. The pattern of staining that is obtained when methanol-fixed sections are used for Tg antibodies is characteristic and has a floccular "puffy" appearance.

Radioimmunoassay is also rarely used. Many of the RIA procedures are now being superseded with enzyme immunoassay techniques.

The prevalence of Tg autoantibodies varies with the sensitivity of the assay from 25% using IIF up to 100% in very sensitive hemagglutination tests, ELISA, or RIA tests (13). These antibodies are found in individuals with chronic thyroiditis, myxedema, Graves' disease, goiter, thyroid tumors, and other polyendocrine disorders. The highest titers are seen in patients with autoimmune thyroid disorders. Low titers of Tg antibodies may be found in normal individuals. The prevalence of such antibodies in subjects without overt thyroid disease is higher in women. The incidence also increases with age, so that 18% of women over 40 years old may have antibodies to Tg. Total Tg antibody is not a specific marker of autoimmune thyroiditis as so many other conditions also show the presence of this antibody. Recent evidence suggests, however, that there may be disease-related epitope specificity of the autoantibody (12). The disease-related antibodies were detected by competitive inhibition ELISA experiments of murine monoclonal antibodies.

Thyroid Peroxidase (TPO) of Thyroid Epithelial Cells, Formerly Known as Microsomal Antigen

Thyroid peroxidase was identified as an antigen that reacts with human antimicrosomal antibodies (14,15). However, purified TPO is not readily available for use in diagnostic tests. The most commonly used tests for the microsomal autoantibodies are IIF using primate thyroid tissue, a commercially available hemagglutination assay, and now ELISA and at least one RIA. One commercial test now uses chemiluminescence as its read-out. A microsomal antibody standard is also available through the National Institute for Biological Standards and Control. The address is mentioned.

Recent studies have provided some information on the biochemical and immunochemical character of the antigen. Problems have been encountered in purifying the antigen, since, after isolation and solubilization of the microsomes, contaminating Tg has been found (16–19). Despite this problem, two independent groups of investigators used immunoprecipitation (18,19) and Western immunoblotting (19) techniques to identify a protein with a molecular weight of about 105 kDa that binds to antimicrosomal antibody from patients with autoimmune disease. Intrachain disulfide bonds may be present, since the investigators (18) found a difference in the mobility of the antigen in polyacrylamide gel electrophoresis when comparing reducing versus nonreducing conditions. At least two epitopes bind antibodies from patient sera. One of the antigenic sites is a sequential epitope, while the other may be a conformational epitope dependent upon the integrity of the intrachain disulfide bonds. Two recent reviews discuss the immunologic and molecular characteristics of the TPO autoantigen (20) and the TPO antibodies (21).

Historically, the test of choice for many years for the detection of microsomal antigens was the complement fixation test using an optimal dilution of thyrotoxic thyroid extract (22). The immunofluorescence method that replaced this test was found to be more sensitive, and IIF remains one of the commonly used tests for microsomal autoantibody. The substrate consists of frozen human or monkey thyroid tissue that is air dried and unfixed. A positive test of patient's sera on unfixed slides appears as bright fluorescence of the cytoplasm of the follicular epithelial cells. Commercially available HA tests are now supplanting the IIF test because of the speed of the HA and its increased sensitivity. The increased sensitivity, however, can lead to reduced specificity, as a small group of normal individuals may also exhibit these autoantibodies.

Titers of microsomal antigen by IIF can reach 1200 or higher. Titers of microsomal antibody obtained by hemagglutination can reach well over 25,000. The antibodies to the microsomal antigens belong predominantly to the IgG class and, when detected by IIF, stain the cytoplasm of thyroid cells. The IIF test for antibodies to thyroid microsomal antigens is positive in approximately 70% to 90% of patients with chronic thyroiditis. It is also positive in 64% of patients with primary hypothyroidism, 50% of patients with thyrotoxicosis, 10% of patients with simple goiters, and 17% of patients with thyroid tumor. It can also be found in normal individuals at a low frequency and titer.

Indirect Immunofluorescence

Briefly, serum is placed on a tissue section (frozen section, 4 μ thick). If autoantibodies are present, they will bind to the appropriate antigen. Excess serum is washed away. A second reagent, antihuman immunoglobulin conjugated to a fluorescent dye (usually fluorescein isothiocyanate, abbreviated as FITC), is then incubated with the tissue section. Unbound reagent is again washed away. Autoantibodies are detected by microscopes (transmission or incident light illumination) with an appropriate light source (usually mercury vapor or halogen quartz) and a filter system that will enable the fluorescent markers to be seen.

The most important variables involved in producing a standardized technique are 1) type of substrate, including source, storage, and preparation; 2) duration of staining and washing; and 3) specificity and sensitivity of the conjugate. An essential part of each test is the incorporation of known positive and negative reactive sera as controls.

The most readily available substrate tissue for IIF is primate thyroid. Primate thyroids are available through animal supply firms. They should be shipped and stored as frozen specimens. A word of caution should be given, however, as not all thyroids are appropriate. If three are ordered, usually one is satisfactory. Another option is to buy precut slides from a company that supplies autoimmune reagents. These slides work out well.

Rabbit or goat antisera, prepared by immunization with human globulin or with individual isotypes of immunoglobulins (e.g., heavy chain or subclass specific) and conjugated to FITC, are used to detect the site of the reaction between tissue substrate and antibody from the patient's serum.

Each conjugated antiserum should be characterized for sensitivity and specificity. Sensitivity is dependence on the degree of fluorescein labeling and the potency of the antiserum. The number of fluorescein groups per protein molecule is known as the F/P ratio. Most conjugates for IIF have an F/P ratio that ranges between 1.0 and 4.5. An F/P ratio that is too high can result in nonspecific staining; if it is too low, staining intensity is poor. If the specific antibody content is known (as a titer or mg Ab/mL), the conjugate can be diluted to a standard concentration of antibody; otherwise the appropriate concentration must be determined empirically or by a checkerboard titration.

Commercially available antiglobulin conjugates are satisfactory. However, different lots, even from the same company, may vary. Therefore, each conjugated antiserum must be tested to determine the optimum dilution for maximum fluorescent staining without significant nonspecific staining. To do this, an IIF is performed that contains a checkerboard titration of multiple dilutions of a positive patient's serum against several dilutions of the FITC-conjugated antiserum. A further check would be to perform parallel staining of the old conjugate compared to the new conjugate.

Generally, commercially available conjugates come in lyophilized form and can be stored for long periods of time. Once reconstituted, they will remain potent for weeks if stored at 4°C. However, it is best to divide the conjugate into small aliquots and store them at −20°C; in this manner potency will be retained for several months. Once the reconstituted conjugate has been diluted, however, the life span of the reagent is limited to a few days. Treatment and storage of these conjugates may be different with different manufacturers, and therefore careful reading of the package inserts is essential.

Plasma is less useful for use in IIF, because the fibrinogen causes considerable nonspecific fluorescence of tissue substrate; therefore, only serum is the sample of choice. Since concentrated serum will also cause nonspecific staining and unclear results, an initial serum dilution of 1:10 or greater is recommended, depending on the sensitivity of the assay. Screening of patient sera can be performed initially using two or more dilutions. Positive sera should be retested using serial dilutions until an end point is reached. Until standard sera are generally available, each laboratory will have to establish its own set of standards regarding quantitation.

Each assay run should include controls for autofluorescence of tissue, for conjugate specificity, as well as known positive sera for each recognized pattern (described below), and known negative sera. Fluorescein isothiocyanate conjugate combined with an optional counterstain of rhodamine B-BSA (Rh B-BSA) will provide good contrast to the FITC conjugate alone. Reconstituted Rh B-BSA, 10 to 20 μL, is added per milliliter of the appropriate dilution of FITC-conjugated antiserum. The amount of the counterstain can be adjusted to account for the different tissues. Evans blue is frequently used as an alternative counterstain.

Indirect IF is less sensitive, but reportedly can detect nonagglutinating antibodies that are missed by other procedures. It can also detect antibodies to CA2, which are undetectable by hemagglutination.

Commercially Available Kits

Several kits for TPO–microsomal autoantibodies are available, either as hemagglutination or ELISA. One word of caution: Some tests may be called TPO but actually use a microsomal preparation for coating. These preparations of "TPO" from human tissue invariably contain Tg contaminants. Manufacturers try to mitigate these contaminants by adding an anti-Tg reagent to the diluent. However, a false positive could result if the sample contains a high titer of Tg autoantibodies. The tests that use recombinant antigen are not subject to this potential failing.

Again, with any kit, it is essential to follow the manufacturer's instructions exactly. When changing lots or changing techniques for evaluation of autoantibodies, parallel testing of the old and the new is also necessary. Documentation of the parallel testing should be maintained.

Thyrotropin Receptor

Autoantibodies that bind to the thyrotropin (TSH) receptor on the surface of thyroid epithelial cells are the primary cause of the hyperthyroidism of Graves' disease. The thyroid-stimulating autoantibodies bind near to or with the TSH receptor and mimic TSH activity, resulting in uncontrolled stimulation since there is no negative feedback control. Tests for TSAb are primarily of two types, bioassays or binding assays. Each of these tests are highly complex and require specialized reagents. Most bioassays have limited utility because they are cumbersome and require scarce materials, such as viable slices of fresh human thyroid tissue. Bioassays evaluate functional aspects of the antibodies as their end point. Binding assays are based on competition between ^{125}I-labeled TSH and patient autoantibodies for binding to thyroid preparations. However, these assays do not discriminate among the heterogeneous types of autoantibodies that may be bound (i.e., stimulating vs blocking). Different specificities of autoantibodies to the thyroid epithelial cell surface on or near the TSH receptor may be represented. A true value of the TSAb may not be represented. These antibodies and their tests have recently been reviewed (4,5).

The detection of thyroid-stimulating antibodies in patients with Graves' disease ranges from 55% to 95% depending on the assay. The TSAb assay is of greatest utility in conditions in which conventional test results are equivocal or where clinical signs and symptoms are not readily apparent (e.g., ophthalmopathology in the absence of other features). Moreover, the TSAb assay is usually negative in patients with thyrotoxicosis in association with thyroid nodules, with cancer, or in patients with subacute thyroiditis. Therefore, a positive test confirms a diagnosis of Graves' diseases with a high degree of confidence. The assay can be used to monitor patient therapy, as successful treatment of Graves' disease with propylthiouracil can result in lowering levels of TSAb antibodies. The assay has also proved useful in the diagnosis of neonatal thyrotoxicosis.

Laboratory Methods for the Detection of Other Endocrine Organs

Autoantibodies to endocrine organs share certain characteristics. Antibodies bind to antigens associated with the cytoplasm of cells, usually to unidentified antigens. The antibodies belong predominantly to the IgG class and, in general, have rather low titers (not higher than 100) and are rarely found in normal individuals. IIF is the predominant and, in most cases, only method of autoantibody detection.

The presence of antibodies to these endocrines suggests that the disease is idiopathic, potentially of immune origin, and not of malignant, infectious, or other nature. However, it is not uncommon for patients with autoantibodies to one endocrine organ to have multiple endocrine reactivities. Furthermore, not all patients with a particular disorder have the autoantibodies, so that a negative test obviously does not exclude a particular diagnosis. On the other hand, a positive test is not necessarily diagnostic, in that the patient might have other autoantibodies to endocrine organs without clinical disease.

Adrenal

The idiopathic form of primary adrenocortical insufficiency (Addison's disease) is frequently associated with autoimmune phenomena. Autoantibodies to the adrenal cortex can be demonstrated by indirect immunofluorescence on primate adrenal tissue substrate in approximately 50% of these patients (38–64% in various studies). In patients with forms of Addison's disease due to exogenous etiology (e.g., tuberculosis), these antibodies infrequently develop.

The same reagents and procedures previously described for the general IIF test are used. Frozen, unfixed, and air-dried sections of monkey adrenal are used as tissue substrate. Because titers of antibody are low and are rarely found in the normal population, starting dilutions can be as low as 1:2. However, it is important to include a negative control serum at the same dilution. Nonspecific binding is high at these concentrations of sera. Based on prospective studies, the presence of adrenal autoantibodies in "normal" individuals may serve as a predictive sign of incipient adrenal failure (23).

The autoantibodies may react with individual zones or with all three zones of the cortex. Most sera stain the whole cortex, with a brighter fluorescence in the glomerulosa zone. A few sera stain only the fasciculata and reticularis zones, and not the glomerulosa zone. The latter pattern has been reported with sera that also stain the interstitial cells of the testis and the theca interna cells of the ovary. Idiopathic Addison's disease is frequently associated with other autoimmune conditions and their respective autoantibodies. In certain patients the autoantibodies cross-react with steroid-secreting cells of the theca interna of the ovary or with the interstitial cells of the testes. In patients with Addison's disease and in those with primary ovarian failure, clinical evidence of ovarian failure is correlated with the presence of these autoantibodies

Other Endocrine Organs

Autoantibodies to antigens of ovary, testis, placenta, and parathyroid can be detected by IIF using frozen sections of the respective primate or human tissue.

Autoantibodies that stain the cytoplasm of cells of the theca interna, interstitial and corpus luteum cells of the ovary, interstitial cells of the testis, and the trophoblast of the placenta have been detected in the sera of patients with Addison's disease and those with premature ovarian failure (5). The antigens involved have not been very well characterized, and the test itself is at present more of research than of diagnostic interest.

Autoantibodies to parathyroid tissue are found in sera from patients with idiopathic hypoparathyroidism (IHP). These antibodies have been detected by IIF on sections of normal human parathyroid tissue obtained at autopsy (5). They are not directed against parathyroid hormone, but against cytoplasmic antigens of parathyroid cells. These autoantibodies to parathyroid cells are found in the serum of approximately 38% of patients with IHP, 26% of indviduals with idiopathic Addison's disease, 12% of patients with chronic thyroiditis, and 6% of control subjects (5). Since approximately 60% of patients with IHP do not have demonstrable parathyroid antibodies, a negative test obviously does not exclude IHP. On the other hand, a positive test, while indicating IHP, is not necessarily diagnostic, in that the patient might have adrenal insufficiency or thyroiditis, alone or in combination.

Laboratory Methods for the Detection of Gastric Parietal Cells

Indirect immunofluorescence is the method of choice for detection of parietal cell autoantibodies. These autoantibodies are readily detected by IIF with sections of rodent stomach (mucosa) as tissue substrate. Mouse stomach is preferred over rat stomach because many human sera contain heterophil antibodies that react to the mucosal cells of rat stomach (24). The pattern of staining resembles that seen with mitochondrial antibodies; therefore, a control test on kidney should also be performed. A true parietal cell will not react to kidney tissue, while mitochondrial autoantibodies will react to both. Parietal cell antibodies are found in 90% or more of patients with pernicious anemia. Recently, the autoantigen has been identified as the alpha and beta subunits of gastric H/K adenosine triphosphatase (ATPase) (25). Although an ELISA that uses this enzyme and a Western blotting technique that uses gastric extracts have been reported, these are not yet available commercially. These antibodies are also present in a number of other conditions, such as chronic thyroiditis (33%), Sjögren's sicca syndrome (15%), atrophic gastritis (60%), gastric ulcer (22%), and others. The test is frequently used to distinguish autoimmune-associated gastritis from that caused by *Helicobacter pylori*–associated gastritis. This type of gastritis is rarely associated with autoimmune responses (25). The antibodies are also found in the normal population, with an incidence that varies according to age and sex, that is, from 2% in subjects younger than 20 years to 16% in individuals older than 60 years. The antibodies are seen more frequently in women than in men.

REFERENCES

1. Witebsky E, Rose NR, Terplan K, et al. Chronic thyroiditis and autoimmunization. JAMA 1957; 164:1439–1447.
2. Braverman LE, Utiger RD. The thyroid. 7th ed. New York: Lippincott-Raven, 1996.
3. Stagnaro-Green A. Postpartum thyroiditis: prevalence, etiology, and clinical implications. Thyroid 1993;16:1–12.
4. Volpe R. Thyrotropin receptor autoantibodies. In: Peter JB, Shoenfeld Y, eds. Autoantibodies. Amsterdam: Elsevier, 1996:822–829.
5. Bigazzi PE, Burek CL, Rose NR, et al. Endocrinopathies. In: Rose NR, DeMacario E, Folds JD, et al, eds. Manual of clinical laboratory immunology. 5th ed. Washington, DC: American Society for Microbiology, 1997:972–988.
6. Kuppers RC, Outschoorn IM, Hamilton RG, et al. Quantitative measurement of human thyroglobulin-specific antibodies by use of a sensitive enzyme-linked immunoassay. Clin Immunol Immunopathol 1993;67:68–77.
7. Voller A, Bidwell D, Bartlett A. Enzyme-linked immunosorbent assay. In: Rose NR, Friedman H, eds. Manual of clinical immunology. 2nd ed. Washington, DC: American Society for Microbiology, 1980:359–371.
8. Voller A, Bidwell DE, Burek CL. An enzyme-linked immunosorbent assay (ELISA) for antibodies to thyroglobulin. Proc Soc Exp Biol Med 1980;163:402–405.
9. Bigazzi PE, Burek CL, Rose NR. Antibodies to tissue-specific endocrine, gastrointestinal, and surface-receptor antigens. In: Rose NR, DeMacario E, Fahey JL, et al, eds. Manual of clin-

ical laboratory immunology. 4th ed. Washington, DC: American Society for Microbiology, 1992: 765–774.

10. Parkes AB, McLachlan SM, Bird P, Rees-Smith B. The distribution of microsomal and thyroglobulin antibody activity among the IgG subclasses. Clin Exp Immunol 1984;57:239–243.
11. Rose NR, Outschoorn IM, Burek CL, Kuppers R. IgG subclass distribution of anti-Tg antibodies among thyroid disease patients and their relatives and in high and low responder mouse strains. In: Pinchera A, Ingbar SH, McKenzie JM, Fenzi GF, eds. Thyroid autoimmunity—thirtieth anniversary: memories and perspectives. New York: Plenum, 1987:189–198.
12. Bresler HS, Burek CL, Hoffman WH, Rose NR. Autoantigenic determinants on human thyroglobulin: II. Determinants recognized by autoantibodies from patients with chronic autoimmune thyroiditis compared to autoantibodies from healthy subjects. Clin Immunol Immunopathol 1990;54:76–86.
13. Burek CL, Rose NR. Thyroglobulin autoantibodies. In: Peter JB, Shoenfeld Y, eds. Autoantibodies. Amsterdam: Elsevier, 1996:810–815.
14. Portmann L, Hamada N, Heinrich G, Degroot LJ. Anti-thyroid peroxidase antibody in patients with autoimmune thyroid disease: possible identity with anti-microsomal antibody. J Clin Endocrinol Metab 1985;61:1001–1003.
15. Czarnocka B, Ruf J, Ferrand M, et al. Purification of the human thyroid peroxidase and its identification as the microsomal antigen involved in autoimmune thyroid diseases. FEBS Lett 1985;190:147–152.
16. Mariotti S, Pinchera A, Marcocci C, et al. Solubilization of human thyroid microsomal antigen. J Clin Endocrinol Metab 1979;48:207–212.
17. Goodburn R, Williams DL, Marks V. The preparation of thyroid microsomal antigen for use in the indirect micro-ELISA method for the detection of anti-thyroid microsomal autoantibody. Clin Chim Acta 1982;119:291–297.
18. Banga AP, Pryce G, Hammond L, Roitt IM. Structural features of the autoantigens involved in thyroid autoimmune disease. Mol Immunol 1985;22:629–642.
19. Hamada N, Grimm C, Mori H, Degroot LJ. Identification of a thyroid microsomal antigen by Western blot and immunoprecipitation. J Clin Endocrinol Metab 1985;61:120–128.
20. Banga JP, Barnett PS, McGregor AM. Immunological and molecular characteristics of the thyroid peroxidase autoantigen. Autoimmunity 1991;8:335–343.
21. Rapoport B, McLachlan S. Thyroid peroxidase autoantibodies. In: Peter JB, Shoenfeld Y, eds. Autoantibodies. Amsterdam: Elsevier, 1996:816–821.
22. Holborow EJ, Brown PC, Roitt IM, Doniach D. Cytoplasmic localization of "complement-fixing" auto-antigen in human thyroid epithelium. Br J Exp Pathol 1959;40:583–588.
23. Betterle C, Zannette F, Zanchetta R, et al. Complement-fixing adrenal autoantibodies as a marker for predicting onset idiopathic Addison's disease. Lancet 1983;1:1238–1241.
24. Dawkins RL, Pummer SC, Krueger RG, Hollingsworth PN. Heterophile antibodies. In: Peter JB, Shoenfeld Y, eds. Autoantibodies. Amsterdam: Elsevier, 1996;351–356.
25. Gleeson PA, van Driel IR, Toh B. Parietal cell autoantibodies. In: Peter JB, Shoenfeld Y, eds. Autoantibodies. Amsterdam: Elsevier, 1996:600–606.

CHAPTER 25

Autoimmune Markers of Type I Diabetes Mellitus

DORLINDA VARGA HOUSE
MASAMICHI NAKAMURA
WILLIAM E. WINTER

With the development of epifluorescent microscopy using indirect fluorescence, in 1974 Bottazzo and colleagues first described the presence of islet cell autoantibodies (ICA) in patients with autoimmune polyglandular syndromes (1). Since that time researchers have sought to address several important questions: 1) Which autoantibody markers are present at the time of diagnosis of type I (insulin-dependent) diabetes mellitus? 2) Which autoantibody markers are predictive of the development of type I diabetes mellitus? 3) How can autoantibody markers be used in the prevention of type I diabetes mellitus?

The goal of this chapter is to address these questions. The term *insulin-dependent diabetes mellitus* (IDDM) is used to denote the clinical presentation and subsequent clinical course of type I ("autoimmune") diabetes. The term *non–insulin-dependent diabetes mellitus* (NIDDM) is used to designate the clinical presentation and subsequent clinical course of type II diabetes.

Autoantibody Markers Present at the Time of Diagnosis of Type I (Insulin-Dependent) Diabetes Mellitus

The autoantibodies that have been detected in new-onset patients with type I diabetes are listed in **Table 25-1**. T cells from diabetic patients have been used to detect other autoantigens (**Table 25-2**). For some autoantigens, such as glutamic acid decarboxylase (GAD), both autoantibodies and T-cell responses have been described. Indeed, type I diabetes results from chronic autoimmune destruction of the insulin-producing beta cells (25,26).

The four most useful markers are 1) islet cell autoantibodies (ICA), 2) insulin autoantibodies (IAA), 3) glutamic acid decarboxylase autoantibodies (GADA), and 4) ICA512/IA-2A. Their approximate frequency of occurrence in patients with new-onset type I diabetes is given in **Table 25-3**. The biology of each marker is discussed below.

ICA Biology

Islet cell autoantibodies are detected by indirect immunofluorescence on blood group O human pancreas (27). Fresh pancreata from cadaveric organ donors are collected by the transplantation service and delivered to the ICA laboratory chilled on ice. The tissue is cut into approximately 1-cm^3 portions that are snap-frozen in isopentane that has been cooled in a dry-ice acetone bath. The resulting blocks of tissue can be immediately mounted on a chuck for cryostatic sectioning, or the blocks can be placed in a 50-mL screw-top container at −70 to −80°C for future use within 24 months.

The 4-μm sections are transferred from the microtome blade to the glass slide by placing the room temperature slide against the tissue. The tissue then instantly adheres to the slide. It is important to make sure that the tissue does not fold. Neat (undiluted) patient's serum is placed upon the tissue and allowed to

TABLE **25-1**

Autoantibodies Detected in New-Onset Patients with Type I Diabetes

Anti-carboxypeptidase-H autoantibodies (2)
51-kDa aromatic L-amino acid decarboxylase autoantibodies (3)
Chymotrypsinogen-related 30-kDa pancreatic autoantibodies (4)
Deoxyribonucleic acid (DNA) topoisomerase II autoantibodies (5)
Glima 38 autoantibodies (6)
Glutamic acid decarboxylase autoantibodies (GADA) (7)
Glycolipid autoantibodies (8)
GLUT2 autoantibodies (9)
Heat shock protein (HSP) autoantibodies* (10)
IA-2β autoantibodies (IA-2βA)
ICA512/IA2 autoantibodies (ICA512/IA-2A) (11)
ICA69 autoantibodies* (12,13)
Insulin autoantibodies (IAA) (14)
Insulin receptor autoantibodies (15)
Islet cell (cytoplasmic) autoantibodies (ICA) (1)
Islet cell–specific 38-kDa autoantibodies (16)
Islet cell surface autoantibodies (17,18)
Proinsulin autoantibodies (19)
Rubella-related autoantibodies (20)
37,000/40,000 M(r) islet tryptic fragment autoantibodies (21)

*Note: controversial.

TABLE **25-2**

Autoantigen Responses by T cells from Patients with Type I Diabetes

Glutamic acid decarboxylase (22)
Imogen 38 (23)
Insulin secretory granule proteins (24)

TABLE **25-3**

Frequency of Occurrence of Autoantibody Markers in Patients with New-Onset Type I Diabetes

ICA	70–80%
IAA	≤50%
GADA	70–80%
ICA512/IA-2A	70–80%

incubate. After incubation and washing with phosphate-buffered saline (PBS), fluorescein-isothiocyanate–labeled goat antihuman immunoglobulin G (IgG) conjugate is applied to the slide. After washing again with PBS, surplus liquid is eliminated and glycerol is applied followed by a cover slip.

Islet cell autoantibody titers have been standardized into JDF (Juvenile Diabetes Foundation) units (28). Low titers are less than 10 JDF units with the lowest reported positive being 5 JDF units. Stronger titers are 20 JDF units or greater. In nondiabetic individuals, sera with low JDF titers may revert to negative. However, with JDF titers of 20 units or more, reversion to negative is rare.

Blood group O pancreata are used to avoid the potential confusion of isohemagglutinins reacting with tissue ABO antigens. Likewise, using unfixed tissue avoids the potential problem of detecting insulin antibodies or autoantibodies. With fixed pancreas tissue, insulin is retained in the tissue. However, with unfixed tissue, insulin is washed away by the many PBS wash steps.

Variations in ICA methodology (29) have involved prolonged incubation times (e.g., overnight incubation), use of nonhuman tissue substrate (e.g., mouse or monkey), counterstaining of alpha cells to identify islets, and use of horseradish peroxidase (HRP)–labeled second antibodies. While each variation may offer a potential advantage, most research laboratories use the same basic technique that was described by Bottazzo et al in 1974 (1).

A question of great concern is: "What cytoplasmic autoantigens are detected by ICA-positive sera?" When blocking studies are performed, ICA react with islet sialoglycoconjugates, GAD (30), and recombinant IA2 (31). This will be of great importance in the discussion of strategies to screen for "prediabetes."

In equal frequency to the detection of ICA in the general school-aged population (~1 in 250 children) (32), autoantibodies to the glucagon-secreting alpha cells are detected. Alpha cell autoantibodies are not associated with either progression to type I diabetes or with hypoglucagonemia (33).

Islet cell autoantibodies are present in about three fourths of whites with new-onset type I diabetes (27). In contrast, only about 40% of African-Americans with the clinical diagnosis of insulin-dependent diabetes express ICA (27). This suggests heterogeneous etiologies of youth-onset diabetes in African-Americans (34). Presumably because the autoantigens detected by ICA are lost from the islet by islet cell destruction with subsequent loss of stimulation of the immune system, ICA become undetectable after 5 to 10 years of disease. Persistent

ICA are seen most commonly in patients with autoimmune polyglandular syndromes.

Islet cell autoantibodies are also found in 10% to 15% of patients with type II diabetes (35–38). Patients with clinical non–insulin-dependent diabetes with ICA have a higher rate of reversion to insulin treatment, lower C-peptide levels, and higher frequencies of HLA-DR3 and DR4, which are type I diabetes-associated human leukocyte antigen (HLA) alleles. Because type II diabetes is nine times as common as type I diabetes, there are as many patients with "autoimmune" type II diabetes as there are patients with type I diabetes. Therefore, immunointervention trials should target individuals at risk for autoimmune type II diabetes as well as those at risk for type I diabetes (so-called prediabetic individuals).

While high-titer ICA do fix complement, ICA are not pathogenic, as they are directed against antigens that are predominantly intracellular. It is important to note that ICA react with *all* cells of the islet, including beta and alpha cells. This provides further evidence that ICA are not pathogenic, as hyperglucagonemia is a consequence of beta cell failure and there is no evidence of permanent alpha cell hypofunction.

IAA Biology

Insulin autoantibodies were first described by Palmer and colleagues (14). While it was well known that antibodies to insulin develop *after* insulin treatment, it was a surprise to the diabetes community in 1983 when Palmer detected autoantibodies to soluble insulin *before* the administration of exogenous insulin. Insulin is the only autoantigen discovered to date that is beta cell specific.

Insulin autoantibodies are detected by the ability of patients' sera to immunoprecipitate ^{125}I-labeled A14 monoiodinated insulin (39). Basically, patient serum is incubated with ^{125}I-labeled A14 insulin in the presence of an excess of cold (unlabeled) insulin. After incubation, PEG (polyethylene glycol) is added to precipitate immune complexes. After centrifugation, the radioactivity in the resulting pellet is counted and is expressed as a percent of the total radioactivity. The upper limit of normal is usually expressed as the control range plus three standard deviations. Knowing the quantitative amount of radiolabeled insulin allows IAA concentrations to be expressed in nanograms of insulin precipitated. In the University of Florida Autoantibody laboratory, IAA are present when more than 125 ng of insulin is precipitated.

Enzyme-linked immunosorbent assays (ELISA) measure insulin antibodies that are not necessarily associated with type I diabetes (40,41). Therefore ELISA assays should not be used to measure IAA.

Insulin autoantibodies are seen more commonly in children than in adults, as up to 50% of children will be positive for IAA at the time of diagnosis of type I diabetes (39). Once insulin therapy is initiated, IAA can no longer be detected, as exogenous insulin will induce insulin antibodies that cannot be differentiated from insulin *auto*antibodies. However, insulin antibody titers are much higher than IAA titers. IAA can be found in autoimmune conditions other than type I diabetes such as Hashimoto's thyroiditis.

GADA

Autoantibodies found in the sera of patients with type I diabetes that immunoprecipitated ^{35}S-methionine–labeled islet proteins of 64,000 mW (64 kDa) were first described by Baekkeskov et al in 1982 (42). Similar autoantibodies have also been described in biobreeding (BB) rats (43) and nonobese diabetic (NOD) mice (44).

In 1990, Baekkeskov et al (7) discovered that the 64-kDa autoantigen was glutamic acid decarboxylase. This enzyme catalyzes the conversion of glutamic acid to the inhibitory neurotransmitter gamma-aminobutyric acid (GABA). There are two forms of GAD, each coded for by a unique gene: GAD65 (molecular weight: 65 kDa) and GAD67 (molecular weight: 67 kDa) (45). GADA are predominantly directed against GAD65 (46,47). GAD is found in abundance in the nervous system. Outside of the nervous system, GAD is found in the kidney and pancreatic islets. Alpha, beta, and delta (somatostatin-producing) cells all express GAD (48).

GADA are found in the neurologic disease stiff-man syndrome (7). Presumably a deficiency of the inhibitory neurotransmitter GABA impairs the ability of the patient to relax voluntary muscles. One third of patients with stiff-man syndrome have or will eventually develop type I diabetes. In contrast to type I diabetes, in which GADA are in relatively low titer and react with conformational determinants, GADA in stiff-man syndrome are in very high titer and react with linear and conformational determinants (49). For example, GADA in patients with stiff-man syndrome can be detected using Western blot assays with denatured GAD, while such assays are routinely negative for GADA when the sera are from patients with type I diabetes.

Most GADA assays detect the ability of patients' sera to immunoprecipitate GAD (50). There are several major approaches to the measurement of GADA:

1. GAD is radioactively labeled with ^{35}S, ^{125}I, or ^{3}H and the radioactivity in the precipitate is expressed as a percent of total radioactivity. Immune complexes can be precipitated with PEG or antihuman immunoglobulin antibodies.
2. The enzymatic activity of immunoprecipitated GAD is measured by the conversion of radioactively labeled glutamic acid to $^{14}CO_2$.
3. A sandwich ELISA is carried out where GAD is spaced out from the wall of the well by sheep antibodies to GAD (e.g., GAD6) and patients' sera supply GADA. After washing, HRP-labeled goat antihuman immunoglobulin antibodies are added. After substrate addition, the level of GADA is proportional to the color change.
4. A well is coated with anti-GAD antibodies. GAD labeled with horseradish peroxide (GAD-HRP) is in solution. Addition of patients' sera leads to GADA binding to GAD-HRP, depleting the test mixture of GAD-HRP that would otherwise bind to the anti-GAD antibody that is fixed to the wall of the well. Decreased signal from decreased amounts of GAD-HRP indicates that the patients' sera contained GADA. Because GAD-HRP is depleted in such a solid-phase assay, the assay is termed a "depletion" ELISA technique (or DELISA).

ICA512/IA-2A

Sequencing of a clone from a lambda gt11 human islet expression library that was identified using human diabetic sera revealed the neuroendocrine islet autoantigen ICA512 (islet cell antigen 512) (51). Using Northern blot analysis, ICA512 is expressed in brain and pancreas.

ICA512 is included within IA-2, which is a 106-kDa intrinsic transmembrane protein that belongs to the protein tyrosine phosphatase (PTP) family (52). Protein tyrosine phosphatases comprise a family of receptor-like and cytoplasmic signal-transducing enzymes. These enzymes catalyze the dephosphorylation of phosphotyrosine residues and are characterized by homologous catalytic domains. Other members of the PTP family are listed in **Table 25-4**.

The IA-2 cDNA was isolated from a human insulinoma subtraction library (ISL-153) (53). With a total length of 3.6 kilobases (kB), the complementary DNA (cDNA) included a 2937-bp open reading frame, predicting a 979 amino acid protein with an isoelectric point (pI) of 7.09. By Northern analysis, IA-2 is found in brain, pituitary, pancreas, and brain tumor cell lines.

Sequencing of ICA512-3, a cDNA with a 1644-bp open reading frame, reveals a transmembrane protein with a single membrane-spanning segment and a cytoplasmic domain (54). This is similar to the first intracellular (catalytic) domain of CD45, the T cell protein tyrosine phosphatase. ICA512 is expressed in secretory granules of beta cells as well as other peptide-secreting endocrine cells and neurons

TABLE **25-4**

Representative Members of the Protein Tyrosine Phosphatase (PTP) Family

CD45	Located on lymphocytes
RPTP alpha	Receptor protein tyrosine phosphatase alpha
PTP-NP	PTP–neural and pancreatic
LMW-PTP	Low M(r) phosphotyrosine protein phosphatase
PTP-SL	A brain-specific PTP
PTPD1	Skeletal muscle
PTPH1	Expressed in a variety of tissues
PTPMEG1	Expressed in a variety of tissues
R-PTP kappa	Central nervous system
PTP-PEST	Expressed in a variety of cell lines
SH-PTP3	Expressed in a variety of tissues
PTP zeta	Brain
PTP1B	
LRP	
PTP beta	
PTP delta	
PTP epsilon	
LAR	

that contain neurosecretory granules (55). Following exposure at the cell surface, ICA512 is cleaved at its luminal domain to be transported to the Golgi complex and resorted into new secretory granules.

Recent work has identified a second transmembrane protein tyrosine phosphatase: IA-2β (56). Tryptic digestion of radiolabeled islet cell proteins indicates that IA-2 provides a 37-kDa fragment while IA-2β contributes a 40-kDa fragment (56–58). Previously, Christie et al (21) showed that autoantibodies against these fragments were more predictive of the development of type I diabetes than autoantibodies against the 64-kDa autoantigen that was later identified as GAD. IA-2 and IA-2β share several common epitopes while other epitopes are unique to each molecule.

Radiolabeling of ICA512/IA-2 has allowed the assay to be performed in a semi-automated mode. Some assays have used fragments of ICA512, for example, the ICA512bdc assay that detects autoantibodies to amino acid residues 256-979 of the IA-2 molecule that includes the intracellular domain (59).

Autoantibody Markers Predictive of the Development of Type I Diabetes Mellitus

Either alone or in combination, when ICA (32,60–66), GADA (21,47,59,67), or ICA512/IA-2A (59,68) is present in nondiabetic individuals, such markers are highly predictive of the later development of type I diabetes when combined with low first-phase insulin response (FPIR) to intravenous glucose administration. The intravenous glucose tolerance test (IVGTT) is the most sensitive metabolic measure of beta cell dysfunction (61–66). In patients who eventually manifest type I diabetes, the IVGTT will become abnormal months to years before the oral glucose tolerance test (OGTT) becomes abnormal. Once the OGTT is abnormal in an autoantibody marker–positive individual, clinical insulin-dependent diabetes mellitus will become manifest within 1 to 2 years if not sooner. The copresence of IAA with ICA, GADA, and/or ICA512/IA-2A further increases the risk for type I diabetes. However, by itself, IAA is not a strong predictor of type I diabetes.

The only prospective trials to assess the utility of autoantibody markers to predict type I diabetes involve the use of ICA with or without IAA (32,60). Such studies have targeted high-risk individuals, for example, relatives of patients with type I diabetes, as well as individuals in the general pediatric population who are positive for ICA. Riley et al (60), in studies of first-degree relatives of patients with type I diabetes, and Schatz et al (32), in studies of a general school-aged population, showed that ICA, when combined with low FPIR (e.g., <1st percentile) in response to a bolus of intravenous glucose, predicts type I diabetes with an accuracy of greater than 50% over 5 years of follow-up. For relatives of type I diabetes patients, this figure is near 65%. Furthermore, by 10 years of follow-up, essentially all such high-risk individuals are predicted to develop type I diabetes.

When reviewing the literature, it is important to be critical of the use of the term *prediabetic* when authors discuss autoantibody-positive nondiabetic individuals. Prediabetic individuals are those who are prospectively followed until the time when clinical insulin-dependent diabetes mellitus actually develops. Until this time the individual is properly referred to as "autoantibody-marker positive, nondiabetic."

If first-degree relatives of patients with type I diabetes are screened for ICA, approximately 3% will be ICA positive. This is a reasonable figure, as the empiric risk of type I diabetes in first-degree relatives is about 5%. The potential advantage of ICA over GADA and ICA512/IA-2A is that ICA frequency in the general population is quite low at only approximately 0.4%. In contrast, the frequency of GADA and ICA512/IA-2A in the general population is considerably higher at 1% to 3%.

The Use of Autoantibody Markers in the Prevention of Type I Diabetes Mellitus

Studies initiated in the 1980s addressed the question: "Can beta cell function be salvaged in new-onset type I diabetes patients with the use of immunosuppressive therapy?" (69). A tremendous variety of therapies were attempted to effect beta cell rescue (**Table 25-5**). While cyclosporin A and azathioprine could induce a remission in type I diabetes in about half of new-onset patients so treated, none of the remissions were permanent. Remission was

TABLE 25-5

Previous Immunotherapeutic Approaches to the Treatment of New-Onset Type I Diabetes

Anti-CD5 antibody conjugated to the ricin A chain (70)
Antithymocyte globulin (71)
Azathioprine (72–74)
Bacillus Calmette-Guérin (BCG) (75)
Buffy coat transfusions (76)
Ciamexone (77)
Cyclosporin A (78–83)
Interferon (84,85)
Intravenous immunoglobulin (86)
Levamisole (87)
Plasmapheresis (88–90)
Prednisone (91,92)
Thymopentin (93)

often defined solely on the basis of C-peptide secretion regardless of whether the patient was insulin dependent or independent at that particular time. Few patients remained off insulin for more than 1 year after the diagnosis of type I diabetes. All patients eventually became clinically insulin dependent within months of discontinuing immunosuppressive therapy. With cyclosporin A there was a significant risk of nephrotoxicity (94). From studies of patients receiving kidney transplants who were treated with azathioprine, a reversible lymphoma developed in approximately 1 in 1000 such individuals and this risk was expected in new-onset type I diabetes patients so treated.

Because of the limited efficacy of immunosuppression in the treatment of newly diagnosed patients with type I diabetes, the therapeutic emphasis has now been placed on *preventing* beta cell destruction before the development of frank glucose intolerance. When discussing interventions in nondiabetic individuals, the side effects described above for cyclosporin A and azathioprine are unacceptable. Therefore, therapeutic approaches to prevent type I diabetes must be very innocuous, as such interventions will be applied to clinically *asymptomatic* individuals although such individuals would be autoantibody marker positive and will likely display an abnormal FPIR (95). New therapies may attempt to 1) prevent environmental exposure to diabetogenic triggers, 2) improve beta cell resistance to autoimmune attack by free radicals, and 3) induce tolerance to beta cell autoantigens and rest the beta cells. Researchers in Finland are poised to begin a trial of cow's milk avoidance in early infancy in an effort to prevent type I diabetes. While several epidemiologic studies suggest that breast feeding is protective of the development of type I diabetes (96–100), the most recent data do *not* support a protective role for breast feeding (101,102).

Nicotinamide can act as a free-radical scavenger and inhibitor of the DNA repair enzyme poly (ADP-ribose) polymerase (103). These actions could maintain intracellular levels of NAD^+ preventing beta cell death. Several studies are planned or are in progress [e.g., the ENDIT trial: *E*uropean *N*icotinamide *I*ntervention *T*rial, which also includes Texas and Canada (e.g., CANENDIT)], which will attempt to show a preventative benefit when marker-positive nondiabetic individuals ingest nicotinamide (104). However, several papers have disputed the claim that nicotinamide is of any benefit in preventing or treating type I diabetes (105).

The last approach is the subject of the Diabetes Prevention Trial 1 (DPT-1), which is funded by the National Institutes of Health (NIH) and the JDF International. In the DPT-1 trial, first-degree relatives of patients with type I diabetes are screened for ICA. Confirmed marker-positive individuals undergo an IVGTT every 6 months. When two of three IVGTTs reveal deficient FPIRs indicating a risk for type I diabetes of greater than 50%, the consenting individual is randomized to no therapy or twice-daily subcutaneous insulin injections at a total dose of about 0.25 units/kg/day. This is approximately one fourth of the usual daily dose of insulin used to treat type I diabetes. The goal of DPT-1 is to delay the onset of type I diabetes while it is hoped that small doses of exogenous insulin will also be able to prevent type I diabetes.

Subcutaneous insulin could rest the beta cell, allowing time for beta cell repair. At the same time, suppression of endogenous insulin secretion could decrease surface autoantigen expression and/or decrease autoantigen peptide presentation by beta cell class I major histocompatibility complex (MHC) molecules to CD8 Tk cells. Insulin may also act as a tolerogen to induce anergy to insulin and possibly other islet cell autoantigens (106–110). Data from Shah et al (111) indicate that intensive treatment of humans with insulin during the first year after the diagnosis of type I diabetes prolongs C-peptide secretion. Furthermore, there are preliminary data concerning the value of insulin treatment of autoantibody marker–positive humans in the prevention of type I diabetes (112).

In the DPT-1 trial for individuals with a lower risk for type I diabetes (e.g., 25–50%), oral insulin is being administered. A similar approach has been used to treat patients with multiple sclerosis where myelin basic protein is taken orally (113,114). Because autoimmune type II diabetes may affect as many individuals as does type I diabetes, trials of oral insulin therapy in patients with newly diagnosed type II diabetes are planned. The DIPP (*Di*abetes *P*rediction and *P*revention) trial in Finland is administering nasal insulin to induce beta cell autoantigen tolerance.

As these trials get under way, researchers are wrestling with the next problem: Once we know how to prevent type I diabetes, what is the best screening strategy? For the general population, several researchers have suggested initial genetic screening of cord blood for high-risk HLA alleles such as HLA DR3 and DR4 and/or DQB1*0302 and HLA DQB1*0201. This is based upon the numerous studies that show associations between specific HLA alleles and risk for type I diabetes (115–134). The advantage of genetic screening is that such studies need only be undertaken once. This would considerably limit the number of children who would then need to undergo periodic autoantibody marker screening. Some studies suggest that with the appropriate DQB1 type (heterozygosity for DQB1*0302 and HLA DQB1*0201), risk for type I diabetes may approach 1 in 3 (~33%). **Table 25-6** provides comparative data for risk of type I diabetes according to family history and HLA serotype. The DAISY (*D*iabetes *A*uto*i*mmunity *S*tudy in *Y*outh) project is a prospective assessment of risk for type I diabetes based on cord blood HLA screening. So far, more than 9000 cord bloods have been tested, with approximately 2% of samples high risk (DR3/DR4, DQB1*0302). As non-HLA genetic markers of susceptibility are better defined (e.g., the insulin gene locus, IDDM-2) (135,136), testing for such markers can be added to the HLA algorithm to identify patients at high genetic risk for type I diabetes (137,138).

Human leukocyte antigen (HLA) type as an indication for autoantibody screening would miss at least 5% of patients with potential type I diabetes but would preclude the need to screen the entire school-aged population repeatedly throughout childhood and adolescence. HLA typing would target screening to the individuals at highest risk for type I diabetes, making the program more cost effective.

Screening for high-risk HLA alleles could be performed using filter paper samples at a reasonable cost (e.g., <$10–$20/sample) given that neonatal screening programs exist in all 50 states. Likewise, individuals with HLA DR2, DRB1*1501, and DQB1*0602, regardless of marker status, almost never develop type I diabetes and could be excluded from further testing.

Whether or not genetic screening is performed, the question remains as to which autoantibody markers would be used in a general population screening program. Clearly, ICA would not be suitable for screening three to four million children every year (the number of births each year in the United States) because the ICA test is extremely labor intensive, is impossible to automate, and is very difficult to perform accurately on a long-term, repetitive basis. While IAA could be automated, IAA frequency in new-onset type I diabetes is too low to be used as the sole screening test for potential cases of prediabetes. Because the GAD and ICA512/IA-2 autoantigens have been cloned, assays for GADA and ICA512/IA-2A can be automated to provide high throughput, precision, and accuracy. Indeed, using these

TABLE **25-6**

Risk of Developing Type I Diabetes According to Family History and HLA Serotype

	Absolute Risk	**(%)**
General population	1:500	(0.2%)
DR3 (+)	1:400	(0.25%)
DR4 (+)	1:400	(0.25%)
DR3/DR4 (+)	1:40	(2.5%)
Mother with type I diabetes	1:50	(2%)
Father with type I diabetes	1:14	(7%)
First-degree relative with type I diabetes	1:20	(5%)
HLA identical sibling	1:7	(14%)
Share DR3/DR4 with diabetic sibling	1:4	(25%)
Twin with type I diabetes	1:3–1:2	(33–50%)

assays separately or combined in the same test tube, at least 80% and as many as 90% of individuals in the general population who are destined to develop type I diabetes could be identified.

It is not precisely known at what ages autoantibody markers appear in the serum and therefore several screening samples for GADA and ICA512/IA-2A would need to be collected (139). Autoantibody marker screening might be performed at ages 2, 4, 8, and 10 years. The screenings at ages 2 and 4 years would be to identify the youngest children, in whom type I diabetes develops near age 5, while the 8- and 10-year-old screenings would be to detect children destined to develop type I diabetes during adolescence. The BABY-DIAB study indicated that serologic evidence of beta cell autoimmunity can arise very early in life (139). The efficiency of screening could be pushed still higher if IAA were added to the GADA and ICA512/IA-2A assays (e.g., "triple" testing) (140).

For screening purposes, testing for all three autoantibodies (GADA, IAA, ICA512/IA-2A) in a single tube ("simultaneous" triple testing) could offer significant cost advantages over performing individual assays. Simultaneous triple testing for GADA, IAA, and ICA512/IA-2A by immunoprecipitation could use a common autoantigen label (e.g., ^{125}I or ^{35}S), or each autoantigen could be individually labeled with a unique fluorescent tag (e.g., europium or terbium) yet measured in the same tube. If a common label were employed, positives would be rescreened with individual assays for GADA, IAA, and ICA512/IA-2A. Positive screens would also undergo confirmatory ICA testing. It has been suggested that, like ICA, IA-2βA (autoantibodies to IA-2β) could serve as a confirmatory marker of beta cell autoimmunity. Not all autoantibody markers appear in the same time sequence in all individuals. Some researchers have proposed that IAA and GADA may be the earliest autoantibody markers to become positive while ICA512/IA-2A may be a later marker of humoral beta cell autoimmunity and a better predictor of actual progression to insulinopenia. As the number of positive markers increases in an individual, so does his or her risk for type I diabetes (141,142).

Autoantibody marker–positive individuals would be offered periodic metabolic testing by IVGTT. If beta cell function did decline, oral or subcutaneous autoantigen therapy would be initiated to induce tolerance and suppress beta cell autoimmunity and beta cell attack, averting the development of clinically evident insulin-dependent diabetes mellitus. Such approaches have been effective in NOD mice (143). While insulin is being used in the DPT-1 study, future studies might also administer GAD or ICA512/IA-2, or both, in an attempt to induce tolerance (144).

In addition to autoantigen tolerization, another approach to prevent type I diabetes involves cytokine, anticytokine, or anticytokine receptor administration to shift the immune response from a Th1 to a Th2 response (145). CD4 Th1 clones secrete predominantly interleukin-2 (IL-2), interferon gamma (IFN-γ), tumor necrosis factor alpha (TNF-α), and TNF-β. CD4 Th2 clones secrete predominantly IL-4, IL-5, IL-10, and TGF-β. Both types of clones secrete GM-CSF and IL-3. The hypothesis is that downregulation of Th1 cells would be beneficial, as cell-mediated immune responses stimulated by Th1 cells are responsible for insulitis and the autoimmune destruction of beta cells in type I diabetes. On the other hand, while Th2 cells would foster autoantibody production (especially from CD5+ B cells), autoantibodies in type I diabetes are not pathogenic. **Table 25-7** lists approaches that might shift the balance of the immune response from Th1 to Th2 cells (146).

TABLE **25-7**

Therapeutic Approaches that Could Theoretically Encourage a Th2 Immune Response Over a Th1 Immune Response

Monoclonal antibodies that block Th1 products
Anti–IL-2 monoclonal antibody
Anti–IFN-γ monoclonal antibody
Anti–TNF-α monoclonal antibody
Anti–TNF-β monoclonal antibody
Monoclonal antibodies that block receptors for Th1 products
Anti–IL-2 receptor monoclonal antibody
Anti–IFN-γ receptor monoclonal antibody
Anti–TNF receptor monoclonal antibody
Administer cytokines that inhibit Th1 cells
IL-10
Tumor growth factor beta (TGF-β)
Administer cytokines that foster Th2 response
IL-4
IL-5
IL-6

Summary and Conclusions

Over the last two decades, researchers have defined a number of autoantibody markers that are predictive of the development of type I diabetes (147–160). An abnormal IVGTT in the face of positive autoantibody markers is highly predictive of type I diabetes (32,60,161,162).

The major research challenge now involves developing safe and efficacious strategies that can routinely prevent type I diabetes. Immunointervention trials in newly diagnosed patients with clinical insulin-dependent diabetes mellitus are no longer indicated (163) other than to evaluate the safety of potential therapies. Avoidance of environmental triggers (102,164), strengthening the beta cell against attack (103–105,165–168), and use of autoantigen tolerization (113,146) are three promising approaches to the prevention of insulitis (169–173) and beta cell destruction (25,26). With recent advances in our understanding of the immune system (174,175), preventative therapies should be ready within one to two decades. *However, in the meantime, testing nondiabetic individuals for autoantibody markers of beta cell autoimmunity should be restricted to the research setting.* In patients with diagnosed diabetes, either insulin dependent or non–insulin dependent, finding ICA, GADA, ICA512/IA-2A, or IAA (in the absence of previous insulin treatment) indicates an autoimmune etiology for the diabetes.

Once preventative therapies are perfected for type I diabetes, genetic prescreening (e.g., cord blood HLA typing) and periodic autoantibody marker screening of the pediatric population who are genetically at risk for type I diabetes can be undertaken. It is not unreasonable to believe that type I diabetes will be one of the first autoimmune diseases to be prevented in our lifetime.

Acknowledgments

Doctor House was a fellow in Pediatric Endocrinology and Diabetes and was supported by NIH National Research Service Award 1F32 DK09207-01. She is now in private practice in Lake Mary, Florida with the Pediatric Endocrine and Diabetes Specialists of central Florida. Doctor Nakamura was a Postdoctoral Research Fellow and was supported by Fujita Health University of Aichi, Japan.

REFERENCES

1. Bottazzo GF, Florin-Christensen A, Doniach D. Islet-cell autoantibodies in diabetes mellitus with autoimmune polyendocrine deficiencies. Lancet 1974;2:1279–1283.

2. Castano L, Russo E, Zhou L, et al. Identification and cloning of a granule autoantigen (carboxypeptidase-H) associated with type I diabetes. J Clin Endocrinol Metab 1991;73: 1197–1201.

3. Rorsman F, Husebye ES, Winqvist O, et al. Aromatic-L-amino-acid decarboxylase, a pyridoxal phosphate-dependent enzyme, is a beta-cell autoantigen. Proc Natl Acad Sci USA 1995;92:8626–8629.

4. Kim YJ, Zhou Z, Hurtado J, et al. IDDM patients' sera recognize a novel 30-kD pancreatic autoantigen related to chymotrypsinogen. Immunol Invest 1993;22:219–227.

5. Chang YH, Hwang J, Shang HF, Tsai ST. Characterization of human DNA topoisomerase II as an autoantigen recognized by patients with IDDM. Diabetes 1996;45:408–414.

6. Aanstoot HJ, Kang SM, Kim J, et al. Identification and characterization of glima 38, a glycosylated islet cell membrane antigen, which together with GAD65 and IA2 marks the early phases of autoimmune response in type 1 diabetes. J Clin Invest 1996;97:2772–2783.

7. Baekkeskov S, Aanstoot HJ, Christgau S, et al. Identification of the 64K autoantigen in insulin-dependent diabetes as the GABA-synthesizing enzyme glutamic acid decarboxylase. Nature 1990;347:151–156.

8. Cabrera-Rode E, Diaz-Horta O, Fernandez LE, et al. Glycolipids as the major autoantigens of cytoplasmatic islet cell antibodies. Autoimmunity. 1995;20:145–151.

9. Johnson JH, Crider BP, McCorkle K, et al. Inhibition of glucose transport into rat islet cells by immunoglobulins from patients with new-onset insulin-dependent diabetes mellitus. N Engl J Med 1990;332:653–659.

10. Atkinson MA, Holmes LA, Scharp DW, et al. No evidence for serological autoimmunity to islet cell heat shock proteins in insulin dependent diabetes. J Clin Invest 1991;87:721–724.

11. Rabin DU, Pleasic SM, Shapiro JA, et al. Islet cell antigen 512 is a diabetes-specific islet

autoantigen related to protein tyrosine phosphatases. J Immunol 1994;152:3183–3188.

12. Pietropaolo M, Castaño L, Babu S, et al. Islet cell autoantigen 69 kD (ICA69): molecular cloning and characterization of a novel diabetes-associated autoantigen. J Clin Invest 1993;92:359–371.
13. Lampasona V, Ferrari M, Bosi E, et al. Sera from patients with IDDM and healthy individuals have antibodies to ICA69 on western blots but do not immunoprecipitate liquid phase antigen. J Autoimmun 1994;7:665–674.
14. Palmer JP, Asplin CM, Raghu PK, et al. Anti-insulin antibodies in insulin dependent diabetes before insulin treatment—a new marker for autoimmune B cell damage. Diabetes 1983;32:76A.
15. Maron R, Elias D, DeJongh BM, et al. Autoantibodies to the insulin receptor in juvenile onset insulin-dependent diabetes. Nature 1983;303:817–818.
16. Pak CY, Cha CY, Rajotte RV, et al. Human pancreatic islet cell specific 38 kilodalton autoantigen identified by cytomegalovirus-induced monoclonal islet cell autoantibody. Diabetologia 1990;33:569–572.
17. Lernmark A, Freedman ZR, Hofmann C, et al. Islet-cell-surface antibodies in juvenile diabetes mellitus. N Engl J Med 1978;299:375–380.
18. Maclaren NK, Huang S-W. Antibody to cultured human insulinoma cells in insulin-dependent diabetes. Lancet 1975;1:997–999.
19. Bohmer K, Keilacker H, Kuglin B, et al. Proinsulin autoantibodies are more closely associated with type 1 (insulin-dependent) diabetes mellitus than insulin autoantibodies. Diabetologia 1991;34:830–834.
20. Karounos DG, Thomas JW. Recognition of common islet antigen by autoantibodies from NOD mice and humans with IDDM. Diabetes 1990;39:1085–1090.
21. Christie MR, Tun RY, Lo SS, et al. Antibodies to GAD and tryptic fragments of islet 64K antigen as distinct markers for development of IDDM. Studies with identical twins. Diabetes 1992;41:782–787.
22. Atkinson MA, Kaufman DL, Campbell L, et al. Response of peripheral blood mononuclear cells to glutamate decarboxylase in insulin-dependent diabetes. Lancet 1992;339:458–459.
23. Arden SD, Roep BO, Neophytou PI, et al. Imogen 38: a novel 38-kD islet mitochondrial autoantigen recognized by T cells from a newly diagnosed type 1 diabetic patient. J Clin Invest 1996;97:551–561.
24. Roep BO, Arden SD, de Vries RRP, Hutton JC. T-cell clones from a type-1 diabetes patient respond to insulin secretory granule proteins. Nature 1990;345:632–634.
25. Atkinson MA, Maclaren NK. What causes diabetes? Sci Am 1990;262:62–71.
26. Thai A-C, Eisenbarth GS. Natural history of IDDM. Diabetes Rev 1993;1:1–14.
27. Neufeld M, Maclaren NK, Riley WJ, et al. Islet cell and other organ-specific autoantibodies in U.S. Caucasians and Blacks with insulin-dependent diabetes mellitus. Diabetes 1980;29:589–592.
28. Gleichmann H, Bottazzo GF. Progress toward standardization of cytoplasmic islet cell-antibody assay. Diabetes 1987;36:578–584.
29. Nayak RC, Omar MAK, Rabizadeh A, et al. Cytoplasmic islet cell antibodies. Diabetes 1985;34:617–619.
30. Atkinson MA, Kaufman DL, Newman D, et al. Islet cell cytoplasmic autoantibody reactivity to glutamate decarboxylase in insulin-dependent diabetes. J Clin Invest 1993;91:350–356.
31. Lan MS, Wasserfall C, Maclaren NK, Notkins AL. IA-2, a transmembrane protein of the protein tyrosine phosphatase family, is a major autoantigen in insulin-dependent diabetes mellitus. Proc Natl Acad Sci USA 1996;93:6367–6370.
32. Schatz D, Krischer J, Horne G, et al. Islet cell antibodies predict insulin-dependent diabetes in United States school age children as powerfully as in unaffected relatives. J Clin Invest 1994;93:2403–2407.
33. Winter WE, Maclaren NK, Riley WJ, et al. Pancreatic alpha cell autoantibodies and glucagon response to arginine. Diabetes 1984;33:435–437.
34. Winter WE, Maclaren NK, Riley WJ, et al. Maturity-onset diabetes of youth in Black Americans. New Engl J Med 1987;316:285–291.
35. Winter WE. Atypical diabetes in Blacks. Clin Diabetes 1991;9:49–56.
36. Irvine WJ, McCallum CJ, Gray RS, Duncan LJP. Clinical and pathogenic significance of pancreatic islet-cell antibodies in diabetics treated with oral hypoglycemic agents. Lancet 1977;1:1025–1027.
37. Di Mario U, Irvine WJ, Borsey DQ, et al. Immune abnormalities in diabetic patients not

requiring insulin at diagnosis. Diabetologia 1983; 25:392–395.

38. Niskanen L, Karjalaienen J, Sarlund H, et al. Five year follow-up of islet-cell antibodies in type 2 (non–insulin dependent) diabetes mellitus. Diabetologia 1991;34:402–408.

39. Atkinson MA, Maclaren NK, Riley WJ, et al. Are insulin autoantibodies markers for insulin-dependent diabetes mellitus? Diabetes 1986;35: 894–898.

40. Greenbaum CJ, Palmer JP, Kuglin B, Kolb H. Insulin autoantibodies measured by radioimmunoassay methodology are more related to insulin-dependent diabetes mellitus than those measured by enzyme-linked immunosorbent assay: results of the Fourth International Workshop on the Standardization of Insulin Autoantibody Measurement. J Clin Endocrinol Metab 1992;74:1040–1044.

41. Levy-Marchal C, Bridel MP, Sodoyez-Goffaux F, et al. Superiority of radiobinding assay over ELISA for detection of IAAs in newly diagnosed type I diabetic children. Diabetes Care 1991;14: 61–63.

42. Baekkeskov S, Nielson JH, Marner B, et al. Autoantibodies in newly diagnosed diabetic children immunoprecipitate human pancreatic islet cell proteins. Nature 1982;298:167–169.

43. Baekkeskov S, Dryberg T, Lernmark A. Autoantibodies to a 64-kilodalton islet cell protein precede the onset of spontaneous diabetes in the BB rat. Science 1984;224:1348–1350.

44. Atkinson MA, Maclaren NK. Autoantibodies in nonobese diabetic mice immunoprecipitate 64,000-M_r islet antigen. Diabetes 1988;37:1587–1590.

45. Kaufman DL, Erlander MG, Clare-Salzler M, et al. Autoimmunity to two forms of glutamate decarboxylase in insulin-dependent diabetes mellitus. J Clin Invest 1992;89:283–292.

46. Christie MR, Hollands JA, Brown TJ, et al. Detection of pancreatic islet 64,000 M(r) autoantigens in insulin-dependent diabetes distinct from glutamate decarboxylase. J Clin Invest 1993;92:240–248.

47. Luhder F, Schlosser M, Mauch L, et al. Autoantibodies against GAD65 rather than GAD67 precede the onset of type 1 diabetes. Autoimmunity 1994;19:71–80.

48. Vives Pi M, Somoza N, Vargas F, et al. Expression of glutamic acid decarboxylase (GAD) in the alpha, beta and delta cells of normal and diabetic pancreas: implications for the pathogenesis of type I diabetes. Clin Exp Immunol 1993;92: 391–396.

49. Richter W, Seissler J, Northemann W, et al. Cytoplasmic islet cell antibodies recognize distinct islet antigens in IDDM but not in stiff man syndrome. Diabetes 1993;42:1642–1648.

50. Clare-Salzler M, Kaufman D, Tobin A. Glutamate decarboxylase on IDDM autoantigen. Diabetes Care 1992;15:132–135.

51. Gianani R, Rabin DU, Verge CF, et al. ICA512 autoantibody radioassay. Diabetes 1995;44: 1340–1344.

52. Lan MS, Wasserfall C, Maclaren NK, Notkins AL. IA-2, a transmembrane protein of the protein tyrosine phosphatase family, is a major autoantigen in insulin-dependent diabetes mellitus. Proc Natl Acad Sci USA 1996;93:6367–6370.

53. Lan MS, Lu J, Goto Y, Notkins AL. Molecular cloning and identification of a receptor-type protein tyrosine phosphatase, IA-2, from human insulinoma. DNA Cell Biol 1994;13:505–514.

54. Rabin DU, Pleasic SM, Shapiro JA, et al. Islet cell antigen 512 is a diabetes-specific islet autoantigen related to protein tyrosine phosphatases. J Immunol 1994;152:3183–3188.

55. Solimena M, Dirkx R Jr, Hermel JM, et al. ICA 512, an autoantigen of type I diabetes, is an intrinsic membrane protein of neurosecretory granules. EMBO J 1996;15:2102–2114.

56. Lu J, Li Q, Xie H, et al. Identification of a second transmembrane protein tyrosine phosphatase, IA-2beta, as an autoantigen in insulin-dependent diabetes mellitus: precursor of the 37-kDa tryptic fragment. Proc Natl Acad Sci USA 1996;93:2307–2311.

57. Bonifacio E, Lampasona V, Genovese S, et al. Identification of protein tyrosine phosphatase–like IA2 (islet cell antigen 512) as the insulin-dependent diabetes-related 37/40K autoantigen and a target of islet-cell antibodies. J Immunol 1995;155:5419–5426.

58. Payton MA, Hawkes CJ, Christie MR. Relationship of the 37,000- and 40,000-M(r) tryptic fragments of islet antigens in insulin-dependent diabetes to the protein tyrosine phosphatase–like molecule IA-2 (ICA512). J Clin Invest 1995; 96:1506–1511.

59. Verge CF, Gianani R, Kawasaki E, et al. Prediction of type I diabetes in first-degree relatives using a combination of insulin, GAD, and

ICA512bdc/IA-2 autoantibodies. Diabetes 1996; 45:926–933.

60. Riley WJ, Maclaren NK, Krischer J, et al. A prospective study of the development of diabetes in relatives of patients with insulin-dependent diabetes. N Engl J Med 1990;323:1167–1172.

61. Gorsuch AN, Spencer KM, Lister J, et al. Evidence for a long prediabetic period in type I (insulin-dependent) diabetes mellitus. Lancet 1981;2:1363–1365.

62. Srikanta S, Ganda OP. Chronic progressive beta cell dysfunction in relatives of patients with type 1 diabetes. Diabetes 1983;32:51A.

63. Srikanta S, Ganda OP, Eisenbarth GS, Soeldner JS. Islet-cell antibodies and beta-cell function in monozygotic triplets and twins initially discordant for type I diabetes mellitus. N Engl J Med 1983;308:322–325.

64. Srikanta S, Ganda OP, Jackson RA, et al. Type 1 diabetes mellitus in monozygotic twins: chronic progressive beta cell dysfunction. Ann Intern Med 1983;99:320–326.

65. Srikanta S, Ganda OP, Jackson RA, et al. Pretype 1 (insulin-dependent) diabetes: common endocrinological course despite immunological and immunogenetic heterogeneity. Diabetologia 1984;27:146–148.

66. Srikanta S, Ganda OP, Gleason RA, et al. Pretype 1 diabetes, linear loss of beta cell response to intravenous glucose. Diabetes 1984;33:717–720.

67. Atkinson MA, Maclaren NK, Scharp DW, et al. 64,000 M_r autoantibodies as predictors of insulin-dependent diabetes. Lancet 1990;335:1357–1360.

68. Bonifacio E, Genovese S, Braghi S, et al. Islet autoantibody markers in IDDM: risk assessment strategies yielding high sensitivity. Diabetologia 1995;38:816–822.

69. Winter WE, Maclaren NK. Type I insulin dependent diabetes: an autoimmune disease that can be arrested or prevented with immunotherapy. In: Barness L, ed. Advances in pediatrics. Chicago: Year Book, 1985:159–175.

70. Skyler JS, Lorenz TJ, Schwartz S, et al. Effects of an anti-CD5 immunoconjugate (CD5-plus) in recent onset type I diabetes mellitus: a preliminary investigation. The CD5 Diabetes Project Team. J Diabetes Complications 1993;7:224–232.

71. Silverstein J, Riley W, Barrett D, et al. Immunosuppressive therapy (IT) for newly diagnosed insulin dependent diabetes mellitus (IDD) with antithymocyte globulin (ATG) and prednisone (pred.). Pediatr Res 1984;71:295A.

72. Harrison LC, Colman PG, Dean B, et al. Increase in remission rate in newly diagnosed type I diabetic subjects treated with azathioprine. Diabetes 1985;34:1306–1308.

73. Riley WJ, Maclaren NK, Spillar RS. Reversal of deteriorating glucose tolerance with azathioprine in pre-diabetes. Transplant Proc 1986;18: 819–822.

74. Silverstein J, Maclaren N, Riley W, et al. Immunosuppression with azathioprine and prednisone in recent-onset insulin-dependent diabetes mellitus. N Engl J Med 1988;319:599–604.

75. Shehadeh N, Calcinaro F, Bradley BJ, et al. Effect of adjuvant therapy on development of diabetes in mouse and man. Lancet 1994;343: 706–707.

76. Cavanaugh J, Chopek M, Binimelis J, et al. Buffy coat transfusions in early type I diabetes. Diabetes 1987;36:1089–1093.

77. Usadel KH, Teuber J, Schmeidl R, et al. Management of type I diabetes with ciamexone. Lancet 1986;2:567. Letter.

78. Stiller CR, Dupre J, Gent M, et al. Effects of cyclosporin immunosuppression in insulin-dependent diabetes mellitus of recent onset. Science 1984;223:1362–1367.

79. Assan R, Feutren G, Debray-Sachs M, et al. Metabolic and immunological effects of cyclosporin in recently diagnosed type I diabetes mellitus. Lancet 1985;1:67–71.

80. Feutren G, Papoz L, Assan R, M, et al. Cyclosporin increases the rate and length of remissions in insulin-dependent diabetes of recent onset. Results of a multicentre double-blind trial. Lancet 1986;2:119–124.

81. Dupre J, Stiller CR, Gent M, et al. Clinical trials of cyclosporin in IDDM. Diabetes Care 1988;11(suppl 1):37–44.

82. Bougneres PF, Carel JC, Castano L, et al. Factors associated with early remission of type I diabetes in children treated with cyclosporine. N Engl J Med 1990;318:663–670.

83. Chase HP, Butler-Simon N, Garg SK, et al. Cyclosporine A for the treatment of new-onset insulin-dependent diabetes mellitus. Pediatrics 1990;85:241–245.

84. Rand KH, Rosenbloom AL, Maclaren NK, et al. Human leukocyte interferon treatment of

two children with insulin-dependent diabetes. Diabetologia 1981;21:116–119.

85. Koivisto VA, Aro A, Cantell K, et al. Remissions in newly diagnosed type I (insulin-dependent) diabetes: influence of interferon as an adjunct to insulin therapy. Bull Int Study Group for Diabetes in the Young 1984;10:16.

86. Pocecco M, De-Campo C, Cantoni L, et al. Effect of high doses of intravenous IgG in newly diagnosed diabetic children. Helv Paediatr Acta 1987; 42:289–295.

87. Cobb WE, Molitch M, Reichlin S. Levamisole in insulin-dependent diabetes mellitus. N Engl J Med 1980;303:1065–1066.

88. Leslie RDG, Pyke DA. Immunosuppression of acute insulin-dependent diabetes. In: Irvine WJ, ed. The immunology of diabetes. Edinburgh: Tevoit Scientific, 1980:345–347.

89. Ludvigsson J, Heding L, Lernmark A, Lieden G. An attempt to break the autoimmune process at the onset of IDDM by the use of plasmapheresis and high doses of prednisolone. Bull Int Study Group for Diabetes in the Young 1982; 6:11–12.

90. Ludvigsson J, Heding L, Gudrun L, et al. Plasmapheresis in the initial treatment of insulin-dependent diabetes mellitus in children. Br Med J 1983;286:176–178.

91. Elliott RB, Crossley JR, Berryman CC, Hames AG. Partial preservation of pancreatic β-cell function in children with diabetes. Lancet 1981; 2:1–4.

92. Jackson R, Dolinar R, Srikanta S, et al. Prednisone therapy in early type I diabetes: immunological effects. Diabetes 1982;31:48A.

93. Giordano C, Panto F, Amato MP, et al. Early administration of an immunomodulator and induction of remission in insulin-dependent diabetes mellitus. J Autoimmun 1990;3:611–617.

94. Martin S, Schernthaner G, Nerup J, et al. Follow-up of cyclosporin A treatment in type 1 (insulin-dependent) diabetes mellitus: lack of long-term effects. Diabetologia 1991;34:429–434.

95. Muir A, Ramiya V. New strategies in oral immunotherapy for diabetes prevention. Diabet Metabol Rev 1996;12:1–14.

96. Beppu H, Winter WE, Atkinson MA, et al. Bovine albumin antibodies in NOD mice. Diabetes Res 1987;6:67–69.

97. Mayer EJ, Hamman RF, Gay EC, et al. Reduced risk of IDDM among breast-fed children. The Colorado IDDM Registry. Diabetes 1988;37: 1625–1632.

98. Virtanen SM, Rasanen L, Aro A, et al. Infant feeding in Finnish children less than 7 yr of age with newly diagnosed IDDM. Childhood Diabetes in Finland Study Group. Diabetes Care 1991;14:415–417.

99. Karjalainen J, Martin J, Knip M. A bovine albumin peptide as a possible trigger of insulin-dependent diabetes mellitus. N Engl J Med 1992;327:302–307.

100. Savilahti E, Saukkonen TT, Virtala ET, et al. Increased levels of cow's milk and β-lactoglobulin antibodies in young children with newly diagnosed IDDM. The Childhood Diabetes in Finland Study Group. Diabetes Care 1993;16: 984–989.

101. Atkinson MA, Bowman MA, Kao KJ, et al. Lack of immune responsiveness to bovine serum albumin in insulin-dependent diabetes. N Engl J Med 1993;329:1853–1858.

102. Maclaren NK, Atkinson MA. Is insulin-dependent diabetes mellitus environmentally induced? N Engl J Med 1992;327:347–349.

103. Elliott RB, Chase HP. Prevention or delay of type 1 (insulin-dependent) diabetes mellitus in children using nicotinamide. Diabetologia 1991; 34:362–365.

104. Manna R, Migliore A, Martin LS, et al. Nicotinamide treatment in subjects at high risk of developing IDDM improves insulin secretion. Br J Clin Pract 1992;46:177–179.

105. Herskowitz RD, Jackson RA, Soeldner JS, Eisenbarth GS. Pilot trial to prevent type I diabetes: progression to overt IDDM despite oral nicotinamide. J Autoimmun 1989;2:733–737.

106. Daniel D, Wegmann DR. Protection of nonobese diabetic mice from diabetes by intranasal or subcutaneous administration of insulin peptide B-(9-23). Proc Natl Acad Sci USA 1996;93:956–960.

107. Atkinson MA, Maclaren NK, Luchetta R. Insulitis and diabetes in NOD mice reduced by prophylactic insulin therapy. Diabetes 1990;39:933–937.

108. Zhang ZJ, Davidson L, Eisenbarth G, Weiner HL. Suppression of diabetes in nonobese diabetic mice by oral administration of porcine insulin. Proc Natl Acad Sci USA 1991;88:10252–10256.

109. Muir A, Peck A, Clare-Salzler M, et al. Insulin immunization of nonobese diabetic mice

induces a protective insulitis characterized by diminished intraislet interferon-gamma transcription. J Clin Invest 1995;95:628–634.

110. Thivolet CH, Goillot E, Bedossa P, et al. Insulin prevents adoptive cell transfer of diabetes in the autoimmune non-obese diabetic mouse. Diabetologia 1991;34:314–319.

111. Shah SC, Malone JI, Simpson NE. A randomized trial of intensive insulin therapy in newly diagnosed insulin-dependent diabetes mellitus. N Engl J Med 1989;320:550–554.

112. Keller RJ, Eisenbarth GS, Jackson RA. Insulin prophylaxis in individuals at high risk of type I diabetes. Lancet 1993;341:927–928.

113. Weiner HL, Friedman A, Miller A, et al. Oral tolerance: immunologic mechanisms and treatment of animal and human organ-specific autoimmune diseases by oral administration of autoantigens. Annu Rev Immunol 1994;12:809–837.

114. Sosroseno W. A review of the mechanisms of oral tolerance and immunotherapy. J R Soc Med 1995;88:14–17.

115. Cudworth AG, Woodrow JC. Genetic susceptibility in diabetes mellitus: analysis of the HLA association. Br Med J 1976;2:846–848.

116. Cudworth AG, Wolf E. The genetic susceptibility to type I (insulin-dependent) diabetes mellitus. Clin Endocrinol Metab 1982;11:389–407.

117. Owerbach D, Lernmark A, Platz P, et al. HLA-D region beta-chain DNA endonuclease fragments differ between HLA-DR identical healthy and insulin-dependent diabetic individuals. Nature 1983;303:815–817.

118. Owerbach D, Hagglof B, Lernmark A, Holmgren G. Susceptibility to insulin-dependent diabetes defined by restriction enzyme polymorphism of HLA-D region genomic DNA. Diabetes 1984;33:958–965.

119. Sheehy MJ, Rowe JR, MacDonald MJ. A particular subset of HLA-DR4 accounts for all or most of the DR4 association in type I diabetes. Diabetes 1985;34:942–944.

120. Todd JA, Bell JI, McDevitt HO. HLA-DQβ gene contributes to susceptibility and resistance to insulin-dependent diabetes mellitus. Nature 1987;329:599–604.

121. Henson V, Maclaren N, Riley W, Wakeland EK. Polymorphisms of DQβ genes in HLA-DR4 haplotypes from healthy and diabetic individuals. Immunogenetics 1987;25:152–160.

122. Michelsen B, Lernmark A. Molecular cloning of a polymorphic DNA endonuclease fragment associates insulin-dependent diabetes mellitus with HLA-DQ. J Clin Invest 1987;79:1144.

123. Maclaren N, Riley W, Skordis N, et al. Inherited susceptibility to insulin-dependent diabetes is associated with HLA-DR1, while DR5 is protective. Autoimmunity 1988;1:197–205.

124. Fletcher J, Mijovic C, Odugbesan O, et al. Transracial studies implicate HLA-DQ as a component of genetic susceptibility to type 1 (insulin-dependent) diabetes. Diabetologia 1988;31:864–870.

125. Horn GT, Bugawan TL, Long CM, Erlich HA. Allelic sequence variation of the HLA-DQ loci: relationship to serology and insulin-dependent diabetes susceptibility. Proc Natl Acad Sci USA 1988;85:6012–6016.

126. Owerbach D, Gunn S, Ty G, et al. Oligonucleotide probes for HLA-DQA and DQB genes define susceptibility to type 1 (insulin-dependent) diabetes mellitus. Diabetologia 1988;31:751–757.

127. Morel PA, Dorman JS, Todd JA, et al. Aspartic acid at position 57 of the HLA-DQ chain protects against type I diabetes: a family study. Proc Natl Acad Sci USA 1988;85:8111–8115.

128. Sheehy MJ, Scharf SJ, Rowe JR, et al. Diabetes-susceptible HLA haplotype is best defined to a combination of HLA-DR and DQ alleles. J Clin Invest 1989;83:830–835.

129. Nepom GT. A unified hypothesis for the complex genetics of HLA associations with IDDM. Diabetes 1990;39:1153–1157.

130. Baisch JM, Weeks T, Giles R, et al. Analysis of HLA-DQ genotypes and susceptibility in insulin-dependent diabetes mellitus. N Engl J Med 1990;322:1836–1841.

131. Bognetti E, Meschi F, Malavasi C, et al. HLA-antigens in Italian type 1 diabetic patients: role of DR3/DR4 antigens and breast feeding in the onset of the disease. Acta Diabetol 1992;28:229–232.

132. Gutierrez-Lopez MD, Bertera S, Chantres MT, et al. Susceptibility to type 1 (insulin-dependent) diabetes mellitus in Spanish patients correlates quantitatively with expression of HLA-DQ alpha Arg 52 and HLA-DQ beta non-Asp 57 alleles. Diabetologia 1992;35:583–588.

133. Heimberg H, Nagy ZP, Somers G, et al. Complementation of HLA-DQA and -DQB genes confers susceptibility and protection to insulin-

dependent diabetes mellitus. Hum Immunol 1992;33:10–17.

134. Khalil I, Deschamps I, Lepage V, et al. Dose effect of cis- and trans-encoded HLA-DQ alpha beta heterodimers in IDDM susceptibility. Diabetes 1992;41:378–384.

135. Julier C, Hyer RN, Davies J, et al. Insulin-IGF2 region on chromosome 11p encodes a gene implicated in HLA-DR4–dependent diabetes susceptibility. Nature 1991;354:155–159.

136. Bain SC, Prins JB, Hearne CM, et al. Insulin gene region–encoded susceptibility to type 1 diabetes is not restricted to HLA-DR4–positive individuals. Nat Genet 1992;2:212–215.

137. Winter WE, Obata M, Muir A, Maclaren NK. Heritable origins of type I, insulin dependent diabetes mellitus. Growth Genet Hormones 1991;7:1–6.

138. Winter WE, Chihara T, Schatz DA. The genetics of autoimmune diabetes. Am J Dis Child 1993;147:1282–1290.

139. Roll U, Christie MR, Fuchtenbusch M, et al. Perinatal autoimmunity in offspring of diabetic parents. The German Multicenter BABY-DIAB Study: detection of humoral immune responses to islet antigens in early childhood. Diabetes 1996;45:967–973.

140. Verge CF, Gianani R, Kawasaki E, et al. Prediction of type I diabetes in first-degree relatives using a combination of insulin, GAD, and ICA512bdc/IA-2 autoantibodies. Diabetes 1996;45:926–933.

141. Schatz D, Krischer J, Wasserfall C, et al. ICA, GAD_{65}A, IAA and IA-2 to screen for IDD in schoolchildren and unaffected relatives. Diabetes 1996;45(suppl 2):80A.

142. Bonifacio E, Genovese S, Braghi S, et al. Islet autoantibody markers in IDDM: risk assessment strategies yielding high sensitivity. Diabetologia 1995;38:816–822.

143. Tisch R, Yang XD, Liblau RS, McDevitt HO. Administering glutamic acid decarboxylase to NOD mice prevents diabetes. J Autoimmun 1994;7:845–850.

144. Marx J. Testing of autoimmune therapy begins. Science 1991;252:27–28.

145. Harrison LC, Honeyman MC, DeAizpurua HJ, et al. Inverse relation between humoral and cellular immunity to glutamic acid decarboxylase in subjects at risk of insulin-dependent diabetes. Lancet 1993;341:1365–1369.

146. Hancock WW, Polanski M, Zhang J, et al. Suppression of insulitis in non-obese diabetic (NOD) mice by oral insulin administration is associated with selective expression of interleukin-4 and -10, transforming growth factor-beta, and prostaglandin-E. Am J Pathol 1995;147:1193–1199.

147. Lendrum R, Walker G, Gamble DR. Islet-cell antibodies in juvenile diabetes mellitus of recent onset. Lancet 1975;1:880–883.

148. Lendrum R, Walker G, Cudworth AG, et al. Islet-cell antibodies in diabetes mellitus. Lancet 1976;2:1273–1276.

149. Irvine WJ, Gray RS, McCallum CJ. Pancreatic islet-cell antibody as a marker for asymptomatic and latent diabetes and prediabetes. Lancet 1976;2:1097–1102.

150. Betterle C, Zanette F, Tiengo A, Trevisan A. Five-year follow-up on non-diabetes with islet-cell antibodies. Lancet 1982;1:284–285.

151. Riley WJ, Spillar RP, Waltz J, Brody B. Predictive value of islet cell autoantibodies (ICA)—6 years experience. Diabetes 1984;33:44A.

152. Lernmark A, Baekkeskov S. Islet cell antibodies—theoretical and practical implications. Diabetologia 1981;21:431–435.

153. Ziegler AG, Herskowitz RD, Jackson RA, et al. Predicting type I diabetes. Diabetes Care 1990; 13:762–765.

154. Landin-Olsson M, Palmer JP, Lernmark A, et al. Predictive value of islet cell and insulin autoantibodies for type 1 (insulin-dependent) diabetes mellitus in a population-based study of newly-diagnosed diabetic and matched control children. Diabetologia 1992;35:1068–1073.

155. Palmer JP. Predicting IDDM: use of humoral immune markers. Diabetes Rev 1993;1:104–115.

156. Tuomi T, Groop LC, Zimmet PZ, et al. Antibodies to glutamic acid decarboxylase reveal latent autoimmune diabetes mellitus in adults with a non–insulin-dependent onset of disease. Diabetes 1993;42:359–362.

157. Atkinson MA, Maclaren NK. Islet cell autoantigens in insulin-dependent diabetes. J Clin Invest 1993;92:1608–1616.

158. Schott M, Schatz D, Atkinson M, et al. GAD65 autoantibodies increase the predictability but not the sensitivity of islet cell and insulin autoantibodies for developing insulin dependent diabetes mellitus. J Autoimmun 1994;7:865–872.

159. Christie MR, Genovese S, Cassidy D, et al. Antibodies to islet 37k antigen, but not to glutamate

decarboxylase, discriminate rapid progression to IDDM in endocrine autoimmunity. Diabetes 1994;43:1254–1259.

160. Verge CF, Gianani R, Yu L, et al. Late progression to diabetes and evidence for chronic beta-cell autoimmunity in identical twins of patients with type I diabetes. Diabetes 1995;44:1176–1179.

161. Vardi P, Crisa L, Jackson RA. Predictive value of intravenous glucose tolerance test insulin secretion less than or greater than the first percentile in islet cell antibody positive relatives of type 1 (insulin-dependent) diabetic patients. Diabetologia 1991;34:93–102.

162. Yassin N, Seissler J, Gluck M, et al. Insulin autoantibodies as determined by competitive radiobinding assay are positively correlated with impaired beta-cell function—the Ulm-Frankfurt Population Study. Klin Wochenschr 1991;69:736–741.

163. Drash AL. Is it time to draw the curtain on immune intervention trials in newly diagnosed patients with IDDM? Diabetes Care 1995;18:1499–1501.

164. Atkinson MA, Winter WE, Skordis N, et al. Dietary protein restriction reduces the frequency and delays the onset of insulin dependent diabetes in BB rats. Autoimmunity 1988;2:11–20.

165. Rabinovitch A. Roles of cytokines in IDDM pathogenesis and islet β-cell destruction. Diabetes Rev 1993;1:215–240.

166. Lewis CM, Canafax DM, Sprafka JM, Barbosa JJ. Double-blind randomized trial of nicotinamide on early-onset diabetes. Diabetes Care 1992;15:121–123.

167. Vague P, Picq R, Bernal M, et al. Effect of nicotinamide treatment on the residual insulin secretion in type 1 (insulin-dependent) diabetic patients. Diabetologia 1989;32:316–321.

168. Pozzilli P, Visalli N, Boccuni ML, et al. Randomized trial comparing nicotinamide and nicotinamide plus cyclosporin in recent onset insulin-dependent diabetes (IMDIAB 1). The IMDIAB Study Group. Diabet Med 1994;11:98–104.

169. Gepts W. Pathologic anatomy of the pancreas in juvenile diabetes mellitus. Diabetes 1965;14:619–633.

170. Gepts W, Lecompte PM. The pancreatic islets in diabetes. Am J Med 1981;70:105–115.

171. Foulis AK, Stewart JA. The pancreas in recent-onset type 1 (insulin-dependent) diabetes mellitus: insulin content of islets, insulitis and associated changes in the exocrine acinar tissue. Diabetologia 1984;26:456–461.

172. Bottazzo GF, Dean BM, McNally JM, et al. In situ characterization of autoimmune phenomena and expression of HLA molecules in the pancreas in diabetic insulitis. N Engl J Med 1985;313:353–360.

173. Foulis AK, Liddle CN, Farquharson MA, et al. The histopathology of the pancreas in type 1 (insulin-dependent) diabetes mellitus: a 25-year review of deaths in patients under 20 years of age in the United Kingdom. Diabetologia 1986;29:267–274.

174. Sinha AA, Lopez MT, McDevitt HO. Autoimmune diseases: the failure of self tolerance. Science 1990;248:1380–1388.

175. Janeway CA. How the immune system recognizes invaders. Sci Am 1993;269(3):72–79.

CHAPTER 26

Autoimmune Liver Disease

WAYNE R. HOGREFE
HARRY E. PRINCE

The association of immunologic autoreactivity and liver disease has been recognized for many years. The earliest correlation of autoimmunity and liver disease was identified in systemic lupus erythematosus patients who demonstrated hepatic involvement together with their systemic collagen vascular disease. This hepatic disease was originally described as "lupoid hepatitis" (1,2). Nearly 20 years prior to these reports, hepatic disease similar to lupoid hepatitis had been reported by Cullinan (3). Currently three liver diseases are categorized as autoimmune: "autoimmune" chronic active hepatitis (AI-CAH), primary biliary cirrhosis (PBC), and primary sclerosing cholangitis (PSC). Although immune mechanisms are suspected in the pathogenesis of these diseases, the role of either cell-mediated or antibody-mediated immunity as an effector mechanism in any of these diseases has not been proven. The tissue pathology, whether immunologically mediated or not, involves hepatocytes for AI-CAH and bile-duct epithelial cells for PBC and PSC.

Numerous autoantibodies have been identified in AI-CAH, including antinuclear antibody (ANA), anti-smooth-muscle antibody (SMA), liver-kidney microsomal (LKM) antibody types 1, 2, and 3, soluble liver antigen (SLA) antibody, liver-specific membrane lipoprotein/liver-specific protein (LSP) antibody, and many others. This discussion will focus on the most relevant of these autoantibodies.

Although the diagnosis of AI-CAH requires the presence of at least one or more autoantibodies, the specificity and sensitivity of these autoantibodies in AI-CAH is quite variable. Of the two autoimmune diseases involving bile duct epithelium, PBC is more commonly associated with autoantibodies. The most common antibody detected in PBC is antimitochondria antibody, although ANA, smooth muscle antibody, reticulin antibody, and rheumatoid factor may also be present. The only autoantibody detected in PSC is the antineutrophil cytoplasmic antibody of the perinuclear type.

As the diagnosis of autoimmune liver disease, in particular AI-CAH and PBC, includes the presence of autoantibodies, the immunology laboratory is actively involved in establishing the diagnosis. This chapter discusses the autoantibodies most commonly detected in the three autoimmune liver diseases.

Autoimmune Chronic Active Hepatitis

The development of chronic active hepatitis (CAH) has various etiologies including infectious agents, autoimmune disorders, drug-induced disorders, enzyme deficiency (i.e., α_1-antitrypsin), and Wilson's disease (4). The most common causes of CAH are infectious agents, including viral hepatitis B, C, and D. The second most common cause of CAH is believed to be autoimmune mechanisms, which are separated into three types and described below.

Classifications of AI-CAH

The pathology and subsequent clinical progression of CAH is demonstrated by varying degrees of hepatocellular inflammation, focal to lobular necrosis, and in many cases, development of cirrhosis (5). Classifying the causes of CAH into either viral, drug-induced, or autoimmune is accomplished by defining the clinical history of the patient and detecting either viral antibodies or autoantibodies. The accurate classification of CAH allows for the use of appropriate therapy for each disease presentation; for example, interferon alpha (IFN-α) is used for the treatment of viral hepatitis, and corticosteroids or cytotoxic agents are used for AI-CAH (6).

The most common cause of CAH is viral infection, of which hepatitis B (HBV), hepatitis C (HCV), or hepatitis D (HDV) is the most common; cytomegalovirus (CMV) infection may rarely occur. The diagnosis of chronic hepatitis due to either hepatitis B, C, or D requires the detection of HBs antigen or DNA, HCV antibody or RNA, or HDV antibody or RNA, respectively. The diagnosis of AI-CAH is based not only on the clinical history of the patient and no identifiable viral or drug-induced etiology, but also on the presence of autoantibodies. Numerous autoantibodies have been reported in AI-CAH and are summarized in **Table 26-1**.

Traditionally, AI-CAH has been classified as either type 1 or type 2 based on the antibody profile detected (4). Recently a revised classification proposed adding a type 3 AI-CAH, which again is based on the antibody profile of the patient (7,8). However, the inclusion of type 3 AI-CAH has not been universally accepted at this time.

Lastly, *cryptogenic AI-CAH* is the term used for CAH patients with no identifiable infectious agent or autoantibody marker. All AI-CAH patients have a clinical and histologic appearance of chronic liver disease, but the classification (typing) is determined serologically.

Type 1 AI-CAH

Type 1 (classic) AI-CAH has been defined as CAH with the presence of either ANA and/or SMA (4,6). Although both ANA and SMA are sensitive markers of type 1 AI-CAH, the specificity of these autoantibodies is low to moderate, respectively. Anti-actin antibodies (AAA), in particular antibodies to actin F, were originally thought to reflect the specific epitope for SMA (9,10), but now it is known that actin F antibody is only present in 50% to 80% of type 1 AI-CAH patients (4,11). Other autoantibodies detected in type 1 AI-CAH (with the published percent of incidence) include perinuclear-type antineutrophil cytoplasmic antibody (pANCA) (50% to 90%) (12), and antibody to nuclear lamins A/C (75%) (13).

Antibody to LSP is present in up to 90% of patients with either type 1 or type 2 AI-CAH (4,14). To date the only specific epitope of the complex LSP antigen to be characterized is the hepatic asialoglycoprotein receptor (ASGPR), where between 50% to 83% of AI-CAH patients are positive for ASGPR antibody (15,16). The

TABLE **26-1**

Autoantibodies Associated with Autoimmune Chronic Active Hepatitis

Autoantibody	AI Type	Sensitivity (%)	Specificity	Reference
ANA	1	95–100	Low	(4,6)
ASMA	1	95–100	Moderate	(4,6)
Anti-actin	1	50–80	High	(4,11)
pANCA	1	50–90	Low	(12)
Nuclear lamina A/C	1	75	Moderate	(13)
LSP	1/2	80	Moderate	(14)
ASGPR	1/2	50–83	Moderate	(15,16)
LKM-1	2	95–100	High	(4,6,17)
P450 2D6	2	85	High	(19)
rhP450 2D6	2	74–95	High	(21)
GOR	2	65	High	(24)
LKM-2	2	NA	High	(25)
LKM-3	2	NA	High	(26,27)
SLA	3	35–40	Low	(7,8,29)
Cytokeratin	3	30	High	
Liver/Pancreas	3	<10	Unknown	

LSP and ASGPR antibodies have a high degree of sensitivity for CAH, especially in untreated patients or patients in relapse. However, these antibodies are also present in up to 15% of patients with PBC, liver cancer, connective tissue diseases, and viral hepatitis (16).

Type 2 AI-CAH

Type 2 AI-CAH is classified by the presence of liver-kidney microsomal 1 (LKM-1) antibody (4,6,17). LKM-1 was first described in 1973 by its characteristic immunofluorescent staining pattern on multiple tissues, which is still considered the gold standard for the detection of LKM-1 (18). In 1988 the dominant antigen of LKM-1 was defined as cytochrome P450dbl which was later clarified to be cytochrome P450 2D6 (19). A 33-amino-acid sequence thought to be the epitope for LKM-1 has been defined and will detect 85% of LKM-1-positive sera; an 8-amino-acid sequence will detect 50% of the LKM-1 sera (20).

A recombinant cytochrome P450 2D6 has been produced that will detect 74% and 95% of LKM-1 samples by enzyme-linked immunosorbent assay (ELISA) and Western blot analysis, respectively (21). Using the first-generation HCV serology tests, a high percentage of LKM-1-positive sera were also positive for HCV antibody (22). However, with the second-generation HCV ELISA kits and confirmation using recombinant immunoblot assays (RIBA), the percent of LKM-1-positive sera that were also positive for HCV antibody dropped to 50% (21,23,24).

Patients who are both LKM-1 and HCV positive tend to be older, have a less aggressive disease, and have a clinical course and response to therapy more typical of a HCV-induced CAH. Patients positive for LKM-1 antibody only are younger (2 to 14 years old), predominantly female, and respond to corticosteroids.

An antibody that may be a useful marker for LKM-1/HCV-positive samples is the anti-GOR antibody. GOR (GOR 47-1) is a fusion protein obtained from a cDNA library derived from a chimpanzee with non-A/non-B hepatitis. Sixty to seventy percent of the LKM-1/HCV-positive patients possess anti-GOR antibody (24), whereas GOR antibody is rarely detected in LKM-1-negative/HCV-positive samples. The clinical significance of GOR antibody has yet to be defined.

Other LKM antibodies have been identified, including LKM-2, which is present in tienilic acid–induced hepatitis (25), and LKM-3, which is present in approximately 15% of hepatitis BsAg-positive patients with chronic delta infections (26). The epitope of LKM-3 had been identified as one family of uridine diphosphate glucuronosyltransferases (27). According to a recently published study, LKM-1 antibody is rarely encountered in the United States, but up to 25% of sera classified as antimitochondrial-positive were actually LKM-1 positive, not AMA positive (28).

Type 3 AI-CAH

Recently, it was proposed to separate type 1 AI-CAH patients with antibodies to SLA and/or liver-pancreas antibody (LP) into their own subtype, type 3 AI-CAH (8). SLA antibody is detected in 38% of CAH patients, and may be a sensitive marker of cryptogenic CAH (7,8,29,30). Although the type 1 antibodies (ANA, SMA) are typically present with SLA antibodies, up to 23% of CAH sera will contain only SLA antibodies (7,29).

The most common epitopes bound by SLA antibodies are the liver cytokeratins 18 and 8 (29,30). LP antibody is detected in 9% of AI-CAH patients, with LP antibody being the only antibody detected in one-third of these sera (8,31).

Test Selection for AI-CAH

As outlined above, many autoantibodies are detected in AI-CAH; however, many of these autoantibodies are either not well defined or are detected in a limited number of AI-CAH patients. This section outlines the autoantibodies that have been well defined in their predictive value as well as in their ability to best define the various types of AI-CAH.

The classic definition of type 1 AI-CAH requires either an ANA or SMA together with the appropriate clinical presentation. Although ANA is detected in nearly all type 1 patients, the specificity of ANA for AI-CAH is very low, and thus we will not discuss it further. The most reliable marker for type 1 AI-CAH is SMA. Because no reliable ELISA method has been developed to date, the test of choice for SMA remains the indirect immunofluorescent assay (IFA).

The gold standard for diagnosing type 2 AI-CAH is the detection of LKM-1 antibody by IFA, as it is both highly sensitive and specific. The identification of at least one specific epitope of LKM-1, cytochrome P450 2DL, has made it feasible to perform an enzyme-based assay to detect type 2 AI-CAH, albeit at a lower sensitivity.

Lastly, the detection of antibody to SLA is proposed as one assay that will be used to define type 3 AI-CAH in the absence of other autoantibodies. The sensitivity is low for AI-CAH, and SLA antibody may be detected in all three types of AI-CAH, both with and without other antibodies.

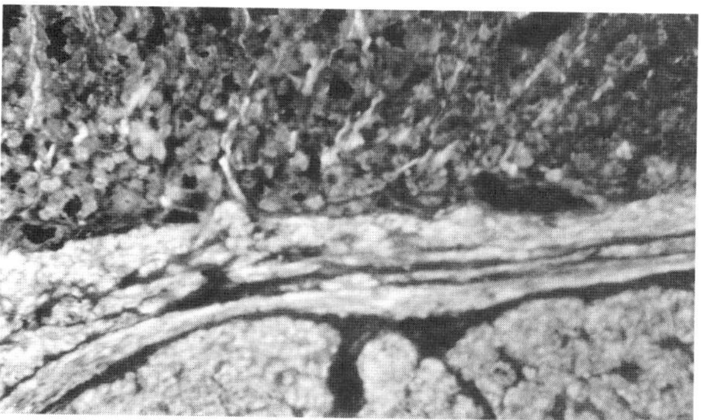

FIGURE **26-1**

Smooth muscle antibody. The smooth muscle bundles of the mucosa muscularis are intensely positive, whereas the mucosa at the top of the figure is negative.

Smooth Muscle Antibody (SMA) by Indirect Immunofluorescent Assay (IFA)

The detection of smooth muscle antibody (SMA) by indirect immunofluorescent assay (IFA) has been well documented for over 20 years. Typically, rodent stomach is the substrate of choice, because antibody binding to the muscularis mucosa is easily discriminated from the adjacent mucosa, rendering the presence of SMA easily discernible. The 4-μm frozen sections of stomach are cut cross-sectionally with either the tissue "flat" with the mucosa exposed or with the tissue rolled around itself. After air drying, the tissue is fixed in acetone for up to 10 minutes. Many commercial sources of rodent stomach are now available, and each should be tested for background reactivity prior to use. The differences in background reactivity are typically due to the fixation process. Serum is the sample of choice to perform this test.

The dilution scheme may start as low as 1:10 in phosphate buffered saline; however, specificity for AI-CAH is low at this titer and high background fluorescence may be present in normal sera. Because SMA can be present transiently at low titers (1:10 to 1:40) in normals and after acute viral infection, especially with CMV, screening for SMA at 1:40 is recommended. Titers of SMA in AI-CAH patients with active disease are typically 1:160 or greater. **Figure 26-1** demonstrates the SMA pattern using rodent stomach.

The SMA IFA method is quick and reliable once the microscope operator is trained to recognize the specific SMA pattern from the background fluorescence seen with some normal sera. Background fluorescence may be minimized by adding 0.0025% Evans blue to the conjugate and by starting the serum dilution scheme at 1:40.

Numerous commercial sources of defined SMA-positive sera are available, and proficiency testing is offered through the College of American Pathologists (CAP) immunology proficiency program, module S2.

Liver-Kidney Microsomal 1 (LKM-1) Antibody

The association of liver-kidney microsomal (LKM) antibody with autoimmune hepatitis was first described in 1973 (18), and it remains the gold standard for detecting type 2 AI-CAH. Subsequent to this first description of LKM antibody, two other LKM antibody patterns were described in conjunction with drug toxicity and infection. The IFA pattern of LKM for AI-CAH remains as originally described, and now is designated LKM-1.

Three tissues are required to discriminate accurately the LKM-1 IFA pattern from the pattern of the anitmitochondrial antibody (AMA) which is present in primary biliary cirrhosis. The three tissues required are liver, kidney, and stomach. The original description of LKM used both human and rodent liver and kidney with equal success, but only stomach of human origin was used in the original studies. Today, rat tissues are used for the detection of LKM-1, because the LKM-3 antibodies present in hepatitis delta infections are only detected using human or primate liver and kidney, and

LKM-2 antibodies present in tienilic acid–induced hepatitis require male mouse liver (25,26).

Although the 4-μm frozen sections of each tissue were originally used without acetone fixation, acetone fixation is preferred because it preserves the integrity of the of the tissues throughout the IFA process. Serum is the preferred sample and is typically screened at 1:10. As with SMA, low screening titers (1:10) present problems with both high background fluorescence with normal sera and possible prozone effect with high-titered LKM sera. The use of Evans blue as a counterstain with the FITC conjugate will help decrease background reactivity. A titer of 1:40 is an appropriate screening dilution for optimal results.

The difficulty of LKM-1 antibody detection by IFA lies in discriminating the LKM-1 IFA pattern from the IFA pattern of AMA. **Table 26-2** outlines the IFA pattern differences between the two antibodies. The LKM-1 antibody primarily binds to the proximal tubules in the kidney and does not bind to any cells of the gastric mucosa, whereas the AMA primarily binds the distal tubules and the loops of Henle in the kidney and strongly reacts with the gastric parietal cells. Both antibodies bind to hepatocytes in the liver with near equal intensity. The microscope operator must become familiar with both patterns to efficiently and accurately discriminate LKM-1 from AMA. Recently, it was reported that many LKM-1-positive sera may be incorrectly interpreted as AMA-positive sera; thus the incidence of type 2 AI-CAH as determined by the presence of LKM-1 antibody may actually be higher than previously believed (28).

Many commercial sources of rat tissues and LKM-1-positive sera are now available. To ensure accurate IFA pattern interpretation, both AMA- and LKM-1-positive sera should be used to evaluate the rodent tissues and to train the microscope operators. No proficiency programs are available for determination of LKM-1 antibody; however, Dr. Rudolf Gruber (Institut für Immunologie, Goethestr. 31, D-80336 München, Germany) has made available well-characterized sera specific for LKM-1, as well as sera specific for AMA (M2 fraction) and for antibody to SLA. Proficiency testing for AMA by IFA is available from the College of American Pathologists (CAP) immunology program, module S2.

TABLE 26-2

IFA Pattern for LKM-1 and AMA

Tissue	LKM-1	AMA
Liver	++	+
Kidney	++ Proximal	++ Distal
Stomach		
Parietal cells	−	++
Chief cells	−	+

Adapted from Rizzetto M, Swana G, Doniach D. Microsomal antibodies in active chronic hepatitis and other disorders. Clin Exp Immunol 1973;15:331–344.

Human Cytochrome P450 2D6/LKM-1 ELISA

Several experimental approaches have been used to develop an enzyme-based method for the detection of LKM-1 antibodies. These methods include the purification of the microsome fraction of hepatocytes (29) and more recently defining cytochrome P450 2D6 as the major epitope for LKM-1 antibodies (19,21). The P450 2D6 has been produced as a recombinant fusion protein, and has been evaluated by both Western blot and ELISA (21). The sensitivity and specificity of ELISA-based systems using both recombinant and purified native P450 2D6 (50-kd protein by Western blot) are high and approach that of LKM-1 identified by IFA (see Table 26-1). Commercial products using either the purified native antigen or the recombinant antigen are available; however, the performance of these kits has not yet been critically evaluated.

Soluble Liver Antigen (SLA) Antibody

The use of soluble fractions of hepatocytes to detect autoantibodies in patients with CAH was first described 10 years ago by Manns and colleagues (7). Originally, CAH patients with SLA antibody were all thought to be LKM-1 and ANA negative by IFA. Today the percent of SLA-positive sera that also contain LKM-1 and SMA antibodies ranges up to 50% (7,8,29). These discrepancies probably reflect the different antigen preparations used, assay conditions at each laboratory, and the type of patients tested. These different results make it difficult to assess the true sensitivity and specificity of this test in relation to other antibody tests available.

Two proteins are believed to be primarily responsible for the SLA reactivity, and they are 48- and 52-kd proteins designated cytokeratin 18 and 8, respectively (8,30). It is apparent that a subgroup of AI-CAH patients only contain SLA antibody and are negative for ANA, LKM-1, and to a lesser degree negative for SMA. The utility of SLA has yet to be determined, but it may truly represent another subgroup of CAH.

Primary Biliary Cirrhosis

Primary biliary cirrhosis (PBC) is a disease of unknown etiology that is characterized by a slowly progressive destruction of small intrahepatic bile ducts, ultimately leading to cirrhosis. Surrounding the damaged bile ducts is a cellular reaction that includes lymphocytes, plasma cells, eosinophils, and histiocytes. Noncaseating granulomas form as the bile ducts are destroyed; periportal inflammation, piecemeal necrosis, fibrosis, and ultimately biliary cirrhosis develop as the disease progresses to the late stages. PBC is a disease with a female : male predominance of 9 : 1 that manifests primarily in the fifth decade of life. As the disease progresses, functional impairment, often subclinical, is seen in the pancreas, thyroid, kidney, salivary, and lacrimal glands. Systemic disease involvement may also include rheumatologic disease features such as the CREST syndrome or the sicca syndrome (15,32).

In the past, a liver needle biopsy was often used to confirm PBC, although the characteristic pathology may not be apparent in the small tissue sampling if it is taken during the early stages of the disease. The discovery of a serologic test that would aid in the diagnosis of PBC was first published by Walker et al. in 1965 when they described the IFA pattern of antimitochondria antibodies (AMA) present in PBC patients (33). Several years later Rizzetto et al. (18) further characterized the similar IFA patterns of AMA and LKM using multiple tissues. Now the specific epitopes of AMA have been well characterized, and purified antigens and recombinant proteins to detect AMA are available in a variety of assay formats, including ELISA and Western blot. With the increased specificity and sensitivity of AMA testing resulting from these advances, the immunology laboratory can provide critical diagnostic results that will diminish the need for liver biopsy to diagnose PBC.

A separate category of AMA-negative PBC patients has been proposed by Goodman et al. (34). This patient group, designated as having "autoimmune cholangitis," has a clinical picture similar to PBC; however, these patients are AMA negative and may be SMA or ANA positive. Other investigators consider autoimmune cholangitis as a variant of AI-CAH that predominantly affects the bile ducts (32). Further characterization of this patient group awaits further studies.

Test Selection for PBC

Three groups of autoantibodies have been associated with PBC: AMA with identification of nine different mitochondrial antigens (M1–M9), antinuclear antibodies with a multiple nuclear dot pattern (MND-ANA), and keratin (cytoskeletal) antibodies. Keratin antibodies are present in only 2% of PBC patients (35) and will not be discussed further.

The reported occurrence of the multiple nuclear dot pattern in PBC has varied between 13% and 44% (36). This variation depends on the cell line used in the IFA procedure and the patient population selected for study. The most consistent estimate is that approximately 15% of PBC patients have MND-ANA (37,38). The MND-ANA-positive PBC patients frequently include those whose clinical picture includes a sicca syndrome. Although one report indicates that MND-ANA is not specific for PBC (39), most others report a high but not exclusive relationship between the presence of MND-ANA and PBC. The MND-ANA reacts with two sets of proteins at 78- to 92-kd and 96- to 100-kd as determined by Western blot studies (38). The latter protein has now been identified as Sp100, a cell growth suppression/transcription-activating protein that can be upregulated by interferon (40,41). Antibody to Sp100 is present in approximately the same percent of PBC patients as MND-ANA (15%). Extensive studies on the specificity of Sp100 antibodies have not been published to date; however, Sp100 antibodies are rarely present alone in PBC patients (40).

Antimitochondrial antibodies have been established as the most reliable serologic marker for PBC. The sensitivity of AMA as detected by the IFA procedure is consistently between 90% to 95% (4,42). AMA by the IFA method is present in 25% of CAH patients and in 25% to 30% of cryptogenic cirrhosis patients

(4). AMA is occasionally present in infectious diseases, but is rarely present in the normal population.

The specific epitopes of AMA have been well defined by Western blot (43) and molecular techniques (35,44). Nine separate AMA specificities have been identified and are labeled sequentially M1 to M9 (35). Four specific mitochondrial antigens are associated with PBC: M2 (pyruvate dehydrogenase complex), M4 (sulfite oxidase), M8 (unknown), and M9 (glycogen phosphorylase). The other five antigen specificities of AMA are associated with antibodies from patients with syphilis, myocarditis, drug allergies, and occasional forms of collagen disorders. M2 is the most dominant of the four mitochondrial antigens associated with PBC. The use of purified M2 (pyruvate dehydrogenase complex) in an ELISA format consistently demonstrates high sensitivity (88% to 96%) and high specificity (>95%) for PBC (29,32,35,36). Antibody to the M4 and M8 antigens are always present together with M2 antibodies. Antibodies to the M9 antigen are present together with M2 antibodies in most PBC patients. However, antibodies to M9 may be the only AMA detected in up to 8% of PBC patients (35).

The subunits of the M2 antigen have been further characterized by Western blot (44) and molecular methods (36,42,44,45). Recombinant proteins which represent the 70-kd (E2 subunit of PDH complex) and the 51-kd (E2 subunit of the branched chain 2 oxy-acid dehydrogenase complex) when used together in an ELISA format have a sensitivity of 93% to 96% for PBC (42,46). Three other immunodominant proteins of M2 are detected at 56kd, 45kd, and 36kd by Western blot. The use of purified M2 or a cocktail of the relevant recombinant proteins of M2 subunits has proven highly sensitive and specific for PBC.

MND-ANA

The standard ANA substrate of HEp-2 cells is adequate for the detection of MND-ANA. Serum is used at the standard initial dilution of 1:40. The pattern is 3 to 8 discrete dots within the nucleus, which is quite distinct from either the coarse-speckled ANA pattern or the centromere ANA pattern (**Fig. 26-2**). Most but not all the nuclei will be positive. Only 15% of PBC patients will be positive and the specificity is not well defined. No proficiency samples are available, though commercial sources of MND-ANA are available.

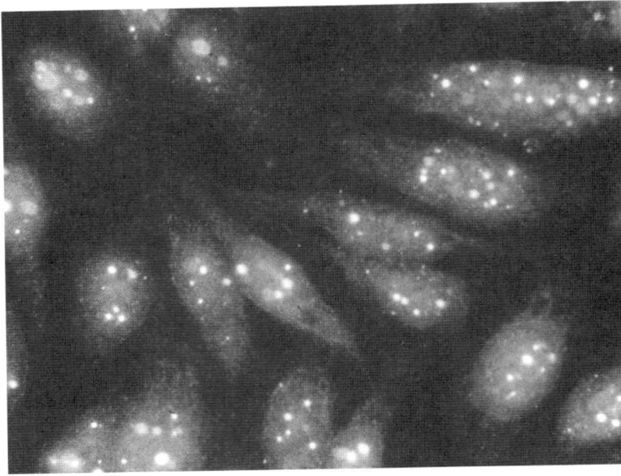

FIGURE 26-2

Multiple nuclear dots. HEp-2 nuclei with 3 to 8 dots per cell from serum of a primary biliary cirrhosis (PBC) patient. (Courtesy of Dr. W. Binder, INOVA Diagnostics.)

AMA by IFA

The tissue of choice to detect AMA is rodent kidney, where serum is screened at either a 1:10 or 1:40 dilution with more than 50% of the PBC sera having AMA titers greater than 1:160. The staining pattern on rodent kidney shows prominent staining of the distal tubules and loops of Henle with lesser staining of the proximal tubules (**Fig. 26-3**). The AMA IFA staining pattern must be distinguished from LKM antibody using multiple tissues (liver, kidney, and stomach) as described previously. The most obvious difference in the AMA and LKM IFA patterns is the staining of parietal cells in the gastric mucosa by AMA sera but not by LKM sera (**Fig. 26-4**).

There are numerous commercial sources of rodent tissues and AMA-positive sera. Proficiency samples from the College of American Pathologists (CAP) are also available.

AMA by ELISA

With the discovery of the M2-antigen specificity of AMA for PBC patients, the use of purified M2 antigen or cocktails of recombinant M2 antigens has allowed the development of Western blot and ELISA methods very specific for PBC. The

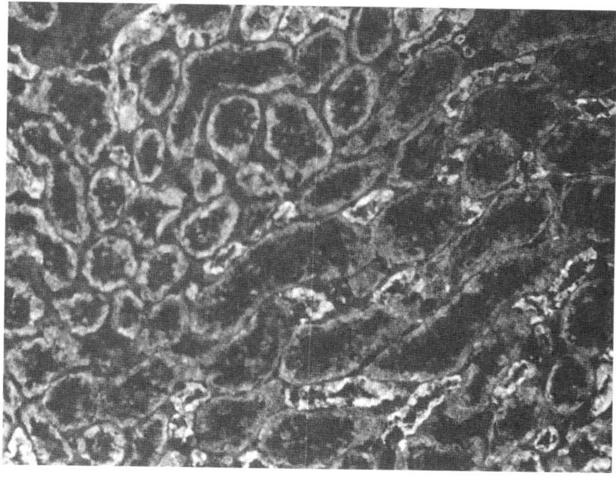

FIGURE 26-3

Antimitochondrial antibody. The cytoplasm of the tubule epithelium of the rat kidney bind AMA. Note the distal tubules (smaller) to the left are more intensely positive than the proximal tubules (larger) to the right with AMA sera. LKM-1 antibodies preferentially bind to the proximal tubule epithelium.

FIGURE 26-4

Parietal cell binding by AMA. AMA bind to the parietal cells of the stomach, whereas LKM-1 antibodies do not bind to parietal cells.

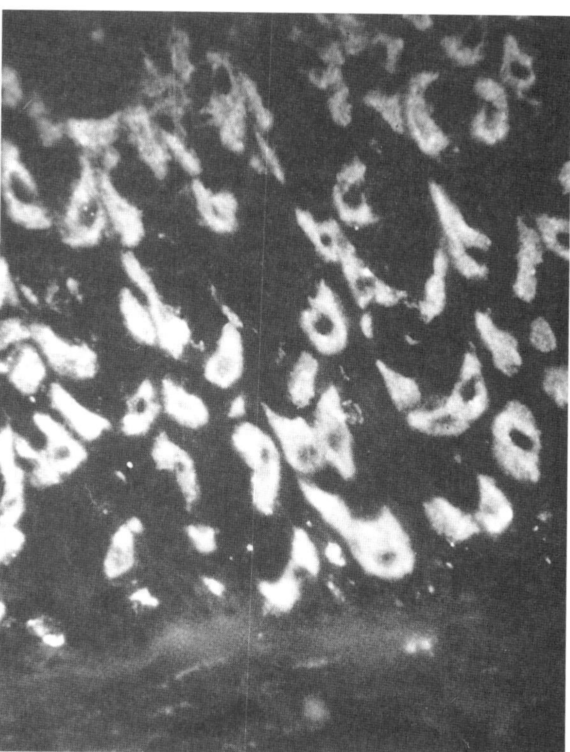

assays using either purified native or recombinant M2 proteins are more specific than the IFA assay. The increased specificity is due to the lack of M2-specific antibodies in chronic active hepatitis or cryptogenic cirrhosis, diseases that have AMA as detected by IFA.

Several commercial sources of the M2 ELISA are now available using either purified M2 or recombinant M2. Kits using recombinant M2 should include more than one recombinant protein (i.e., the E2 subunit of PDH only), as otherwise the sensitivity of the kit may be low. Serum samples are the most appropriate samples to run, and proficiency samples are available through the College of American Pathologists (CAP).

Primary Sclerosing Cholangitis

Primary sclerosing cholangitis (PSC) is a chronic liver disease characterized by inflammation and fibrosis of both intrahepatic and extrahepatic bile ducts. Early in disease, morphological findings include a mononuclear cell (predominantly lymphocytic) infiltrate and the characteristic "onion skin" periductal fibrosis. In later stages, inflammation becomes more extensive, leading to narrowing and obliteration of small bile ducts and eventually cirrhosis. Approximately one-third of PSC patients have a rapid course and die of liver failure or require liver transplant (4,47,48).

PSC occurs primarily in young men, but may also be found in children and older adults. The major symptoms are fatigue, pruritis, hyperpigmentation, xanthelasma (lipid deposits in the skin of the eyelids), and jaundice (48). Approximately 70% of PSC patients exhibit concurrent ulcerative colitis (UC) (47,49). PSC is associated with HLA-B8, HLA-DR3, and HLA-DRw52, suggesting a genetic basis for the disease (4).

Test Selection for PSC

For many years, theories of an autoimmune basis for PSC were questioned because of the relative lack of autoantibodies in sera from PSC patients. AMA is very rare, and only about 10% of patients exhibit anti-LSP and anti-ASGPR antibodies (4). In 1986, however, Chapman and coworkers (50) provided evidence for autoimmune involvement in PSC. They found that

62.5% of PSC patients had circulating antibodies reactive with an antigen in portal tracts of liver from patients with bile duct obstruction. Additional experiments revealed that the antigen recognized by these antibodies was associated with the nuclei of tissue neutrophils (51). Subsequent studies by several investigators have shown that this antibody represents a pANCA (reviewed in 47). Most pANCA in PSC are atypical, producing a "very perinuclear" staining pattern, in contrast to the central nuclear staining pattern typical of myeloperoxidase (MPO) specific pANCA (47).

Measurements of the sensitivity of pANCA for PSC are remarkably similar across studies, ranging from 62% to 87% (47). The presence of pANCA is not specific for PSC among autoimmune liver diseases; however, pANCA is detected in 30% to 50% of AIH patients and approximately 30% of PBC patients (49,52,53). Most investigators agree that the presence of pANCA in PSC patient sera does not correlate with disease activity, duration, severity, or treatment (reviewed in 47).

In light of the concomitant occurrence of UC in a large proportion of PSC patients, the discovery that the atypical pANCA pattern that characterizes PSC is found in approximately 75% of patients with UC (49,52,55,56) generated great interest. However, pANCA is not restricted to the subset of PSC patients with UC; similar percentages of patients in PSC-only and PSC-plus-UC groups exhibit pANCA (49,52,55). Likewise, pANCA is detected at similar percentages in UC patients with no PSC (47).

The common occurrence of pANCA in PSC and UC suggests a possible immunopathogenic relationship between these two diseases. Supporting this hypothesis are data demonstrating that PSC pANCA is more closely related to UC pANCA than to AIH pANCA. PSC and UC pANCA react only with neutrophils, whereas AIH pANCA react with both neutrophils and monocytes (12,54,55,57).

Although PSC, UC, AIH, and PBC are all characterized by the frequent detection of pANCA, three lines of evidence indicate that the epitopes generally recognized by PSC pANCA are different from those recognized by pANCA found in the other three diseases.

First, studies examined pANCA reactivity with ethanol-fixed versus methanol-fixed neutrophils (56). Using either substrate, 87% of PSC sera exhibited pANCA reactivity. In contrast, 78% of UC sera were pANCA-positive with ethanol-fixed cells, but only 17% were positive with methanol-fixed cells. Similarly, only 13% of sera from AIH patients and 16% of sera from PBC patients exhibited pANCA reactivity using methanol-fixed cells. Thus, antigenic determinants recognized by PSC pANCA were not affected by methanol fixation, whereas determinants recognized by pANCA in most UC, AIH, and PBC sera were destroyed by methanol treatment.

Second, studies of pANCA reactivity by Western blotting used sonicated neutrophil preparations as antigen (52,56). The sonication conditions that were used ruptured the cell membrane but left the granules intact, and the gel was run in the absence of reducing agent. Under these conditions, 80% of PSC sera reacted with at least one band; in contrast, only 9% of UC sera, 13% of AIH sera, and 11% of PBC sera showed blot reactivity. It is unclear whether the absence of pANCA reactivity associated with UC, AIH, and PBC reflected epitope unavailability due to the method of cell preparation or epitope inactivation by the electrophoretic process. Whatever the reason, epitopes recognized by most PSC pANCA were not similarly affected.

Third, studies examined the effect of DNAse treatment of ethanol-fixed neutrophils on pANCA reactivity (57). Specimens selected for study were PSC (without UC) sera, UC sera, and AIH sera that were pANCA-positive with ethanol-fixed neutrophils (no PBC sera were studied). DNAse treatment of neutrophils led to complete loss of pANCA reactivity in 30% of PSC sera and 14% of AIH sera, compared to 70% of UC sera. The remaining sera in each patient group (70%, 86%, and 30%, respectively) gave a homogeneous cytoplasmic staining pattern with DNAse-treated neutrophils. Additional experiments showed that UC pANCA sera did not react with double-stranded DNA or ethanol-fixed neutrophils pretreated with trypsin.

These findings suggest that the antigen recognized by most UC pANCA is a protein either directly complexed with DNA or requiring intact DNA to maintain its integrity. In contrast, the PSC and AIH pANCA antigen appears to be granule proteins that interact with DNA via charge differences artifactually induced by ethanol treatment, much in the same way MPO-directed antibodies produce a pANCA staining pattern (47,57).

Definitive identification of the neutrophil cytoplasmic antigen(s) recognized by PSC pANCA has not been accomplished. Investigators agree that the antigen is not proteinase 3 (PR3), elastase, or cathepsin G. Similarly, less than 20% of PSC pANCA sera show reactivity with MPO, lactoferrin, or lysozyme (49,53,55,58). The most common antigenic specificity for PSC pANCA identified thus far is bactericidal/permeability-increasing protein (BPI), an endotoxin-binding protein found in azurophilic granules. Stoffel et al. (58) found that 44% of PSC pANCA-positive sera and 18% of PSC pANCA-negative sera (36% of total PSC sera) reacted with BPI. It seems apparent that additional uncharacterized neutrophil cytoplasmic proteins are recognized by PSC pANCA. Identification of these additional neutrophil antigens remains an area of intense investigation.

Until the antigenic specificity of PSC pANCA has been identified, the routine IFA for ANCA remains the most sensitive laboratory test for PSC. One should bear in mind, however, that roughly a quarter of PSC patients do not exhibit pANCA. Also one should remember that pANCA is observed in other autoimmune liver diseases and in UC; thus, it is of low specificity for PSC. As expected from these observations, the positive predictive value of pANCA for PSC is also low.

ANCA Assay Method

The ANCA IFA employs ethanol-fixed neutrophils attached to microscope slides. The slides are incubated with serum diluted with phosphate buffered saline (starting dilutions vary from 1:8 to 1:40), washed, and then incubated with fluorescein-labeled $F(ab')_2$ antihuman immunoglobulin or IgG. Cell-associated fluorescence is then assessed via microscopy. Nuclear or perinuclear staining is indicative of pANCA. As noted above, most pANCA reactivity associated with PSC is of the "very perinuclear" type (**Fig. 26-5**). Positive sera are titered to end point using serial twofold or fourfold dilutions.

Sera for ANCA testing should be free of hemolysis and lipid. If delays of greater than 24 hours between serum collection and testing are expected, it is recommended that the serum be frozen then thawed immediately before testing. Repeated freeze/thaw cycles should be avoided.

Each assay setup should contain a negative serum and a positive serum of known titer as controls. Unfortunately, well-characterized reference preparations for pANCA are not readily available.

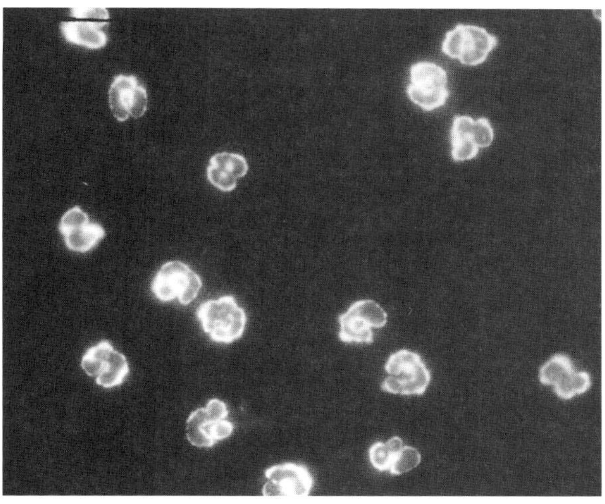

FIGURE **26-5**

pANCA pattern on human neutrophils. The pANCA detected in PSC and AI-CAH sera will stain human neutrophils with accentuation of staining at the periphery and central clearing of neutrophil nuclei.

Slides containing ethanol-fixed neutrophils are commercially available from several vendors at a cost of $2 to $3 per well (usually in a 6-well or 12-well format). The assay requires approximately 2 hours of setup time. Prepared slides should be read by a medical technologist with general experience in immunofluorescence and specific experience in ANCA interpretation.

A caveat of this procedure is the possible misinterpretation of an antinuclear antibody (ANA) as pANCA. Although an ANA pattern is not likely to be confused with the atypical pANCA pattern of PSC, it is nevertheless good practice to test pANCA-positive sera on rodent liver or kidney tissue or HEp-2 cells to distinguish ANA reactivity from pANCA reactivity. A false-positive pANCA on ethanol-fixed neutrophils caused by ANA will be positive on tissue or HEp-2 preparations.

A confirmatory step in identifying MPO-directed pANCA reactivity is the analysis of reactivity on formalin-fixed neutrophils. Using this substrate, MPO-directed pANCA produces a cytoplasmic ANCA (cANCA) pattern. The majority of PSC pANCA also give a cANCA pattern on formalin-fixed cells, but approximately 15% of PSC pANCA do not stain formalin-fixed neutrophils at all. Thus, confirmatory testing of PSC pANCA on formalin-fixed neutrophils is of questionable value due to decreased sensitivity.

As mentioned in an earlier section, approximately 75% of PSC sera exhibit pANCA reactivity. The specificity of pANCA for PSC is low, because this antibody is also found in UC and AIH, and PBC. Predictive values must be determined by each laboratory for the unique patient makeup of its client base.

Laboratories performing ANCA testing should participate in some type of proficiency testing program. ANCA proficiency testing is available through the College of American Pathologists (CAP) Diagnostic Immunology Survey, Series 2. The Clinical Laboratory Improvement Act (CLIA) requires participation in interlaboratory comparisons on an on-going basis for researchers not involved in CAP survey testing.

In the future, the newly recognized distinctions of PSC pANCA reactivity in modified ANCA IFA and Western blot procedures may lead to testing systems with increased specificity for PSC versus other autoimmune liver diseases and UC. For example, an algorithm involving ANCA testing with some combination of ethanol-fixed neutrophils, methanol-fixed neutrophils, DNAse-treated neutrophils, and Western blot may enable the clear distinction of PSC from UC, AIH, and PBC. The development of such an algorithm will require the analysis of a large number of sera from well-characterized patients under strict quality assurance conditions. In the long term, identification and characterization of the neutrophil antigen(s) recognized by pANCA in various disease states is needed for the development of highly sensitive and specific laboratory tests for PSC.

REFERENCES

1. Joshe RA, King WE. The "L-E cell" phenomenon in active chronic viral hepatitis. Lancet 1955;ii: 477–479.
2. Mackay IR, Taft LI, Cowling DC. Lupoid hepatitis. Lancet 1956;ii:1323–1326.
3. Cullinan ER. Idiopathic jaundice (often recurrent) associated with subacute necrosis of the liver. St Bartholomew's Hosp Rev 1936;69:55–142.
4. McFarlane IG, Farrant JM, Eddleston ALWF. Autoimmune liver disease. In: Lachmann PJ, Peters DK, Rosen FS, Walport MJ, eds. Clinical aspects of immunology. Boston: Blackwell Science, 1993;3:1969–1986.
5. Desmet VJ, Gerber M, Hoofnagle JN, et al. Classification of chronic hepatitis: diagnosis, grading, and staging. Hepatology 1994;19:1513–1520.
6. Krawitt EL. Autoimmune hepatitis: classification, heterogeneity and treatment. Am J Med 1994; 96(1A):23S–26S.
7. Manns M, Gerken G, Kyriatsoulis H, et al. Characterization of a new subgroup of autoimmune chronic active hepatitis by autoantibodies against a soluble liver antigen. Lancet 1987;i: 292–294.
8. Stechemesser E, Klein R, Berg PA. Characterization and clinical relevance of liver-pancreas antibody in autoimmune hepatitis. Hepatology 1993; 18:1–9.
9. Zauli D, Crespi C, Miserocchi F, et al. Comparison of various cell types as substrates for the detection of antiactin antibodies in chronic liver disease. Diag Clin Immunol 1987;5:184–187.
10. Lidman K, Biberfield G, Fagraeus H, et al. Antiactin specificity of human smooth muscle antibodies in chronic active hepatitis. Clin Exp Immunol 1976;24:266–272.
11. Leiborvitch L, George T, Levi Y, et al. Anti-actin antibodies in sera from patients with autoimmune liver diseases and patients with carcinomas by ELISA. Immunol Lett 1995;48:129–132.
12. Targan SR, Landers C, Vidrich A, Czaja AJ. High-titer antineutrophil cytoplasmic antibodies in type 1 autoimmune hepatitis. Gastroenterology 1995;108:1159–1166.
13. Wesierska-Gadik J, Penner E, Hitchman E, Sauermann G. Antibodies to nuclear lamins in autoimmune liver disease. Clin Immunol Immunopathol 1988;49:107–115.
14. McFarlane IG, Williams R. Liver membrane antigens. J Hepatol 1985;1:381–390.
15. McFarlane BM, McSorley CG, Vergani D, et al. Serum antibodies reacting with the hepatic asialoglycoprotein receptor (hepatic lectin) in acute and chronic liver disorders. J Hepatol 1986;3:196–205.
16. Treichel V, Poralla T, Hess G, et al. Autoantibodies to human asialoglycoprotein receptor in autoimmune type chronic hepatitis. Hepatology 1990;11:606–612.
17. Homberg JC, Abuaf N, Bernard O, et al. Chronic active hepatitis associated with antiliver/kidney

microsome antibody type 1: a second type of "autoimmune" hepatitis. Hepatology 1987;7: 1333–1339.

18. Rizzetto M, Swana G, Doniach D. Microsomal antibodies in active chronic hepatitis and other disorders. Clin Exp Immunol 1973;15:331–344.
19. Zanger UM, Houri HP, Laeper J, et al. Antibodies against human cytochrome P-450dbl in autoimmune hepatitis type II. Proc Natl Acad Sci USA 1988;85:8256–8260.
20. Manns MP, Griffin KJ, Sullivan KF, Johnson EF. LKM-1 autoantibodies recognize a short linear sequence in P450IID6, a cytochrome P-450 monoxygenase. J Clin Invest 1991;88:1370–1378.
21. Seelig R, Renz M, Bünger G, et al. Anti-LKM-1 antibodies determined by use of recombinent P4502D6 in ELISA and Western blot and their association with anti-HCV and HCV-RNA. Clin Exp Immunol 1993;92:373–380.
22. Lenzi M, Ballardini G, Fusconi M, et al. Type 2 autoimmune hepatitis and hepatitis C virus infection. Lancet 1990;335:258–259.
23. Durazzo M, Philipp T, Van Pelt FNAM, et al. Heterogeneity of liver-kidney microsomal autoantibodies in chronic hepatitis C and D virus infection. Gastroenterology 1995;108:455–462.
24. Michel G, Ritter A, Gerken G, et al. Anti-GOR and hepatitis C virus in autoimmune liver diseases. Lancet 1992;339:267–269.
25. Homberg JC, Andre C, Abuaf N. A new liver-microsome antibody (anti-LKM2) in tienilic acid-induced hepatitis. Clin Exp Immunol 1984;55: 561–570.
26. Crivelli O, Lavarinis C, Chiaberge E, et al. Microsomal autoantibodies in chronic infection with the HBsAg associated delta (δ) agent. Clin Exp Immunol 1983;54:232–238.
27. Philipp T, Durazzo M, Trautwein C, et al. Recognition of uridine diphosphate glucuronosyl transferases by LKM-3 antibodies in chronic hepatitis D. Lancet 1994;344:578–581.
28. Czaja AJ, Manns MP, Homburger HA. Frequency and significance of antibodies to liver/kidney microsomes type 1 in adults with chronic active hepatitis. Gastroenterology 1992;103:1290–1295.
29. Gruber E, Felber E, Pope GR, et al. Detection of autoantibody against M2, LKM-1, and SLA in liver disease by standardized uniform ELISA-techniques. J Clin Labor Anal 1994;8:284–292.
30. Wächter B, Kyriatsoulis A, Lohse AW, et al. Characterization of liver cytokeratin as a major target antigen of anti-SLA antibodies J Hepatol 1990; 11:232–239.
31. Klein R, Stechemesser E, Berg PA. Characterization of anti-liver-pancreas (LP) antibodies in autoimmune chronic active hepatitis (CAH) by Western blotting (WB) (abstract). Hepatology 1992;16:556.
32. Sherlock S. Primary biliary cirrhosis: clarifying the issues. Am J Med 1994;96(1A):27S–33S.
33. Walker JG, Doniach D, Roitt M, Sherlock S. Serologic tests in diagnosis of primary biliary cirrhosis. Lancet 1965;1:827–831.
34. Goodman ZD, McNally PR, Davis DR, Ishak KG. Autoimmune cholangitis: a variant of primary biliary cirrhosis. Dig Dis Sci 1995;40:1232–1242.
35. Berg PA, Klein R. Antimitochondrial antibody in primary biliary cirrhosis and other disorders: definition and clinical relevance. Dig Dis Sci 1992;10:85–101.
36. Bassendini MF, Yeaman JJ. Serological markers of primary biliary cirrhosis: diagnosis, prognosis and subsets. Hepatology 1992;15:545–548.
37. Fritzler MJ, Valencia DW, McCarty GA. Speckled pattern antinuclear antibodies resembling anti-centromere antibodies. Arthritis Rheum 1985;27: 92–96.
38. Fusconi M, Cassani F, Govani M, et al. Anti-nuclear antibodies of primary biliary cirrhosis recognize 78–92 kD and 96–100 kD proteins of nuclear bodies. Clin Exp Immunol 1991;83:291–297.
39. Pawlotsky JM, Andre C, Metreau JM, et al. Multiple nuclear dots antinuclear antibodies are not specific for primary biliary cirrhosis. Hepatology 1992;16:127–131.
40. Sternsorf T, Guldner HH, Szostecki C, et al. Two nuclear dot-associated proteins, PML and Sp100, are often co-autoimmunogenic in patients with primary biliary cirrhosis. Scand J Immunol 1995; 42(2):257–268.
41. Grotzinger T, Jensen K, Guldner HH, et al. A highly amplified mouse gene is homologous to the human interferon-responsive Sp100 gene encoding an autoantigen associated with nuclear dots. Mol Cell Biol 1996;16(3):1150–1156.
42. van de Water J, Cooper P, Surk CD, et al. Detection of autoantibodies to recombinant mitochondrial proteins in patients with primary biliary cirrhosis. N Engl J Med 1989;320:1377–1380.
43. Fusconi M, Baum H, Caselli A, et al. Demonstration of peptide specific and cross-reactive

epitopes in proteins reacting with antimitochondrial antibodies in primary biliary cirrhosis. J Hepatol 1992;15:162–169.

44. Gershwin ME, Mackey IR, Sturgess D, Coppel RL. Identification and specificity of a cDNA encoding the 70 kDa mitochondrial antigen recognized in primary biliary cirrhosis. J Immunol 1987;138:3525–3531.

45. Yeaman J, Fussey SPM, Danner DJ, et al. Primary biliary cirrhosis: identification of two major M2 mitochondrial autoantigens. Lancet 1988;2:1067–1070.

46. Leung PSC, Iwazama T, Prindiville T, et al. Use of designer recombinant mitochondrial antigens in the diagnosis of primary biliary cirrhosis. Hepatology 1992;15:367–372.

47. Goeken JA. ANCA in inflammatory bowel and liver diseases: new evidence for an autoimmune etiology? Clin Immunol Newslett 993;13:119–125.

48. James SP, Strober W, Greenspan JS. Gastrointestinal, hepatobiliary, and orodental diseases. In: Stites DP, Terr AI, Parslow TG, eds. Basic and clinical immunology. 8th ed. Norwalk, CT: Appleton and Lange, 1994:457–477.

49. Hardarson S, LaBrecque DR, Mitros FA, et al. Antineutrophil cytoplasmic antibody in inflammatory bowel and hepatobiliary diseases. Am J Clin Pathol 1993;99:277–281.

50. Chapman RW, Cottone M, Selby WS, et al. Serum autoantibodies, ulcerative colitis and primary sclerosing cholangitis. Gut 1986;27:86–91.

51. Snook JA, Chapman RW, Fleming K, Jewell DP. Anti-neutrophil nuclear antibody in ulcerative colitis, Crohn's disease and primary sclerosing cholangitis. Clin Exp Immunol 1989;76:30–33.

52. Seibold F, Weber P, Klein R, et al. Clinical significance of antibodies against neutrophils in patients with inflammatory bowel disease and primary sclerosing cholangitis. Gut 1992;33:657–662.

53. Mulder AHL, Horst G, Haagsma EB, et al. Prevalence and characterization of neutrophil cytoplasmic antibodies in autoimmune liver diseases. Hepatology 1993;17:411–417.

54. Saxon A, Shanahan F, Landers C, et al. A distinct subset of antineutrophil cytoplasmic antibodies is associated with inflammatory bowel disease. J Allergy Clin Immunol 1990;86:202–210.

55. Duerr RH, Targan SR, Landers CJ, et al. Neutrophil cytoplasmic antibodies: a link between primary sclerosing cholangitis and ulcerative colitis. Gastroenterology 1991;100:1385–1391.

56. Klein R, Eisenberg J, Weber P, et al. Significance and specificity of antibodies to neutrophils detected by Western blotting for the serological diagnosis of primary sclerosing cholangitis. Hepatology 1991;14:1147–1152.

57. Vidrich A, Lee J, James E, et al. Segregation of pANCA antigenic recognition by DNase treatment of neutrophils: ulcerative colitis, type 1 autoimmune hepatitis, and primary sclerosing cholangitis. J Clin Immunol 1995;15:293–299.

58. Stoffel MP, Csernok E, Herzberg C, et al. Anti-neutrophil cytoplasmic antibodies (ANCA) directed against bactericidal/permeability increasing protein (BPI): a new seromarker for inflammatory bowel disease and associated disorders. Clin Exp Immunol 1996;104:54–59.

CHAPTER 27

Autoimmune Neuropathies

DAVID F. CARNEY

The existence of a number of autoantibodies to selected central and peripheral nervous system components in association with a variety of neurologic diseases is well recognized (1–4). This chapter focuses on an important subset of this antibody group, namely autoantibodies to gangliosides and sulfated-carbohydrate antigens associated with autoimmune neuropathies. A number of other autoantibodies associated with neurologic diseases also exist that are not covered in this chapter, including antibodies found in paraneoplastic syndromes, phospholipid antibodies, antineurofilament antibodies, and systemic lupus erythematosus–related antibodies such as antiribosomal P and anti-Ki (3).

Gangliosides belong to a family of acidic glycolipids that are composed of a ceramide and a carbohydrate moiety that may contain up to four sialic acids (2) (**Table 27-1**). The gangliosides differ in the number and location of sialic acid residues, with the letters M, D, and Q constituting one, two, and four sialic acids per molecule, respectively (see Table 27-1). Gangliosides are located in the plasma membrane of neuronal cells and processes, where they are believed to participate in a variety of cellular and membrane functions (2). Antiganglioside antibodies associated with autoimmune neuropathies include those directed against GM1, asialo-GM1, GD1b, GD1a, and GQ1b (1,5–7). The antigenic epitope in gangliosides has been localized to the Gal β1–3 GalNAc portion of the carbohydrate moiety (5,8). It is believed that differences in antibody specificities to the different gangliosides are due to steric effects contributed by the sialic acid groups, though in some cases, antibodies specifically directed against the sialic acids can also occur (9). Specific neuropathy syndromes associated with high titer antiganglioside antibodies are summarized in **Table 27-2**.

There are a number of autoantibodies against sulfated carbohydrate-containing neural antigens that are associated with autoimmune neuropathies. Sulfated galactose-containing glycolipids (sulfatides) constitute one of the major glycolipids of this class of antigens (10). Sulfatides contain the antigenic epitope SO_4-3-galactose, which is attached to a ceramide (see Table 27-1). Heterogeneity among the sulfatides is due to differences in the composition of the fatty acid portion of the cerebroside. Another important group of glycolipids in this class are the sulfated glucuronic-containing glycolipids, particularly sulfoglucuronyl paragloboside (SGPG) and sulfoglucuronyl lactosaminyl paragloboside (see Table 27-1) (11,12). The glycoproteins MAG and P_0 presumably also belong to this antigen class, based on the observation that antibodies that bind to the glucuronyl sulfate epitope of SGPG also cross-react with MAG and P_0 (13,14). These results suggest that SGPG, MAG, and P_0 contain an epitope with common structural features. Neuropathies associated with high titer autoantibodies against this group of antigens are summarized in Table 27-2.

Rationale of Test Selection for the Diagnosis, Evaluation, and Monitoring of Specific Diseases or Conditions

Categorization of a neuropathy as an autoimmune disorder is important for ruling out other

TABLE **27-1**

Structures of Antigens Involved in Autoimmune Neuropathies

Neural Antigen	**Structure**
GM1	Galβ1-3GalNAcβ1-4(NeuAcα2-3)Galβ1-4Glcβ1-1′Cer
Asialo-GM1	Galβ1-3GalNAcβ1-4Galβ1-4Glcβ1-1′Cer
GD1a	NeuAcα2-3Galβ1-3GalNAcβ1-4(NeuAcα2-3)Galβ1-4Glcβ1-1′Cer
GD1b	Galβ1-3GalNAcβ1-4(NeuAcα2-8NeuAcα2-3)Galβ1-4Glc1-1′Cer
GQ1b	Galβ1-3GalNAcβ1-(NeuAcα2-8NeuAcα2NeuAcα2-8NeuAcα2)4Galβ1-4Glc1-1′Cer
Sulfatide	SO_4-3Galβ1-1′Cer
SGPG	SO_4-3GlcAβ1-4GlcNAcβ1-3Galβ1-4Glcβ1-1Cer

Abbreviations: *Cer*, ceramide; *Gal*, galactose; *GalNAc*, N-acetylgalactosamine; *Glc*, glucose; *GlcA*, glucuronic acid; *GlcNAc*, N-acetylglucosamine; *NeuAc*, N-acetylneuraminic acid; *SGPG*, sulfoglucuronyl paragloboside.

TABLE **27-2**

Neuropathies Associated with High Titer Autoantibodies to Neural Antigens

Antibody	**Neuropathy**	**Reference**
GM1	MMN, SMN, LMND, GBS, ALS	(1,16,27,30)
Asialo-GM1	MMN, SMN, LMND, GBS	(1,2,26)
GD1b	PSN, MMN, SMN, LMND, GBS	(1,4,5)
GD1a	GBS	(7)
GQ1b	MFS, GBS, PSN	(6,36)
Sulfatide	PSN, SMN, GBS, CIDP	(10)
MAG	PSDN, SMDN	(10)
P_0	PSDN, SMDN	(13)

Abbreviations: *ALS*, amyotrophic lateral sclerosis; *AMN*, acute motor neuropathy; *CIDP*, chronic inflammatory demyelinating polyneuropathy; *GBS*, Guillain-Barré syndrome; *LMND*, lower motor neuron disease; *MAG*, myelin-associated glycoprotein; *MFS*, Miller-Fisher syndrome; *MMN*, multifocal motor neuropathy; *PSDN*, predominantly sensory demyelinating neuropathy; *PSN*, predominantly sensory neuropathy; *SMDN*, sensorimotor demyelinating neuropathy; *SMN*, sensorimotor neuropathy.

causes of neuropathy, including inherited disorders, systemic diseases such as diabetes, deficiency states, toxins, ischemia, paraneoplastic disorders, and inflammatory demyelination (15). In addition, high titer antibodies to specific neural antigens in patients have been shown to correlate with specific neuropathy syndromes (see Table 27-2) (1,2,5,10,16). Further, some patients who present with neurologic symptoms and demonstrate high titer autoantibodies may have a monoclonal gammopathy, which may or may not be associated with malignancies such as multiple myeloma, Waldenström's macroglobulinemia, and B-cell lymphoma or chronic lymphocytic leukemia (4). Patients with high titer anti-GM1 or anti-MAG have monoclonal gammopathies in approximately 10% or 50% of these cases, respectively (17). Therefore, all patients that present with high titer autoantibodies to neural antigens should be evaluated for monoclonal gammopathies, as clinically indicated.

Some autoimmune-mediated neuropathy patients have shown clinical improvement when treated with immunosuppressive therapy (6,18,19). Neuropathy patients with high titers of anti-GM1, MAG, or GQ1b exhibited reductions in titer and clinical improvement when treated with cyclophosphamide, or plasmapheresis, or both (6,18,19). Repeat assays for autoantibodies to neural antigens in patients undergoing these treatments may be useful for monitoring the immunosuppressive effectiveness of therapy (18,19).

Assay Methods

Thin-Layer Chromatography

The immunoassay method of choice for autoantibodies associated with neuropathy syndromes depends on the antigen used in the assay. For most of the glycolipids, including the gangliosides and sulfated galactose and glucuronic-containing glycolipids, the two immunoassay methods of choice are enzyme-linked immunosorbent assay (ELISA) and thin-layer chromatography (TLC) immuno-overlay (20,21). ELISA is usually preferred over TLC because of the advantages of high sensitivity and specificity, simplicity, and low cost. TLC offers the advantage that highly purified antigen preparations are not required and only a single lane can be used to screen each patient serum for antibodies to multiple neural antigens that become separated during the chromatographic process. The TLC method suffers from the disadvantages of being relatively labor intensive and requiring the use of large quantities of highly volatile organic solvents.

ELISA

Although a number of ELISA assays using glycolipid antigens have been reported with a variety of modifications, most methods share many common features (22–24). Sulfatides and many of the gangliosides are available commercially in purified form, and thus can be directly coated onto ELISA plates. Sulfated glucuronic-containing glycolipids are not available commercially in purified form and must be purified from neural tissues such as cauda equina or sciatic nerve using organic solvents (25). For the glycolipid antigens, hydrophobic plates such as Falcon 3915 and Immunolon-3 are preferred because they give low nonspecific binding as well as higher specificity among closely related epitopes, as compared to hydrophilic plates (24). Glycolipid antigens are dissolved and coated in ELISA wells in an organic solvent such as methanol, ethanol, chloroform, or various mixtures of these solvents (22,24). Antigen titrations are required to find the minimum saturating concentration. The most common antigen coating concentration is 500 ng/well, but various laboratories have used a range of between 10 to 4000 ng/well (22,24). After solvent evaporation, a blocking step is included, which usually consists of incubating antigen-coated wells with 1% to 3% bovine serum albumin (BSA) (22,24). Some laboratories have suggested the use of human serum albumin or histone H3 as an alternative to BSA for the purpose of detecting nonspecific binding (2,26). Serum patient samples are preferred, but citrated or EDTA plasma can also be used for antibody detection. No special sample handling is required, and in our hands antibody reactivity was retained in samples stored at −20°C or lower for at least 2 years.

There are inconsistencies among various laboratories concerning the use of detergents in wash buffers in ELISA assays using glycolipid antigens (22,24). Tween-20 (0.05%) is reported to significantly reduce nonspecific binding of serum antibodies to glycolipid antigens (16,22,23). Because low nonspecific reactivity is observed when detergent washes are used, some laboratories that use detergent do not include wells for nonspecific binding (20). However, detergents also dramatically reduce specific antibody binding in addition to lowering nonspecific binding (22,23). For example, anti-GM1 titers are up to 3 to 10 times higher when detergent is avoided (2). In a recent survey of the literature on ELISA of antiganglioside antibody methods, about half of the laboratories surveyed (10 of 21) did not use detergent in the assay (24).

Several strategies have been reported for evaluating the significance of elevated serum antibody levels against neuronal glycolipid antigens. Results are most often expressed as a titer and less often as an arbitrary unit value (5,27–29). Many laboratories define the absolute titer for antiglycolipid antibodies as the highest serial dilution of patient serum at which the OD is 0.05 to 0.1 OD units above the nonspecific binding control (28). Although the use of this method is acceptable for initially defining titer units, the routine use of this method for patient samples may be unreliable due to variabilities inherent in the ELISA assay related to antigen coating, detecting reagents, washing steps, and reaction times and temperatures. Incorporation of a standard curve or calibrator using a patient serum with an assigned titer (or arbitrary unit value) may be preferable to correct for plate-to-plate and day-to-day variations in the assay.

Interpretation of neuropathy autoantibody titers is typically accomplished by comparing patient titers to titers obtained from a panel of disease-free, healthy donors (6,7,30,31). Some laboratories consider a titer as positive when the value is above the highest normal value obtained (27). Statistical methods are more reliable for obtaining the cutoff value to distinguish negative (normal) titers from titers significantly elevated above normal. According to the National Committee for Clinical Laboratory Standards, patient values above the 97.5th percentile of the distribution of healthy normal individuals are considered statistically elevated above normal (32,33). Alternatively, investigators have set the cutoff for antibody titers at 2 to 3 standard deviations above the mean value obtained from a panel of normal individuals (6,7,30,31). Using this method, the cutoff titer is typically above the highest normal value.

We and others have observed that differences exist in the cutoff titer among different antiglycolipid antibodies, ranging from as low as 1:100 or less to as high as 1:1600 or more (1,28,33). Therefore, cutoff titers should be established independently for each antigen. In addition, cutoff titers for antibodies to a single antigen can differ for different antibody isotypes by as much as sixfold (26). Most laboratories perform both IgM and IgG (and less frequently IgA) isotyping for most of the neuropathy autoantibodies. Therefore, cutoff titers should be established independently for each antibody isotype.

Western Blot

Assays for MAG are typically done by Western blot, although improved methods for MAG purification have justified the availability of an ELISA assay for MAG detection (34). For the Western blot method, proteins in purified human myelin are separated by polyacrylamide electrophoresis and blotted onto nitrocellulose. The blotted nitrocellulose membranes are incubated with diluted patient sera and immunostained by standard techniques. Anti-MAG detection by ELISA offers many obvious advantages over Western blot. Unfortunately, minor contaminants that can cause false-positive reactions in the ELISA assay may be present in purified MAG preparations. Unless these contaminants are removed, detection of anti-MAG activity by ELISA should be confirmed by Western blot (34).

Interpretation of Tests

High titers of many of the neuropathy autoantibodies correlate with specific neuropathy syndromes, whereas low to intermediate titers are less predictive of specific neuropathy syndromes (1,2,5,10,16). Of the autoantibodies associated with neuropathy, high anti-GM1 has shown the best correlation with specific neuropathy syndromes (1,16). Greater than 80% of patients with high titer anti-GM1 have either multifocal motor neuropathy or lower motor neuron syndromes (1,2,23). Although high anti-GM1 titers are very specific for these neuropathies, high titers are present only in 20% to 50% of these cases, the remainder of which have low to intermediate GM1 titers (1,23,35). Other neuropathies associated with high titer anti-GM1 are summarized in Table 27-2. Whereas high GM1 titers are relatively specific for some neuropathy syndromes, low anti-GM1 titers are observed in 20% to 30% of patients with other neurologic diseases as well as non-neurologic diseases (16,35). We have observed low to intermediate titers of IgM anti-GM1 in some motor or sensorimotor neuropathies as well as in a variety of other related and nonrelated disease groups (**Fig. 27-1**). Of interest is that approximately 10% of patients with high GM1 titers have monoclonal gammopathies (4), and these patients should be evaluated accordingly, as clinically indicated.

Asialo-GM1 has shown similar antigenic specificity to GM1, with high titer antibodies to asialo-GM1 occurring in up to 36% of patients with lower motor neuron syndromes (1). Anti-GQ1b has shown high specificity for Miller-Fisher syndrome, and the highest GQ1b titers in these patients are observed when the assay is performed on acute phase serum (6,36). About one-quarter to one-third of patients with predominantly sensory or sensorimotor neuropathy have high titer antisulfatide or anti-MAG, and about 20% of these patients will have both antibodies (10). In one report, 56% of patients with neuropathy and monoclonal gammopathy had high titer anti-MAG, and 5% of these patients had high titer antisulfatide (28).

Quality Assurance

Internal

Replacement of current standards with new lots of standards should be parallel tested against the current standards. The original standards used for validating the assay should be included in the parallel testing, when feasible. New controls should be phased in and new control values accepted only if the current controls are within predefined range limits. Library samples acquired during the validation process that consist of low, medium, and high antibody titers

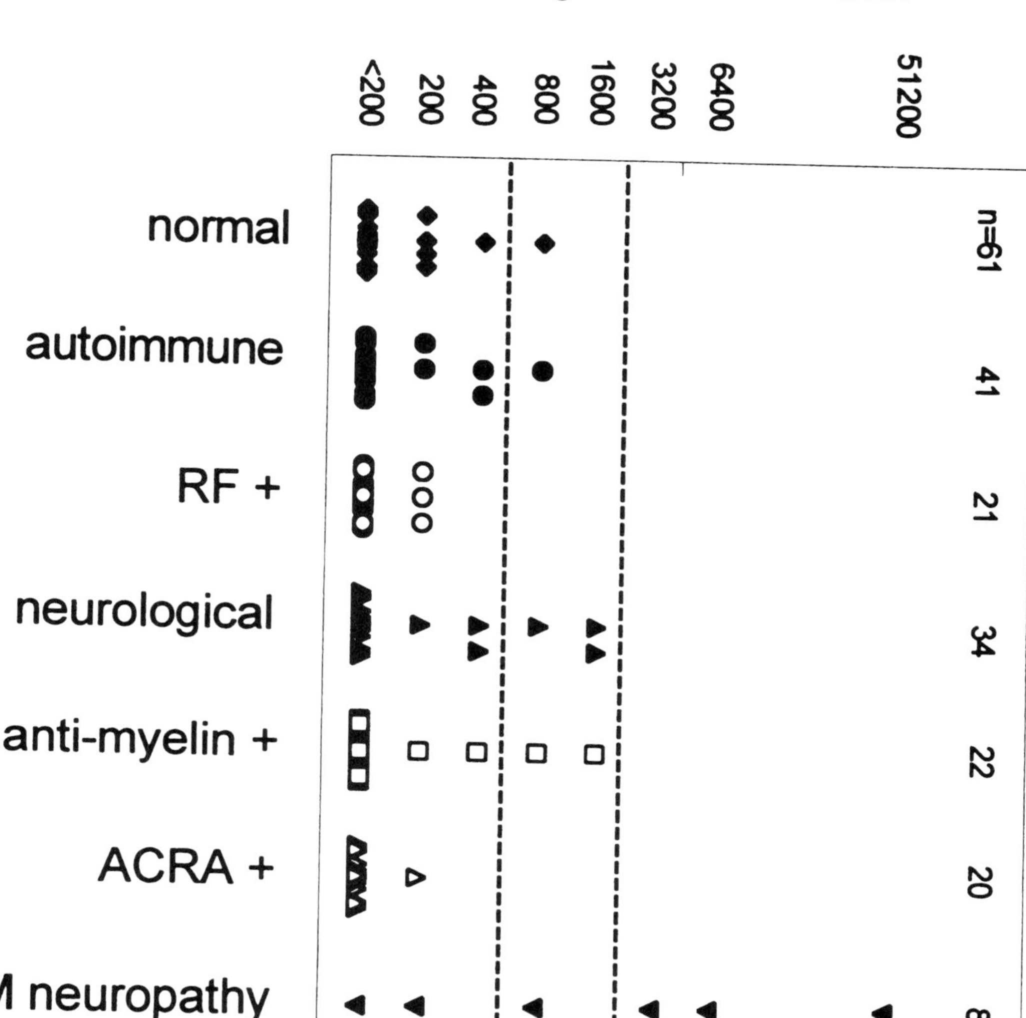

FIGURE **27-1**

IgM anti-GM1 titers obtained from patients in various disease groups: 1) *normal*—healthy, disease-free volunteers; 2) *autoimmune*—includes patients with systemic lupus erythematosus, Sjögren's syndrome, or rheumatoid arthritis; 3) *RF* +—rheumatoid-factor positive; 4) *neurological*—includes neurologic disorders other than SM neuropathies; 5) *antimyelin* +—determined by indirect immunofluorescence microscopy; 6) *ACRA* +—acetylcholine receptor antibody positive determined by immunoprecipitation; 7) *SM neuropathy*—patients with sensorimotor or motor neuropathy. Patients with titers below the 97.5th percentile of the titer distribution of normal individuals (<1:800) are negative for IgM anti-GM1. Titers between 1:800 to 1:1600 (demarcated with dashed lines) are intermediate positive titers. Titers in this category do not correlate with specific neuropathy syndromes. High titers of ≥1:3200 show a positive correlation with SM neuropathies. The GM1 ELISA method used at the SRL was the same as in Table 27-3.

should be run periodically (i.e., every 6 months), and values should agree with the original values within defined guideline limits set by each laboratory. New lots of antigen and detecting reagents should be parallel tested against current lots, prior to replacement in the assay. If patient antibody titer values are determined from a standard curve, positive sera should periodically be titered out to end point and the results compared to that obtained from the standard curve.

External

Two independent studies have performed interlaboratory comparison for determination of anti-GM1 (22,23). Both studies found good correlation for sera with high and low titers, but significant variation was observed for titers intermediate between these two ranges. We found similar results when we compared the results of our GM1 assay with those of several other laboratories (**Table 27-3**). Controlled proficiency surveys would be helpful as an initial step toward standardization of these assays. None are as yet available for autoantibodies associated with neuropathies.

TABLE **27-3**

IgM Anti-GM1 Titer Correlation Among Clinical Laboratories

Sample No.	SRL[b]	IgM Anti-GM1 Titer[a]			
		Lab 1	**Lab 2**	**Lab 3**	**Lab 4**
1	51,200	3200		68,000	
2	6400	3200	25,600	39,000	
3	6400		1600		
4	3200				HI POS
5	1600	800		3700	
6	1600	<800			
7	800	800	1600		
8	800	1600	400		
9	800	800			
10	800	800	200		
11	800	<800			
12	400	<800			
13	400	<800	800		
14	400	<800	100		
15	<400	<800			
16	<400	<800	400		
17	<400	<800	200		
18	<400		200		
19	<400		100		
20	<400		NEG		
21	<400		NEG		
22	<400		NEG		
23	<400		100		
24	<400		NEG		
25	<400	<800	NEG		
26	<400	<800			
27	<400				NEG
28	<400				NEG
29	<400				NEG
30	<400				NEG
31	<400				NEG

[a] The anti-GM1 assay performed at the SRL was done as follows. ELISA wells were coated with 500 ng of GM1 in methanol and then blocked with 1% BSA. Diluted patient sera were added to wells with and without GM1 and incubated at room temperature for 90 min. All washes were performed without detergent. Antibody binding was detected with peroxidase conjugated goat anti-human IgM and 2,2′-azino-di-[3-ethylbenzthiazoline sulfonate]. Specific anti-GM1 binding for each patient was calculated by subtracting the OD_{490} values of wells without GM1 from the values of wells coated with GM1 for each patient. These values were compared to a standard curve consisting of a patient serum with a known anti-GM1 titer to assign titer values for each patient.

[b] *SRL*, Scripps Reference Laboratory.

Comments

The detection and monitoring of high titer autoantibodies associated with autoimmune neuropathies is useful diagnostically because many of these diseases are treatable with conventional immunosuppressive therapy (6,18,19). It is apparent that several significant modifications are in use for immunoassays that detect autoantibodies in neurologic disease (22–24). Based on the variability in test results observed in interlaboratory comparative studies (see Table 27-3) (22,23), standardization of these assays needs to be encouraged.

Another area of concern is the variable assignment of titer values or arbitrary unit values, indicating the need for establishment of WHO international standards or their equivalent. The use of an internal calibrator or standard curve for ELISAs is encouraged to adjust for plate-to-plate and day-to-day variations, as well as reagent lot-to-lot differences.

Finally, the assignment of disease correlations for patients with low to intermediate titer assignments should be carefully considered due to the lack of disease specificity (5,27,33,35).

REFERENCES

1. Pestronk A, Chaudhry V, Feldman EL, et al. Lower motor neuron syndromes defined by patterns of weakness, nerve conduction abnormal-

ities, and high titers of antiglycolipid antibodies. Ann Neurol 1990;27:316–326.

2. Pestronk A. Invited review: motor neuropathies, motor neuron disorders, and antiglycolipid antibodies. Muscle Nerve 1991;14:927–936.
3. Zeballos RS, McPherson RA. Update of autoantibodies in neurologic disease. Clin Lab Med 1992;12:61–83.
4. Latov N. Pathogenesis and therapy of neuropathies associated with monoclonal gammopathies. Ann Neurol 1995;37:S32–S42.
5. Sadiq SA, Thomas FP, Kilidireas K, et al. The spectrum of neurologic disease associated with anti-GM1 antibodies. Neurology 1990;40:1067–1072.
6. Yuki N, Sato S, Tsuji S, et al. Frequent presence of anti-GQ1b antibody in Fisher's syndrome. Neurology 1993;43:414–416.
7. Yuki N, Yamada M, Sato S, et al. Association of IgG anti-GD1a antibody with severe Guillain-Barré syndrome. Muscle Nerve 1993;16:642–647.
8. Shy ME, Heiman-Patterson T, Parry GJ, et al. Lower motor neuron disease in a patient with autoantibodies against Gal(β1-3)GalNAc in gangliosides GM1 and GD1b: improvement following immunotherapy. Neurology 1990;40:842–844.
9. Ben Younes-Chennoufi A, Léger J-M, Hauw J-J, et al. Ganglioside GD1b is the target antigen for a biclonal IgM in a case of sensory-motor axonal polyneuropathy: involvement of *N*-acetylneuraminic acid in the epitope. Ann Neurol 1992;32:18–23.
10. Pestronk A, Li F, Griffin J, et al. Polyneuropathy syndromes associated with serum antibodies to sulfatide and myelin-associated glycoprotein. Neurology 1991;41:357–362.
11. McGinnis S, Kohriyama T, Yu RK, et al. Antibodies to sulfated glucuronic acid containing glycosphingolipids in neuropathy associated with anti-MAG antibodies and in normal subjects. J Neuroimmunol 1988;17:119–126.
12. Rowland LP, Sherman WL, Hays AP, et al. Autopsy-proven amyotrophic lateral sclerosis, Waldenström's macroglobulinemia, and antibodies to sulfated glucuronic acid paragloboside. Neurology 1995;45:827–829.
13. Bollensen E, Steck AJ, Schachner M. Reactivity with the peripheral myelin glycoprotein P0 in serum from patients with monoclonal IgM gammopathy and polyneuropathy. Neurology 1988;38:1266–1270.
14. Ariga T, Kohriyama T, Freddo L, et al. Characterization of sulfated glucuronic acid containing glycolipids reacting with IgM M-proteins in patients with neuropathy. J Biol Chem 1987;262:848–853.
15. Bosch EP, Mitsumoto H. Disorders of peripheral nerves, plexuses in neurology in clinical practice: the neurological disorders. In: Bradley WB, Daroff RB, Fenichel GM, Marsden DS, eds. Neurology in clinical practice. Boston MA: Butterworth-Heinemann, 1991:1719–1804.
16. Adams D, Kuntzer T, Burger D, et al. Predictive value of anti-GM1 ganglioside antibodies in neuromuscular diseases: a study of 180 sera. J Neuroimmunol 1991;32:223–230.
17. Ilyas AA, Cook SD, Dalakas MC, Mithen FA. Anti-MAG IgM paraproteins from some patients with polyneuropathy associated with IgM paraproteinemia also react with sulfatide. J Neuroimmunol 1992;37:85–92.
18. Pestronk A, Cornblath DR, Ilyas AA, et al. A treatable multifocal motor neuropathy with antibodies to GM1 ganglioside. Ann Neurol 1988;24:73–78.
19. Blume G, Pestronk A, Goodnough LT. Anti-MAG antibody-associated polyneuropathies: improvement following immunotherapy with monthly plasma exchange and IV cyclophosphamide. Neurology 1995;45:1577–1580.
20. Freddo L, Yu RK, Latov N, et al. Gangliosides GM1 and GD1b are antigens for IgM M-protein in a patient with motor neuron disease. Neurology 1986;36:454–458.
21. Gregson NA, Jones D, Thomas PK, Willison HJ. Acute motor neuropathy with antibodies to GM1 ganglioside. J Neurol 1991;238:447–451.
22. Marcus DM, Latov N, Hsi BP, et al. Measurement and significance of antibodies against GM1 ganglioside. Report of a Workshop, 18 April 1989, Chicago, IL (conference report). J Neuroimmunol 1989;25:255–259.
23. Kornberg AJ, Pestronk A. The clinical and diagnostic role of anti-GM1 antibody testing. Muscle Nerve 1994;17:100–104.
24. Ravindranath MH, Ravindranath RMH, Morton DL, Graves MC. Factors affecting the fine specificity and sensitivity of serum antiganglioside antibodies in ELISA. J Immunol Methods 1994;169:257–272.
25. Chou DKH, Ilyas AA, Evans JE, et al. Structure of sulfated glucuronyl glycolipids in the nervous system reacting with HNK-1 antibody and some

IgM paraproteins in neuropathy. J Biol Chem 1986;261:11717–11725.

26. Kornberg AJ, Pestronk A. Chronic motor neuropathies: diagnosis, therapy, and pathogenesis. Ann Neurol 1995;37:S43–S50.

27. van den Berg LH, Marrink J, de Jager AEJ, et al. Anti-GM1 antibodies in patients with Guillain-Barré syndrome. J Neurol Neurosurg Psychiatr 1992;55:8–11.

28. Nobile-Orazio E, Manfredini E, Carpo M, et al. Frequency and clinical correlates of anti-neural IgM antibodies in neuropathy associated with IgM monoclonal gammopathy. Ann Neurol 1994; 36:416–424.

29. von Wulffen H, Hartard C, Scharein E. Seroreactivity to *Campylobacter jejuni* and gangliosides in patients with Guillain-Barré syndrome. J Infect Dis 1994;170:828–833.

30. Pestronk A, Adams RN, Clawson L, et al. Serum antibodies to GM1 ganglioside in amyotrophic lateral sclerosis. Neurology 1988;38:1457–1461.

31. van den Berg LH, Lankamp CLAM, de Jager AEJ, et al. Anti-sulphatide antibodies in peripheral neuropathy. J Neurol Neurosurg Psychiatr 1993; 56:1164–1168.

32. Sasse EA, Aziz KJ, Harris EK, et al. Analysis of reference values. In: How to define and determine reference intervals in the clinical laboratory; approved guideline. Villanova, PA: National Committee for Clinical Laboratory Standards, 1995:15–25.

33. García Guijo C, García-Merino A, Rubio G. Presence and isotype of anti-ganglioside antibodies in healthy persons, motor neuron disease, peripheral neuropathy, and other diseases of the nervous system. J Neuroimmunol 1995;56:27–33.

34. Pestronk A, Li F, Bieser K, et al. Anti-MAG antibodies: major effects of antigen purity and antibody crossreactivity on ELISA results and clinical correlation. Neurology 1994;44:1131–1137.

35. Nobile-Orazio E, Carpo M, Legname G, et al. Anti-GM1 IgM antibodies in motor neuron disease and neuropathy. Neurology 1990;40: 1747–1750.

36. Jacobs BC, Endtz HP, van der Meché FGA, et al. Serum anti-GQ1b IgG antibodies recognize surface epitopes on *Campylobacter jejuni* from patients with Miller Fisher syndrome. Ann Neurol 1995;37:260–264.

CHAPTER 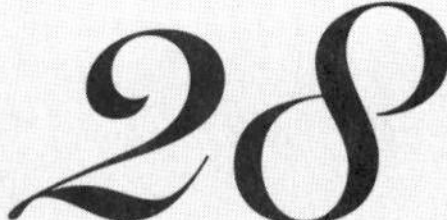

Antineutrophil Cytoplasmic Antibodies in Vascular Inflammatory Diseases

DAVID E. NORMANSELL

Systemic necrotizing vasculitides of medium and small vessels include Wegener's granulomatosis, microscopic polyangiitis, Churg-Strauss syndrome, and necrotizing and crescentic glomerulonephritis in which vasculitis is limited to the kidney. These diseases are marked by inflammation of and damage to blood vessels, leading to local necrosis, granuloma formation, and ischemia (1–3). Antineutrophil cytoplasmic antibodies (ANCAs) have been noted in the circulation of patients with these diseases, and are an accepted diagnostic aid, especially for Wegener's granulomatosis (4–15). ANCAs are autoantibodies directed against antigens located mostly in the azurophilic or primary granules of neutrophils and in some monocyte granules; the main autoantigens are proteinase 3 (PR3) and myeloperoxidase (MPO) (6–8).

The gold standard for ANCA detection is an indirect immunofluorescence assay using ethanol-fixed human neutrophils as substrate. Two major fluorescence patterns have been described: a cytoplasmic pattern mainly due to autoantibodies to PR3 and a perinuclear pattern mainly due to autoantibodies to MPO (6,9,10,15). A third, and rarer, atypical ANCA pattern is due to autoantibodies to cellular antigens other than PR3 and MPO, including elastase, lactoferrin, cathepsin G, bactericidal/permeability-increasing protein (BPI), lysozyme, and possibly others (10–12,15–18).

The two major staining patterns are illustrated in **Figure 28-1**:

1. **cANCA.** The cytoplasmic pattern (cANCA) is characterized by fine granular staining of the neutrophil cytoplasm, especially close to the nucleus and within the nuclear lobes, and with a definite diminution of staining intensity closer to the plasma membrane. The nucleus is not stained and the rounded shape of the cell is clearly delineated. The major cANCA antigen, PR3, is a serine protease that remains associated with the granules following ethanol fixation.
2. **pANCA.** The perinuclear pattern (pANCA) is characterized by nuclear fluorescence in a peripheral or rim pattern, and the overall shape of the cell is not clearly distinguishable. The major pANCA antigen, MPO, is cationic, and when the membranes are disrupted by ethanol fixation it redistributes to the negatively charged DNA in the nucleus, and may also bind to the nucleus of an adjacent cell. A similar redistribution may occur with other cationic components of the granules. Unfortunately, the pANCA pattern is similar to that seen with some antinuclear antibodies (ANAs), which can lead to confusion. Fixation of the slides with formaldehyde prevents redistribution of the MPO antigen, and the anti-MPO antibodies then give a cytoplasmic

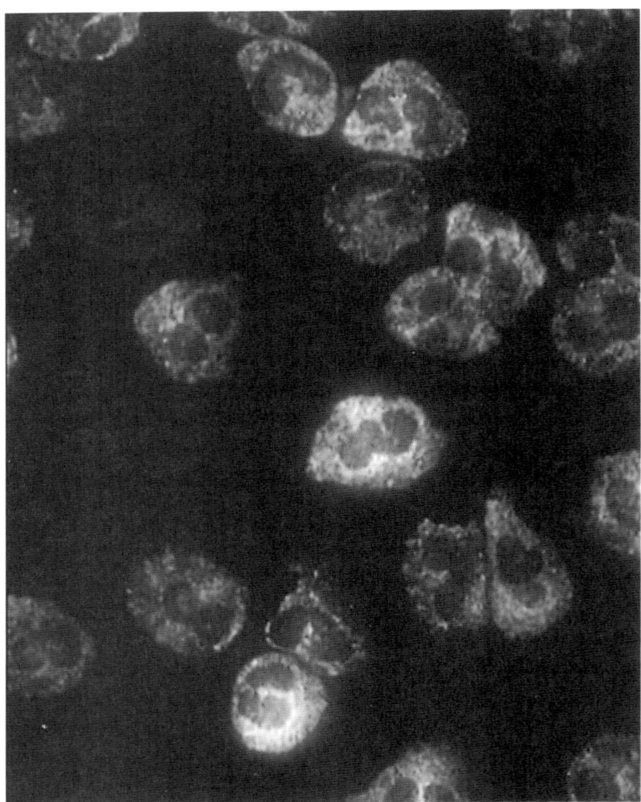
A

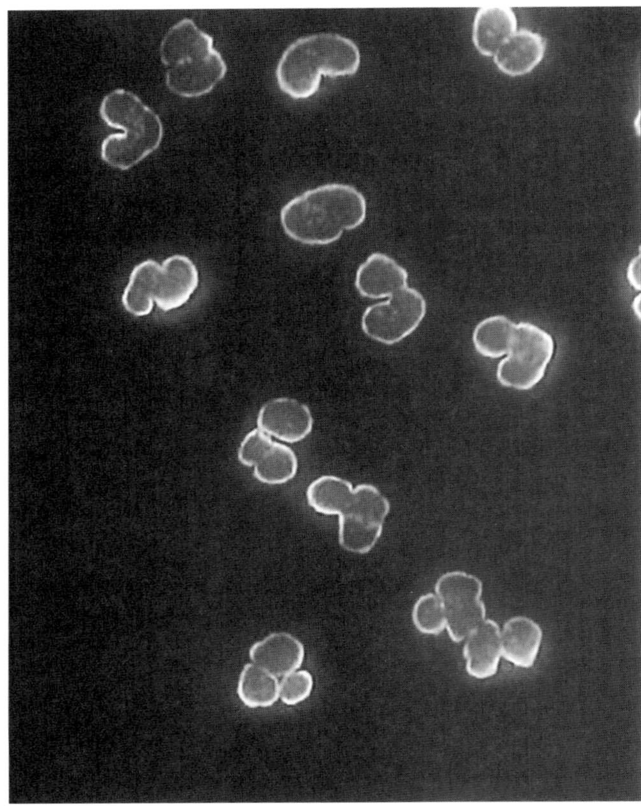
B

FIGURE 28-1

Major indirect immunofluorescence patterns of ANCAs. (A) cANCA. (B) pANCA. (Photographs courtesy of INOVA Diagnostics, Inc., San Diego, CA 92121.)

fluorescence pattern very similar to the cANCA pattern. An ANA usually will not bind to the nucleus of a formaldehyde-fixed cell.

The atypical ANCA pattern on ethanol-fixed slides may be a granular cytoplasmic staining without the diminution of staining from nuclear to plasma membrane regions that is seen in a cANCA pattern, or it may be a strong perinuclear pattern. ANCA-positive sera are almost always monospecific, showing a single staining pattern (12).

Clinically, a positive ANCA is useful in the detection of necrotizing vasculitis, and may provide information on the extent of the disease process. For example, patients with active Wegener's granulomatosis usually have positive cANCA titers of 1:320 or even higher (5,6,13,14,19,20). The test becomes negative on successful treatment with immunosuppressive drugs. Monitoring of the treated patient is necessary, because relapses are common and recurrence of a positive cANCA anti-PR3 titer, or an increase in titer, precedes reactivation of the disease (13,21–24), especially for IgG3 anti PR3 antibodies (25).

The pANCA pattern is also seen in Wegener's granulomatosis, but less frequently than cANCA. The perinuclear pattern is more likely to be seen in idiopathic or vasculitis-associated necrotizing crescentic glomerulonephritis (6), Churg-Strauss syndrome, or microscopic polyangiitis (15). Atypical pANCA patterns (strong perinuclear staining) may be seen in inflammatory bowel disease, especially ulcerative colitis (18,26–28).

The sensitivity of the cANCA pattern for active Wegener's granulomatosis is estimated to be 90% to 95%, with a specificity of 95% to 98%

(5,6,14,21), but substantially lower figures than these have been reported (29).

The Indirect Immunofluorescence Test

Fixed human neutrophils are incubated with dilutions of test sera, washed, and bound antibodies are detected by incubating the slides with fluorescein-labeled goat anti-human immunoglobulins. In our laboratory the majority of the sera tested for ANCAs is negative, so it is cost effective to screen the test sera on formaldehyde-fixed slides prior to testing on ethanol-fixed slides. Absence of cytoplasmic staining on a formaldehyde-fixed slide indicates that the serum is most probably ANCA negative, and further testing is not performed unless clinically indicated.

Homogeneous cytoplasmic staining without any granulation is not an ANCA; it is most probably due to nonspecific binding of overlabeled fluorescent antibody to cell components, or binding of IgG complexes in the test serum to Fc gamma receptors on the cell membrane. Another non-ANCA response, indicating poorly fixed cells, shows a coarse speckled stain, a "starry sky" pattern that includes the nucleus. This test should be repeated on a new batch of fixed cells.

All ANCA positive sera are retested on ethanol-fixed slides to determine the pattern and titer of the antibody. This protocol does not eliminate all problems with antinuclear antibodies (ANAs), because an ANA can obscure a pANCA pattern and might prevent a titer from being determined. Thus, ANA testing is still necessary for pANCA-positive sera. Laboratories that do not use formaldehyde-fixed slides *must* test all pANCA positive sera for ANAs.

Substrate slides may be prepared in the laboratory using neutrophils from normal donors (5,6,11,13,14,30). These slides have the advantage of having both neutrophils and lymphocytes on the slide. The presence of an ANA in the test serum will be apparent on a majority of the lymphocytes, whereas an ANCA will not stain a lymphocyte, except when cationic antigens migrate from a neutrophil to an adjacent cell. Substrate slides are also available commercially, prepared from short-term cultures of human neutrophils (INOVA Diagnostics, San Diego, CA).

The test protocol preferred in my laboratory is as follows:

1. Patient sera are diluted 1:20 with phosphate buffered saline (PBS) buffer (0.01 M (molar) potassium phosphate buffer, pH 7.2, containing 0.15 M (molar) sodium chloride). Commercial positive (4+) and negative controls are used undiluted. An inhouse weak-positive control, previously titered and aliquotted, is thawed ready for use; this should be a 1+ positive at a 1:40 dilution.
2. Sufficient formaldehyde-fixed slides are allowed to warm to room temperature in a humidified atmosphere. Control sera and test sera (20^{4} µL) are added to separate wells and the slides incubated at room temperature in a moist atmosphere for 20 minutes.
3. The slides are washed twice for 5 minutes with PBS, then pretitered fluorescein conjugated goat anti-human immunoglobulins (20 µL) is added to each well. The slides are then incubated at room temperature in a moist atmosphere in the dark for 20 minutes.
4. The slides are washed twice for 5 minutes with PBS, excess moisture is removed, and mounting medium (polyvinyl alcohol) and a coverslip are added. Slides are viewed in a fluorescent microscope (using the appropriate filter combinations for fluorescein) as soon as possible; they may be stored in the dark at 4°C for up to 12 hours.

Sera positive for ANCAs on formaldehyde-fixed slides are retested on ethanol-fixed slides for pattern and titer; they are diluted twofold serially, from 1:20 to 1:640, and the procedure described above is repeated. Each slide should contain positive (both cANCA and pANCA) and negative controls, and each run must also contain weak-positive and PBS controls. Sera still positive at a dilution of 1:640 are retested at higher dilutions.

Quality Control

The undiluted positive control should give bright 3+ to 4+ fluorescence; the negative and PBS controls must give no fluorescence. These controls serve as tests of the antigen, the fluorescent antibody, and the overall procedure. The weak-positive control serves as a sensitivity control for both the fluorescent antibody and the fluorescent microscope. Each batch of fluorescent antibody must be checked for appropriate titer using known positive and negative patients. Thus, a bank of appropriate sera must be acquired that can be used for these quality control steps. The sera should be titered and diluted to appropriate concentrations, then frozen in small aliquots. A fresh aliquot is used for each batch of fluorescent antiserum and the results are compared with previous results obtained with the control sera. A consistent performance with the known sera confirms that the test is maintaining its specificity and sensitivity through changes in reagents.

With each new lot of slides, inhouse controls or fluorescent antibody, old and new reagents are tested side by side to prove continuity of performance. A record of each of these overlap assays must be kept for certification purposes. If a reference serum linked to a standard serum is included in the test, results may be expressed in international units and compared directly with other laboratories (31).

Availability of Standard Sera for Quality Control

An international reference standard ANCA-positive serum is available from the Laboratory of Autoimmune Serology, Statens Seruminstitute, DK-2300, Copenhagen, Denmark (30,32). This serum has a cANCA titer of 1:320, and has no other detectable autoantibodies. It is supplied in 200 μL aliquots, lyophilized in a glass ampoule, for 600 DKR. The same serum can be used in PR3 ANCA tests (see below).

Solid Phase Assays

Although the indirect immunofluorescence test provides information on the major ANCA patterns, it is a subjective test and interpretations can vary between laboratories. To increase the specificity of the test it has become popular to follow the indirect immunofluorescence test with a solid phase assay against specific antigens, such as purified PR3 and MPO antigens, and thus define the antibodies more specifically. In theory, a solid phase assay will eliminate false-positive reactions due to other neutrophil antigens and should also eliminate interference due to ANAs. A solid phase assay may be the only way to resolve difficult or atypical fluorescence patterns.

Several procedures for the preparation of PR3 and MPO antigens have been described (summarized in 33). Wieslander and Wiik have published extensive details on the structure and characteristics of PR3 and MPO (34,35), but the epitopes with which the autoantibodies react have not been defined in detail and are thought to be both linear and conformational (36–39). Inhibition studies have defined several different epitopes for both PR3 and MPO (40), but the epitope specificity seems to be restricted within a given patient (41). It is not known whether the epitope specificity changes during the disease process in a given patient. The direct coating of purified PR3 or MPO antigens on to plastic wells may lead to denaturation of the proteins and destruction of some epitopes (42).

Several solid phase assay protocols have been published (43–50), and Hagen et al. (33) have compared assays in different laboratories based on different antigen preparations. This work showed that the purity and physical nature of the antigen were crucial to the performance of each assay, and that a standardized methodology was essential if a low coefficient of variation (CV) was to be obtained for the assay.

The generally accepted procedure for antigen preparation begins with isolated human neutrophils which are "exploded" by nitrogen cavitation; the granules are then collected using a Percoll gradient. Ion exchange chromatography is used to separate the granule proteins and affinity chromatography provides the final purification step (33). Polyacrylamide gel electrophoresis is used to monitor the product: PR3 has a molecular weight of 29,000 daltons on reduced or nonreduced gels, and usually shows as a triple band due to different levels of glycosylation; MPO should be a single band at 140,000 daltons (nonreduced), 73,000 daltons (partially reduced), or 59,000 and 13,500 daltons (fully reduced). Other granule antigens can be isolated by similar procedures (8).

Purified PR3, MPO, and other pertinent antigens are available from Wieslab AB in Lund, Sweden (Professor Jorgen Wieslander, Solvegatan 41, Ideon, S-223 70 Lund, Sweden). MPO is also available from Calbiochem, La Jolla, California, but the purity should be checked prior to use as it may contain lactoferrin (7).

A standard assay procedure similar to that detailed by Hagen et al. (33) is described here:

1. High binding microtiter wells are coated with antigen at a concentration of between 0.1 and 1.0 μg/mL in 100 μL 0.05 M[5] sodium carbonate buffer pH 9.6 for 1 to 2 hours at 37°C or overnight at 4°C.
2. The wells are emptied and then blocked by filling with "blotto" (PBS containing 1% bovine serum albumin, 0.1% Tween-20, and 0.1% dry milk powder) for 1 hour at room temperature.
3. The wells are washed 3 times with PBS containing 0.1% Tween-20 (PBST), and dilutions of test sera (100 μL) in PBST are added in duplicate. The plates are incubated for 2 hours in a moist atmosphere at room temperature and washed 4 times with PBST.
4. One-hundred microliters of a suitable dilution of enzyme labeled anti-human-antibody are added; the plates are incubated at room temperature for 2 hours in a dark moist atmosphere; they are washed 5 times with PBST; and substrate solutions are added.
5. The reaction is stopped after color development by addition of acid (if the enzyme label is horseradish peroxidase) or alkali (if the enzyme label is alkaline phosphatase), and the optical density (OD) is read. The level of antigen coating and the dilution of the labeled antibody must be established by prior experimentation. The test serum dilution should begin at 1:50.

The controls needed include the following:

- Uncoated but blocked wells to detect any antibodies that react with the "blotto" or that bind to the plate.
- A bank of normal sera to provide an initial background and normal cutoff OD.
- A bank of sera drawn from patients with other inflammatory diseases, such as rheumatoid arthritis and systemic lupus erythematosus (i.e., sera that can be expected to contain increased levels of IgG).
- Known positive sera, one a reasonably strong positive, and one a weak positive.

The cutoff value is calculated from the normal donor sera. At least 15 normal sera should be assayed, at a dilution of 1:50, and the mean OD and standard deviation (SD) determined. The cutoff is the mean OD plus two SDs. All of the normal sera should lie below this value.

The ELISA is repeated using at least 15 sera from patients with other inflammatory diseases, which should also be negative at a 1:50 dilution. If any are positive, or just above the cutoff value, and a clinical review confirms their diagnosis, then the cutoff value must be increased. The increased level of IgG in these sera presents a problem; this IgG may be "sticky" and may lead to nonspecific binding of the labeled antibody. In addition, some of these inflammatory sera may have low affinity antibodies to impurities in the antigen preparation, or to the blocking reagent. Thus, it may be necessary to increase the ionic strength of the diluent by adding potassium chloride (to 0.05 M), or to add a neutral human protein (1% pooled normal human albumin) to the diluent.

The weak-positive and strong-positive sera should have OD values that are just above (weak) and well above (strong) the "gray zone" which is the OD range between 2 and 3 SDs above the mean. These sera should be aliquoted and stored at −80°C, and a freshly thawed aliquot should be used for each run to ensure consistency from run to run. Strongly positive test sera (OD > 2) should be diluted and rerun.

The problem with this assay is that there is very little correlation between laboratories. The study by Hagen et al. (33) highlighted difficulties in the assay and emphasized the need for a standard methodology—only then could CVs of 20% (anti-PR3) and 34% (anti-MPO) be obtained. Clearly, standard antigen preparations and standard ANCA sera are needed.

The reference serum for anti-PR3 antibodies (from the Statens Seruminstitute, Denmark, see above) (30,32) can be used as a standard in the anti-PR3 ELISAs. A suitable reference serum for anti-MPO antibodies is not yet available.

Correlation between indirect immunofluorescence and the solid phase assays has been reported to be only 80% to 90% (51,52). The difference is ascribed either to antibodies to antigens other than PR3 or MPO (fluorescence positive and generally a pANCA pattern), or to loss of epitopes when the antigen is coated onto the plastic surface. One comparison between indirect immunofluorescence and a commercially available ELISA for anti-PR3 and anti-MPO antibodies (SCIMEDX/Euro Diagnostica) has been published (53). These authors found good correlation between the two assay procedures (99.2% for cANCA, 98.9% for pANCA), and similar sensitivity and specificity between indirect immunofluorescence and ELISA. They concluded that the commercial ELISA performed as well as the indirect immunofluorescence assay for the detection of ANCAs. The authors did not provide details of the antigen preparations used, but noted that they were purified fractions from neutrophil alpha granules using a published technique (44). The results of this study are at variance with the prevailing view in the literature that both immunofluorescence tests and ELISAs are needed because some sera are positive by one of the tests and negative by the other (51,52,54). Clearly, more studies of this type are needed.

Sera that are positive in the indirect immunofluorescence test but negative for anti-PR3 and anti-MPO antibodies may be atypical ANCAs. These antibodies are associated with cystic fibrosis (IgA anti-BPI), rheumatoid vasculitis and some lupus patients (antilactoferrin), some lupus patients (antineutrophil elastase), and inflammatory bowel disease (antilactoferrin, anticathepsin G, and antibodies to a DNAse-sensitive antigen in the neutrophil nucleus) (55). Much more work is needed on these atypical ANCAs to determine their diagnostic usefulness. There are no current standards for their detection.

Little, if any, correlation exists between indirect immunofluorescence titers and ELISA ODs (54). The reason for this is not clear.

ELISA Capture Assays

To avoid possible loss of epitopes when antigens are coated directly onto a solid phase, the plate can be coated with one or more specific antibodies to "capture" the antigen (52,56). Of course, the capture will obscure some epitopes, either by direct reaction with important epitopes or by holding the antigen in such a way as to prevent access by the patient's antibodies. Either polyclonal or monoclonal capture antibodies can be used, but monoclonal antibodies will provide a more consistent assay. A mixture of two antibodies of equal affinity, directed against opposite sides of the antigen molecule, should provide an efficient capture system.

Baslund et al. (52) showed that, for a group of 170 sera, all possible anti-PR3 ANCAs were detected when two monoclonal antibodies were used as capture antibodies. Details of affinity or site specificity of the monoclonal antibodies were not provided, but the general principle clearly works, and it should be easy to establish combinations of monoclonal antibodies to permit detection of all possible ANCA specificities.

The general method used for capture ELISAs follows that for direct ELISAs detailed above, with the exception of the initial capture antibody coating step. This step would probably be more efficiently performed by using an initial coating of goat anti-mouse immunoglobulins followed by a mixture of monoclonal antibodies to form the capture layer. The amounts of antibodies to use in this step have to be established, but the capture assay is clearly the method of choice. The reference serum for anti-PR3 antibodies (30,32) can be used as a standard in the anti-PR3 capture ELISA. Monoclonal antibodies to PR3 and MPO are available from Wieslab AB (Lund, Sweden).

Baslund et al. (52) showed that their capture assay was more efficient than using both indirect immunofluorescence and a direct ELISA for detecting anti-PR3 ANCAs in Wegener's granulomatosis sera, but this finding needs to be confirmed by others with a larger series of patients. The capture step increases the cost of the assay, so this increase must be set against the assay improvements. Much more work needs to be done to establish the specificity and steric arrangement of the epitopes with which ANCAs react so that the capture assay can be tailored for maximum sensitivity and specificity.

Other Tests

Immunoblots using natural or recombinant antigens, or synthesized epitopes need to be investigated as possible methods for detecting ANCAs. A specific response to one or more particular epitopes may be indicative of autoimmune disease, whereas a response to other epitopes may be normal (57). If "disease epitopes" do indeed exist, it may be possible to design a rapid single-step assay to detect such diagnostically important autoantibodies.

REFERENCES

1. Savage COS, Lockwood CM. Systemic vasculitides. In: Lachmann PJ, Peters K, Rosen FR, Walport MJ, eds. Clinical aspects of immunology.

5th ed. Boston: Blackwell Science, 1993;2:1205–1216.

2. Jennette JC, Falk RJ. Clinical and pathological classification of ANCA-associated vasculitis: what are the controversies? Clin Exp Immunol 1995; 101(suppl 1):18–22.
3. Jennette JC. Antineutrophil cytoplasmic autoantibody-associated diseases: a pathologist's perspective. Am J Kidney Dis 1991;18:164–170.
4. Davies DJ, Moran JE, Niall JF, Ryan GB. Segmental necrotizing glomerulonephritis with antineutrophil antibody: possible arbovirus etiology? Brit Med Bull 1982;285:606.
5. van der Woude FJ, Rasmussen N, Lobatto S, et al. Autoantibodies against neutrophils and monocytes: tool for diagnosis and marker of disease activity in Wegener's granulomatosis. Lancet 1985;1:425–429.
6. Falk RJ, Jennette JC. Anti-neutrophil cytoplasmic autoantibodies with specificity for myeloperoxidase in patients with systemic vasculitis and idiopathic necrotizing and crescentic glomerulonephritis. N Engl J Med 1988;318:1651–1657.
7. Kallenberg CGM, Brouwer E, Weening JJ, Cohen Tervaert JW. Anti-neutrophil cytoplasmic antibodies: current diagnostic and pathophysiological potential. Kidney Int 1994;46:1–15.
8. Borregaard N, Kjeldsen L, Lollike K, Sengelov H. Granules and secretory vesicles of the human neutrophil. Clin Exp Immunol 1995;101(suppl 1):6–9.
9. Jennette JC, Wilkman AS, Falk RJ. Anti-neutrophil cytoplasmic autoantibody-associated glomerulonephritis and vasculitis. Am J Pathol 1989;135: 921–930.
10. Wiik A, Stumman L, Kjeldsen L, et al. The diversity of perinuclear antineutrophil cytoplasmic antibodies (pANCA) antigens. Clin Exp Immunol 1995;101(suppl 1):15–17.
11. Lock RJ. Detection of autoantibodies to neutrophil cytoplasmic antigens. J Clin Pathol 1994; 47:4–8.
12. Lesavre P. Antineutrophil cytoplasmic autoantibodies antigen specificity. Am J Kidney Dis 1991; 18:159–163.
13. Cohen Tervaert JW, van der Woude FW, Fauci AS, et al. Association between active Wegener's granulomatosis and anticytoplasmic antibodies. Arch Intern Med 1989;149:2461–2465.
14. Nolle B, Specks U, Ludemann J, et al. Anticytoplasmic autoantibodies: their immunodiagnostic value in Wegener's granulomatosis. Ann Intern Med 1989;111:28–40.
15. Kallenberg CGM. Antineutrophil cytoplasmic autoantibodies with specificity for myeloperoxidase. In: Peter JB, Schoenfeld Y, eds. Autoantibodies. Amsterdam: Elsevier, 1996:53–60.
16. Cohen Tervaert JW, Mulder AHL, Stegeman CA, et al. Occurrence of autoantibodies to human leukocyte elastase in Wegener's granulomatosis and other inflammatory disorders. Ann Rheum Dis 1993;52:115–120.
17. Zhao MH, Jones SJ, Lockwood CM. Bactericidal/permeability-increasing protein (BPI) is an important antigen for anti-neutrophil cytoplasmic antibodies (ANCA) in vasculitis. Clin Exp Immunol 1995;99:49–56.
18. Murphy LK, Targan SR. Antineutrophil cytoplasmic antibodies in inflammatory bowel diseases. In: Peter JB, Shoenfeld Y, eds. Autoantibodies. Amsterdam: Elsevier, 1996:47–52.
19. Gross WL, Ludemann G, Kiefer G, Lehmann H. Anticytoplasmic antibodies in Wegener's granulomatosis. Lancet 1986;1:806.
20. Ludemann G, Gross WL. Autoantibodies against cytoplasmic structures of neutrophil granulocytes in Wegener's granulomatosis. Clin Exp Immunol 1987;69:350–357.
21. Cohen Tervaert JW, Huitema MG, Hene RJ, et al. Prevention of relapses in Wegener's granulomatosis by treatment based on antineutrophil cytoplasmic antibody titer. Lancet 1990;336:709–711.
22. Specks U, Wheatley CL, McDonald RM, et al. Anticytoplasmic autoantibodies in the diagnosis and follow-up of Wegener's granulomatosis. Mayo Clin Proc 1989;64:28–36.
23. Gaskin G, Savage COS, Ryan JJ, et al. Antineutrophil cytoplasmic antibodies and disease activity during long-term follow-up of 70 patients with systemic vasculitis. Nephrol Dial Transplant 1991;6:689–694.
24. Jayne DRW, Gaskin G, Pusey CD, Lockwood CM. ANCA and predicting relapse in systemic vasculitis. Quart J Med 1994;88:127–133.
25. Cohen Tervaert JW, Mulder AHL, Kallenberg CGM, Stegeman CA. Measurement of IgG3 levels of anti-proteinase 3 antibodies (aPR3) is useful in monitoring disease activity in Wegener's granulomatosis. J Am Soc Nephrol 1994;5:828.
26. Jennette JC, Falk RJ. The coming of age of serologic testing for anti-neutrophil cytoplasmic

autoantibodies (editorial, comment). Mayo Clin Proc 1994;69:908–910.

27. Zhao M-H, Lockwood CM. Antineutrophil cytoplasmic autoantibodies with specificity other than PR3 and MPO (X-ANCA). In: Peter JB, Shoenfeld Y, eds. Autoantibodies. Amsterdam: Elsevier, 1996:68–73.

28. Hertervig E, Wieslander J, Johansson C, et al. Anti-neutrophil cytoplasmic antibodies in chronic inflammatory bowel disease. Scand J Gastroenterol 1995;30:693–698.

29. Davenport A, Lock RJ, Wallington TB, Feest TG. Clinical significance of anti-neutrophil cytoplasm antibodies detected by a standardized indirect immunofluorescence assay. Quart J Med 1994; 87:291–299.

30. Wiik A. Antineutrophil cytoplasmic antibodies. In: Rose NR, Conway de Macario E, Folds JD, et al., eds. Manual of clinical laboratory immunology. 5th ed. Washington, DC: ASM Press, 1997: 954–959.

31. Feltkamp TEW. Standards and reference preparations. In: van Venrooij WJ, Maini RN, eds. Manual of biological markers of disease. Dordrecht: Kluwer Academic, 1993;A11:1–12.

32. The international serum standard of anti-neutrophil cytoplasm antibodies (ANCA) according to the 1st international workshop on ANCA, 1988. APMIS 1989;97(suppl 6):30.

33. Hagen EC, Andrassy K, Csernok E, et al. Development and standardization of solid phase assays for the detection of anti-neutrophil cytoplasmic antibodies (ANCA). A report on the second phase of an international cooperative study on the standardization of ANCA assays. J Immunol Methods 1996;196:1–15.

34. Wieslander J, Wiik A. ANCA antigens: proteinase 3. In: van Venrooij WJ, Maini RN, eds. Manual of biological markers of disease. Dordrecht: Kluwer Academic, 1994;B7.1:1–9.

35. Wieslander J, Wiik A. ANCA antigens: myeloperoxidase. In: van Venrooij WJ, Maini RN, eds. Manual of biological markers of disease. Dordrecht: Kluwer Academic, 1994;B7.2:1–9.

36. Falk RJ, Becker M, Terrell R, Jennette JC. Anti-myeloperoxidase autoantibodies react with native but not denatured myeloperoxidase. Clin Exp Immunol 1992;89:274–278.

37. Bini P, Gabay JE, Teitel A, et al. Antineutrophil cytoplasmic antibodies in Wegener's granulomatosis recognize conformational epitope(s) on proteinase 3. J Immunol 1992;149:1409–1415.

38. Williams RC Jr, Staud R, Malone CC, et al. Epitopes on proteinase-3 recognized by antibodies from patients with Wegener's granulomatosis. J Immunol 1994;152:4722–4737.

39. Roberts DE, Peebles C, Curd JG, et al. Autoantibodies to native myeloperoxidase in patients with pulmonary hemorrhage and acute renal failure. J Clin Immunol 1991;11:389–397.

40. Huang Z, Zhao M-H, Lockwood CM. Epitope mapping on the protease 3 molecule using monoclonal antibodies and sera from patients with Wegener's granulomatosis. Clin Exp Immunol 1995;101(suppl 1):50.

41. Short AK, Moguilevsky N, Lockwood CM. Restricted specificity of anti-MPO antibodies in systemic vasculitis: implications for therapy. Clin Exp Immunol 1995;101(suppl 1):38.

42. Pesce AJ, Michal JG. Artifacts and limitations of enzyme immunoassay. J Immunol Methods 1992; 150:111–119.

43. Rasmussen N, Sjolin C, Isaksson B, et al. An ELISA for the detection of anti-neutrophil cytoplasm antibodies. J Immunol Methods 1990;127:139–145.

44. Rasmussen N, Ludemann J, Utecht B. ELISA examination for IgG-ANCA in sera submitted for the 1st international workshop on ANCA. APMIS 1989;97(suppl 6):21–22.

45. Savage COS, Winearls CG, Jones S, et al. Prospective study of radioimmunoassay for antibodies against neutrophil cytoplasm in diagnosis of systemic vasculitis. Lancet 1987;1:1389–1393.

46. Ludemann J, Utecht B, Gross WL. Detection and quantitation of anti-neutrophil cytoplasm antibodies in Wegener's granulomatosis by ELISA using affinity-purified antigen. J Immunol Methods 1988;114:167–174.

47. Niles JL, Pan GL, Collins AB, et al. Antigen-specific radioimmunoassays for anti-neutrophil cytoplasmic antibodies in the diagnosis of rapidly progressive glomerulonephritis. J Am Soc Nephrol 1991;2:27–36.

48. Goldschmeding R, Cohen Tervaert JW, Dolman KM, et al. ANCA: a class of vasculitis-associated autoantibodies against myeloid granule proteins: clinical and laboratory aspects and possible pathogenetic implications. Adv Exp Med Biol 1991;297:129–139.

49. Ulmer M, Rautman A, Gross WL. Immunodiagnostic aspects of autoantibodies against

myeloperoxidase. Clin Nephrol 1992;37:161–168.

50. Rasmussen N, Daha MR. Concluding remarks on solid phase assays. Neth J Med 1990;36:143–145.

51. Wieslander J. How are antineutrophil cytoplasmic autoantibodies detected? Am J Kidney Dis 1991;18:154–158.

52. Baslund B, Segelmark M, Wiik A, et al. Screening for anti-neutrophil cytoplasmic antibodies (ANCA): is indirect immunofluorescence the method of choice? Clin Exp Immunol 1995;99:486–492.

53. Godbole MS, Valenzuela R, Deodhar SD, et al. Comparative study of ELISA and indirect immunofluorescence for the detection of anti-neutrophil cytoplasmic antibodies. Am J Clin Pathol 1995;104:667–672.

54. Gross WL, Csernok E, Szymkowiak CH. Anti-neutrophil cytoplasmic autoantibodies with specificity for proteinase 3. In: Peter JB, Schoenfeld Y, eds. Autoantibodies. Amsterdam: Elsevier, 1996:61–67.

55. Billing P, Tahir S, Calfin, B, et al. Nuclear localization of the antigen detected by ulcerative colitis-associated perinuclear antineutrophil cytoplasmic antibodies. Am J Pathol 1995;147:979–987.

56. Goldschmeding R, van der Schoot CE, ten Bokkel Huinink D, et al. Wegener's granulomatosis autoantibodies identify a novel diisofluorophosphate-binding protein in the lysosomes of normal human neutrophils. J Clin Invest 1989;84:1577–1587.

57. Burek CL, Rose NR. Thyroglobulin autoantibodies. In: Peter JB, Shoenfeld Y, eds. Autoantibodies. Amsterdam: Elsevier, 1996:810–815.

CHAPTER 29

Standardized Anticardiolipin Testing

E. NIGEL HARRIS
SILVIA S. PIERANGELI

Anticardiolipin tests are important in diagnosis of a disorder termed the "antiphospholipid syndrome" (APS) (1). Patients affected with APS are subject to recurrent episodes of thrombosis in arteries and/or veins, pregnancy loss (probably secondary to thrombosis of vessels in the placenta), and thrombocytopenia. Diagnosis is based on finding a "moderate to high" positive anticardiolipin test and/or a positive lupus anticoagulant test with any one of the characteristic clinical features presented above (2). Both tests measure autoantibodies specific for phospholipids, phospholipid binding proteins, or a complex of these molecules. In addition to APS, anticardiolipin tests are positive in a variety of disorders, including connective tissue diseases, infectious disorders such as syphilis (3,4), Q fever, AIDS (5,6), and some drug-induced disorders (7). It is generally believed that anticardiolipin antibodies are clinically significant only when present in APS; thus, there have been continuous attempts to modify the assay to make it more specific for APS. Based on an early observation that patients with high positive IgG anticardiolipin tests were more likely to have APS (8), efforts were devoted to quantifying the anticardiolipin ELISA test in a standardized manner. At the time those efforts were started, there were no published methods for standardizing ELISA tests for autoantibody measurement. This chapter will discuss how a series of anticardiolipin workshops have been used to validate and improve measurement of anticardiolipin antibodies, as well as resolve issues concerning anticardiolipin specificity.

History

In 1983, a group of investigators at the Hammersmith Hospital in London, England, were interested in a subgroup of patients with systemic lupus erythematosus (SLE) who had an unusual coagulation abnormality called the "lupus anticoagulant" (9,10). Plasma samples from these patients had prolonged clotting times determined by the Partial Thromboplastin Time (PTT) test. What was puzzling about these patients was that instead of experiencing bleeding abnormalities, as might be predicted by prolonged clotting times, these patients were subject to thrombosis (9). The lupus anticoagulant phenomenon was known to be caused by an autoantibody (11). The autoantibody was believed to bind phospholipids, because they inhibited two phospholipid-dependent coagulation reactions in the clotting cascade—the prothrombin-thrombin conversion and factor X activation (11). About 25% to 50% of patients with the lupus anticoagulant reaction also had a biological false-positive test for syphilis (BFP-STS), and antibodies responsible for the BFP-STS were known to bind cardiolipin, a negatively charged phospholipid. In addition, one group had also demonstrated that a monoclonal antibody with lupus anticoagulant activity bound negatively charged phospholipids such as phosphatidylserine (12). The lupus anticoagulant reaction was a functional assay affected by a number of variables, including how plasma samples were prepared and stored, as well as what reagents were used for testing. In addition, the test lacked sensitivity and could not be readily standardized. Characterizing the autoantibody for studies of disease pathogenesis was also difficult.

The group in London reasoned that use of a solid phase immunoassay with cardiolipin as antigen might be one way of detecting antibodies with lupus anticoagulant activity (13). They hypothesized that such a test would have the advantages of greater sensitivity, more reproducibility, better quantitation, and the possibility of standardization. The group succeeded in establishing a solid phase radioimmunoassay with cardiolipin as antigen, and the antibodies were termed "anticardiolipin antibodies" (13). The test proved more sensitive than the lupus anticoagulant assay and enabled diagnosis of a much larger number of patients with the antiphospholipid syndrome (APS). What proved surprising was that only about 80% of the lupus anticoagulant positive samples were anticardiolipin positive, and some high positive anticardiolipin samples were lupus anticoagulant negative, suggesting that although the antibodies might be related, some of their characteristics varied. Also noteworthy was the determination that anticardiolipin antibodies cross-reacted with negatively charged phospholipids, such as phosphatidylserine and phosphatidylglycerol (14,15). Thus, the name "anticardiolipin" antibodies was changed to "antiphospholipid" antibodies (16), and the disorder with which these antibodies were associated was called the "antiphospholipid syndrome" (APS) (2).

Widespread adoption of the solid phase anticardiolipin assay led to several potential problems. These antibodies were soon reported in several disorders such as syphilis (3,4), AIDS (5,6), connective tissue diseases, as well as in normal individuals who did not have features of the disorder. "False" positive tests in the aforementioned conditions could best be explained by the sensitivity of the anticardiolipin test. However, methods of performing the test also varied and results were questionable in some instances. Fortunately, it was recognized that the majority of patients with APS tended to have high anticardiolipin antibody levels, usually of the IgG isotype (however, some patients were only IgM positive). To ensure that the anticardiolipin test would retain its value in diagnosis APS, it would be necessary to identify antibodies by isotype and to quantify results using some reliable unit of measurement. There was also a need to establish which testing methods were valid as well as standard procedures for performing the solid phase immunoassay. To achieve these goals, an international standardization workshop was first conducted in 1986 (17).

The First Anticardiolipin Standardization Workshop

The goals of the first workshop to standardize anticardiolipin methodology included validation of assay methods to detect anticardiolipin antibodies, establishment of a unit of measure that would be reproducible in other laboratories, and development of standard samples which would enable individual laboratories to validate their own testing methods. At the time, autoantibody tests were often validated simply by one or a small group of "authoritative" laboratories distributing a few selected samples to other laboratories, and asking participants to identify which of the samples were positive. The goals of the first anticardiolipin workshop were more complex.

Six specially prepared samples were distributed to 30 laboratories (17). These samples were prepared in such a way that a determination could be made as to which laboratories had valid assays. A very high positive IgG sample and a very high positive IgM sample were mixed with varying quantities of normal human serum. Each of the mixtures was tested in the anticardiolipin assay at 1/50 dilution. Six mixtures were selected so that they covered the full optical density range of the anticardiolipin assay. Each of the six samples was assigned a unit value based on the calculated quantity of IgG and IgM anticardiolipin antibody present. The calculation was performed as described in **Table 29-1**. When the optical density readings of the six samples were plotted against their calculated values using a log-log plot, a straight line correlation was obtained and a correlation coefficient could be determined (**Fig. 29-1**) (17). We predicted that laboratories with valid assays would have statistically significant correlations between optical density readings and anticardiolipin values. In contrast, laboratories with nonvalid assays would show no correlation between optical density readings and sample concentrations (see Fig. 29-1).

The 30 participating laboratories were asked to run the samples on three different days and report their optical density readings; IgG

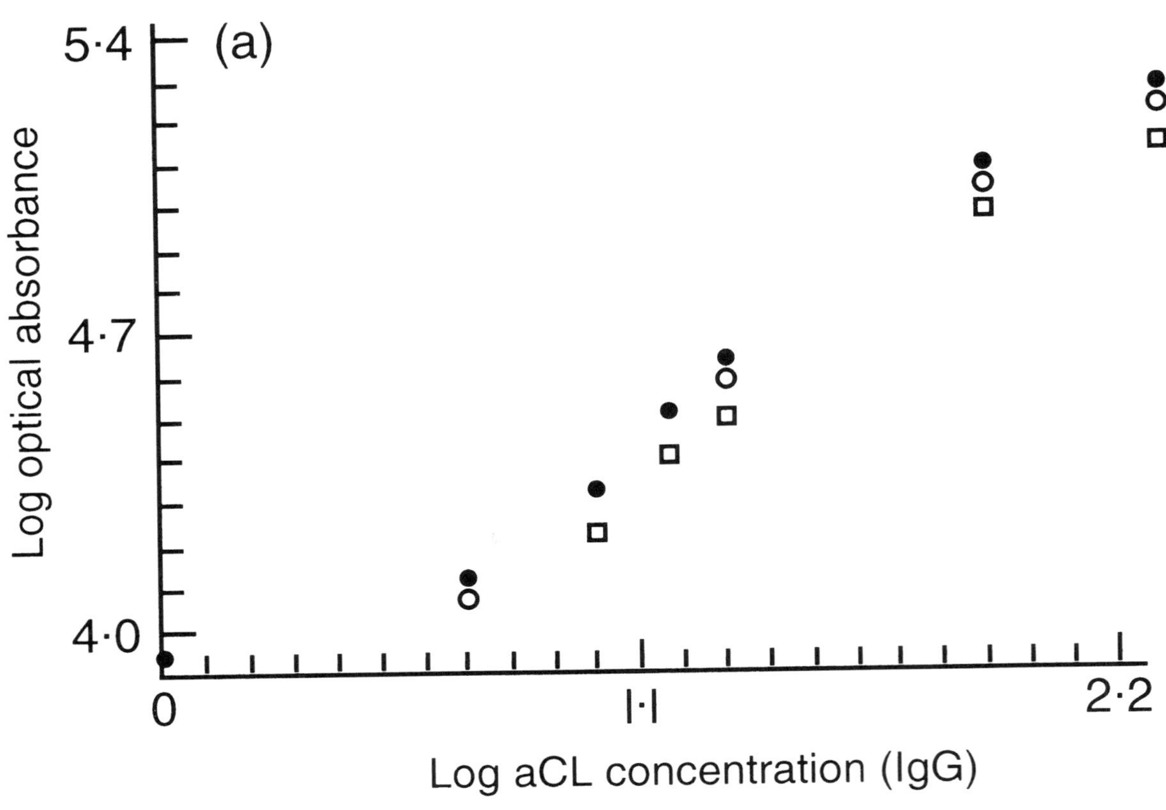

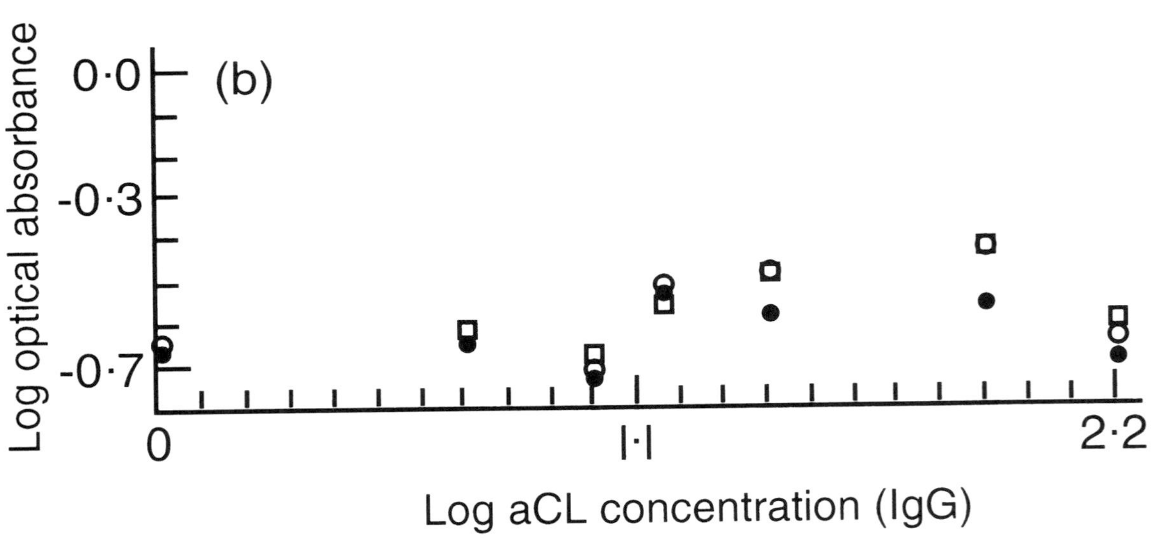

FIGURE **29-1**

Example of approximate linear relationship between logarithmic values of optical absorbance and logarithmic values of IgGaCL concentrations encompassed by the seven standard samples for (a) a laboratory with a valid assay and (b) a laboratory with an assay that was not valid. (a) (●) day 1, (○) day 2, (□) day 3; R^2 = 98.7%, F regression = NS, $\log_e Y = -1.365 + 0.071 \times \log_e(X)$. (Reproduced by permission from Harris EN, Gharavi AE, Patel S, Hughes GRV. Evaluation of the anti-cardiolipin antibody test: report of an international workshop held 4 April 1986. Clin Exp Immunol 1987;68:215–222.)

TABLE 29-1

Calculation of Anticardiolipin Levels in the Six Samples Distributed to Participating Laboratories in the First Anticardiolipin Standardization Workshop

Step 1.	A high positive IgG anticardiolipin serum sample was assigned a value based on the quantity of affinity purified anticardiolipin antibody isolated from it. The sample was estimated to contain 300 μg/mL of IgG anticardiolipin and it was assigned a value of 300 GPL units (thus, 1 μg/mL of IgG anticardiolipin was defined as 1 GPL). A high positive IgM anticardiolipin sample was assigned a value in MPL units using the same method
Step 2.	Mixtures of the high positive samples and normal human serum (negative for IgG anticardiolipin) were prepared, and values of IgG and IgM anticardiolipin calculated for each mixture based on the proportion of positive sample present. Thus a 1:1 mixture of positive sample and normal human serum had a value of 300 ÷ 2 = 150 GPL units; a 1:4 mixture would have a value of 300 ÷ 5 = 60 GPL units. (The IgM sample was incorporated into the mixtures and values of IgM cardiolipin in MPL units were calculated using the same method.)
Step 3.	Each of the mixtures was diluted 1/50 in 10% adult bovine serum/PBS (v/v) and these were run in the anticardiolipin assay.
Step 4.	Six mixtures were selected that spanned the optical density range of the IgG and IgM anticardiolipin assay (17). These mixtures were distributed to participating laboratories.

and IgM anticardiolipin were to be run separately. Laboratories were "blinded" with respect to the concentration of IgG and IgM anticardiolipin in the individual samples (indeed, they had no knowledge about how the samples were prepared). Twenty-three of the 30 participating laboratories were shown to have valid assays (17). Laboratories using nonvalid methods were found to be using gelatin/PBS or PBS alone as sample diluents. Laboratories with valid assays used 10% adult or fetal calf serum in PBS (v/v), or 1% bovine serum albumin (BSA) in PBS (w/v). In addition, the use of Tween in the assay, or warming cardiolipin-coated plates at 37°C were also shown to yield nonvalid results (17). These findings were confirmed in subsequent studies (18).

The workshop's findings enabled the six samples to be used more widely to validate anticardiolipin tests. These samples could also be used to construct a calibration curve for routine assays (**Fig. 29-2**). A subsequent study showed that the relationship of optical density readings to IgG or IgM anticardiolipin concentrations was best expressed by a log-logit rather than a log-log relationship (**Fig. 29-3**).

Another result of the workshop was that it enabled levels of anticardiolipin antibodies to be expressed in units that could be adopted by all laboratories ("GPL" for IgG antiphospholipid; "MPL" for IgM antiphospholipid). Other laboratories went on to confirm that patients with moderate to high antibody levels, particularly IgG, were more subject to recurrent thrombosis and pregnancy losses (19,20). The most detailed demonstration of this relationship was reported by Escalante and colleagues (21). Units of measure of anticardiolipin positivity were also used to establish laboratory criteria for diagnosis of the APS (2).

Problems with Anticardiolipin Standardization

A number of problems became evident within a few years of completion of the first anticardiolipin standardization workshop. One of the first was that there was much variation in individual measurements of antibody levels, despite considerable care in performance of the assay. Thus, readings of 50 GPL units might vary anywhere from 35 to 65 GPL units. Because of this, laboratories were urged not only to report absolute anticardiolipin levels, but also to define them semiquantitatively as low, medium, or high, since use of semiquantitative measures might achieve better interlaboratory agreement than use of absolute values. Our laboratory also uses an "inhouse standard" in addition to calibrators to improve reproducibility—if the value of the inhouse standard was outside of a defined range (±2 standard deviations of the mean value), the run was repeated. Use of a defined standard, in addition to calibrators, has also been adopted by one commercial ELISA kit (Louisville APL Diagnostics Inc., Louisville, Kentucky). We also found that in the final step of the assay, stopping the color reaction when a sample of about 80 to 90 GPL or MPL units reached a reading of 1.0 offered better reproducibility (22).

Another difficulty was that some laborato-

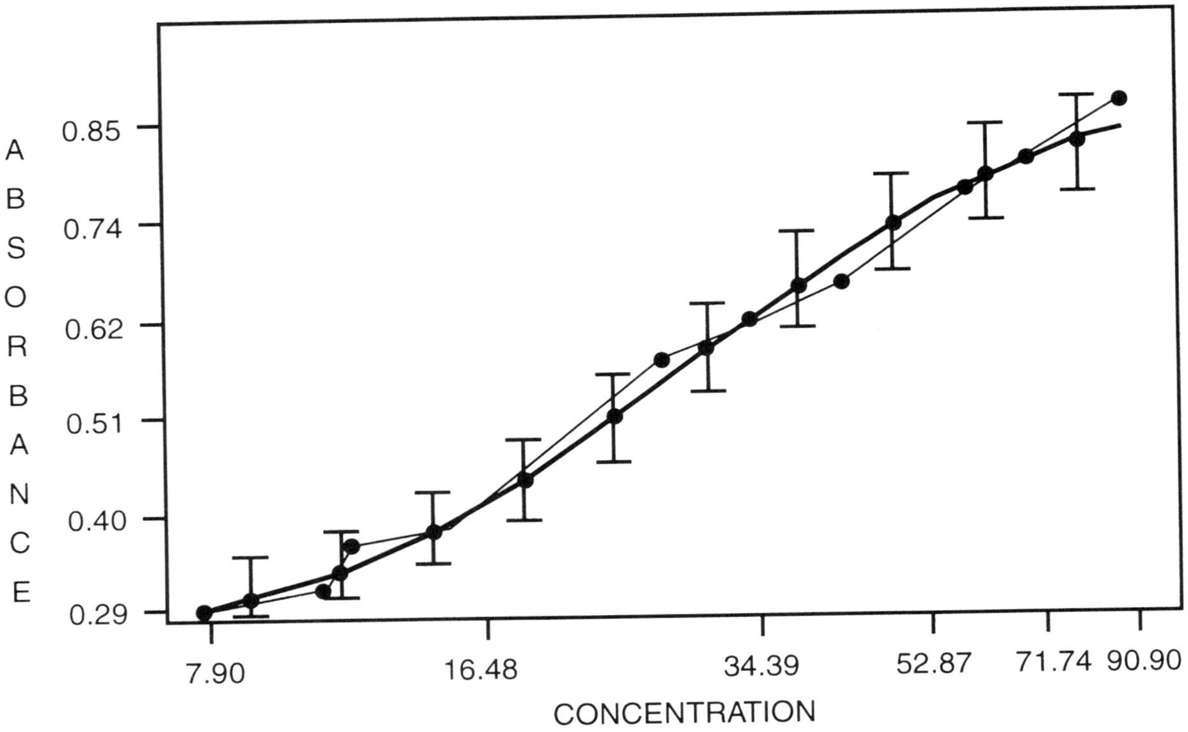

FIGURE **29-2**

The relationship between optical density (absorbance) and level of aCL antibody (concentration) best fits a log-logistical curve. Such a curve can be constructed (by computer) by running 5–7 standards with known aCL levels on each ELISA plate. aCL levels of unknown samples run on the same plate can be derived from this curve. aCL level and isotype appear to correlate with risk of complications. Curve fit: Absorbance = (0.2561 − 0.8856)/[1 + (Conc./30.5094)1.9834] + 0.8856. Standard error: 0.0343 abs. (Reprinted with permission from Harris EN, Pierangeli S. The anticardiolipin ELISA. In: Techniques in Diagnostic Pathology, vol 2; Academic Press Ltd., 1991.)

ries never adopted the new units of measure, preferring instead to use optical density readings or standard deviations to express results—both of the latter units of measurements vary considerable even in a single laboratory. Another method of calculating anticardiolipin levels that proved unreliable was calculating concentration by determining the ratio of the optical density (OD) reading of a sample to that of a single standard with known GPL or MPL units [Concentration of unknown sample = (Optical density unknown sample ÷ Optical density standard) × Units of standard]. The above calculation would be acceptable if the relationship of optical density readings to concentration was linear, but this is the case only over a narrow range of the assay. In addition, the optical density readings of any two samples may vary significantly in opposite directions, making measurements of ratios between two samples even more unreliable. The second anticardiolipin workshop discussed below highlighted the unreliability of use of a single reference standard to calculate anticardiolipin levels (23).

The Second Anticardiolipin Workshop

The goals of the second workshop were quite different from the first. Essentially, this exercise sought to determine the level of agreement between laboratories if a semiquantitative measure of anticardiolipin antibody levels was used (23). All participating laboratories were given samples designated as G1, G2, and G3 for IgG, and M1, M2, and M3 for IgM. These samples helped define semiquantitative levels

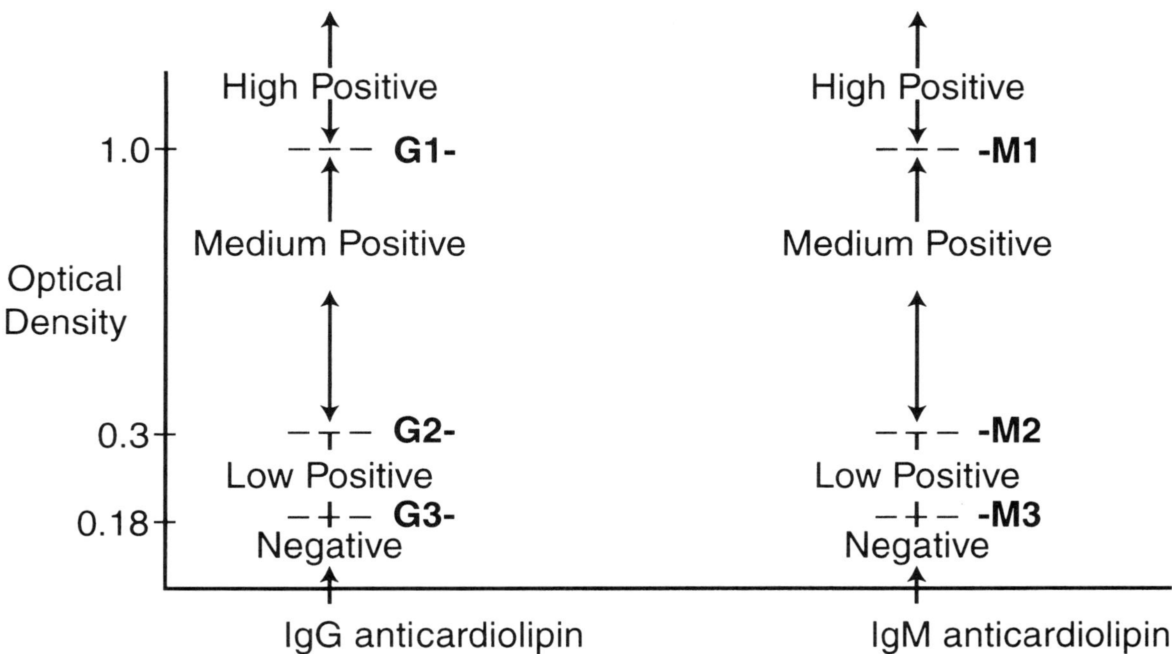

FIGURE 29-3

Samples were defined as high, medium, low, or negative based on their optical density (OD) relative to the optical densities of the reference samples run on the same ELISA plate. For the IgG assay, high positive samples were those with OD above G1; medium positive samples had OD between G1 and G2; low positive samples between G2 and G3, and negative samples and OD less than G3. The same principle was used for IgM samples. (Reproduced by permission from Harris EN. The second international anticardiolipin standardization workshop/ the Kingston Antiphospholipid Antibody Study (KAPS) group. Am J Clin Pathol 1990;94:476–484.)

of positivity. Thus G1 was used to define the border between "high" and "medium" levels—samples with OD readings above G1 were defined as "high" and samples below G1 but above G2 defined as "medium" (see Fig. 29-3). G2 was used to distinguish "medium" from "low" and G3 used to distinguish "low" from "negative." Participating laboratories were subdivided into regions, and laboratories in each region were asked to distribute samples between themselves which they would define as "high," "medium," "low," or "negative." The results of the workshop showed good interlaboratory agreement for "high" and "medium" positive samples, but "low-negative" distinctions were not as good (23).

The findings of this workshop prompted the Antiphospholipid Standardization Laboratory (currently at Morehouse School of Medicine, Atlanta, Georgia) to extend the number of calibrators used for the assay. A set of 9 rather than 5 calibrators was introduced, with more calibrators being used below 20 GPL and MPL units. It was hoped that use of more calibrators below 20 units would enable better definition of the low positive range of the assay and would allow better distinction between low positive and negative. Unfortunately, there is so little change of optical density readings with anticardiolipin concentrations at low levels that use of more calibrators in this region did not improve precision significantly. However, better precision in the low positive range of the assay may not be important anyway, as it is generally observed that most patients with APS have "moderate" to "high" rather than "low" positive levels (8,19–21). Nevertheless, a recent study suggests that low positive anticardiolipin results have some value in predicting features of APS (24).

The second standardization workshop still did not achieve uniform success in establishing reproducible measurement of anticardiolipin levels. Some subsequent reports continued to find variations between laboratories reporting anticardiolipin results, even when semiquantitative measures of antibody levels were determined (25). The latter findings may be partially explained by continued resistance to use of standard methods for performing the test as well as use of a single reference standard rather than a calibration curve to calculate anticardiolipin levels.

The Third Anticardiolipin Workshop

β_2-Glycoprotein 1

Soon after introduction of the anticardiolipin assay, some investigators noted that use of 10% fetal calf or adult bovine serum to dilute patient sera resulted in enhanced cardiolipin binding activity, when compared to 1% BSA/PBS (w/v) or 0.3% gelatin/PBS (w/v) as diluents (26). Indeed, the first standardization workshop demonstrated that use of 10% fetal or bovine serum enabled more valid measurement of anticardiolipin levels (17). In 1990, three laboratories reported that the "factor" responsible for enhanced binding activity was β_2-glycoprotein 1 (β_2GP1) (27–30). β_2GP1 is a 50kd protein present in serum. This protein avidly binds negatively charged phospholipids. The function of the protein is unknown, but because it can inhibit phospholipid-dependent coagulation reactions (e.g., prothrombin-thrombin conversion), it is believed to act as a natural anticoagulant. The observation that β_2GP1 enhanced anticardiolipin binding activity had possible pathogenic implications. Investigators hypothesized that the anticoagulant function of β_2GP1 might be neutralized by anticardiolipin antibodies, which would favor thrombosis (27,28). A second observation reported with respect to β_2GP1 was that presence of the protein appeared to *decrease* binding of anticardiolipin antibodies from patients with syphilis, contrasting with enhancement of binding of sera from patients with APS (29,30).

Within a few years of the initial reports regarding β_2GP1, some (31–35) but not all (30,36–38) laboratories reported that β_2GP1 alone could be used as antigen. For example, Matsuura and colleagues reported that when ELISA plates were oxidized by gamma irradiation, then coated with β_2GP1, there was binding of anticardiolipin antibodies to the β_2GP1 in the absence of cardiolipin (33). In addition, they reported that binding to β_2GP1 was specific to APS sera and was not evident when sera from patients with syphilis and other infectious disorders were examined. They reasoned that anticardiolipin antibodies recognize "neo-epitopes" on β_2GP1 that are exposed when β_2GP1 binds negative surfaces such as cardiolipin or oxidized polystyrene plates. The observations of Matsuura and colleagues were tested in the fourth anticardiolipin workshop, results of which will be discussed below. Although other laboratories reported binding to β^2GP1, there was much variation in methods used and differences existed particularly with respect to the assay plates used (33,39).

In another observation of interest with respect to β_2GP1, Gharavi and colleagues reported that mice immunized with β_2GP1 alone developed both anticardiolipin and anti-β_2GP1 antibodies (40). These two populations of antibodies did not appear to be cross-reacting. A follow-up study by Pierangeli and colleagues confirmed that immunization of mice with β_2GP1 induced anticardiolipin (and anti-β_2GP1) antibodies, but those investigators also found that immunization of mice with purified human anticardiolipin antibodies also induced formation of murine anticardiolipin antibodies (41). They reasoned that phospholipid-binding proteins (such as β_2GP1 and human anticardiolipin antibodies) complex with circulating phospholipids such as those present in circulating lipoproteins. The complex of "foreign" proteins with phospholipids serve as immunogens which result in generation of antiphospholipid antibodies (41). Subsequent studies suggest that these antibodies induced in mice are separately specific for cardiolipin, β_2GP1, as well as both antigens (42,43). This latter observation was also suggested in a recent study in which murine monoclonal antibodies were raised with specificities for cardiolipin alone, β_2GP1 alone, and both cardiolipin and β_2GP1 (44).

The Third Workshop

Controversy surrounding the role of β_2GP1 in anticardiolipin assays and a need to analyze anticardiolipin kits prompted a third anticardiolipin workshop in 1994 (45). The workshop sought to test several controversial questions. One was whether anticardiolipin antibodies could bind cardiolipin in the absence of β_2GP1. Another objective was to compare performance of selected commercial ELISA kits with the standard anticardiolipin bench method.

The main findings of this workshop were that immunoglobulins from APS patients did bind cardiolipin and phosphatidylserine *in the absence* of β_2GP1, but addition of β_2GP1 increased binding activities of the samples to both phospholipid antigens (45). No binding to polystyrene ELISA plates coated with β_2GP1 alone was demonstrated—which left unresolved the issue of antibody binding to β_2GP1. Finally, there was excellent correlation demonstrated between the anticardiolipin kits tested and the bench method, suggesting that *some* kits could provide results comparable to the bench method (only a few of the many ELISA anticardiolipin kits that were commercially available were tested in this workshop).

The Fourth Anticardiolipin Workshop

Which Test Is More Specific for Identification of APS Samples?

In September 1996, a fourth anticardiolipin workshop was conducted (46). The objective of this most recent workshop was to compare four techniques for measurement of anticardiolipin antibodies to determine which was more specific for identification of APS. Samples tested were eight APS, four anticardiolipin positive syphilis, two anticardiolipin positive (one obtained from a patient with Q fever and the other from a patient with SLE, neither of whom had features of APS), and six from normal healthy controls. Techniques evaluated were the anticardiolipin bench method; two commercial anticardiolipin ELISA kits (INOVA Diagnostics, Inc., and INCSTAR Corporation); an antiphospholipid kit in which a mixture of phospholipids was used as antigen (APhL ELISA Kit, Louisville APL Diagnostics, Inc., Louisville, Kentucky); a recent anti-β_2GP1 kit in which gamma-irradiated plates are coated with β_2GP1 (INOVA Diagnostics, Inc.); and a flow cytometric technique in which IgG and IgM antibodies to cardiolipin and to phosphatidylserine can be determined simultaneously (thus obtaining four measurements—IgG and IgM anticardiolipin and IgG and IgM antiphosphatidylserine).

The results obtained by this workshop were noteworthy. All techniques tested were 90–100% sensitive, correctly identifying almost all sera from patients with APS. However, results varied with respect to specificity. The APhL ELISA Kit (Louisville APL Diagnostics, Inc., Louisville, KY) using a mixture of phospholipids as antigens was most specific (100% specific); the anti-β_2GP1 (INOVA Diagnostics, Inc.) was nearly as specific, with only the Q fever sample (but not the syphilis or SLE samples) "falsely" identified as positive. The flow cytometer method with phosphatidylserine as antigen showed the third best specificity, "falsely" identifying only two samples. None of the anticardiolipin assays, whether bench method, ELISA kit, or flow cytometric methods, proved to be specific: the syphilis, Q fever, and SLE samples were all reported as positive.

The workshop also sought to compare anticardiolipin measurements between the commercial kits and bench method. There was good correlation between the bench method and the anticardiolipin ELISA kits. However, there was no correlation of anticardiolipin and anti-β_2GP1 levels, even when kits prepared by the same company were compared.

Anticardiolipin Workshops: Reflections on Their Significance

Over the past 10 years, anticardiolipin workshops served a variety of purposes. In the first workshop, the assay methods that enabled valid measurements of anticardiolipin antibody levels were determined. In addition, units of measurement were established, and six calibrator standards were introduced to assist laboratories worldwide in establishing the anticardiolipin assay. The second workshop demonstrated that semiquantitive measures of anticardiolipin antibody levels enabled the best agreement between laboratories. The third and fourth workshops sought to settle controversial issues regarding anticardiolipin specificity, but also sought to examine some of the newly introduced commercial kits. Together, these workshops have demonstrated that investigators working collaboratively can contribute to improvement in testing methods, and to greater understanding of scientific issues such as those related to anticardiolipin specificity.

Acknowledgments

We wish to thank Ms. Trina White for her expert typing of this manuscript.

REFERENCES

1. Harris EN. Antiphospholipid syndrome. In: Klippel JH, Dieppe PA, eds. Rheumatology. London: Mosby-Year Book, 1994: Section 6;32.1–32.6.
2. Harris EN. Syndrome of the black swan. Br J Rheumatol 1987;26:324–326.
3. Moritsen S, Hoier-Madson M, Wiik A, et al. The specificity of anti-cardiolipin antibodies from syphilis patients and from patients with systemic lupus erythematosus. Clin Exp Immunol 1989; 76:178–183.
4. Harris EN, Gharavi AE, Wasley GD, Hughes GRV. Use of an enzyme-linked immunosorbent assay and of inhibition studies to distinguish between antibodies to cardiolipin from patients with syphilis or autoimmune disorders. J Infect Dis 1988;157:23–31.
5. Intrator L, Oksenhendler E, Desforges L, P.B. Anticardiolpin antibodies in HIV infected patients with or without autoimmune thrombocytopenic purpura. Br J Haematol 1988;67:269–270.
6. Canoso RT, Zon LI, Groopman JE. Anticardiolpin antibodies associated with HTLV-III infection. Br J Haematol 1987;65:495–498.
7. Canoso RT, Sise HS. Chlorpromazine-induced lupus anticoagulant and associated immunologic abnormalities. Am J Hematol 1982;13:121–129.
8. Harris EN, Chan JKH, Asherson RA, et al. Thrombosis, recurrent fetal loss and thrombocytopenia. Predictive value of the anti-cardiolipin antibody test. Arch Intern Med 1986;146:2153–2156.
9. Boey MD, Colaco CB, Gharavi AE. Thrombosis in SLE: striking association with the presence of circulating "lupus anticoagulant." BMJ 1983;287: 1021–1023.
10. Hughes GRV. Thrombosis, abortion, cerebral disease and the lupus anticoagulant. BMJ 1983; 287:1088–1089
11. Shapiro SS, Thiagarajan P. Lupus anticoagulant. Prog Haemostas Thromb 1982;6:263–285.
12. Thiagarajan P, Shapiro SS, DeMarco L. Monoclonal immunoglobulin Mλ coagulation inhibitor with phospholipid specificity: mechanism of a lupus anticoagulant. J Clin Invest 1980;66:397–405.
13. Harris EN, Gharavi AE, Boey ML, et al. Anticardiolipin antibodies: detection by radioimmunoassay and association with thrombosis. Lancet 1983;II:1211–1214.
14. Harris EN, Gharavi AE, Tincani A, et al. Affinity purified anti-cardiolipin and anti-DNA antibodies. J Clin Lab Immunol 1985;17:155–162.
15. Harris EN, Gharavi AE, Loizou S, et al. Crossreactivity of anti-phospholipid antibodies. J Clin Lab Immunol 1985;16:1–6.
16. Harris EN, Gharavi AE, Hughes GRV. Antiphospholipid antibodies. Clin Rheum Dis 1985;11:591–609.
17. Harris EN, Gharavi AE, Patel S, Hughes GRV. Evaluation of the anti-cardiolipin antibody test: report of an international workshop held 4 April 1986. Clin Exp Immunol 1987;68:215–222.
18. Gharavi AE, Sammaritano LR, Wen J, Elkon KB. Induction of antiphospholipid antibodies by immunization with anticardiolipin cofactor (abstract). Arthritis Rheum 1991;34(suppl):S43.
19. Alving BM, Barr CF, Tank DB. Correlation between lupus anticoagulants and anticardiolipin antibodies in patients with prolonged activated partial thromboplastin times. Am J Med 1990;88:112–116.
20. Silver RM, Draper ML, Scott JR, et al. Clinical consequences of antiphospholipid antibodies: an historic cohort study. Obstet Gynecol 1994;83: 372–377.
21. Escalante A, Brey RL, Mitchell BD, Dreiner U. Accuracy of anticardiolipin antibodies in identifying a history of thrombosis among patients with systemic lupus erythematosus. Am J Med 1995;98:559–567.
22. Gharavi AE, Harris EN, Asherson RA, Hughes GRV. Anticardiolipin antibody isotype distribution and phospholipid specificity. Ann Rheum Dis 1987;46:1–6.
23. Harris EN. The second international anticardiolipin standardization workshop/the Kingston Antiphospholipid Antibody Study (KAPS) group. Am J Clin Pathol 1990;94:476–484.
24. Silver RM, Porter TF, Leeuwen IV, et al. Anticardiolipin antibodies: clinical consequences of "low titers." Obstet Gynecol 1996;87:494–500.
25. Peaceman AH, Silver RK, MacGregor SN, Socol ML. Interlaboratory variation in antiphospholipid antibody testing. Am J Obstet Gynecol 1992;144: 1780–1784.

26. Tincani A, Meroni PL, Brucato A, et al. Antiphospholipid and anti-mitichondrial type M5 antibodies in systemic lupus erythematosus. Clin Exp Rheumatol 1985;3:321–326.

27. Galli M, Comfurius P, Maasen C, et al. Anticardiolipin antibodies (ACA) directed not to cardiolipin but to a plasma protein cofactor. Lancet 1990;336:1544–1547.

28. McNeil HP, Simpson RJ, Chesterman CN, Krillis S. Anti-phospholipid antibodies are directed against a complex antigen that includes a lipid-binding inhibitor of coagulation: β_2 glycoprotein 1 (apolipoprotein H). Proc Natl Acad Sci USA 1990;87:4120–4124.

29. Matsuura E, Igarashi Y, Fujimoto M. Anticardiolipin antibodies directed not to cardiolipin but to a plasma protein co-factor. Lancet 1990; 336:1547.

30. Sammaritano LR, Lockshin MD, Gharavi AE. Antiphospholipid antibodies differ in aPL cofactor requirement. Lupus 1992;1:51–56.

31. Arvieux J, Pouzol P, Roussel B, et al. Measurement of anti-phospholipid antibodies by ELISA using β_2 glyoprotein 1 as an antigen. Br J Haematol 1992;81:568–573.

32. Viard JP, Amoura Z, Bach JF. Association of anti-β_2 glycoprotein with lupus circulating anticoagulant and thrombosis in SLE. Am J Med 1992;93: 181–186.

33. Matsuura E, Igarashi Y, Yasuda T, et al. Anticardiolipin antibodies recognize beta(2)-glycoprotein 1 structure altered by interacting with an oxygen modified solid phase surface. J Exp Med 1994;179(2):457–462.

34. Martinuzzo ME, Forastriero RR, Carreras LO. Anti-β(2) glycoprotein 1: detection and association with thrombosis. Br J Haematol 1995;89: 397–402.

35. Cabiedes J, Cabral A, Alareon-Segovia D. Clinical manifestations of the antiphospholipid syndrome in patients with systemic lupus erythematosus associate more strongly with anti-β_2 glycoprotein 1 than with antiphospholipid antibodies. J Rheumatol 1995;22:1899–1906.

36. Pierangeli SS, Harris EN, Davis SA, DeLorenzo G. β_2 glycoprotein 1 enhances cardiolipin binding activity but is not the antigen for antiphospholipid antibodies. Br J Haematol 1992;82:565–570.

37. Pierangeli SS, Goldsmith GH, Krnic S, Harris EN. Differences in functional activity of anticardiolipin antibodies from patients with syphilis and the antiphospholipid syndrome. Infect Immun 1994;62(9):4081–4084.

38. Gharavi AE, Harris EN, Sammaritano LR, et al. Do patients with antiphospholipid syndrome have antibodies to β_2 glycoprotein 1? J Lab Clin Med 1993;122(4):426–431.

39. Roubey RAS, Eisenberg RA, Harper MF, Winfield JB. "Anticardiolipin" antibodies recognize β_2 glycoprotein 1 in the absence of phospholipid. J Immunol 1995;154:954–960.

40. Gharavi AE, Sammaritano LR, Wen J, Elkon KB. Induction of antiphospholipid antibodies by immunization with β_2 glycoprotein 1. J Clin Invest 1992;90:1105–1109.

41. Pierangeli SS, Davis SA, Harris EN. Induction of phospholipid binding antibodies in mice and rabbits by immunization with human β_2 glycoprotein 1 or anticardiolipin antibodies alone. Clin Exp Immunol 1993;93(2):269–272.

42. Kouts S, Wang MX, Adelstein S, Krilis SA. Immunization of a rabbit with β_2 glycoprotein 1 induces charge-dependent crossreactive antibodies that bind amonic phospholipids and have similar reactivity autoimmune antiphospholipid antibodies. J Immunol 1995;155; 958–966.

43. Gharavi AE, Sammaritano LR, Bovastro JL, Wilson WA. Specificities and characterisitics of β_2 glycoprotein 1 induced antiphospholipid antibodies. J Lab Clin Med 1995;125:775–778.

44. Gharavi AE, Pierangeli SS, Gharavi EE, et al. Chromobogenic properties of antiphospholipid antibodies do not depend on their binding to β_2 glycoprotein 1 alone. Lupus 1998 (in press).

45. Harris EN, Pierangeli SS, Birch D. Anticardiolipin wet workshop report: Vth International Symposium on Antiphospholipid Antibodies. Am J Clin Pathol 1994;101(5):616–624.

46. Pierangeli SS, Stewart M, Silva LK, Harris EN. Report of an anticardiolipin wet workshop during the VIIth International Symposium on antiphospholipid antibodies. J Rheumatol 1998; 25:156–162.

CHAPTER 30

Quality Assurance and Standardization in the Diagnostic Allergy Laboratory

ROBERT G. HAMILTON

Laboratory quality assurance may be defined as a group of plans, policies, and procedures that are used to maximize quality of analytical measurements. This chapter focuses on quality assurance and more specific quality control practices that may be employed in the diagnostic allergy laboratory to ensure maximal overall assay performance with minimal variation in the test specimen, reagents, and assays, and minimum error associated with final analytical result.

Human Allergic Disease

Allergic rhinitis, extrinsic asthma, atopic dermatitis, and allergic gastroenteropathy are allergic diseases that share a common pathophysiology (1). Initial exposure of an immunologically naive, genetically predisposed individual to a foreign substance (allergen) may elicit the production of allergen-specific human immunoglobulin E (IgE) antibody. Once generated, IgE circulates in the blood and eventually binds onto epsilon-Fc receptors resident on the surface of effector cells, such as mast cells and basophils, that contain and produce vasoactive mediators. Once the individual is IgE antibody positive, he or she is classified as "sensitized" and subsequent reexposure to the same offending allergen may, but does not always, trigger the release of vasoactive mediators. The route of exposure (inhalation, ingestion, skin contact, or injection) and level of allergen exposure influences the type and severity of the allergic symptoms that are observed in a sensitized individual. **Table 30-1** lists some of the allergic disease classifications and symptoms that are commonly reported by allergic individuals. **Table 30-2** summarizes the analytes that are measured in the diagnostic allergy laboratory.

In the diagnosis of allergic disease, IgE antibodies of defined allergen specificities in the skin and serum are considered the primary diagnostic marker. Total serum IgE is a secondary diagnostic analyte that is frequently measured but does not possess the same inherent diagnostic value as allergen-specific IgE antibody. The reasons for this relate to the wide overlap in the total serum IgE levels between atopic and nonatopic populations (2) and the fact that the percentage of an individual's total IgE which is specific for any given allergen specificity may vary over time within the same individual and among individuals who are allergic to the same allergen.

Allergic diseases can be managed by avoidance, pharmacotherapy, immunotherapy, or a combination of these therapies. Of these, avoidance or the separation of the allergic individual from the allergen is considered by some investigators to be the most effective and possibly the least costly alternative. However, to avoid an allergen source, one must know its location and relative level in relation to risk targets for further sensitization and symptom induction. The diagnostic immunology laboratory participates in the avoidance therapy program by both

TABLE 30-1

Allergic Diseases and Symptoms Associated with Type 1 (IgE Antibody-Mediated) Hypersensitivity

Disease Classifications
- Allergic rhinitis (hay fever)
- Asthma (extrinsic)
- Atopic dermatitis
- Allergic gastroenteropathy
- Anaphylaxis
- Urticaria and angioedema
- Allergic vasculitis

Selected Allergic Symptoms*
- Skin: hives, rash, swelling, itching, redness, irritation
- Eyes: itching, tearing, watery, redness
- Upper airway (mouth, nose, throat): runny nose, itching and/or tight throat, swelling, sneezing
- Lungs: asthma, wheezing, cough, shortness of breath, chest discomfort
- Stomach (gastrointestinal): nausea, vomiting
- Heart (cardiovascular): chest pain, palpitations, low blood pressure, lightheadedness, fast pulse

*The symptoms noted in this table can be differentially expressed in a number of allergic diseases, depending on the particular individual.

TABLE 30-2

Diagnostic Allergy Laboratory Analytes

Analytes Used in Diagnosis
- Total serum IgE
- Allergen-specific IgE antibody
  - Individual allergen specificities
  - Multi-allergen screens

Analytes Used in Management
- Allergen-specific IgG antibody
- Aeroallergen levels in environmental specimens
  - Dust mite allergen (Der p 1, Der f 1)
  - Cat allergen (Fel d 1)
  - Dog allergen (Can f 1)
  - Cockroach allergen (Bla g 1, Bla g 2)
- Viable mold spores
- Cotenine (serum/urine metabolite of nicotine)

Research Analytes
- Eosinophil cationic protein
- Mast cell tryptase
- Vasoactive mediators (histamine, prostaglandins, leukotrienes)
- Cytokines (IL-4)

identifying sources (location and type) of allergen and quantifying their levels in an environment, such as a home or workplace or in household and medical products. Cotenine, a serum/urine marker for direct and passive exposure to smoke (nicotine), is an indirect environmental measurement that can be useful with asthmatics in developing their avoidance program.

Finally, specialized diagnostic allergy laboratories measure analytes that are useful to researchers. These include a marker of eosinophil activation (eosinophil cationic protein), mast cell degranulation (mast cell tryptase), vasoactive mediators (histamine, prostaglandins, leukotrienes), and cytokines. Due to space constraints, IgE antibodies and aeroallergens are the only analytes examined in this chapter.

Laboratory Tests Useful in the Diagnosis and Management of Allergic Disease

Historically, the skin test has been used by allergists as a primary diagnostic tool for identifying IgE antibodies in skin. A positive skin test supports a clinical history that is suggestive of an IgE-mediated allergy. However, in cases where antihistamines or other medications compromise the validity of the skin test results, dermatographism actually precludes skin testing, or the individual is simply apprehensive about potential adverse reactions from direct exposure to allergen, a serological immunoassay for IgE antibody is considered an efficacious alternative diagnostic test for the detection of IgE antibodies. There are also occasions when allergen extracts used for skin testing vary in their potency as a result of being infrequently used, suboptimally stored, or inherently unstable (e.g., food, mold extracts). In these situations, serological testing of individuals for allergen-specific IgE represents a useful alternative to the skin test in the diagnosis of human allergic disease in that it employs stable, highly quality controlled allergen-containing reagents.

Once an individual has been diagnosed as having an allergy, the laboratory can aid the patient in planning his or her avoidance program by measuring allergens in indoor environments, outdoor air, and consumer and medical products (3–5). Indoor "indicator" aeroallergens produced by dust mites, cats, dogs, and cockroaches are readily measured by monoclonal-antibody–based immunoassays to identify environments that place allergic individuals with these sensitivities at risk for either symptoms or increased sensitization.

Tree, grass, and weed pollen and mold spore levels provided by certified stations through the United States Aerobiology Network also give the allergic patient information about the type and quantity of clinically important allergens in the outdoor air. These daily measurements can identify periods when it may be unhealthy for severely allergic individuals to venture outdoors.

The relative quantity of allergen can also be measured in consumer and medical products using competitive inhibition assays that use human IgE antibody as a reagent. Two recent illustrations of this analysis include the detection of potent peanut allergen in a suspected unlabeled food that was eaten just before a severe allergic reaction in a peanut-allergic child, and the detection of natural rubber latex in unlabeled medical and consumer products (e.g., rubber catheter tips, latex condoms, latex examination gloves, toy balloons, or latex dental dams) to identify safe alternatives for use by the latex-allergic individual.

Specific IgG antibody has been used clinically as a marker for antigenic exposure to selected drugs such as penicillin, protamine, and insulin, and as a marker for reduced risk for reactions in Hymenoptera venom–allergic patients who are on venom immunotherapy (6). Otherwise, allergen-specific IgG antibody levels have not been shown to be generally clinically useful.

Finally, the allergy laboratory has served an important function in the monitoring of the serum levels of select therapeutic drugs such as the bronchodilator Theophylline in allergy patients because of their narrow safe therapeutic dosing regimen. However, presently, therapeutic drug monitoring is not a common activity for the diagnostic allergy laboratory because of the relative safety and wide therapeutic ranges of the available drugs used to treat patients with asthma and allergies.

Assay Methods

Total and Allergen-Specific IgE

In the mid-1960s, two groups identified IgE as the immunoglobulin that possesses reaginic activity and mediates the erythema reaction (7–8). In 1967, Wide et al. (9) reported the first immunoassay for the detection of allergen-specific IgE antibody in serum. Their radioallergosorbent test (RAST) employed a paper disk solid phase on which allergens were covalently coupled and used to bind specific antibodies from human serum. Following a buffer wash to remove unbound serum proteins, bound IgE antibody was detected with a radiolabeled anti-human IgE.

Over the years, many commercial versions of the RAST assay have been developed. Most of these are two-site immunoassays that employ an allergen-containing reagent and an anti-human IgE reagent to detect allergen-specific IgE. However, the emergence of highly diverse commercial IgE antibody assays has created a number of practical problems in terms of standardization and quality assurance. First, the quality of allergens that are used for manufacturing allergen-containing reagents have varied widely. Therefore, results from any two IgE antibody immunoassays are currently not directly comparable because each assay detects a different subset of the IgE antibody specificities within a given patient's serum. Second, commercial immunoassays have evolved using different relative calibration schemes to estimate antibody quantity. Therefore, direct comparison of IgE antibody results generated by commercially available clinical assays is not currently possible, except in limited qualitative terms (e.g., positive vs. negative, low vs. moderate vs. high). Finally, until recently, there has been no consensus on methods for defining the quality of assay reagents, the comparative performance of assay methods, or the accuracy and clinical utility of the generated IgE antibody results. Many of these issues have been examined by the National Committee on Clinical Laboratory Standards (NCCLS) guideline, which has developed a consensus on evaluation methods and desired analytical performance characteristics for immunologic assays that measure human IgE antibodies of defined allergen specificities (10).

Aeroallergen Levels in Environmental Specimens

Within the past few years, two-site immunoenzymetric assays have been developed that employ monoclonal antibodies specific for potent aeroallergens that are released into indoor environments by dust mites, cats, dogs, mice, rats, and cockroaches. These assays use buffer extracts of fine (sieved) dust as biological test specimens. Unknown aeroallergen levels are interpolated from a reference curve in nanograms or units of allergen per milliliter, depending on the degree of reference material calibration, and then converted to nanograms or units per gram of fine dust.

Because this is in fact considered an environmental analysis, rigorous expectations for assay performance and quality assurance are typically not placed on these measurements by licensing agencies. Moreover, despite of the rather recent emergence of these assays and the limited sources of specific monoclonal antibody reagents and standardized calibrators, wide interlaboratory variation has been observed with Der f 1 levels, the group 1 allergen produced by *Dermatophagoides farinae* (dust mite), in one international proficiency survey conducted by investigators from New Zealand.

Quality Assurance and Quality Control Issues

Specimen Considerations

Two general types of specimens are used in the assays discussed in this chapter: human serum and extracts of fine house dust. Once received in the laboratory, all serum or crude dust specimens are given a specimen number, cross-checked against the paperwork for inconsistencies and missing information, processed as discussed above, and frozen until the time of analysis. The laboratory quality assurance program has detailed procedures in place for each of these processes, including verification of the information to ensure minimal transcription errors. Moreover, a quality assurance program should take a number of specific issues into consideration with regard to test specimen quality.

Serum is the primary test specimen in the total IgE and allergen-specific IgE antibody assays. Anticoagulants added to collect plasma can interfere with the quantification of IgE in some assays when less than the required amount of blood is drawn into the collection device. Other fluids such as culture supernatants and research-derived secretions including tears, nasal, and lung lavages can be analyzed in the IgE assays, but this is uncommon. Any blood specimen that is grossly hemolyzed, icteric, or lipemic should in general not be used in any serological assay due to possible interference which can produce nonparallelism and high nonspecific binding levels. Sera or plasma should be routinely frozen ($-20°C$) if they are to be used more than 8 hours after collection; freezing at lower temperatures is not considered necessary, but is not detrimental to IgE antibody immunoreactivity unless repeatedly frozen and thawed. All human blood specimens should be considered infectious and be treated with universal precautions.

Dust collected from indoor home and work environments is a heterogeneous mixture of organic matter (human and animal dander, insect parts, food particles) and inorganic matter (dirt, sand). In most studies, dust is retrieved using a defined vacuuming protocol and one of several commercially available vacuum collectors designed to collect particles $\geq 1\,\mu m$ in diameter. Areas that are sampled for defined periods of time include sites such as the bedroom, living room, and kitchen, the rooms where the allergic individual spends the majority of his or her time.

Once it is submitted to the laboratory, the crude dust specimen is processed through a 50 mesh sieve (50 wires per inch; 0.009 inch in diameter), which allows particles smaller than $250\,\mu m$ through the 0.011-inch opening onto waxed laboratory weighing paper. This process produces a homogeneous fine dust, which can be sampled reproducibly for quantitative allergen measurement. With this procedure, virtually all of the allergenic material remains in the sieved dust specimen. Because dust is an environmental specimen, it may also contain residual cleaning solvents, freshener powders, and other potentially interfering substances that are applied to household carpets and upholstered furniture. Moreover, the type of outdoor environment surrounding the home or workplace (e.g., rocky vs. sandy, rural vs. urban) can cause highly variable dust specimen matrices. Fortunately, the microtiter plate-based immunoenzymetric assays appear to be very insensitive to interference from these highly variable sample matrices.

Finally, the dust is extracted in a physiological buffer by the addition of 100 mg of fine dust to 2 mL of filtered borate- or phosphate-buffered saline containing irrelevant protein (bovine serum albumin). Following end-over-end rotation overnight (16 to 18 hours), the specimen is centrifuged and the supernatant is filtered (0.22 μm) to remove any fine particles. Levels of dust mite, cat, dog, and cockroach allergen as detected by immunoassay do not appear to be measurably altered by up to 20 repeated freeze thaw cycles.

IgE Assay Reagents

The majority of total serum IgE assays used today employ solid phase anti-human IgE to capture IgE antibodies from serum. Allergen-specific IgE antibody immunoassays use a solid phase allergen-containing reagent (allergosorbent) to bind specific antibodies from serum. Following this first incubation, both assays share the remaining supplies, assay buffers and the anti-human IgE detection reagent in common. The anti-IgE and allergen-containing reagents have special considerations that need to be considered in a quality assurance program.

Anti-IgE Reagents Because IgE concentrations in serum are the lowest of all the human immunoglobulin isotypes (typically 0.004% of total immunoglobulins), the anti-human IgE reagent must possess no detectable cross-reactivity (<0.001%) with epitopes on human IgG1-4, IgA1-2, IgM, and IgD or other non-IgE human serum proteins (10). Polyclonal, monoclonal, and mixtures of both have been successfully used in commercial assays to detect capture and detect bound IgE. Documentation of the specificity of the anti-human IgE reagent requires the use of highly purified immunoglobulin proteins of all known human isotypes and allotypes in either a direct binding (dilutional analysis) study or competitive inhibition analysis (10).

In the direct binding studies, unlabeled anti-human IgE antiserum or finalized labeled anti-human IgE reagents are evaluated for their ability to bind to highly purified and potentially cross-reactive human immunoglobulins. In one proposed quality control scheme, 10 dilutions of anti-human IgE reagent bracketing the final proposed working strength are added to replicate tubes containing molar excess amounts of solid phase human IgE and solid phase non-IgE antigens. The reaction time, temperature, pH, diluent, and other assay conditions should closely mimic the reagent's use in the final assay. After a buffer wash to remove unbound material, bound anti-IgE is detected and a percentage cross-reactivity is computed as the relative concentration of anti-human IgE reagent that produces a 25% maximal response when binding to solid phase non-IgE versus IgE protein (see Appendix C of the NCCLS guideline 10).

In the competitive inhibition assay, one proposed approach has been to add defined quantities of up to 10 dilutions of each homologous (IgE) and heterologous (non-IgE) soluble inhibitor protein in a serum protein matrix to different tubes containing a fixed amount of human serum (IgE antibody source) and solid phase human IgE. The goal is to evaluate the ability of non-IgE proteins to competitively inhibit the binding of either unlabeled or labeled anti-human IgE to solid phase human IgE. The reagent addition can be either sequential or simultaneous. Following a final buffer wash and detection of bound anti-human IgE, the percentage of cross-reactivity is computed in an analogous manner to the direct binding assay approach.

Allergen-Containing Reagent The allergen is the single most important component reagent in IgE antibody assays. Several hundred clinically important allergen specificities have been identified from among the pollens (weed, grasses, trees), animal epidermis, mold, house dust mite, insects, drugs, occupational allergens, and foods. Most of these allergen specificities are highly complex, heterogeneous mixtures of proteins.

There are many reasons for allergen-containing reagent heterogeneity among the commercially available reagents. The same allergen source material collected during two time periods may be misidentified, contaminated, or its allergenic content may simply vary as a function of inherent biological variation. The extraction process may differ among or within manufacturers, causing intra-lot, inter-lot, or inter-manufacturer differences in allergen composition. There may be variable stability of the allergen during storage. Internal allergen reference standards used in quality control may not be available or they may vary in their composition. The quality control human serum pools are known to contain a heterogeneous mixture of IgE antibody specificities that will vary with each pool. Finally, the validation and acceptance criteria for the final allergen-containing reagents differ among manufacturers.

The quality assurance program for allergen-containing reagents begins with clear designation of the allergen source, based on identity testing performed by the supplier and a written description of its common and scientific names (genus and species). At present, only five of the hundreds of allergen extracts (timothy grass, common ragweed, birch tree, dog hair/dander, and house dust mite) have been given World Health Organization (WHO) standard status and three (Bermuda grass, rye grass, and *Alternaria* extract) are pending. For many more allergens, major allergenic molecules to which more than 50% of sensitized persons react have been purified and immunochemically characterized. Each crude allergen mixture and purified allergen component has its unique designation, as defined by the World Health Organization/International Union of Immunological Societies (WHO/IUIS) Allergen Nomenclature Subcommittee based on their genus and species (common ragweed, *Ambrosia artemisiifolia* group 1 allergen = Amb a 1). These have been assembled into the Allergen Nomenclature Addendum of the NCCLS Guideline (10), along with known cross-reactivities among the many allergen specificities and the molecular weight of the primary allergens that have been isolated and characterized.

Manufacturers of allergen-containing reagents conduct an extensive quality control testing program to validate the allergen source material and document the potency of the original allergen extract. A variety of testing methods are used in this process that vary among manufacturers. These include nonimmunologic tests (total protein, amino acid analyses, isoelectric focusing (IEF), SDS polyacrylamide gel electrophoresis), immunochemical assays (RAST inhibition, immunoelectrophoresis, Western blot analysis, IEF immunoblot analysis, radial immunodiffusion), and cellular and in vivo assays (basophil histamine release, skin test titration). Once the allergen-containing reagent has been manufactured, it is tested for its binding capacity, immunoreactivity, specificity, inter-lot reproducibility, and real-time stability. All these results are inserted into a product certification sheet which should be available to the end-user of the allergen-containing reagent upon request.

Quality Control Serum Pools

Pools of IgE antibody-containing sera are prepared by diagnostic allergy laboratory personnel as quality control reagents to evaluate intra- and inter-assay variation and occasionally inter-method or laboratory variation. The theoretical goal in the preparation of a serum pool is to maximize IgE antibody heterogeneity so that the pool mimics, as closely as achievable, the distribution and relative levels of the various IgE antibody specificities present in the general population of subjects allergic to that allergen specificity.

Ideally, potential allergic candidates would be identified for inclusion based on their clinical history and a positive skin test. However, because in practice it is very difficult to obtain volumes of serum containing IgE antibody specific for most of the hundreds of clinically important allergen specificities, inclusion often occurs randomly on the basis of the presence of detectable levels of IgE antibody in the test immunoassay. Other practical difficulties include:

- The collection of multi-liter quantities of serum so that the serum pool can be used over an extended period of time.
- The dilution of minor IgE antibody specificities.
- Overrepresentation of major allergen specificities by mixing equivalent volumes of multiple sera.

Ideally, the final serum pool should contain IgE antibody specific for all preselected allergen specificities of clinical interest.

Standards and Reference Preparations

Several types of reference materials are used in the diagnostic allergy laboratory. For all clinically used total serum IgE assays, test specimen results are interpolated from a calibration curve constructed with a standard that has been cross-standardized to international human IgE standard (WHO 75/502). Most assays are also cross-verified with a secondary IgE reference preparation (US Standard for human serum IgE, NIAID-NIH/BOB-FDA Cat A-699-001-500). Results of currently available total serum IgE assays are reported in IU/mL (international units per milliliter) where 1 IU/mL is equivalent to approximately 2.44 ng/mL. This rigorous international standardization has allowed excellent concordance among the available total serum IgE assays, as evidenced by the low variance reported in the College of American Pathologists SE (Diagnostic Allergy) Proficiency Survey (11).

In comparison to total serum IgE assays, the current state of IgE antibody assays standardization is relatively poor. Consensus has not been reached among the manufacturers as to the best method for standardizing the units of IgE antibody results generated by commercially available assays. Ideally, a reference serum would be available that has a defined mass/volume concentration of IgE antibody specific for each of the several hundred allergen specificities. In rare cases, reference sera that have been calibrated in mass per volume units for antibody content to a specific allergen (e.g., ragweed) have been produced in research laboratories (12). However, due to the almost impossible task of preparing comparable serum pools containing known amounts of IgE antibody specific for each of the clinically important allergen specificities, alternative strategies for calibration of the IgE antibody assay have been adopted.

Unfortunately, the heterogeneity of calibration schemes and their associated reference sera have created problems for the allergist and patient who must interpret the finalized IgE antibody results. At the present time, levels of IgE antibody specific for a particular allergen and generated from any 2 of the 19 different assays are not directly comparable. Of greatest concern, they have different arbitrary units that have no relationship to each other. This difficult state of affairs was the primary motivation for convening of a group of scientists from academia, industry, and government under the auspices of the NCCLS to establish recommendations for future consensus on calibration and IgE antibody assay standardization. It is hoped that the 1998 guideline (10) will lead to a single consensus calibration method for IgE antibody assays.

Calibration Methods

As indicated above, the presence of IgE antibody in the skin or serum is diagnostic for sensitization to allergen. To this end, a variety of qualitative response or dose units have evolved in IgE antibody assays that employ a positive/negative threshold above which the specimen is considered IgE positive and the patient can be classified as sensitized to the allergen. The most common method of reporting IgE results is in relative "classes," typically ranging from 0 to 5, or 0 to 6. A class result is generated based on the relative magnitude of the response or dose level in relationship to the positive threshold, with class 0 as negative, and higher levels of IgE antibody assigned higher class designations. This system should be intuitively understandable to allergists who use a similar semiquantitative system to grade their skin tests based on the size of the observed wheal and erythema.

More recently, investigators have begun to study if the actual quantity of IgE antibody in the serum rather than just its presence provides a better marker of the degree of sensitivity and the magnitude of the symptoms that might be experienced by the allergic individual as a result of allergen exposure. Because absolute quantitation of the level of IgE antibody in serum is not presently routine, the answer to the question about the relationship between serum IgE antibody levels and the magnitude of symptoms experienced by the patient has remained unclear. At present, there appears to be no clearly definable correlation between the level of measured IgE antibody and the clinical response. This relationship is, however, complicated by many confounding variables, such as the route and magnitude of the allergen exposure and the genetic predisposition of the individual for serious allergic reactions. In any case, the future trend in laboratory measurement of IgE antibody is toward more quantitative measurements. Two quantitative calibration approaches have been considered for IgE antibody assays: homologous and heterologous interpolation.

Homologous interpolation involves the preparation of individual serum pools containing IgE antibody of known mass per volume quantities for each of the clinically relevant allergen specificities. By constructing a dose-response calibration or reference curve with the reference serum, test specimen results can be interpolated in ng/mL of IgE antibody for that particular allergen specificity. Unfortunately, over the years many well-intentioned investigators have shown this approach to be quantitatively elegant, but entirely impractical. It has simply not been possible to find enough patients with allergies to the less common allergen specificities to prepare large serum pools. The size of the serum pool is important, because IgE antibodies are present in such low ng/mL concentrations and the serum must often be used undiluted. Hundreds of allergy laboratories perform assays every day, resulting in rapid consumption of precious serum pools. Therefore, calibrated serum pools have remained restricted to the research laboratory, where they are used to define the "absolute" quantity of antibody in patient's sera for special research studies. Calibration of the content of specific antibody in these pools by depletion methods, elution techniques, or saturation analysis has also remained technically challenging (12–13).

The *heterologous calibration* scheme involves the construction of a single common reference curve with a calibrated IgE antibody-containing serum in each assay and interpolation of all antibody specificities from that single reference curve. Thus, an IgE anti-ragweed standard curve constructed in ng/mL or IU/mL of antibody may be used to interpolate results from a single assay where IgE anti-dust mite, anti-cat, anti-insulin, anti-cockroach, anti-peanut, and so on are also analyzed by simply using different allergosorbents in a separate part of the assay. Results for all the IgE antibody measurements are interpolated in IgE anti-ragweed nanogram per milliliter equivalents. The one requirement for this system is that the dilution curves for the various IgE antibody specificities are all parallel to the chosen reference curve. This ensures that the same interpolated result will be computed after correction for dilution, no matter if a serum is analyzed undiluted or at a high dilution. Engineered chimeric (human-mouse) IgE anti-nitrophenyl (NP) antibodies have also been proposed for use as a generic reference reagent for constructing heterologous IgE antibody standard curves using an NP-solid phase in the calibration portion of the assay (14).

One useful heterologous interpolation scheme for clinical IgE antibody assays was first introduced in the Pharmacia-Upjohn CAP System. In this assay, a total serum IgE calibration curve is generated using a serum with known amounts of total serum IgE in kIUa/L and a solid phase anti-human IgE capture antibody. In the body of the assay, individual allergosorbents with different allergen specificities are used at the same time to bind IgE antibodies of the desired specificities from test patients' sera. Following the first serum incubation, the whole assay is washed, and bound IgE in the calibration and test sera portions of the assay are detected with the same conjugated anti-human IgE reagent. In this manner, IgE anti-cat dander can be interpolated from the total serum IgE calibration curve in kIUa/L of IgE based on the WHO IgE reference serum in the same manner as IgE anti-ragweed and any other IgE antibody specificity. From a practical point of view, this approach appears to have merit because it can be employed by manufacturers of other commercially available assays and it is traceable to the WHO IgE reference preparation. Although good parallelism has been shown between the total IgE reference curve and the specific IgE portion of the CAP System assay, it still remains to be shown whether other assay methods can achieve the same degree of parallelism with this heterologous interpolation system.

Once the individual component reagents are assembled, performance of the intact assay needs to be evaluated in terms of intra- and inter-assay variation (precision), detection limit (lowest level distinguishable from a "zero concentration" specimen), and dilution recovery or parallelism. Detailed procedures for evaluating each of these parameters are provided in the appendices of the NCCLS guideline (10). Other variables that may be considered include the linear or working range of the assay, stability of the calibration curve, potential interferences, and cross-reactivity issues.

Intra-Laboratory Quality Control

Internal laboratory quality control practices are required for laboratory licensure. The strategies employed in diagnostic allergy laboratories can vary; however, several principles may be generalized. For highly standardized assays such as those that measure total serum IgE, commonly three control sera are analyzed which cover the low (1–10 IU/mL), medium (50–100 IU/mL), and high (1000–2000 IU/mL) regions of the assays' working range. If one of the control serum values is out of the mean ±2 SD range, as defined by results from 10 to 15 previous assays, a problem with the reagents or technical performance needs to be investigated. In addition, Levey Jennings plots and the use of defined rules for assay acceptance can be employed to maximize assay quality (15).

For less well-standardized quantitative assays such as those used to measure allergen-specific IgE antibody, other issues need to be considered. In one strategy, each allergosorbent (of a different specificity) may be considered a separate reagent that needs its own quality control testing by the laboratory using its own human serum pool containing relevant specific IgE antibody. This approach would require laboratories to keep an extensive serum bank of IgE-positive sera for every allergen specificity, which is costly and impractical.

The other extreme would be to accept the concept that the allergen-specific IgE assay uses several hundred different allergen-containing reagent components, each of which is purchased by the user in a pre-quality-controlled state. By accepting the manufacturer's quality control data and using the reagent before it expires, further quality control testing of each allergosorbent becomes unnecessary. In this case, only the calibration portion of the assays needs to be quality controlled in each assay. This is readily accomplished in a manner similar to the total serum IgE assay by analyzing low, medium, and high level quality control sera. In addition to evaluating the calibration curve, some laboratories have elected to prepare serum pools for 5 to 10 allergen specificities where large amounts of IgE-containing serum are available. By rotating among these specificities and analyzing one in each assay, an abbreviated quality control of the allergosorbent component of the assay can be accomplished.

External Inter-Laboratory Proficiency Testing

All federally licensed clinical laboratories that perform diagnostic allergy testing are required to participate in at least one external proficiency testing program. One such well-subscribed program is conducted by the College of American Pathologists (CAP). In this program, five sera are sent to each participating laboratory 3 times a year at 17-week intervals. The laboratory is requested to measure total serum IgE and IgE antibody to five predefined allergen specificities. The sera sent to the participants typically contain total serum IgE levels that vary from low nonatopic range (10 IU/mL) to high atopic range (15,000 IU/mL). During a year period, the 15 total serum IgE measurements are graded based on per group (same assay) performance. Laboratories exceeding the 3 SD range are notified that they have failed the challenge and need to review their procedures and assays for problems. These laboratories also can lose their federal clinical laboratory license (under CLIA, the Clinical Laboratory Improvement Act) due to poor technical performance.

The total serum IgE is a graded analyte, but the allergen-specific IgE measurement is presently not graded for purposes of evaluating laboratory performance for licensure. As discussed above, the IgE antibody results cannot be directly compared between assays because of large differences in the allergen-containing reagent that cause each assay to detect a different subpopulation of IgE antibody. Moreover, units of the final results generated by different assays are not comparable. Also, there are often only a small number of laboratories that perform some of the assays, which makes it impossible to compare laboratories even within an assay peer group. Therefore, the qualitative class results are the primary form of results provided back to the participant in a summary.

Laboratories can only judge their performance in terms of detecting IgE antibody in sera from subjects with a positive clinical history and skin test for the appropriate allergen-specificity. The class 1 result is a problem because it is considered negative by some laboratories and allergists and a borderline positive by others. Thus, interpretation of weakly positive results is difficult. Moreover, the relative value of a class 2, 3, 4, or 5 result varies among the methods, and thus only negative and positive results can clearly be critiqued among different assays.

In the United States, 19 different versions of allergen-specific IgE assays are used, which makes the proficiency data very heterogeneous. In contrast, the laboratories that participate in the European Diagnostic Allergy Scheme essentially use a single quantitative assay method. The European coordinating center computes proficiency data in a manner analogous to that used for total serum IgE in the CAP survey, and laboratories that exceed the 3 SD range are considered outliers. With the NCCLS committee evaluation and performance guideline, it is hoped that eventually all assays will converge on a similar calibration method and unitage for IgE antibody. This would make the evaluation of the diagnostic allergy proficiency survey results more meaningful for participants.

As a result of the undisputed clinical utility of IgE antibody measurements in the diagnosis of allergic disease (16), IgE antibodies are poised to be among the first group of antibodies that will be rigorously scrutinized when human antibodies eventually reach a federally regulated analyte status.

Summary

Analytical methods used in the diagnostic allergy laboratory remain in a constant state of evolution that mirrors improvements in reagents and technology. Although the state of standardization is good for the total serum IgE assay, it has remained limited for present day allergen-specific IgE antibody assays. Consensus guidelines for performance evaluation and standardization as proposed by an NCCLS committee will serve to promote uniformity of calibration schemes, reported units, and the quantitative nature of future IgE antibody assays.

During the past decade, we have also seen a new group of monoclonal antibody-based immunoenzymetric assays emerge into the diagnostic allergy laboratory for the measurement of primary "indicator" allergens in dust specimens from indoor environments. These new assays have created a new mission for the allergy laboratory that involves evaluation of homes and work places for promotion of avoidance therapy and more effective monitoring of remediation.

REFERENCES

1. Saxon A, Diaz-Sanchez D, Zhang K. The allergic response in host defense. In: Rich RR, ed. Clinical immunology: principle and practices. St Louis: Mosby, 1995;1:847–876.
2. Hamilton RG, Adkinson NF Jr. Measurement of total serum IgE and allergen-specific IgE antibody. In: Manual of clinical laboratory immunology. In: Rose HR, Macario EC de, Fahey JL, et al., eds. Washington, DC: American Society for Microbiology, 1992:689–701.
3. Hamilton RG, Chapman MD, Platts-Mills TAE, Adkinson NF Jr. House dust aeroallergen measurements in clinical practice: a guide to allergen-free home and work environments. Immunol Allergy Pract 1992;14:96–112.
4. American Academy of Allergy, Asthma and Immunology. Aeroallergen monitoring network: pollen and spore report 1995, 1996:1.
5. Yunginger JW, Jones RTG, Fransway AF, et al. Extractable latex allergens and proteins in disposable medical gloves and other rubber products. J Allergy Clin Immunol 1994;93:836–842.
6. Golden DBK, Lawrence ID, Hamilton RG, et al. Clinical correlation of the venom specific IgG antibody level during maintenance venom immunotherapy. J Allergy Clin Immunol 1992;90: 386–393.
7. Ishizaka K, Ishizaka T, Hornbrook MM. Physicochemical properties of human reaginic antibody. IV. Presence of a unique immunoglubiln as a carrier of reaginic activity. J Immunol 1966;97: 75–85.
8. Johansson SGO, Bennich H. Immunological studies of an atypical (myeloma) immunoglobulin. Immunology 1967;13:381–394.
9. Wide L, Bennich H, Johansson SGO. Diagnosis of allergy by an in vitro test for allergen antibodies. Lancet 1967;2:1105.
10. Matsson P, Hamilton RG, Adkinson NF Jr, et al. Evaluation methods and analytical performance characteristics of immunological assays for human IgE antibody of defined allergen specificities. NCCLS Guideline Vol. 16. Wayne, PA: National Committee on Clinical Laboratory Standards, 1998:1/LA20-A.
11. Participant Summary, Diagnostic Allergy Survey 1996, Set SE-C. Northfield, IL: College of American Pathologists, 1996.
12. Gleich GJ, Jacob GL, Yunginger JW, Henderson LL. Measurement of the absolute levels of IgE antibodies in patients with ragweed hay fever. Effect of immunotherapy on seasonal changes and relationship to IgG antibody. J Allergy Clin Immunol 1977;60:188–198.
13. Butler JE, Hamilton RG. Quantitation of specific antibodies: methods of expression, standards, solid phase considerations and specific applications. In: Butler JE, ed. Immunochemistry of solid phase immunoassays. Boca Raton, FL: CRC Press, 1991:chap 9.
14. Hamilton RG. Application of engineered chimeric antibodies to the calibration of human antibody standards. Ann Biol Clin 1991;49:242–248.
15. Westgard JO, Klee GE. Quality assurance. In: Tietz NW, ed. Textbook of clinical chemistry. Philadelphia: WB Saunders, 1986:424–458.
16. Bernstein IL. Proceedings of the task force on guidelines for standardizing old and new technologies used for the diagnosis and treatment of allergic diseases. J Allergy Clin Immunol 1988;82:487–492.

CHAPTER 31

Histocompatibility Assays in Transplantation

NORA C. NUGENT
MILDRED K. FLEETWOOD

The field of histocompatibility is fortunate to have well-defined laboratory standards provided by American Society for Histocompatibility and Immunogenetics (ASHI) (1). ASHI accredits histocompatibility laboratories in specific categories or fields of transplantation such as renal, solid organ other than renal, and bone marrow. The quality assurance standards appear within the ASHI standards (1). ASHI has deemed status from CLIA and is currently applying to JCAHO and the States of New York, Oregon, and Florida for deemed status.

Details of histocompatibility methods are superbly supplied by the ASHI manual (2) and the manual of the Southeastern Organ Procurement Foundation (SEOPF) (3). Other accrediting agencies such as the College of American Pathologists and American Association of Blood Banks (AABB) also have checklists that are helpful in this field. Wang-Rodriguez and Rearden provide a succinct review of the field of histocompatibility and the pertinent immunology (4).

Laboratory Tests

The initial laboratory testing for potential transplant patients involves blood grouping, HLA typing, identifying alloantibody to HLA antigens, and determining of the presence of autoantibody. Once these tests are completed, the patient may be placed on the recipient waiting list for solid organs by blood group, on the local organ procurement organization (OPO) list, and on the national list, the United Network for Organ Sharing (UNOS).

The determination of a suitable recipient for a donor organ is based on the point system devised by UNOS and is specific for each type of organ. The potential renal recipient is allotted points on the basis of HLA match with the donor, level of sensitization to HLA antigens of the recipient, and duration of waiting on the list. When a donor HLA type is entered into the UNOS computer, the computer searches for the recipient with the most points for this donor and for six antigen or phenotypic (no mismatched antigens) matches. Six antigen and phenotypic matches are a mandatory share throughout the United States. If there are no six antigen or phenotypic matches for the donor, the donor organ is first offered to the local OPO list patients with the highest points as determined by the UNOS point system. At this time, HLA matching is not done for other solid organs. However, HLA typing is recommended to provide future information on patient outcome.

One of the problems in finding a suitable donor for a patient is the presence of circulating antibody to HLA antigens. Patients may become sensitized to HLA antigens as a result of pregnancy, blood transfusions, and previous transplants with mismatched antigens. Because the HLA antigens share many epitopes, they can be grouped into cross-reacting epitope groups (CREGS). An example of a CREG is the A1 CREG consisting of A1, 36, 9, 10, and 11. A patient receiving a mismatched A1 CREG transplant could reject that organ and develop broadly reacting antibodies to all the antigens of that group, making it very difficult to find a future compatible donor for that patient. In addition, there are the broad specificities of BW4 and BW6 into one or the other of which all B locus antigens can be defined. If a recipient is homozygous for one of these and is mismatched with the other broad specificity, he or she may make antibody to the broad specificity and thereby be unsuitable for at least 50% of future potential donors.

Matching for CREGS has been suggested as an alternative to the UNOS matching algorithm. This approach may provide greater access to a larger donor pool for recipients and could overcome the difficulty of having to match for less common antigens found predominantly in minority group patients. Should the patient lose the kidney, the development of antibody may be limited; CREG matching makes it easier to find a future compatible donor.

Requirements

Testing for each type of transplant will vary and each center has specific protocols. Bone marrow transplant will require high resolution DNA typing of HLA antigens rather than standard serologic definition.

Test Selection for Evaluation of a New Patient/Recipient

1. Blood group: Matching for blood group is preferred for all solid organ transplants. Blood group compatibility is not required for bone marrow transplant.
2. HLA class I typing: Identifies HLA A, B, C unique antigens of recipient.
3. HLA class II typing: Identifies HLA DR, DQ unique antigens of recipient.
4. Autocrossmatch: Identifies if the recipient has autoantibody.
5. Panel reactive antibody (PRA): Identifies if the recipient has preformed alloantibody. This determination is made by calculating the percentage of cells killed on a cell panel. The panel should consist of enough cells (50 or more) to represent each of the major HLA antigens at least once. The panel could be from selected donors and stored frozen in aliquots or from fresh random sources. Also frozen cell panel trays are available from commercial sources.
6. Crossmatching: Identifies the presence of preformed antibody specific to the potential donor. For living related or living nonrelated transplants a T-cell crossmatch and a B-cell crossmatch are performed for those who are considering donation. A flow cytometry crossmatch is also recommended for living related and living nonrelated donors and for patients receiving second and third organs. A crossmatch with the spouse of female patients is often performed to identify antibody produced as a result of pregnancy.
7. A mixed lymphocyte culture assay: In the case of living related donor transplantation, it gives information about the degree of matching in the D region. Some centers perform this routinely to enhance donor selection and others do not.

Specimen Requirements and Collection

Whole blood is collected with anticoagulant, either sodium heparin (preservative free and not lithium heparin) or acid citrate dextrose. A complete typing and autocrossmatch requires 40 mL of blood. An additional 10 mL of blood collected in plain red top tubes (no additives, no serum separator) is needed for blood grouping, crossmatching, and PRA testing.

Labeling Requirements

Each tube must have:

Full name

Identifying number (medical record or social security number)

Date of collection

Relationship to the recipient for family members

The presence of this information allows one to use the same tube for blood group and type.

Specimen Handling and Storage

Blood collected with anticoagulant is maintained at room temperature and should be processed within 24 hours of collection. Blood should be processed as soon after collection as possible as it becomes increasingly more difficult with time to isolate B lymphocytes needed for class II typing and crossmatching.

Panel Reactive Antibody (PRA)

Blood collected in plain red top tubes for monthly PRA testing is maintained at room temperature and should be received in the lab within 3 days. Beyond that length of time, specimens become more and more hemolyzed and should not be used. Aliquots of patient serum for future crossmatching should be made and stored at −70°C. An inventory system for easy retrieval of these specimens is re-quired. We suggest graphing the results so that it is easy to select peak sera from the inventory of all sera at the time of final crossmatch (**Fig. 31-1**).

Donor Testing

Tests

1. Blood group and subtype for blood group A (BGA) (A1, A2) if blood group is A.
2. Infectious diseases testing:

   RPR

   HIV-1/HIV-2 combo

   HIV antigen

   Hepatitis B surface antigen

   HCV

   HTLV-1/HTLVII

   Hepatitis B core antibody (total and Igm)

   CMV

3. HLA class I typing for A, B, C antigens
4. HLA class II typing for DR, DQ antigen.

For cadaver renal donors, the complete HLA typing (class I and II) is needed to match renal donors with recipients through the UNOS system, and to identify six antigen and phenotypic matches.

Assay Methods

Method standards are defined by the American Society for Histocompatibility and Immunogenetics (ASHI) and by the College of American Pathologists (CAP). Complement-dependent microcytotoxicity assays are used for HLA typing and crossmatching. There are two basic methods and both are used for typing.

1. NIH: No wash step prior to adding complement (2,3).
2. Amos modified: One or more washes performed prior to adding complement (2,3).

Currently, ASHI requires the use of complement-dependent cytotoxicity assays for antibody screening and crossmatching recipients (ASHI Standards H1.100) (1). For crossmatching donor T lymphocytes with recipient sera, an additional method using antiglobulin (anti-human κ light chain, anti-human globulin) is often used (2,3). Crossmatching donor B lymphocytes with recipient sera is highly recommended for patients with high levels of antibody and/or patients with previous transplants. Flow cytometer crossmatching is a non-complement-dependent assay with added sensitivity. Crossmatching techniques must have greater sensitivity than the basic NIH microlymphocytotoxicity assay (ASHI Standard I3.130) (1). The sensitivity of these crossmatch methods varies, and they are ranked accordingly in **Table 31-1**.

Controls for HLA Testing and Cytotoxic Crossmatching

HLA Class I and Class II Typing

Positive Controls

Antilymphocyte serum and anti-B cell serum are used for positive control. Positive control may also be a human serum made from a pooled multispecific anti-HLA serum. The positive control must give an "8" reaction (81–100% cell death).

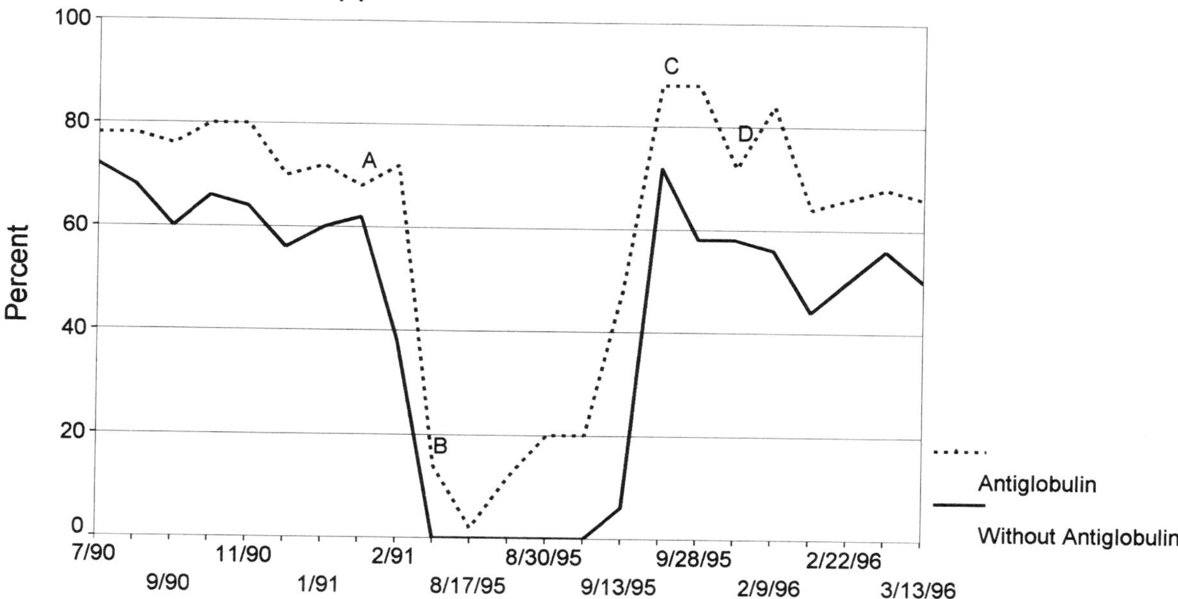

FIGURE **31-1**

Postimmunosuppressant PRA: the changes of % PRA in one patient over time. (A) Date of transplant. (B) Withdrawal of immunosuppressant. (C) Peak PRA after removing immunosuppressant. (D) Nephrectomy. It is customary to obtain sera 2 weeks after nephrectomy to look for rising antibody titers, but it is not common to obtain sera after stopping immunosuppressants. Note that the peak titer (C) occurred 6 months prior to nephrectomy (D). Obtaining weekly samples after stopping immunosuppressants is extremely important, otherwise peak sera may be missed.

TABLE **31-1**

Sensitivity of Crossmatch Methods

Most Sensitive	**Antibody Detected**
1. Flow cytometer crossmatch	Very low level non-complement-fixing and complement-fixing antibody. Ig class specific.
2. Antiglobulin	Low-level non-complement-fixing and complement-fixing antibody. Detects CYNAP* antibody.
3. Amos modified-wash method	Complement-fixing antibody. Detects IgG antibody.
4. NIH with extended incubation times	Complement-fixing antibody. Detects IgG and IgM antibody.
5. NIH no-wash method	Complement-fixing antibody. Detects IgG and IgM antibody.
Least Sensitive	

*CYNAP: Cytotoxicity negative absorption positive.

Negative Controls

Fetal bovine serum or pooled human serum from nontransfused male donors is used for negative control. The negative control must show zero to ten cell death or a "1" reaction.

Typing Controls

Antisera of known specificity are required to reproduce the known specificity with the appropriate cells (4).

Mixed Lymphocyte Controls

Mixed lymphocyte controls require three or more unrelated stimulator cells or two unrelated cells and a pool of at least three other unrelated cells for each responder cell tested.

Unrelated cell controls: usually two

Autologous controls

Radiation controls

Media controls

Cell controls

Cytotoxic Crossmatching Controls

Cytotoxic crossmatching controls include the following:

Positive and negative controls as for class I and class II typing

Complement controls

AHG control: an antiserum specific for one of the donor antigens previously tested and shown to exhibit CYNAP phenomenon

Cell controls

Quality Control

Complement

Quality control for complement is covered in the ASHI standards (E5.310, F5.300) (1). Rabbit complement must be shown to be effective at the working dilution and higher and to retain its effectiveness during storage at −70°C. Often it is necessary to screen several lots of complement to find one that works well under a lab's conditions. Different complements are usually needed for A, B, C typing and for DR, DQ typing. This becomes a major project for histocompatibility labs requiring a great deal of time. Complement should be titered in a checkerboard manner with one strong and one weak antiserum (**Table 31-2**).

It must be tested for toxicity to avoid misleading background cell death. The negative control tested with each dilution of complement can be used to assess toxicity. In addition, frozen cell panel trays can be used for this purpose after a working dilution of complement has been determined by testing the panel with pooled human serum.

Antiglobulin

An effective AHG reagent will detect low titer antibody and non-complement-fixing antibody that will be missed in the standard complement-dependent cytotoxicity assay. However, these reagents often exhibit strong prozone effects and must be titered correctly. The reagent should be tested in parallel without AHG using a known antibody and positive reactions compared by dilution.

Once an effective working dilution has been determined, stock concentrations can be made and stored at −70°C. The reagent is stable for years under these conditions. In our laboratory, AHG is titered quarterly and an AHG control is added to every T-cell crossmatch tray to ensure that the working dilution remains effective.

TABLE **31-2**

Complement: Example of Checkerboard Titration

Complement dilutions	**Positive control**	**Negative control**	**Antiserum**	**Dilutions**		
			1/1	**1/2**	**1/4**	**1/8**
None	8	1	1	2	1	1
1/2	8	1	8	8	1	1
1/3	8	1	8	8	1	1
1/4	8	1	8	8	2	1
1/5	8	1	8	2	1	1
1/6	8	1	8	1	1	1
1/8	8	1	8	1	1	1
Cell control	1	1	1	1	1	1

NOTE: This complement is effective at a 1/4 dilution. The working dilution should be 1/2.

Typing Trays and Sera

The specificity of typing sera and the effectiveness of typing trays must be demonstrated. All typing reagents and trays should be tested in parallel with known reagents. There are several computer programs available to calculate correlation coefficients of typing sera, perform tail analysis, and analyze the overall effectiveness of typing trays.

Reagents

All reagents used in the histocompatibility laboratory must be prescreened for effectiveness and lack of toxicity to live cells. This can be accomplished by testing new reagents on the cell panel along with the regular monthly PRA patient samples. These reagents include but are not limited to tissue culture media, buffers, vital stains, and mineral oil.

Flow Crossmatch Reagents

Positive and negative controls must be screened for effectiveness and lack of background cell death in the case of the negative control. The positive control should be titered in a checkerboard manner with the fluorescent stain tagged anti-human IgG for the working dilutions of each (**Table 31-3**).

The selection of working dilutions for anti-human IgG and positive control is based on channel values and the channel shift from negative to positive control. Choose the lowest background (lowest channel value) for the negative control and the dilution of positive control and antihuman IgG that produces the best separation (channel displacement) from positive to negative. In the example given in Table 31-3, the dilutions to choose are 1/4 for anti-human IgG and 1/16 for the positive control as indicated by the highest channel displacement from negative control.

Mixed Lymphocyte Cultures

Mixed lymphocyte cultures are covered in the ASHI standards (G2.200–G2.500) (1). Serum used in culture medium must be sterile, must support cell growth, and must be tested for absence of cytotoxic antibodies. Each assay must include:

1. An autologous control.
2. Three or more unrelated stimulator cells or two unrelated cells and a pool of at least three other unrelated cells for each responder cell tested.

Practicability

Time Involved in Cell Isolation

Cell isolation from blood: 1 hour

T-cell isolation from blood: 2 hours

B-cell isolation from blood: 2 hours plus 2 hours preincubation to allow antigens to regenerate on the cell surface if nylon wool columns are used. Isolation of B lymphocytes using a nylon wool column strips cells of their surface antigens. Preincubation of approximately 2 hours is required to allow the cells to regenerate their surface antigens. The regeneration of the antigens should be confirmed by running a class II typing tray along with B cell crossmatches.

TABLE **31-3**

Flow Crossmatch Reagents: Example of Checkerboard Titration

	Antihuman	**IgG**	**Dilutions**			
Positive control						
	1/4	1/8	1/16	1/32	1/64	Channel*
1/16	132.47	127.82	125.54	120.87	117.82	Displacement
1/32	124.06	116.14	114.36	116.44	110.96	
1/64	112.11	105.15	103.36	103.23	94.53	Values
Negative control	56.84	59.52	57.52	58.59	59.44	Channel values

*Channel displacement from negative control.

T-cell isolation from node: 1 hour

B-cell isolation from node: 1 hour plus 2 hours preincubation (nylon wool)

T-cell isolation from spleen: 2 hours

B-cell isolation from spleen: 2 hours plus 2 hours preincubation (nylon wool). More rapid isolations of B cells can be done using immunomagnetic beads. This method does not require nylon wool separation or a 2-hour preincubation step.

Assay Times (after Cell Preparation)

Class I typing: 3 hours

Class II typing: 4 hours

T-cell crossmatch: After cell preparation a simple preliminary crossmatch using one serum and no dilution can be completed in 3 hours. The HLA typing can be done simultaneously.

The final crossmatch should test all the recipient's relevant sera in duplicate with titration using two methods, one more sensitive than the other. The time for a final crossmatch ranges from 3 to 5 hours depending on the number of relevant sera.

If the preliminary typing and crossmatching is centralized through the use of shared crossmatch trays, the transplanting laboratory need only do the final crossmatch. A B-cell crossmatch using the recipient's relevant sera with titration takes 4 to 6 hours and a flow crossmatch takes 4 hours. This usually requires an additional technologist, thus limiting the prospective use of the flow crossmatch for cadaver donors to those laboratories that have adequate numbers of technologists to provide 24-hour coverage for both methods.

The times given for these assays are approximate. The need to make fresh cell preparations, particularly from spleen tissue, and a patient history requiring more sera to be tested in both T cell and B cell crossmatches can add up to 4 hours to the assays.

Level of Skill Required to Perform Assays

Performance of these assays requires a great deal of skill and experience. Prolonged training periods (6 months or more) are necessary to prepare a technologist to perform unsupervised in the on-call situation. Competency needs to be documented and reexamined at periodic intervals. The appendix to this chapter provides our training program guide and checklist.

Pitfalls and Troubleshooting

Cost

The cost of these assays is high. The reagents and typing trays are expensive, ranging from \$25 to \$45 per typing tray. Also, the work is labor intensive. A typical typing may require three trays for ABC and three trays for DR.

Typing Trays and Antisera

Typing trays and sera are available from many commercial sources. These reagents are tested for specificity on cell donors of the commercial companies in their laboratories, using their complement and typing methods. However, there is no guarantee that these reagents will perform with exactly the same effectiveness in an individual clinical laboratory. In our laboratory, we find we usually need no less than two basic trays and one extended tray to identify less frequent antigens for class I typing. We like to use a combination of trays from several commercial sources. These technical difficulties are also the case for class II typing as well and are further compounded by the need either for purified B lymphocytes or for different incubation periods for immunomagnetic bead isolation.

Complement

No two complements are alike. When complement is diluted for use in wash step methods, its titer can be observed to deteriorate over time with storage at −70°C. We do not store frozen liquid complement for more than 1 year. This necessitates screening for new lots of complement from several different sources once a year for both class I and class II. One year we screened 11 lots from four companies for class I typing alone before identifying an appropriate lot. All of these lots were tested with fresh and frozen cells from three donors with two different antisera for use in typing and crossmatching or antibody screening.

B lymphocytes are more sensitive to nonspecific toxicity from complement, so the complement used for class I typing and crossmatching is usually not suitable for class II typing and crossmatching. We use a frozen liquid complement screened specifically for class II typing, but we have found that lyophilized, absorbed complement specific for B lymphocytes works best for class II crossmatching.

When crossmatching B lymphocytes at 4°C spurious reactions can sometimes occur if cold-reacting xenoantibodies have not been completely absorbed from the complement used.

Vital Stains

The size of the dye molecule can alter the sensitivity of typing and crossmatching. Eosin is the most common vital stain used, but trypan blue and fluorescent stains such as ethidium bromide are also used.

Antiglobulin Reagents

The major pitfall encountered with antiglobulin reagents (AHG, anti-ϰ light chain) is the determination of the proper working dilution. The titration must be carried out far enough to avoid prozone effects. Several sera and cells should be tested and careful timing is essential.

Cell Isolations

All cytotoxic assays require viable cells for testing. Each step of a cell isolation can damage the membranes of cells making them more susceptible to toxic effects of reagents used and will allow them to nonspecifically take up vital stain. Enzymes such as DNAse or density gradients can be used to remove dead cells from the final preparations. Cell preparations must also be at least 80% to 90% lymphocytes. The testing could yield unreliable results because anti-HLA antibody could be bound to nontarget cells present. Therefore, depending on the source of cells, steps must be taken to remove contaminating platelets, red cells, monocytes, and granulocytes. A method of positive selection such as immunomagnetic beads also can be used.

The skill and experience of the technologist performing cell isolations is extremely important. Viability of the lymphocytes must be documented for each preparation and test performed.

Crossmatching

The major pitfall in crossmatching is the selection of appropriate patient sera to test. Some laboratories choose peak and current sera only. Other laboratories define an appropriate time limit for sera; they do not, for example, find it necessary to test sera that is more than 5 years old. But ASHI recommends using current sera (less than 48 hours old for sensitized patients or within 7 days for unsensitized patients), peak sera, and sera collected 2 weeks after transfusion or nephrectomy or any potentially sensitizing event.

A simple graph showing sensitizing events in relation to PRA values can be an excellent aid to the technologist when selecting patient sera for crossmatch, and we plot a graph for each patient chart (see Fig 31-1).

Interpretation

Wash steps, AHG reagents, choice of complement, and incubation times can increase the sensitivity of typing and crossmatching. The specificity of the reactions is enhanced by knowledge of the patient's history. Have there been sensitizing events? Does the patient demonstrate autoantibody and is the detectable serum antibody sensitive to reducing reagents such as DTT? "Wash" methods tend to detect IgG antibody only. Care should be exercised in interpreting negative crossmatches as a result of DTT treatment of the patient's serum, and the history of the patient's sensitizing events should be considered as newly formed IgM class antibody to HLA antigens may be present.

The interpretation of the results should take into consideration steroid treatment of the donor and the number of transfusions the donor had received. The viability of the donor cells is adversely affected by the length of time the specimens have been stored.

We highly recommend maintaining a complete laboratory file on each patient so that information needed at the time of final crossmatch is included in one place. Our patient file includes the following information:

HLA typing results of patient (spouse and sibs)

Complete PRA history

Transfusion history

Information on pregnancies

Previous crossmatch data

Antibody specificity, if known

Unacceptable antigens

Pertinent clinical notes from transplant committee

Blood group

MLC data

Graph of PRA if highly sensitized (see Fig. 31-1)

All worksheets and reports

TABLE **31-4**

Documentation Checklist

Date:
Time of arrival of tissue:
Recipient:
Medical record number:
Recipient tissue type:
Recipient blood group:
Donor:
UNOS number:
Donor blood group:
Donor tissue type:
Match: **Report Ag Match to Transplant Surgeon**

T-cell crossmatch
  Peak serum PRA:
  Current serum:
  Untested sera:
  Postnephrectomy sera:
  Postimmunosuppressant sera:
B-cell crossmatch
  Peak serum:
  Current serum:
  Postnephrectomy sera:
Recipient sensitization history
  Transfusions:
  Pregnancy:
  Previous transplant:
Serology results
  Recipient CMV:
  Donor CMV:
  Donor RPR:
  Donor HBsAg:
  Donor HIV antigen:
  Donor HIV antibody:
  Donor HTLV-1:
  Donor HCV:
  Donor anti-HB Core IgM (tissue donors):

Time of reporting: ______________________ Date: ______________________

Technologist's signature: ______________________

Director's signature: ______________________ Date: ______________________

On the front cover there is a sheet for the director's signature and space to document reviews of all reports. We use a check list for review at the time of the final crossmatch for renal transplant to document everything that is discussed when the technologist talks to the director prior to every transplant (**Table 31-4**).

Quality assurance in the histocompatibility laboratory is an important part to improving transplant success. Laboratory policies must be under consistent, continuous review and should be modified as new information about the relevance to clinical outcome becomes available. We must continuously strive to do what is best for patient outcome in a manner that is cost effective for all concerned.

REFERENCES

1. American Society for Histocompatibility and Immunogenetics. Accreditation Standards, Inspection Guidelines and Checklist. Lenexa, KS: March 15, 1995.
2. Nikaein A, Cluff D, Phelan D, et al, eds. Laboratory Manual. 3rd ed. Lenexa, KS: American Society for Histocompatibility and Immunogenetics, 1994.
3. Tardif GN, MacQueen JM, eds. Tissue typing reference manual. 3rd ed. Richmond, VA: South-Eastern Organ Procurement Foundation, 1993.
4. Wang-Rodriguez J, Rearden A. Effect of crossmatching on outcome in organ transplantation. Crit Rev Clin Lab Sci 1995;32(4):345–376.

Appendix: Geisinger Medical Center Histocompatibility Laboratory Training Program

When the technologist completes the first 6 months of training for on-call duties, cellular and platelet assays will be introduced, but the schedule and pace of training will be set by the technologist. The training for these assays will not necessarily be completed by the end of 8 months. Training will also be given for the flow cytometer and flow cytometer crossmatch and local tray making. Mandatory safety education includes radiation safety and training on the blood irradiator in addition to the standard mandatory yearly education required in every laboratory. **Table 31-A1** shows our checklist for on-call trainees.

New Technologist Lectures

A. Basics of histocompatibility testing—in lab
B. Basics of immunology and histocompatibility—medical technology lectures

Reading Assignments

1. HLA 1997. Terasaki PI, Gjertson DM, eds. California: UCLA Tissue Typing Laboratory, 1997. (latest edition)
2. SEOPF Tissue Typing Reference Manual
3. ASHI Laboratory Manual
4. GMC tissue typing laboratory procedure manual
5. *Manual of Clinical Laboratory Immunology.* Rose NR, Freidman H, Fahey JL, eds. 5th ed. Washington, DC: ASM Press, 1997.
6. *Basic and Clinical Immunology.* Introduction to Medical Immunology. 2ed. Virella G, Goust J-M, Fudenberg HH, eds. New York: Marcel Dekker, 1990.
7. *Immunology.* Roitt IM, Brostoff J, Male DK. 2nd ed. New York: Gower Medical, 1989.
8. ASHI regional and national meeting material
9. UNOS meeting information
10. ASHI standards and checklist
11. CAP standards (College of American Pathologists—Histocompatibility standards)

First Month

1. Isolation of lymphocytes from normal blood
2. Basics of serological testing: CDC, NIH, Amos modified
3. Panel maintenance: cell freezing
4. Tissue typing of normal individuals: class I
5. Single antigen typing
6. Prepare reagents:
   Veronal buffer

   Trypan blue

   2% EDTA

   DNAse

   Nylon wool

   Complement

   Thrombin

   Tris-ammonium chloride

   PBS: buffers with and without EDTA

TABLE 31-A1

Training Checklist for On-Call

Employee's Name: ______________________________

Procedures	Trainer's Initials	New Technologist's Initials/Date
1. Isolation of lymphocytes from blood; troubleshooting cell preparations		
2. Basics of serological testing: CDC, NIH, Amos modified procedure		
3. Cell freezing; panel maintenance		
4. Class I typing of normal individuals		
5. Single antigen typing; class I disease association		
6. Prepare reagents		
Veronal buffer		
1% trypan blue in PBS		
1% trypan blue in H_2O		
2% EDTA in veronal buffer		
Trypan blue working solution for typing trays		
DNAse		
Thrombin		
Tris-ammonium chloride		
RPMI with PHS		
PHS aliquots		
Complement aliquots		
PBS		
PBS-EDTA		
Mineral/paraffin oil		
Straws		
7. Equipment function checks and operations		
Centrifuges		
Freezers: locations and inventory		
Incubators		
Water baths		
Dry baths		
Autoscope system		
Tray oiler		
Lambda dot (serum plater)		
Lambda jets (cell plater)		
LN2 storage system		
8. PRA		
Serum preparation and storage, log books, patient records		
Test ordering/labels		
Understand organization of cell panel		
Organize tray layouts for screening		
Prelabel trays and oil trays		
Set up Lambda dot; organize patient sera		
Plate trays		
Thaw and prepare cells for screening		
Run trays with and without AHG		
Record results; calculate PRA		
Identify antibody specificities		
Understand cross-reactions and public specificities		
Record results in patients' charts		
Answer in computer		
10. Enter commercial typing trays in autoscope system		
11. Isolate T and B cells from blood, node, and spleen		
12. DR typing: Amos modified		
13. Prepare central lab crossmatch trays		

TABLE **31-A1**
Continued

Procedures	Trainer's Initials	New Technologist's Initials/Date
14. Prepare final crossmatch trays		
Select patient sera		
Titrate and plate patient sera		
Select controls		
Perform standard and AHG T cell crossmatches		
Perform B cell crossmatches		
Understand UNOS point system		
Understand infectious diseases testing required		
Understand reporting of results		
15. Update/maintain list and antigen sheets		
16. Perform autocrossmatches		
17. Patient records		
Review charts		
Tissue typing results		
Sensitization history, chart notes		
Transplant meeting minutes		
Family study information		
PRA history		
Transfusion history		
Crossmatch history		
Work sheets		
18. Family studies: renal		
Potential donors' UAs		
Phenotypes/genotypes/assign haplotypes		
19. Billing		

Employee's signature: ______________________ Date: ______________

Supervisor's signature: ______________________ Date: ______________

Director's signature: ______________________ Date: ______________

RPMI with PHS, Penn-Strep: pooled human serum and penicillin

Streptomycin solution

Mineral oil

Positive control/negative control

7. Equipment

Centrifuges: GLC, Eppendorf, Fisher micro-centrifuge

Freezers: location, inventory, alarm system

Incubators, water baths, dry baths

Liquid nitrogen storage system

Tray oiler, serum plater, cell plater

Hamilton, Terasaki syringes

Autoscope system (computer assisted)

Clinical laboratory computer system

Test

After first 2 weeks.
After second 2 weeks.

Second Month

PRA

Under strict supervision:

1. Serum preparation, storage, logs, patient records
2. Ordering in computer, labels
3. Understand organization of cell panel
4. Organize tray
5. Prelabel and oil trays
6. Set up serum plater
7. Plate trays

8. Thaw cells, prepare for screening
9. Run trays: with and without AHG
10. Record results/calculate PRA
11. Identify antibody specificities
12. Understand cross-reaction and public specificities
13. Record results in patients' charts
14. Answer results in computer

Test

Covering months 1 and 2.

Third Month

Class II Typing

1. Isolate T and B cells from peripheral blood, node, and spleen
2. Perform standard DR typing
3. Perform DR typing using immunomagnetic beads
4. Prepare reagents for immunomagnetic beads

Test

Covering first 3 months.

Fourth Month

Crossmatching

1. Select, titrate, and plate patient sera
2. Perform T-cell crossmatch with and without antiglobulin
3. Perform B-cell crossmatches
4. Perform auto T and B cell crossmatches
5. Perform DTT crossmatches
6. Understand UNOS point system
7. Understand OPO organ allocation system
8. Central lab screening trays

Test

Covering first 4 months. At the end of 4 months the technologist should have a working knowledge of:

HLA class I and Class II antigens—serological definition

WHO nomenclature

Private specificities, splits, and public specificities

Antibodies to HLA antigens, cross-reacting antibodies, causes of antibody stimulation

Complement lability, pathway, fixation

Antiglobulin (anti-κ light chain, AHG) binding and function

Fifth Month

Patient Records, Billing, Family Studies

1. Review chart forms
2. Review transplant lists
3. Family studies

Genotype and Assign Haplotypes

4. Terasaki cell and serum exchange
5. Bill patients for HLA typing, PRA, crossmatches

Test

Covering first 5 months.

Sixth Month

Quality Control

1. Perform class I complement titration
2. Perform class II complement titration
3. Perform antiglobulin titration
4. Review QC logs
5. Review QC on all reagents

Test

Covering 6 months. Assignment to call schedule.

Seventh Month

Cellular Assays

1. Mixed lymphocyte cultures
2. Lymphocyte transformations
3. Radiation safety survey, radioisotope inventory, usage, and disposal reports

Eighth Month

Platelet Assays

1. HLA matched platelets
2. Prepare platelet reagents: PBS-EDTA-Na azide, chloroquine, paraformaldehyde
3. Prepare, fix, and store platelets
4. Prepare avidin and biotin reagents
5. Perform antiplatelet and platelet surface immunoglobulin assays
6. Read on flow cytometer

CHAPTER 32

Serologic Assays for Tumors

MARK E. ASTILL
LORRAINE W. WILSON

Serologic testing of cancer patients has become a powerful tool in the arsenal of modern health care. Since the recognition of the association of Bence Jones proteins with myeloma, there has been a continuous and active search for other biological markers for use in oncology management. The realization that an in vitro measurement could reflect the presence of and process of malignancy was a seminal event.

Cells undergoing neoplastic transformation generate metabolic products associated with mutation. There are tumor markers that reflect and are associated with neoplastic conversion. This process involves two major requirements for cell transformation:

1. There must be a loss of regulated proliferation. Cells must begin to rapidly grow and divide, although this rapid growth by itself is not a neoplastic disease. Indeed, cells that are rapidly growing may be associated with benign hyperplasia, and these benign tumors can remain in a specific location and be relatively low in risk.
2. The second event involves loss of cell differentiation. This reversion back to a more fetal stage can result in the production of the important carcinoembryonic proteins such as carcinoembryonic antigen (CEA). CEA was the first of the fetal protein markers discovered, and research over the last 30 years has provided a wealth of information regarding correlation of tumor marker with the malignant process.

, can either be well or poorly differ- 'en within the same tumor. The het- of tumor tissue is one of the main challenges associated with biopsy and direct microscopic examination of tissue. Further, a malignant transformation may involve the production of proteolytic enzymes, which promote the metastases of cells to other tissue locations. It is this combination of unregulated growth and dedifferentiation coupled with enhanced invasiveness that make these malignant cells so serious.

Types of Diseases

Tumor markers have been identified for several major malignant diseases, including ovarian, pancreatic, gastric, breast, prostatic, hepatic, and colorectal carcinoma. **Table 32-1** lists these cancers and the dominant markers, as well as other cancers with markers currently used. At the heart of the utility of a tumor marker in disease management is the concept of specificity and sensitivity.

Specificity is a measure of the likelihood of a false-positive determination. The percentage of truly negative samples is the ratio of true negatives to the sum of true negatives and false positives. A 100% *specific* assay will identify only those individuals with a specific type of tumor and will exclude those with either benign or other noncancer disorders. Correspondingly, a 100% *sensitive* assay will measure all individuals with a particular type of cancer. It is a ratio of truly positive patients with the sum of true positives and false negatives. An ideal tumor marker has both sensitivity and specificity. However, there are few, if any, single markers that by themselves are effective tools.

Most important is the recognition that a panel of markers is much more useful in a

TABLE **32-1**

Tumor-Associated Markers

Primary Disease	Principal Marker	Secondary Markers
Adrenal pituitary tumors	Cortisol	Free catecholamines, DHEA, 17-ketosteroids, prolactin
B-cell malignancies	B2M	LD
Bladder cancer	Urinary CEA	NMP22, BTA, T-antigen, urokinase inhibitor, TPA, cytokeratins, glycosaminoglycans
Bone cancer	Alkaline phosphatase	Bence Jones protein, total hydroxyproline, serum calcium
Brain tumor	Desmesterol	Polyamines
Breast cancer	CA15-3, CA27-29	CEA, calcitonin, CA549, CA-M26, CK-BB, ferritin, β-hCG, LASA-P, P-21 protein, PS-2, prolactin
Bronchogenic carcinoma	Prolactin	
Carcinoid tumors	Urinary 5-HIAA, serotonin	Histamine, ADH, bradykinin
Cervical cancer	SCC	AG-4 antibodies, CA125, CEA, cytokeratins, HPV, TPA
Choriocarcinoma	hCG	
Colorectal carcinoma	CEA	CA19-5, CA19-9, CA72-4, CK-BB, NSE
CNS	VMA, HVA, CEA	
Cushing's syndrome	ACTH	Endorphin, lipotropin
Duodenal carcinoma	ADH	Pancreatic polypeptide
Endocrine pancreatic tumors	Pancreatic polypeptide	
Ganglioneuroblastoma	HVA, VMA	
Ganglioneuromas	Metanephrines, VMA	
Gastric carcinoma	CA72-4	CA19-9, CA50, CEA, ferritin, CK-BB, hCG, LASA, pepsinogen II, prothrombin
Glucagonoma	Glucagon	
Head and neck tumors	SCC	
Hepatocellular carcinoma	AFP	CEA, ferritin, γGT, ALP, TPA, γ-glutamyltranspeptidase
Hypercalcemia of malignancy	PTH-related peptide	
Insulinoma	Insulin	C-peptide, IGF-I binding protein I
Kidney tumors	CEA	NSE
Lung cancer	NSE	ACTH, CK-BB, calcitonin, CA72-4, CEA, AFP, ferritin, LASA-P, TPA
Medullary thyroid carcinoma	Calcitonin	NSE
Melanoma	Melanoma-associated antigen	NSE, plasma catecholamines, LASA-P, L-dopa
Microadenomas (pituitary)	Prolactin	
Multiple myeloma	Immunoglobulins, heavy and light chain	B2M, IgA, Bence Jones protein
Mesothelioma	Hyaluronic acid	
Multiple endocrine neoplasias	Chromogranin A	
Neuroblastoma	VMA	HVA, NSE, cystathionine, ferritin, metanephrines
Osteosarcomas	Alkaline phosphatase	
Ovarian carcinoma	CA125	UGF, inhibin, AFP, amylase isoenzyme, CEA, CK-BB, hCG, galactosyltransferases, LD, TPA
Pancreatic carcinoma	CA19-9	CA195, CA50, CA72-4, CEA, CK-BB, ADH, ALP, ferritin, galactosyltransferase isoenzyme II, γ-glutamyltranspeptidase
Parathyroid tumors	PTH intact	
Pheochromocytoma	Metanephrine	Chromogranin A, plasma catecholamines
Pituitary tumors	Alpha subunit of pituitary hormones	FSH, LH, prolactin, TSH

TABLE 32-1
Continued

Primary Disease	Principal Marker	Secondary Markers
Placental tumors	hCG	Alpha subunit of hCG
Prostate carcinoma	Free PSA, PSA-ACT, total PSA	PAP, ALP, CEA, CK-BB, TPA
Renal cell carcinoma		Renin, erythropoietin, interleukin-4, prostaglandin A, CA15-3, parathyroid hormone, NSE, prolactin, AFP
Sarcoma	Serum B2M	
Spleen tumors	Ferritin	
Squamous cell cancers, cervix	SCC	
Squamous cell cancers, lung	SCC	
Squamous cell cancers, head and neck	SCC	Ferritin
Stomach carcinoma	CA72-4	CEA, NSE
Teratoblastoma	Ferritin, AFP	hCG
Testicular cancer	hCG	
Testicular cancer, nonseminomatous	AFP	β-hCG, LDH
Uterine cancer	SCC	
Vipoma (pancreas)	VIP	
Waldenström's macroglobulinemia	B2M	Monoclonal IgM
Zollinger-Ellison syndrome	Gastrin	

disease management setting. It is also essential that specific patterns associated with the panel of markers be understood. In a disease management setting, the correlation of markers with detection of recurrent or residual disease is an important issue, as are the prognosis, staging, and classification of the tumor.

Role of the Laboratory in Disease Diagnosis, Evaluation, and Management

Rationale of Test Selection

Screening and Diagnosis

Generally, because of insufficient specificity and sensitivity, tumor markers are not recommended for screening. Moreover, the relatively low frequency of cancer in the general population does not warrant the extraordinary cost associated with population screening. Notable though is the utility of prostate-specific antigen (PSA) in combination with digital rectal examination (DRE) and/or transrectal ultrasound (TRUS) as a screening tool for clinically significant prostate cancer. This screening can potentially save individuals with treatment for an organ-confined disease.

The diagnosis of cancer should not depend solely on the measurement of a tumor marker. Indeed, there are a variety of other diseases that result in the non-neoplastic elevation of tumor markers. Nevertheless, tumor markers are useful as an adjunct method for cancer detection.

Monitoring Therapy

This is likely the most efficient and meaningful use of tumor markers. When there is no other measurable disease the marker(s) can be a means for monitoring the success of therapy by tracking any elevation in concentration. When deciding upon the appropriate marker, the half-life and the range of concentration should be primary considerations, especially in determining the frequency of testing. As there is no single marker with 100% sensitivity, multiple marker panels can aid in the management of therapy.

It is important that baseline measurements of these markers take place before therapy begins. It is generally most useful to choose the marker most elevated above normal as the primary source of disease information.

Recurrence and Prognosis

After surgical removal of a tumor, the level of the tissue-derived marker should drop to "normal" levels presuming a complete loss of tumor tissue. Consequently, this is a powerful method for determining efficacy of surgery and recurrence of disease. Through serial monitoring of patient's sera, marker elevation can precede clinical symptoms often by 3 to 6 months. These types of tests are useful in patients where a history of a marker or panel of markers is well known.

Tumor aggressiveness, invasive ability, and susceptibility to specific treatment are all important considerations in disease prognosis. A good example of this is the panel of markers used in prognosis of breast cancer. After nodal involvement, estrogen and progesterone receptor elevation are predictors of survival as well as response to hormone therapy. Cathepsin D is a lysosomal protease used in predicting tumor aggressiveness and c-*erb*-b2 is a growth factor reflecting tumor activity. The limitation with these assays has been the necessity of testing on biopsied tumor tissue. It has been recently discovered that a 120-kd extracellular domain portion of the c-*erb*-b2 molecule is released into the vascular system. Consequently, it can be measured through sera analysis. Moreover, this extracellular domain seems to correlate with other serum tumor markers.

Staging and Classification

Generally, an elevated tumor marker concentration corresponds to an increasing tumor stage and grade. This is expected as one would assume that any tumor that has metastasized has a greater probability for tumor marker production. Tumor marker assays are especially useful for germ cell–derived tumors. The utility of simultaneous measurement of α-fetoprotein (AFP) and β human chorionic gonadotropin (β-hCG) in discriminating germ cell–derived tumors is well known.

Assay Methods

Important considerations in the development of a tumor marker assay include sensitivity and specificity, concentration range, availability of antibodies, antigen, and potential interference. These can be especially important if significantly elevated levels of a tumor marker are possible and erroneous values from a so-called "hook effect" could occur.

Competitive versus Sandwich Formats

In 1969 Berson and Yalow received the Nobel Prize for the first "immunoassay" described, which was a competitive-binding assay for insulin. In this case, radiolabeled insulin was in competition with unlabeled insulin for anti-insulin binding sites. The amount of insulin present in patient sera was proportional to the amount of radioactivity retained from charcoal separation of antibody bound versus unbound. This system provided for the picogram sensitivity now routinely available in an immunoassay format. The underlying principle described here is the competition between a fixed amount of the radioactively labeled antigen and either patient sera, calibrator, or control. Any interference between this binding reaction will result in a falsely elevated value. A further disadvantage with this system relates to the amount of antigen required. In those assays where the antigen is scarce or difficult to come by, preparation of the radiolabeled product requires significant amounts of scarce material.

A sandwich or double-antibody method overcomes this disadvantage. One of the most important demonstrations of this principle is the enzyme-linked immunosorbent assay (ELISA). The principle here uses a solid-phase adsorbed antibody that is exposed to sample containing the tumor marker of interest. After binding to the immobilized antibody, the marker is sandwiched with a second marker-specific antibody that is coupled with an enzyme. After washing the unbound enzyme away, a colorimetric signal is produced with a suitable substrate. The amount of color is directly proportional to the amount of marker.

Variations on this basic theme abound, with a number of different "reporter" molecules available. Sensitivity has been significantly improved using biotin-avidin amplification protocols as well as various chemiluminescent detection formats. Nevertheless, the colorimetric method is commonly used and remains a workhorse of many clinical laboratories.

A limitation with the sandwich format is the possibility of a so-called "hook" effect. At very high levels of tumor marker, rather than forming a sandwich, all antibody binding sites are occupied in both immobilized and reporter antibodies and the sandwich formed is not proportional to tumor marker concentration. Thus, the sample appears to have a lower concentration of tumor marker than is actually present. Accurate values can only be measured upon dilution of the sample.

Immunoassay Factors

The pioneering work of Kohler and Milstein with murine somatic cell hybridization with antibody producing B cells provided the basis upon which most modern tumor marker assays are predicated. Problems of antibody supplies, poor specificity, lack of uniformity, and lot-to-lot variation have been largely resolved with monoclonal antibody production.

The sensitivity and specificity of most tumor marker assays largely depends on the selection of the monoclonal antibody. Indeed, the new generation of tumor markers is largely due to the ability to produce highly specific monoclonal antibodies to unique epitopes found on tumor-associated molecules. Moreover, the utility of a panel of tumor marker tests is becoming more common. Due to tumor heterogeneity, there is generally not a single product produced by a clone of cells. For example, CA 72-4, Ca 19-9, and CEA immunoassays are complimentary in detecting various carcinomas.

Heterophilic Antibody Interference

The use of monoclonal antibodies has not been limited to in vitro diagnostics. Monoclonal antibodies have also been employed in imaging techniques determining tumor metastases as well as other therapeutic regimens. Consequently, it is not unusual to find individuals who have mounted an immune response against a murine antibody. There may be as many as 15% to 40% of individuals who have some type of heterophilic antibody.

These antibodies can directly interfere with an in vitro test using monoclonal antibodies. Results may be either artificially high or low depending upon the specific format employed. These anti-idiotypic antibodies can easily bind to a monoclonal antibody, soluble or adsorbed, and substantially interfere with the capability for specific antigen binding. It is essential to determine whether the diagnostic method used is susceptible to this type of interference and if steps have been taken to neutralize these impacts. Standard approaches for reducing this interference include addition of nonspecific mouse immunoglobulin or an excess of mouse sera.

Clinical Relevance and Correlation

Reference Preparations

The challenge with tumor marker assays, especially those measured by immunoassay, is the lack of a reference material that will provide uniform, accurate results. Commercial assays ostensibly measuring the same tumor marker can give significantly different results. Furthermore, a single laboratory performing tests using the same method will also give more consistent results than different laboratories. Uniformity of results is essential when tumor markers are being used in monitoring. One needs to be assured that a change in tumor marker concentration is due to tumor activity or size and not a change in manufacturers, laboratories, or procedures.

An excellent example of the problems associated with commercial tumor marker kits and a program to develop a reference preparation is illustrated with prostate-specific antigen (PSA). PSA is likely the best tumor marker thus far identified. It is both specific and sensitive, making it the most useful tumor marker available for the diagnosis and management of prostatic carcinoma. Serum measurement of PSA in combination with either transrectal ultrasonography (TRUS) or digital rectal examination (DRE) has been recommended as a screening tool for detection of clinically significant prostate cancer. PSA measurement has been found to be useful for detecting recurrence of cancer after prostatectomy and for monitoring therapy. Moreover, as knowledge of this marker has expanded, it is now possible to use PSA measurement to help in discrimination of benign versus malignant disease, avoiding costly and painful biopsies.

PSA is a serine protease produced by the

epithelial cells of the prostate gland. Enzymatic activity is regulated by binding to protease inhibitors, including α_1-antichymotrypsin (ACT), α_2-macroglobulin (A2M), and other acute phase proteins. In fact, the majority of PSA exists in the complexed form of PSA-ACT and PSA-A2M. Originally, measurements of PSA were reflections of the "total" amount of PSA in circulation. This included both "free" PSA and PSA-ACT. Both of these markers are measured by sandwich immunoassays employing highly specific monoclonal antibodies directed against epitopes unique to free and complexed forms. PSA-A2M is largely not detected, as the size of A2M at 720kd largely conceals the PSA from antibody recognition.

Total PSA values less than 4.0ng/mL are presumed to be reflective of evidence of no disease or success in therapy. Conversely, concentrations >10.0ng/mL are presumptive of significant disease or metastases. Values in the range of 4 to 10ng/mL lie in a region where TRUS and needle biopsies are often employed to rule out carcinoma. Originally, the polyclonal antibody immunoassays gave results that were higher than the subsequent monoclonal assays.

These improved assays also created significant controversy through lack of agreement of PSA measurement between different manufacturers. Originally, assays between manufacturers could vary by up to 2 to 3 times. However, when a common calibrator was used, much of this difference disappeared. Hence, the need for adoption of an international standard was evident. There are several reasons why differences between PSA values are notable:

1. The immunogen used to elicit the antibody can vary significantly. PSA has up to five isoforms, not including the antiprotease complexed fractions. It logically follows that antibodies react with different affinities to all of the circulating forms.
2. A major influence is the lack of uniformity of calibration. Although a calibrator can be configured to maintain a constant ratio of free versus complexed PSA, this will almost certainly not correspond to that same ratio found in *all* patient sera.
3. A further influence is the format of the assay. Performance and sensitivity have significant influence upon observed values.

The National Committee on Clinical Laboratory Standards (NCCLS) has established a PSA subcommittee to specifically address these issues.

Producing Quality Results for Tumor Marker Testing

Quality Control and Quality Assurance

As tumor marker tests are being used for monitoring the course of a patient's disease over long time periods, several challenges are recognized. Test results must be consistent and present a clear picture of the patient's history in spite of possible changes in the testing laboratory's methods and reporting. It is important that a tumor marker assay produce consistent results with no significant drift of calibration over several years. When methods of measuring tumor markers change, it is necessary to address the possibility that a patient may have a different result using one method as compared to another. Significant changes may occur as a result of calibration changes, antibodies of differing specificities, and vulnerability to clinically associated interferences. Any changes in testing methods which may cause a shift in patient values must be communicated to the physician. Reports listing simply the results of the current testing event are only useful if the physician has easy access to the previous results. A cumulative tumor marker tracking report allowing the charting of several tumor markers along with treatment dates would be the best solution.

To detect any lot-to-lot variability, a separate independent control should be used for each assay in addition to any controls included with each tumor marker kit. The additional control may be prepared from a pool of previously tested samples, or may be purchased from another vendor. In the event that a shift occurs with a new lot of reagents, the cause and extent of the problem must be determined and resolved before the reagents are used for routine testing.

When it is necessary to change testing laboratories or methods for a specific tumor marker, a comparison study between the two methods is necessary. If there is a significant bias or if some patients show significant differences in values between the two methods, it will be necessary to establish a new baseline prior to switching to the new test method. This is generally done by performing both tests simultaneously and reporting both results. It is important to inform the physician of the upcoming method change so that all patients may be scheduled for testing if it is needed.

To ensure a quality result, there must be correct sample collection and handling. Although individual tests may be validated for the use of either serum or plasma, it is important that the same sample type is always used. The ideal situation is for the laboratory to have access to the previous results of each patient. This will allow samples to be diluted prior to assay when appropriate, and will also allow testing to be repeated and varified if a result differs significantly from the previous measurement.

Whenever a result differs markedly from what is expected, the laboratory should be contacted and the testing repeated. If a problem is not identified by rechecking the result, a new sample should be sent to confirm the result. Whenever possible, the problem causing the discrepancy should be identified and steps taken to prevent it from recurring. The laboratory should be prepared to store patient samples for long periods of time.

Proficiency testing is available for most of the commonly ordered tumor markers. The College of American Pathologists (CAP) survey program includes β_2-microglobulin, estrogen and progesterone receptors, AFP, CA-125, CEA, PSA, and PAP. All laboratories performing tumor marker testing should participate in the appropriate programs. For those assays in which proficiency testing is not available a program of internal blind testing should be established. The use of blind sample testing will help to monitor problems with assay stability, sample processing, and daily performance of the assay.

BIBLIOGRAPHY

Bast RC Jr, Klug TL, St. John E, et al. A radioimmunoassay using a monoclonal antibody to monitor the course of epithelial ovarian cancer. N Engl J Med 1983;309:883–887.

Bast RC Jr, Knauf S, Epenetos A, et al. Coordinate elevation of serum markers in ovarian cancer but not in benign disease. Cancer 1991;68:1758.

Baylin SB. Ectopic production of hormones and other proteins by tumors. Hosp Prac 1975;Oct: 117–126.

Bodansky O. Reflections on biochemical aspects of human cancer. Cancer 1974;33:364.

Catalona WJ, Smith DS, Ratliff TL, et al. Measurement of prostate-specific antigen in serum as a screening test for prostate cancer. N Engl J Med 1991;324:1156–1161.

Child JA, Spati B, Illingworth S, et al. Serum beta 2 microglobulin and C-reactive protein in the monitoring of lymphomas. Cancer 1980;45:318–326.

Christensson A, Bjork T, Nilsson O, et al. Serum prostate specific antigen complexed to α1-antichymotrypsin as an indicator of prostate cancer. J Urol 1993;150:100.

Del Villano BC, Brennan SM, Brock C, et al. Radioimmunometric assay for a monoclonal antibody-defined tumor marker, CA 19-9. Clin Chem 1983;29:549–552.

Fidler IJ, Hart IR. Biological diversity in metastatic neoplasms: origins and implications. Science 1982;217:998–1003.

Jacobs I, Bast RC Jr. The CA 125 tumour-associated antigen: a review of the literature. Hum Reprod 1989;4:1.

Kane RE, Penny J, Walder K, et al. Changes in the CA 19-9 antigen and Lewis blood group with pulmonary disease severity in cystic fibrosis. Pediatr Pulmonol 1992;12:221–226.

Knight JA, Wu JT, Miya T, Knight DP. A comparison of biochemical markers between benign and malignant ovarian cysts. Clin Physiol Biochem 1986;4:130–135.

Liotta LA. Biochemical mechanisms of tumor invasion and metastases. Clin Physiol Biochem 1987;5:190–199.

Madersbacher S, Klieber R, Mann K. Free α-subunit, free β-subunit of human chorionic gonadotropin (hCG), and intact hCG in sera of healthy individuals and testicular cancer patients. Clin Chem 1992;38:370.

Milstein C, Cuello AC. Hybrid hybridomas and their use in immunohistochemistry. Nature 1983;305: 537.

Nahm MH, Hoffmann JW. Heteroantibody: phantom of the immunoassay. Clin Chem 1990;36:829.

Safi F, Kohler I, Tottinger E, Beger H-G. The value of the tumor marker CA 15-3 in diagnosing and monitoring breast cancer. Cancer 1991;68: 574–582.

Schnipper LE. Clinical implications of tumor cell heterogeneity. N Engl J Med 1986;314:1423–1431.

Sell S. Cancer markers of the 1990s. Comparison of the new generation of markers defined by monoclonal antibodies and oncogene probes to prototypic markers. Clin Lab Med 1990;10:1–37.

Virje MA, Mercer DW, Herberman RB. Tumor markers in cancer diagnosis and prognosis. Cancer 1988;38:102–126.

von Kleist S. What's new in tumor markers and their measurements? Pathol Res Pract 1988;183:95–99.

Wu JT. Measurement of AFP and its lectin-reactive isoforms in liver diseases and various malignancies. Ann Clin Lab Sci 1990;20:98–105.

Wu JT, Mau E, Knight JA. Interference with carcinoembryonic antigen radioimmunoassays by glycoaminoglycans, and their removal. Clin Chem 1983;29:2049.

Wu JT, Knight JA. Alpha-fetoprotein: Its use in clinical medicine. Clin Chem 1987;27:1.

Wu JT. Expression of monoclonal antibody-defined tumor markers in four carcinomas. Ann Clin Lab Sci 1989;19:17.

Wu JT, Christensen SE. Effect of different test designs of immunoassays on "hook effect" of CA 19-9 measurement. J Clin Lab Anal 1991;5:228.

Wu JT. Assay for prostate specific antigen (PSA): problems and possible solutions. J Clin Lab 1994; 8:51.

Wu JT, Astill ME, Gagon SD. Measurement of c-*erb*B-2 protein in sera from patients with carcinomas and breast tumor tissue cytosols: correlations with serum tumor markers and membrane bound oncoprotein. J Clin Lab Anal 1995;9:151.

CHAPTER 33

Cellular Assays for the Evaluation of Human Tumors

A. BETTS CARPENTER
THERESA L. WHITESIDE

The role of the immune system in control of tumor growth and dissemination of metastases has been intensively investigated in recent years. These studies indicate that tumors induce an immune response, as both tumor-specific antibodies and T-cells specific for tumor-associated antigens are detectable in tumor-bearing hosts. However, it remains uncertain to what extent tumor-specific immune cells and/or antibodies are responsible for or involved in the control of cancer progression. Nonspecific immune responses, including inflammatory cells and mediators as well as natural killer (NK) cells, non-major histocompatibility complex (MHC)-restricted T cells and macrophages, clearly contribute to antitumor activity in tumor-bearing hosts. In addition, tumors, and especially tumor metastases themselves, can exert inhibitory effects on the immune system, modifying local and systemic immune responses (1,2). Thus, complex interactions exist between the tumor and the host immune system, which are not completely understood but which appear to influence, at least in part, tumor progression. It is also important to remember that immune responses are likely to change during the course of tumor development, and that the nature of immune cells and of factors these cells produce may be profoundly influenced by the presence and growth of a tumor.

In view of changes in the immune profile of a tumor-bearing host—which tend to occur during the process of tumor progression and which appear to be modulated by therapy—a broad range of assays have become available to monitor the extent of immunocompetence in the tumor-bearing host (3). Most of these assays are nonspecific in that they do not measure responses induced by or directed at the individual's own tumor but rather a general state of immunocompetence of the tumor-bearing host. With few exceptions, these assays are of limited usefulness in evaluating antitumor activity of the immune cells. The reason is that, quite frequently, general immunocompetence of tumor-bearing individuals is not compromised, but their antitumor responses are. In other words, selective immune defects may be present in such individuals that are subtle, restricted to specific cell subsets, and thus are not detectable using standard cellular immune assays. To look for such selective defects, sensitive tumor-specific tests are necessary, and these are difficult to perform and to evaluate in a clinical laboratory.

One of the major difficulties in implementing monitoring of specific antitumor responses in patients with cancer is the limited availability of autologous tumor (AuTu) or AuTu-derived antigens to serve for in vitro stimulation of immune cells or as targets for immune effector cells. Even when AuTu-peptides are known, as in the case of melanoma-specific peptides of which close to a dozen have been cloned and sequenced recently (4,5), it is not easy to detect peptide-specific effector cells in patients with melanoma. Thus, in vitro expansion of rare precursor cells (an estimated frequency of 10^5 to 10^6 in peripheral blood) is generally necessary to demonstrate the presence of melanoma peptide-specific T-cell responses, followed by a sensitive functional assay employing AuTu or a surrogate target cell expressing the relevant peptide in the context of the appropriate MHC restriction element (5).

Another difficulty in measuring antitumor responses involves the selection of the site in which to look for AuTu-specific effector cells. Although cancer is a systemic disease, measurements of the number or functions of mononuclear cells (MNC) in peripheral blood often does not adequately reflect immunologic events that take place at the site of tumor growth or metastasis. Evidence indicates that specific antitumor effector cells are often enriched at the tumor site, in tumor-draining lymph nodes (LN) or in a tumor-bearing organ as opposed to the peripheral circulation. Hence, the search for AuTu-specific effector cells in the peripheral blood, while most convenient, is not always successful. It is apparent, however, that limitations in acquisition of tissue specimens in patients with cancer or the number of effector cells recovered from parts of specimens available for immunologic assays dictate that these assays be performed with the peripheral blood lymphocytes.

Irrespective of the above-mentioned difficulties with measuring of specific antitumor responses, it has been possible to develop a number of cellular assays, which can provide a reasonable estimate of AuTu reactivity in patients with cancer. In addition, certain non-AuTu-specific cellular assays, including natural killer (NK) and lymphokine-activated killer (LAK) activities, have been found to be useful for longitudinal monitoring of patients with cancer and for evaluation of responses to therapy.

In this chapter we focus on the assays that have been used for monitoring of patients with cancer by clinical laboratories, and for which quality assurance and quality control guidelines have been formulated. A number of other assays that fall in the realm of research are not included, and the reader is referred to basic immunology texts for their description.

Isolation of Lymphocytes from Tumor Sites

To evaluate local or locoregional antitumor responses, immune cells have to be first isolated from tumor, tumor-involved tissues, or organs bearing metastases. In general, immune monitoring of lesions, tissues, or organs involved in disease (including cancer) is likely to yield more informative results than will the same assays performed with peripheral blood MNC of cancer patients. Lymphocytes that accumulate at the site of a tumor or its metastases are considered to be more relevant or more involved in tumor progression than those found in the peripheral circulation.

The obvious problem with this strategy is that in patients with cancer, blood is more readily available for immune testing than tissues. Nevertheless, whenever tumor or tumor-involved tissues become available as a result of surgery or tissue biopsy, they should be procured for processing to recover tumor cells as well as lymphocytes for phenotypic and functional immunologic studies. Ideally, peripheral blood MNC should be obtained from a patient at the same time for parallel studies.

Although separation of serum/plasma or MNC from the peripheral blood are routine laboratory procedures, recovery and fractionation of cells from tissues or body fluids containing tumor or tissue cells is time consuming and requires special expertise and considerable effort (6). Recovery of lymphocytes or tumor cells from freshly harvested tissues follows an established and previously described protocol (6).

Viability of tumor-infiltrating lymphocytes (TIL) is almost always 100%, but that of tumor cells varies. Tumor cells with less than 60% viability by a trypan blue dye exclusion are not useful. To ensure adequate cell viability, the conditions for tumor processing, including enzymatic digestion, have to be optimized, and the specimen dissociation performed according to the established protocol. Care has to be taken to avoid vigorous pipetting and high-speed centrifugations and to establish optimal conditions for cell cryopreservation, storage, and thawing.

The quality of the processed and enriched tumor cell suspensions can be determined by preparation of cell smears for Papanicolaou staining. Evaluation of such smears by a pathologist provides an evaluation of the purity and level of enrichment in TIL or tumor cells of every processed cell suspension. The cytology report as well as the final pathology report for the tissue specimen processed are maintained on file in the laboratory.

The recovery of tumor cells or TIL varies with a tumor type. Some tumor specimens, such as ovarian or renal cell carcinomas and melanomas, yield relatively high numbers of TIL and tumor cells in comparison to breast or liver tumors, which are often a poor source of viable cells. It is important to remember that frequently the recovery of tumor cells and TIL depends more on a degree of tumor necrosis and tumor infiltration by MNC than on the size of the tumor tissue received for processing.

It is advisable that processing of tumor tissues for research and, especially, for immunotherapy of patients with autologous tumor vaccines or adoptively transferred lymphocytes be performed in a laboratory specializing in tissue procurement and processing. This type of laboratory exists in most comprehensive cancer centers recognized by the National Cancer Institute. The tissue procurement laboratory operates in accordance with a peer-reviewed program of quality assurance designed to control procedures, reagents, equipment maintenance, record keeping, and employee training. It is staffed by personnel trained in sterile handling and processing of tissues, and these procedures are performed as detailed in an operation manual and under supervision of a professional who is experienced and is prepared to administer quality control checks of the cell viability and recovery at regular intervals. These centers make daily checks of freezers and water baths, use emergency temperature back-up systems, and keep records to document staff and instrument performance. In addition, the staff has a responsibility for assuring that all operations are approved by the Institutional Review Board (IRB) and implemented in accordance with the IRB guidelines.

Specimen Requirements for Cellular Assays in Tumor-Bearing Individuals

Cellular assays for measurements of immune functions generally require considerable cell numbers (i.e., 5 to 10 × 10^6 per assay), fairly large volumes of blood (i.e., 30 mL or more) or other body fluids if more than one assay is to be performed, and facilities for rapid processing of these samples for the cell recovery. Therefore, attempts have been made to miniaturize cellular assays or to use whole blood instead of separated MNC for testing. Newer, more sensitive technologies, including single-cell assays, electrochemoluminescence, or molecular biology-based assays, have been introduced with the intent of decreasing the required cell numbers or blood volumes, and increasing sensitivity of the assays.

In those instances when the phenotype or functions of individual cell subsets in the tissue-derived or blood-derived MNC population is desired, these cell subsets have to be first isolated and purified. The advantages of studies performed with highly purified subsets of immune cells are obvious, but the methods for purification of such subsets from tumor-infiltrating or even blood lymphocytes are tedious and time consuming. These methods are based on selective reactivity of MNC subsets with antibodies and are available in specialized laboratories.

The lack of uniformly acceptable procedures for cell separations and unpredictable yields of cells recovered from tissues or body fluids of patients with cancer have considerably hampered the use of cell separation techniques in the clinical laboratory. Today, most cellular assays are still performed using unfractionated MNC populations recovered from the blood, other body fluids, and occasionally tissues of cancer patients.

It is often unclear which of the available immunologic assays can be reliably performed with fresh versus cryopreserved MNC. For immunologic assays performed as a part of clinical trials, for example, it would be more practical to use serially harvested batches of cryopreserved immune cells instead of freshly harvested specimens. Using of batched samples eliminates the interassay variability, and it facilitates more economic utilization of AuTu cells, which are often available in limited numbers. Many cellular assays, such as proliferation or cytokine production, can be reliably performed with cryopreserved cells.

However, some cellular assays, including cytotoxicity, are best performed with fresh samples, because cryopreservation of MNC, even using rate-controlled freezing in a Cryomed in the presence of human serum and DMSO, often induces a partial and unpredictable loss of functional attributes. Each clinical laboratory is obliged to compare frozen with fresh MNC to ascertain that the reproducibility and reliability of a cellular assay are not compromised by cryopreservation of cells.

More recently, cellular assays have been performed with whole blood instead of separated MNC. The advantage of whole blood assays is that the processing of specimens can be eliminated, thus reducing a chance for altering functions of antitumor effector cells. As phenotypic markers on immune cells are universally tested in whole blood by flow cytometry, it seems reasonable to assess in parallel functions of the same cells in whole blood. It is expected that correlations between the phenotypic and functional properties of immune cells might improve under these assay conditions.

In our experience, the disadvantage of whole blood assays is that they have to be performed with freshly harvested specimens, as those stored overnight or shipped from distant locations by overnight mail may give unreliable results.

Choice of Cellular Assays for Monitoring of Cancer Patients

The choice of cellular assays for evaluation of patients with cancer depends on the circumstances and purpose of the evaluation. Specifically, for patients on clinical protocols, immunologic monitoring is desirable, involving serial assays performed before, during, and after therapy and selected to answer a hypothesis tested in the trial (7). Monitoring assays require a unique set of quality control guidelines, as discussed later in this chapter.

When immunologic evaluation of patients not on protocols is desired, a decision is necessary as to whether non-tumor-specific immune competence or tumor-specific responses are to be measured. The former involves measures of standard immune parameters (e.g., total number of circulating T cells; ability of T cells to proliferate in response to mitogens or to produce cytokines in response to mitogens or non-tumor antigens), which define general immune competence. The latter requires the availability of individual patient's tumor cells, tumor antigens or purified or synthetic tumor peptides for the performance of functional assays, which can define the state of antitumor immunity in this patient. As indicated above, this type of tumor-specific measurement is difficult and can only be performed under specific circumstances. For example, in cancer patients undergoing vaccination with AuTu or AuTu-derived fractions or peptides, measurements of specific AuTu responses are not only possible but necessary to document the presence of vaccination-induced memory responses.

Cellular assays available for a patient with cancer include both phenotypic and functional measures (**Table 33-1**). Phenotypic assays determine the absolute number or proportion of immune cells or their subpopulations, most often using flow cytometry. These assays are based on the identification of cells expressing a set of surface receptors (phenotypic markers). In contrast, functional assays involve testing the ability of immune cells to perform certain defined functions, such as delayed-type hypersensitivity (DTH), proliferation, cytotoxicity, or cytokine production. Although phenotypic assays are technically less demanding, are readily accessible, and are highly reproducible, they do not substitute for functional assays. It cannot be assumed that phenotypic expression of a marker correlates with the functional capacity of a cell; therefore, functional studies are necessary to confirm its function.

Phenotypic Assays

Phenotypic assays are most often performed on whole blood samples, using flow cytometry (Chapter 19) (8,9), but they can use Ficoll-Hypaque separated peripheral blood mononuclear cells (PBMC) or cells separated from body fluids or tissues. A wide range of monoclonal antibodies (MAbs) are available for two-color, three-color, or multiparameter analysis. One important consideration is the selection of a panel of markers for phenotypic analysis. Despite the temptation to use extensive panels of phenotypic markers, it is important to choose those that are most likely to provide meaningful information in a patient with cancer. Activation markers, expression of co-stimulatory molecules, and the presence of cellular adhesion molecules (CAM) on immune cells, in addition to determining the proportion of T, B, NK cells or their subpopulations, are all likely to provide information relevant to the quality of antitumor responses. In addition, receptors for growth factors or cytokines can be phenotypically quantitated, and the results compared with those of functional assays. This type of flow analysis has been particularly useful in defining freshly isolated human TIL as T lymphocytes expressing activation markers and a variety of

TABLE 33-1

Immunologic Cellular Assays Used for Monitoring of Patients with Cancer

Assay Category	Sample Type
1. Phenotypic assays	
Proportions of cells	Whole blood, tissue, body fluids, PBMC
Absolute numbers of cells	Same as above
Cellular subpopulations	Same as above
2. Functional assays	
In vivo DTH skin test	Visual inspection, biopsy
Signal transduction defects	T, NK cells in body fluids, tissues
Cytotoxicity: ADCC, LAK, NK CTL	PBMC, bone marrow cells, tissue-derived cells, cells in body fluids
Cytokine production	
T_H1 vs. T_H2 cytokine profile	Same as above
Lymphocyte proliferation	
MLTC	Same as above

NOTE: The assays listed above can be performed as non-tumor-specific or AuTu-specific assays, depending on the stimulator or target cells used and the expertise of the laboratory with in vitro generation of AuTu-specific effector cells.

CAMs, either completely unable to mediate or partly deficient in mediating antitumor activities (2).

New assays being developed for flow cytometry include tests to measure intracytoplasmic markers using permeabilized cells, and assays to perform functional assays. Intracytoplasmic proteins, including enzymes, cytokines, signal transduction molecules can be measured in the phenotypically defined cells and can provide useful information about the activation state of individual cells and about their functional attributes (7,10,11). Proliferation and cytotoxicity can be measured by flow cytometry simply and more efficiently than in the familiar radiolabeled assays, simultaneously providing the identity of effector cells at the population or single-cell level. As more experience is obtained with these assays, they are likely to replace some of the standard cellular assays in the clinical laboratory.

To optimally use flow cytometry data in the clinical settings and especially in serial monitoring, stringent quality controls of interassay variability are necessary. Some of the lymphocyte subpopulations only constitute a small proportion of the total lymphocytes tested; and changes in these subpopulations induced by therapy, for example, may be difficult to distinguish from normal assay variability. Good quality control procedures can help in meeting this goal.

In addition, changes in the phenotype of cells should be interpreted in conjunction with any changes observed in the functional assays. Specifically, it is important to consider whether changes in function induced during therapy correlate with changes in the number of effector cells. During the course of any cancer treatment, these changes can be dramatic or subtle, and can occur simultaneously in several subsets of cells. In addition, phenotypic and functional measures may not necessarily correlate, as alterations in the immune cell proportions or absolute numbers may be mediated by different mechanisms. For example, during systemic or locoregional therapy with interleukin 2 (IL-2), an increase in the number of circulating NK cells may occur due to increased blood vessel permeability (7,12). At the same time, IL-2 is likely to upregulate NK activity (7). Furthermore, it is possible that shifts in one but not the other parameter will correlate to clinical response or, more likely, that no significant correlations will be detected, even though profound changes in the immune cell number or function are registered during therapy (12).

Flow cytometry with permeabilized immune cells has been recently used for the definition of their cytokine profile and, more specifically, for the quantitation of the T_H1 and T_H2 subsets of CD4+ T cells (13). Shifts in the proportion of these cells have been reported to occur in cancer and other diseases (14), and this technology offers the possibility of determining the frequency of cytokine-expressing cells, that is, the proportion of CD4+ T cells in the population that co-express IL-2 and INF-γ (T_H1) versus IL-4 and IL-10 (T_H2) proteins (15). The technology relies on in vitro stimulation of immune cells to activate cytokine gene expression, which is carried out in the presence of agents known to disrupt intracellular transport (e.g., brefeldin A or monensin), and staining of the permeabilized cells with anticytokine antibodies (15).

Because of the possibility for nonspecific staining with these antibodies, rigorous specificity controls are essential in this method. Such controls include blocking with a molar excess of the relevant cytokine or of unlabeled anticytokine antibody, as reviewed previously (15). In combination with multiparameter flow cytometry, this method can discriminate between T_H1+ and T_H2+ cell populations in complex cellular mixtures such as TIL, bronchoalveolar lavages obtained from patients with cancer of the upper aerodigestive tract, or ascites of patients with ovarian carcinoma.

Functional Assays

DTH Skin Tests

Delayed-type hypersensitivity (DTH) reactions are an in vivo correlate of cellular immunity and provide a convenient and cost-effective method for its assessment in humans (16). DTH can be combined with a skin biopsy to confirm the nature of the cells infiltrating the skin. Although DTH has been traditionally used as a screen for cellular immunity to commonly encountered antigens, it can also be applicable to evaluate patients with cancer for sensitization to autologous tumor or tumor-derived antigens. The DTH reaction, which is based upon previous antigen exposure, is mediated by presensitized T cells and macrophages, and is clinically characterized by an area of induration peaking at approximately 48 to 72 hours.

Generally, the DTH skin tests correlate with in vitro functional tests of cellular immunity such as lymphocyte proliferation and cytokine assays. A panel of five to six commonly encountered antigens is administered intradermally, and the area of induration measured at 24 and 48 hours. A measurement of greater than 5 mm at 48 hours is considered a positive reaction. A reaction less than 5 mm is considered negative, and the patient is considered anergic to that particular antigen. A change in the DTH skin test from unreactive to reactive as a result of therapy is considered a significant result (16).

There are a variety of pitfalls in the evaluation of DTH skin tests (16). First of all, it is important to ensure that a positive reaction is due to sensitized T cells (48 hours), and not to a preexisting antibody reaction (which peaks much earlier, at 18 to 24 hours). A significant area of induration seen at 24 hours may represent a humoral response related to the presence of circulating preformed antibody reacting with the intradermal antigen and forming immune complexes. Therefore, it is possible for an individual to lack a T-cell response to an antigen but, due to the presence of antibody, develop a positive area of induration. However, because of the difference in the kinetics of the two responses, humoral versus cellular reactions can be differentiated.

It is necessary to be cautious about anaphylactic reactions that may occur in sensitized subjects. These reactions can cause washout of antigen and give a false-negative DTH skin result. If DTH skin tests are planned to evaluate the response to a particular immunotherapy, such as vaccination with tumor-derived peptides, a possibility of the effect of multiple antigen exposures on both the frequency and intensity of the response over time has to be considered. It is feasible to partially control for this by comparing patients and controls at multiple time points. Lastly, it is important to obtain a drug history of patients being tested for DTH, as drugs can cause a false-negative reaction.

Attempts have been made to standardize the reagents used for the DTH skin tests, with the goal of being able to compare results from various patients and centers (7,16). For this reason, it is important to standardize the reagents used in a clinical trial by purchasing or preparing enough material of one lot to last for the entire trial. If a new lot must be used during the trial, crossover studies with normal controls should be instituted to ensure comparable results. Another source of variability relates to the antigen preparations: many require dilution prior to use, and diluted antigens can lose activity over time. Therefore, careful dating and expiration dates should be enforced with the antigen preparations for DTH skin tests.

One method to improve standardization is with the use of commercially available antigen impregnated strips available for DTH skin tests. One system is called the Multitest CMI (Connaught Laboratories, Inc., Swiftwater, PA). The use of this system helps control variability and allows comparison of results between laboratories. However, if DTH skin tests for tumor-derived antigens or peptides are performed, commercially standardized DTH preparations are unlikely to be available, and each investigator is responsible for the quality control of the antigen/peptide preparation used and for determining its reactivity in a group of healthy control individuals.

Because most tumor-derived antigens in humans contain epitopes shared among tumors of the same histologic type and are also expressed on normal tissue cells (4), it is expected that a proportion of normal individuals (i.e., those expressing the appropriate HLA restriction elements) will be responsive to these antigens. On the other hand, most patients with cancer, whose T cells may be specifically unresponsive to these antigens, are likely to be DTH negative. A well-documented conversion from DTH-negative to DTH-positive status as a result of vaccination or therapy is a highly significant event. The key is to have clearly documented evidence of the DTH conversion.

The DTH skin test is the only available in vivo measure of specific antitumor response, and its value in the overall assessment of antitumor competence cannot be overemphasized.

Signal Transduction Defects

The presence of functional unresponsiveness in T cells obtained from patients with advanced malignancies has been reported by numerous investigators (reviewed in 2). Fresh T cells isolated from the tumor site (i.e., TIL) were observed to be particularly compromised in cytotoxicity against autologous tumor as well as proliferative responses to mitogens or antigens relative to circulating T cells obtained from the peripheral blood of these patients or from normal controls (1,2). These functional defects were more recently related to the presence of abnormalities in expression and function of protein kinases responsible for signaling via the T-cell receptor (TCR) complex in lymphocytes of patients with advanced cancer.

Abnormal expression of the zeta chain, $p56^{lck}$, zap70, and other signal-transducing molecules appears to be reversible upon therapy of the patients with certain immunomodulating agents, including IL-2 (17). Furthermore, evidence was obtained indicating that normalization of signaling defects during immunotherapy predicts a favorable clinical response, at least in patients with melanoma (17). The level of abnormal expression of the zeta chain and other TCR-associated protein kinases in circulating T cells varies in different patients with cancer, suggesting that these differences could be useful as a measure of tumor-related immunosuppression. Thus, assays for signaling defects (by Western blot, flow cytometry of permeabilized T cells, or ELISA) based on the use of antibodies specific for these molecules represent a useful new addition to the repertoire of assays for evaluation of immunocompetence in patients with cancer (1,17).

Cytoxicity Assays

Cytotoxicity measurements have occupied a special place in the monitoring of patients with cancer, particularly those treated with immune therapies (18). There is good rationale for monitoring cytotoxicity in clinical trials of biologic agents, as they often tend to augment this effector function in many different cell types. The most commonly used assays for cytotoxicity involve a variety of effector cells: cytotoxic T cells, LAK cells, cells mediating antibody-dependent cellular cytoxicity (ADCC), NK cells, and monocytes (18).

Peripheral blood, body fluids, or bone marrow can be used for cytotoxicity assays. The specimens are generally collected in preservative-free heparin tubes, and MNC are obtained following Ficoll-Hypaque centrifugation. MNC should be used in the cytotoxicity assays as soon after collection as possible. If the separated cells must be stored, they can be held at 40°C for up to 18 hours. For cytotoxicity assays, fresh effector cells are preferred over cryopreserved cell preparations.

Depending on the type of cytotoxicity assay being performed, the separated MNC fraction containing effector cells or effector cell precursors may need additional treatment. For the preparation of cytolytic T cells (CTL), it is necessary to pre-incubate the separated mononuclear cells in the presence of specific antigens or cytokines. For example, one can stimulate PBMC in vitro with low levels of cytokines and antigen in expectation of generating antigen-specific CTL following 7 to 14 days of culture (18). LAK cells can be prepared by incubating cells with IL-2 for various periods of time (18). Separated MNC or purified NK cells (CD3–CD56+CD16+) can be used as effectors in NK activity assays.

Similarly, a variety of cell types, such as PBMC or purified monocytes, can be used for measurements of ADCC, with a caveat that effector cells mediating ADCC express Fc receptors (FcR). In PBMC, NK cells are the main effectors of ADCC. To rule out a monocyte contribution to ADCC, it is best to remove the adherent cells population from the PBMC prior to their use in ADCC assays. On the other hand, ADCC with monocytes works best when the effector cells are isolated from PBMC to prevent interference from other cell populations. A variety of methods based on adherence to plastic or nylon wool or negative selection by immunobeads are used to isolate monocytes (18).

The selection of target cells for cytotoxicity assays will depend on the type of test being performed. To measure CTL activity, autologous tumor cells or transfectants expressing the HLA restriction molecules and pulsed with the relevant antigen or peptide must be available. Non-MHC restricted activity of T cells, on the other hand, can be measured using tumor cell lines obtained from the American Type Tissue Collection (ATTC), fibroblasts, Epstein-Barr virus transformed cell lines, and mitogen-stimulated lymphocytes. For assays of NK activity, targets sensitive to NK killing, such as K562 cells, are generally used. For monocyte assays, a monocyte-sensitive but NK-resistant target is needed such as L929 or WEHI-164. LAK assays require NK-resistant target cells such as the Daudi cell line. For ADCC assays, NK-resistant target cells, such as P815, that have been precoated with tumor-reactive IgG antibodies are used. For most assays, the target cells of choice are radiolabeled with 51Cr; however, it is also possible to use a colorimetric assay in which target cell viability is assessed following incubation with effector cells.

In a standard cytotoxicity assay, a constant number of 51Cr-labeled target cells is co-incubated with varying numbers of effector cells in 96-well U-shaped microtiter plates. Effector to target (E:T) cell ratios range from 50:1 to 6:1. The length of time of incubation varies depending upon the type of assay. NK, CTL, and LAK assays are generally incubated for 4 hours, whereas monocyte assays are incubated longer (e.g., 18 hours). Supernatants are harvested, and counted in a gamma counter. Control wells that are obligatory include target cells alone to measure spontaneous isotope release and target cells lysed with a detergent to give the maximum isotope release. The percentage of isotype released is calculated using a standard formula for specific lysis (19). ADCC assays are set up using two sets of wells: one containing antibody-coated targets, the other containing uncoated targets. The level of ADCC is calculated by comparing the percentages of specific lysis in the two sets of wells.

To assure reliability of cytotoxicity data over time, it is crucial to have the assay conditions optimized and the assay performed under laboratory standard operating procedures (19). To control for daily interassay variability, a pool of cryopreserved PBMC obtained from a normal donor by leukopheresis is included in the daily assay. It is optimal if three donor preparations of cells are used, covering low, intermediate, and high levels of cytotoxic activity. However, selection of normal donors for these controls is not easy, and it necessitates screening of a large number of donors because the PBMC of most individuals do not cryopreserve without a substantial loss of cytotoxicity.

In addition to cryopreserved controls, it is advisable to have available a pool of normal donors willing to donate fresh PBMC as daily cytotoxicity controls (20). One suggested quality control program is to run daily three frozen controls (high, medium, and low) along with a fresh control. Prior to using either frozen or fresh controls, a sufficient number of preliminary assays must be performed to determine the mean plus or minus 2 standard deviations (SD) of the cytotoxicity level for each control cell. These levels are used in evaluating the daily QC program, as follows:

- If the fresh and frozen controls are outside 2 SD of the mean, the daily run is rejected.
- If all the frozen controls are out of range, and the fresh control is in range, the run is

accepted, as this tends to indicate that there is a problem with the frozen cells on that particular day.

- If the frozen controls are in range, and fresh control is out of range, the run is also accepted, because fresh controls can occasionally be out of range secondary to biologic variability, including infections, stress, or other conditions likely to modify immune responses (20).

Cytokine Production Assays

The ability of immune effector cells to produce and release cytokines in response to a stimulatory agent can be used as a monitoring strategy (7,21). This approach calls for incubation of cells alone (spontaneous production) or in the presence of an activating agent (stimulated production) and subsequent quantitation of cytokines in cellular supernatants. The former type of assay allows for the assessment of in vivo activation of cells by measuring spontaneous cytokine release. The latter allows for a measure of immunocompetence, the ability to respond to a universal stimulator by release of cytokines (22). Unlike cytotoxicity assays, which are difficult to perform with cryopreserved effector cells, cytokine production assays appear to be reproducible when either fresh or cryopreserved effector cells are used, allowing for batching of assays. The cytokine production assay can also be performed with separated subsets of PBMC, permitting monitoring of cytokine profiles in these cell subsets, and it lends itself especially well to serial monitoring. It can be performed on a single cell level in a modified version called the ELISPOT (23).

Cytokine quantitation in the supernatants obtained from cytokine production assays can be measured using either immunoassays or bioassays (22). There are a variety of both enzyme-linked immunoassays and radioimmunoassays available for the quantitation of cytokines (see Chapters 15, 35). There are numerous commercial kits available, and these offer the advantages of being easy to perform, reproducible within the same system, easy to standardize, and cost effective. In addition, cytokine production assays are not susceptible to inhibitors, which are often present in sera or body fluids of patients with cancer. Both immunoassays and biologic assays can be performed with cellular supernatants (22). The WHO standards are available, which can be used for standardization of these assays. An important caveat in using these assays is that substantial differences might be observed in the level of cytokine produced with kits obtained from different manufacturers. For this reason, each laboratory is obliged to use the WHO cytokine standards to quantitate the assay performance.

Cytokine bioassays have been available for a number of years and generally use cell lines that are sensitive to particular cytokines in regard to dependence or inhibition of growth and other factors (22). The cell lines can be purchased from the ATTC, but must be maintained in the laboratory. Bioassays detect only the biologically active form of a cytokine, and generally have greater sensitivity than immunoassays. However, they require much more hands-on labor, the results can be affected by inhibitors present in the sample, and they are much more difficult to standardize (24).

Evaluation and interpretation of cytokine production assays is difficult as there are not any universally accepted normal ranges (22,24). Many variables affect the values, including culture conditions, cell isolation methods, the stimulators used, and even the type of culture plates used. Therefore, it is crucial that the immunology laboratory standardize the assay conditions inhouse as much as possible. Normal controls should be run to establish ranges of activity, and a pool of cryopreserved cells should be prepared for control of interassay variability in a way similar to that previously described for cytotoxicity assays. Many variables have been reported as influencing in vitro cytokine production in normal individuals, including HLA-DR antigen expression, diet, medications such as corticosteroids and nonsteroidal anti-inflammatory drugs, and age. All of these factors reinforce the importance of establishing standard protocols and a well-planned and enforced laboratory quality control program.

Lymphocyte Proliferation Assays

These tests have been a part of immunopathology laboratories for many years and can still provide valuable information in the monitoring of patients with cancer (7,25). One of the proliferation assays most widely used for in vitro generation of antitumor effector cells is the mixed lymphocyte-tumor culture (MLTC), in which co-cultures of lymphoid cells obtained from a patient are set up at various E:T ratios and allowed to proliferate in response to irradiated AuTu or to fractionated AuTu antigens presented by appropriate antigen-presenting cells (APC). The assay depends on the presence among these lymphocytes of the tumor antigen-specific precursor T cells and on the ability of either the tumor or APC to process and present the antigen to these T cells in a way promoting their maturation and proliferation. Responding T cells will expand, provided the necessary cytokines are present to support proliferation. The assay may be used as a measure of the T-cell competence to respond to AuTu or as a means for generating tumor-specific CTL. The latter generally requires multiple courses of stimulation with the tumor or tumor-derived antigenic fractions and considerable expertise on the part of the laboratory to establish and maintain long-term lymphocyte cultures (26). Tumor cells may produce immunoinhibitory factors, and the overall success of any MLTC depends on the set of conditions designed to optimize response and diminish tumor-associated anergy.

Traditionally, proliferation assays are performed using Ficoll-Hypaque separated PBMC, in which the cells are stimulated with a variety of antigens, mitogens, or cytokines. Proliferation is generally assessed following the uptake of titrated thymidine as a measure of its incorporation into newly synthesized DNA. Novel additions to the traditional techniques include the use of whole blood assays, which have been shown to provide comparable results and significantly decrease the labor intensity of the assays. In addition, there are a number of non-radioactive methods available, including flow cytometry, which offers the advantage of also being able to determine the phenotype of the proliferating cells.

Proliferation assays are most informative when performed together with cytokine or cytotoxicity assays. As with other cellular assays measuring antitumor immunity, there are no established and expected normal ranges for MLTC or other proliferation assays. A quality control program can be established with cryopreserved and fresh normal control cells and used as previously described in these assays (25).

Quality Assurance in Monitoring of Antitumor Responses

Quality assurance (QA) incorporates a variety of laboratory procedures that monitor the overall ability of the laboratory to meet its quality goals (27). There are a variety of components that contribute to a successful QA program, including technical competence, a good quality control (QC) program, a dedication to quality, facilities, and resources capable of adequately supporting the objective, and the mechanisms for problem solving. Thus, QA does not apply to only one particular testing methodology, but rather the QC program for cellular assays must be part of an overall program in place for the immunopathology laboratory.

Establishing a QA program for cellular assays to evaluate antitumor immune responses is a difficult task (7). When the assays are used serially, as a part of monitoring of cancer patients receiving therapies, there are special challenges. To meet the challenge, a well-designed and rigorously maintained QC program is required in a monitoring laboratory. Such a QC program contains several components: definition of standard operating procedures (SOP), training of personnel, instrument maintenance, and review of quality and proficiency testing.

A variety of factors might affect test performance. For example, preanalytical variables affect all tests performed in any clinical laboratory, and include such factors as patient preparation, proper specimen identification, time of specimen collection, transport to the laboratory, and phlebotomy technique. For immune cellular assays, these variables can prove critical. It is preferable to routinely collect and harvest samples for cellular assays in the morning to avoid diurnal variability. It is important to carefully record the collection and arrival times of samples. The laboratory should have well-defined requirements for sample handling, collection times, and length of time following collection for the specimen to reach the laboratory. If these guidelines are not followed, the sample should be rejected.

As previously discussed, the decision to cryopreserve cells or use fresh cells has to be based on preliminary comparative studies, using fresh and cryopreserved lots of the same normal PBMC. This is a crucial decision for serial monitoring, because selection of the assays that can be batched (i.e., tested at the same time for all cells collected in the course of the clinical trial) will avoid day-to-day variability and considerably decrease the cost of monitoring.

Analytical sources of variability are major areas of concern in immune cellular assays (7,27). Using a comprehensive QC program can help assure good performance and provide a decrease in both random and systematic errors. Standardization of each assay has to be performed prior to offering it for monitoring. The importance of reproducibility of assays used for longitudinal monitoring cannot be overemphasized. The standardization data are generated by repeatedly performing the assay with cells obtained from normal individuals under the invariant and previously optimized experimental conditions to establish the mean, median, 80% normal range, and coefficient of variation.

For adequate determination of quality control parameters, the control materials should be run on at least 20 different days. Control charts can then be generated that are graphical displays of observed values indicating upper and lower control units. For commercially available cytokine immunoassays, it is also advisable to include the laboratory's own internal QC standard, as this can increase the user's confidence in the validity of the test results and uncover batch-to-batch variability in commercial kits. The laboratory performing these assays is encouraged to establish a QC program based on cryopreserved and fresh controls, as highlighted in the section on cytotoxicity assays.

In addition to inhouse QC, it is always advisable for the laboratory to participate in a proficiency testing program such as the one offered by the College of American Pathologists (CAP). However, this is difficult to achieve for immunology laboratories performing immune cellular assays in cancer patients. With the exception of flow cytometry quantitation of cell subpopulations, there are no external proficiency testing programs available. For this reason, it is even more critical that the laboratory establishes its own inhouse QC program.

Postanalytic variables include factors involved in test reporting (legible report, correct patient, etc.) and test interpretation (7,27). In the area of test interpretation, much remains to be accomplished, and this has been one of the most challenging aspects of measuring antitumor immunity. To provide the most meaningful interpretation of the data, clinical information is often needed, and this requires frequent interactions with the clinicians. It is crucial that there is a close working relationship between the clinical immunologist, statistician, and the clinician on the design of monitoring, its execution, and analysis of the data obtained.

Conclusion

Cellular assays for immune monitoring of patients with cancer, who may or may not be treated with immunotherapies, represent a considerable challenge to the laboratory. As the use of these therapies becomes more widespread, there may be increased opportunities for improved standardization, and increased interactions between different centers performing this type of testing. This would be a highly desirable and productive effort. As the use of molecular assays increases along with increased use of the flow cytometer as a way to monitor cellular events, it will become easier to improve assay performance and to develop improved methods for standardization between laboratories.

REFERENCES

1. Lai P, Rabinowich H, Crowley-Nowick PA, et al. Alterations in expression and function of signal transduction proteins in tumor associated NK and T lymphocytes from patients with ovarian carcinoma. Clin Cancer Res 1996;2:161–173.

2. Whiteside TL. Tumor infiltrating lymphocytes in human malignancies. Austin, TX: RG Landes, 1993.

3. Ioannides CG, Whiteside TL. T cell recognition of human tumors: implications for molecular immunotherapy of cancer. Short analytical review. Clin Immunol Immunopathol 1993;66: 91–106.

4. Boon T, van der Bruggen P. Human tumor antigens recognized by T lymphocytes. J Exp Med 1993;183:725–729.

5. Storkus WJ, Lotze MT. Tumor antigens recognized by immune cells. In: De Vita VT, Hellmann S, Rosenberg SA, eds. Biologic therapy of cancer. 2nd ed. Philadelphia: JB Lippincott, 1995:64–77.

6. Elder EM, Whiteside TL. Processing of tumors for vaccine and/or tumor infiltrating lymphocytes. In: Rose NR, de Macario EC, Fahey JL, et al., eds. Manual of clinical laboratory immunology. 4th ed. Washington, DC: American Society of Microbiology, 1992:817–819.

7. Whiteside TL, Hank JA. Monitoring of immunologic therapies. In Rose NR, Conway de Macario E, Folds JD et al., eds. Manual of Clinical Laboratory Immunology, Fifth Edition. Washington, DC: ASM Press, 1997:1065–1073.

8. Keren DF, Hanson CA, Hurtubise PE. Flow cytometry and clinical diagnosis. Chicago: American Society of Clinical Pathologists, 1994.

9. Riley RS, Mahin EJ, Ross W. Clinical applications of flow cytometry. New York: Igaku-Shoin, 1993.

10. Jung T, Schauer U, Heusser C, et al. Detection of intracellular cytokines by flow cytometry. J Immunol Methods 1993;159:197–207.

11. Far DF, Peyron JF, Imbert V, Rossi B. Immunofluorescent quantification of tyrosine phosphorylation of cellular proteins in whole cells by flow cytometry. Cytometry 1994;15: 327–334.

12. Sondel PM, Kohler PC, Hank JA, et al. Clinical and immunological effects of recombinant interleukin 2 given by repetitive weekly cycles to patients with cancer. Cancer Res 2988;48:2561–2567.

13. Elson LH, Nutman TB, Metcalfe DD, Prussin C. Flow cytometric analysis for cytokine production identifies T helper 1, T helper 2 and T helper 0 cells within the CD4+, CD27-lymphocyte subpopulation. J Immunol 1995;154:4294–4301.

14. Romagnani S. Biology of human Th1 and Th2 cells. J Clin Immunol 1995;15:121–129.

15. Prussin C. Cytokine flow cytometry: assessing cytokine production at the single cell level. Clin Immunol Newslett 1996;16:85–91.

16. Smith DL, DeShazo RD. Delayed hypersensitivity skin testing. In: Rose NR, de Macario EC, Fahey JL, et al., eds. Manual of clinical laboratory immunology. 4th ed. Washington, DC: American Society of Microbiology, 1992:202–206.

17. Rabinowich H, Banks M, Reichert T, et al. Expression and activity of signaling molecules in T lymphocytes obtained from patients with metastatic melanoma before and after IL-2 therapy. Clin Cancer Res 1996;2:1263–1274.

18. Whiteside TL, Rinaldo CR, Herberman RB. Cytolytic cell functions. In: Rose NR, de Macario EC, Fahey JL, et al., eds. Manual of clinical laboratory immunology. 4th ed. Washington, DC: American Society of Microbiology, 1992:220–230.

19. Whiteside TL. Measurement of cytotoxic activity of NK/LAK cells. In: Cohigan JE, Krubisbeek AM, Margulies DH, et al., eds. Current protocols in clinical chemistry. John Wiley, 1997: Unit 7.18.

20. Bryant J, Day R, Herberman RB. Natural killer cytotoxicity in the diagnosis of immune dysfunction: criteria for a reproducible assay. J Clin Lab Anal 1990;4:102–114.

21. Whiteside TL. Cytokines and cytokine measurements in a clinical laboratory. Clin Diag Lab Immunol 1994;1:257–260.

22. Friberg D, Bryant J, Shannon W, Whiteside TL. In vitro cytokine production by normal human peripheral blood mononuclear cells as a measure of immunocompetence or the state of activation. Clin Diag Lab Immunol 1994;1:261–268.

23. Tanguay S, Killion JJ. Direct comparison of ELISPOT and ELISA-based assays for detection of individual cytokine-secreting cells. Lymphokine Cytokine Res 1994;13:259–263.

24. Whiteside TL. Cytokine measurements and interpretation of cytokine assays in human disease. J Clin Immunol 1994;14:327–339.

25. Fletcher MA, Klimas N, Morgan R, Gjerset G. Lymphocyte proliferation. In: Rose NR, de Macario EC, Fahey JL, et al., eds. Manual of clinical laboratory immunology. 4th ed. Washington, DC: American Society of Microbiology, 1990: 213–219.

26. Miescher S, Whiteside TL, Carrell S, Von Fliedner V. Functional properties of tumor-infiltrating

and blood lymphocytes in patients with solid tumors: effects of tumor cells and their supernatants on proliferative responses of lymphocytes. J Immunol 1986;136:1899–1907.

27. Westgard JO, Klee GG. Quality management. In: Burtis CA, Ashwood ER. Textbook of clinical chemistry. 2nd ed. Philadelphia: WB Saunders, 1994:548–595.

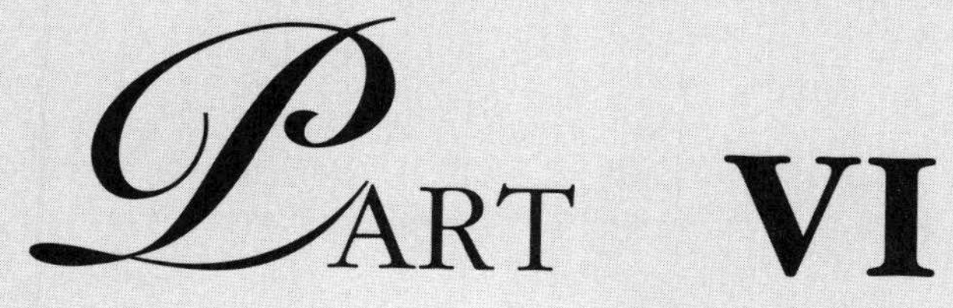

Part VI

Quality Assurance, Quality Control, and Standardization for Infectious Diseases

JOHN L. SEVER, EDITOR

CHAPTER 34

Quality Assurance and Standardization in Clinical Diagnostic Immunology: Immunologic and Molecular Assays for Human Immunodeficiency Virus

NEIL T. CONSTANTINE

Laboratory testing for the investigation of infection by the human immunodeficiency virus (HIV) is well established and has been implemented globally for over a decade. However, no other diagnostic inquiry has required the continual need for care, vigilance, and improvement for the immunology laboratory. The social implications and the medical consequences of classifying individuals as HIV infected have caused an unprecedented necessity for accurate laboratory results. Accordingly, quality assurance, quality control, and quality assessment strategies have been reexamined and refined in an effort to ensure that results are as accurate as the tests allow.

Regulatory agencies have revisited policies and have instituted extraordinary testing requirements to protect the blood supply and injectable therapeutics. In no other diagnostic arena have there been more regulatory agencies (e.g., FDA, AABB, NCCLS, CAP, and CLIA in the United States) tasked with providing guidelines to ensure the accuracy of tests and the testing process. Also, a changing health care system, economic limitations, and more challenging quality assurance requirements have contributed to significant changes in the diagnostic immunology laboratory.

Diagnostics for identifying and monitoring HIV infection continue to evolve, and additional assays have been implemented to address a number of needs for detection and testing effectiveness. In addition to the widely used serological tests, recent licensing by the FDA now offers the use of antigen assays, saliva tests, urine tests, and tests to quantify viral nucleic acids. The identification of a new HIV group (group O) that may be undetected by current serological tests has introduced additional diagnostic dilemmas and has driven manufacturers of test kits to modify tests for increased detection capabilities.

Recent recommendations from the Public Health Service regarding the institution of treatment within 2 hours of exposure have led some laboratories to adopt a rapid HIV assay to decrease turnaround times to be clinically relevant. The quest for maximizing the sensitivity to detect early HIV infection has resulted in efforts to bring new tests to clinical use, as exemplified by recent funding from the National Heart, Lung, and Blood Institute of the National Institutes of Health (NIH) to refine HIV nucleic acid assays for routine use in clinical laboratories (1) in an effort to reduce the window period where HIV infection cannot be detected. The licensing of viral load assays has resulted in a means to predict HIV outcome.

Although these tests contribute to the laboratory's arsenal for identifying, verifying, and monitoring HIV infection, they have introduced an increase in the laboratory's responsibilities. Thus, improvements in diagnostic capabilities, new challenges, and an increase in regulatory requirements have perpetually changed the immunology laboratory.

Characteristics during HIV Infection

Infection by HIV can be defined as the time at which the virus becomes established in the host after exposure. During the following 2 weeks, viremia is thought to increase exponentially until the antibody- and cell-mediated immune responses provide resistance. This time interval, the serological "window period," is characterized by seronegativity, occasionally detectable antigenemia, viremia, and variable CD4 lymphocyte levels. Detection of specific antibody to HIV signals the end of the window period and labels the individual as seropositive. The exact time when antibody can be detected depends on several factors, including the test used, individual host responses, and viral characteristics.

Importantly, antibody may be present at low levels during early infection but not at the detection limit of all assays, yielding an underrepresentation of the time of antibody production. Early generation HIV antibody tests could detect antibody in most individuals by 6 to 12 weeks following infection. Newer generation assays, including the third-generation antigen sandwich assays, can detect antibody in most individuals at about 3 to 4 weeks after infection (2). For testing blood donors, this interval translates to a current risk of acquiring HIV from seroconverting individuals to be between 1 per 440,000 and 1 per 640,000 transfusions (3). Most currently used FDA-licensed screening assays possess equivalent sensitivities, both for detecting persons with established infection (epidemiologic sensitivity) and for detecting low levels of antibody (analytical sensitivity) as occurs during seroconversion.

The detection and characterization of immune responses may also vary depending on individual differences. Most individuals respond in a highly characteristic manner, with antibody production occurring within several weeks to all major HIV core (p15, p17, p24, p55), polymerase (p31, p51, p66), and envelope (gp41, gp120, gp160) antigens. However, qualitative differences occur; some individuals never respond to several antigens (e.g., p17, p31). In most individuals, antibodies to p55 (core precursor) and/or p24 occur initially; however, reactions to these antigens may represent nonspecific reactions found in persons who are not infected (see the discussion of interpretation in "Western blot confirmatory assay").

Similarly, quantitative differences occur, with titers of specific antibodies varying from several-fold to greater than 100,000. In other cases, responses are uncharacteristic, with late responses or perhaps even an absence of antibody responses (4). Rarely, seroreversion has been observed (5), suggesting exposure to nonviable virus and antigens (without infection), or possible clearance of infection. It should also be noted that individuals who have received candidate vaccines will produce responses to those specific antigens without being infected.

Viral characteristics may account for variations in the exhibited immune responses between individuals. This is best exemplified by the classification of poor or absent responses in individuals who are infected but produce seemingly partial responses to viral variants. It has been well described that a number of individuals infected with HIV-2 produce negative or indeterminate results when tested by HIV-1 assays, and vice versa (6). Similarly, a number of serological assays, designed to detect antibodies to HIV-1 and HIV-2 have been shown to produce false-negative results when testing individuals infected with HIV-1 group O (7). This latter issue is responsible for the recent mandate by the US FDA for manufacturers of test kits to address group O by incorporating those antigens in future submissions of HIV test kits for licensure (personal communication).

Thus, the currently available antibody assays may produce misleading results in their effort to identify and characterize immune responses with variants of HIV.

Although HIV p24 antigenemia occurs prior to the appearance of antibody, the detection of antigen is often difficult due to the less than optimal sensitivity of current assays when testing blood (8). However, antigen detection signals infection, and positive results on seronegative individuals can be an effective, though not cost effective, means to identify early infection. Because of recommendations from the FDA, antigen tests are now part of the routine testing of blood targeted for transfusion (9). The institution of this assay in 1995 for screening blood donors in the United States was an attempt to offer a reduction in the window period over the best antibody tests (10). This inquiry can reduce the window period by about 1 week, and is thought to eliminate an additional 5 to 10 units of infected blood per year, resulting in a risk of infection of 1:700,000 (11); four cases of HIV transmission have been documented in antibody-negative individuals (12).

Finally, a new generation of tests is aimed at the detection of nucleic acids (RNA) in plasma by the reverse transcriptase polymerase chain reaction (RT-PCR) and is the newest addition to the diagnostic armamentarium for eliciting HIV infection. Viral RNA is produced shortly after infection is established, and suggests active viral replication. Detection of RNA levels by RT-PCR, although not used routinely for screening or diagnosis, offers the ability to reduce the window period by several additional days prior to antigen and antibody detection, resulting in the elimination of about 10 more infected units per year (13). The recent licensing by the US FDA of a viral load PCR assay now allows the direct quantification of viral RNA levels in plasma. This assay offers a better means to monitor infection during therapy and is a better predictor of disease outcome and death than the CD4 count (see below) (14).

In summary, for the screening of blood or for diagnosis, the current serological window period may be reduced to about 2 weeks if an all-inclusive testing strategy using p24 antigen and RNA detection methods is employed. The kinetic relationship of antibody production, p24 antigenemia, and HIV RNA levels is depicted in **Figure 34-1**. For monitoring HIV infection, antigen levels, RNA levels, and CD4 lymphocyte numbers provide a relatively good estimate of disease progression and outcome. In an infected individual, antigen levels, plasma viremia, and CD4 levels vary considerably during the early stages of infection, but follow predicable kinetics during progression toward AIDS. Antigen and RNA levels increase, while CD4 levels decrease.

The Role of the Immunology Laboratory for Diagnosis, Evaluation, and Monitoring of HIV and AIDS

After a decade of testing, nearly 1 billion tests, and positive results on more than 20 million individuals, the immunology laboratory continues to contribute effectively to the global effort to identify HIV/AIDS (15). The detection of specific antibodies to HIV antigens signals that infection has occurred and is the most widely used means for diagnosis, surveillance, and for protecting the blood supply. In most cases, these antibodies are easily identified in persons with established infection, making the diagnosis easy for the laboratory. However, antibodies may be present and not detectable by all methodologies, as occurs during seroconversion. In addition, antibodies to some HIV antigens may be demonstrable, but may not be qualitatively or quantitatively sufficient to meet the criteria for verification of infection. In these cases, the diagnosis becomes more challenging for the laboratory, and may require the use of ancillary tests and testing strategies.

An increase in vigilance and extraordinary measures in the laboratory, along with a thorough knowledge about antibody, antigen, CD4 levels, and nucleic acid characteristics (16) are essential for laboratory personnel to contribute to the potential for a correct interpretation of results. For example, acknowledgment of an increase in antibody idiotypes over time as demonstrated by paired Western blot testing, or recognition of an increase in the concentration (titer) of particular antibodies over time, can suggest seroprogression which may identify infection even prior to a positive classification using well-established diagnostic test criteria. Similarly, an understanding of test indices (e.g., predictive values) will allow for the proper selection of tests and test strategies for the population being tested, and a background knowledge of test principles allows for trou-

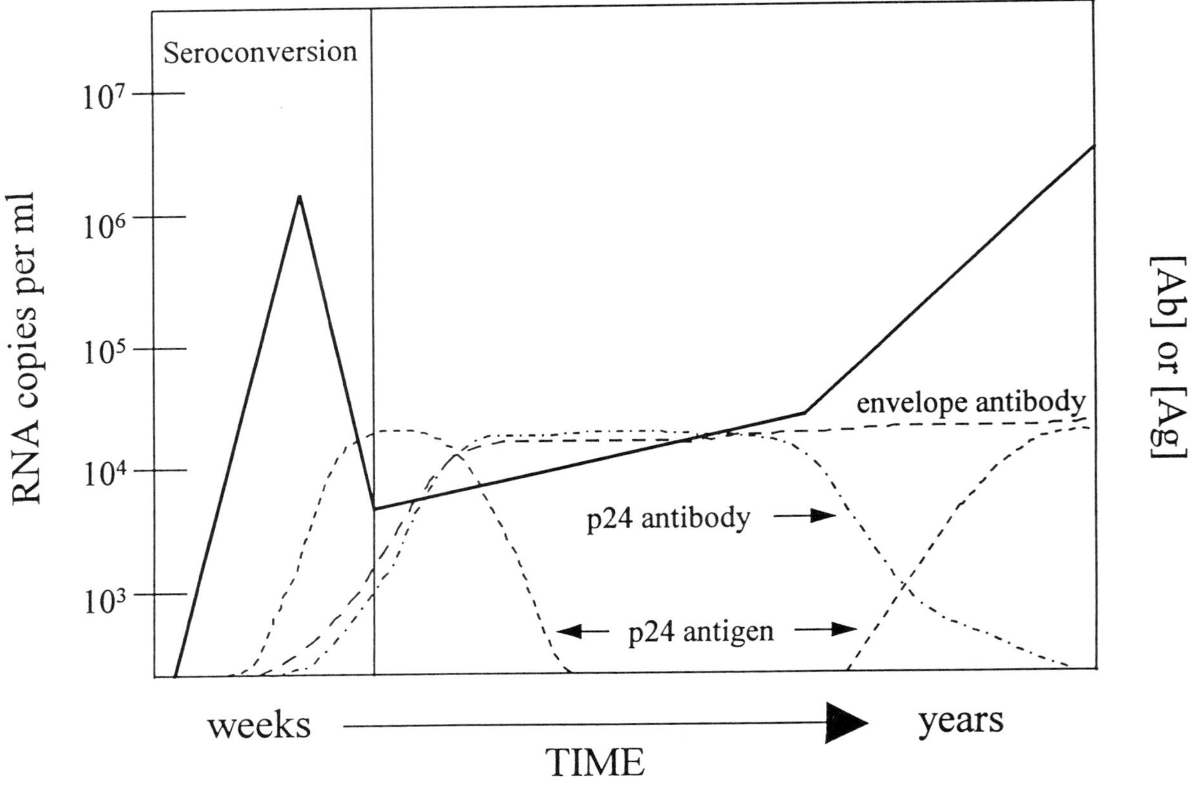

FIGURE 34-1

Kinetic relationships of antibody, antigen, and viral RNA during HIV infection.

bleshooting and the realization of test limitations.

Decisions made by laboratory personnel include the selection of tests, the use of appropriate testing strategies, the choice of criteria for confirming the presence of antibodies, and the extent of incorporation of essential quality assurance and quality control measures. In addition, personnel of the immunology laboratory must consider the adoption of the most cost effective tests depending on the population being tested, and cost effective testing strategies (e.g., for low-volume test situations, HIV-2 ELISA and Western blots should be sent to reference laboratories rather than be offered inhouse). Similarly, because regulations differ when testing blood donors (e.g., limitations for interpreting tests when using external controls, strict adherence to well-defined algorithms), it may not be cost and time efficient to offer blood donor testing, but rather to send these samples out. Finally, with the availability of a large number and variety of methodologies (e.g., saliva, urine, blood spot tests, PCR, antigen testing), it is the role of the laboratory to decide which tests and combination of tests will be the most effective, appropriate, and convenient to use.

Of paramount importance, the immunology laboratory has a responsibility and must take appropriate action to ensure that all measures related to the testing process are controlled and monitored in a way that will maximize the chances that reported results are correct; this includes all preanalytical, analytical, and postanalytical processes.

Rationale of Test Selection

Screening Tests

Immunologic tests must possess both sensitivity (to detect infection) and specificity (to detect noninfection). Tests with low sensitivity produce false-negative results, while tests with low specificity produce false-positive results.

Screening tests are designed to possess exquisite sensitivity to detect all infected individuals, while confirmatory tests possess excellent specificity to rule out noninfection. Algorithms that incorporate this strategy (screening tests followed by confirmatory tests) have been well-established and maximize the chances of obtaining a correct result. In the United States, the convention is to follow this strategy without deviation. In addition, the repeating of screening tests in duplicate prior to confirmatory testing minimizes the chances of technical error. In the United States there is little choice in the use of HIV testing algorithms; only the choice of particular screening and confirmatory methodologies can be made (see below).

Most HIV screening antibody tests currently licensed by the FDA have near-perfect and equivalent degrees of sensitivity for detecting most individuals who are infected with HIV (epidemiologic sensitivity). However, these tests may vary in their ability to detect low levels of antibody (analytical sensitivity) that occur during seroconversion (2). Although tests are available to detect specific HIV IgM antibody produced during early infection, these tests have shown little utility because IgM responses to HIV are not consistently produced during early infection (17). However, the ability of some tests (e.g., third-generation tests) to detect IgM antibody simultaneously with IgG detection may be responsible for their higher analytical sensitivity. The choice of these tests must be weighed against their higher cost and possible higher false-positive rate, and the particular population being tested—that is, blood donors in whom high sensitivity is advisable versus a low risk population in whom the chances of seroconversion are remote for diagnostic purposes. Similarly, the choice for HIV-1 (only) tests can be made for cost-savings in situations where the prevalence of HIV-2 is low.

However, for testing blood donors, screening for HIV-1 and HIV-2 is mandated by the FDA (18), and the choice of an HIV-1/2 combination assay (or individual HIV-1 and HIV-2 tests) is required. For public health, each laboratory must determine whether to use combination assays based on epidemiological data concerning the prevalence of HIV-2, or to offer only HIV-1 testing followed by specific HIV-2 testing on HIV-1 ELISA repeatedly reactive/Western blot negative or indeterminate samples (19). In this case, the selection of an appropriate algorithm must be made based on both epidemiologic and cost issues.

Concerning HIV-1 group O variants, currently licensed HIV screening tests are only about 80% effective in identifying infection by group O (12); therefore, there is little choice to maximize detection of these variants. However, manufacturers have begun to address this issue, and undoubtedly will offer in the near future modified tests designed to detect these variants.

In addition to screening tests that use serum or plasma, FDA-licensed saliva and urine HIV tests are available. Although these tests cannot be selected for screening blood, they offer advantages for diagnosis and epidemiologic investigations. In particular, they are applicable for point-of-care testing situations such as small clinics, physician offices, and in circumstances where phlebotomy is difficult or unavailable.

Similarly, the licensing of an ELISA test for use with blood samples collected via finger-stick allows for simple collection, and has been the basis of the availability of HIV home testing (collection) kits. The blood is collected on filter paper and mailed to a laboratory for ELISA testing. This alternative to conventional media for testing not only simplifies collection and can save on the cost of shipping blood tubes, but also is safer.

The recent recommendation by the Public Health Service for the institution of therapy within 2 hours of exposure to HIV-positive blood or body fluids (20) has underscored the importance of rapid HIV assays. Typical ELISA screening tests require at least 3 hours for completion, while rapid tests can be completed within 10 minutes. The adoption of rapid tests becomes especially attractive if an exposure occurs during hours in which the laboratory is closed, and personnel must be summoned late at night to perform one test on the source patient. However, these tests are more expensive than ELISAs, and their use may be cost effective only in exposure cases or where the total number of HIV tests per day is less than 10; they also may be useful in point-of-care testing situations where instrumentation is unavailable, for determining HIV status of women in labor (for institution of therapy), and for transplants.

Confirmatory Tests

Only a few confirmatory tests are available for verifying HIV infection. In the United States, the choice is between the Western blot and the Indirect Fluorescent Antibody (IFA) test. The selection is based primarily on personal preference; both are equivalent in cost and specificity, and both require subjective interpretation. Most laboratories choose the Western blot because reactivity to specific antigens allows for a careful analysis based on several parameters (e.g., intensity and specific profiles). In addition, expensive equipment (i.e., fluorescent microscope) are not needed. However, the IFA does offer the advantage of allowing resolution of some samples that exhibit indeterminate profiles by Western blot (see below) (21). Unlike screening tests, confirmatory assays do not have to be licensed by the FDA. Only when blood donor reentry is considered is a licensed confirmatory test required.

Monitoring Tests

For monitoring HIV infection, three methodologies are available: the CD4 count, p24 antigen quantitation, and viral load determination. Until recently, p24 antigen levels and CD4 lymphocyte levels were the primary laboratory markers used to monitor treatment effects and to determine prognosis. This has changed recently with the availability of assays to quantify the level of plasma HIV RNA. HIV RNA levels are inversely correlated with CD4 counts, and RNA determination is considered to have greater sensitivity than viral culture and p24 antigen.

Viral RNA concentrations above 100,000 copies per milliliter are considered to be predictive of rapid progression. The expected response following treatment is considered to be <5000 molecules or a >0.5 log decrease (22). It is suggested that the frequency of measurement be at baseline (two measurements at 2-week intervals, and every 3 to 4 months). In summary, the level of HIV RNA is a more powerful predictor of progression than the CD4 count, p24 antigen, and clinical parameters, and has a strong correlation between reduced RNA levels and response to therapy.

Nucleic acid tests are not designed as screening tests due to their inherent propensity for technical error or false results from contamination. However, recently the National Heart, Lung, and Blood Institute of NIH funded proposals to refine nucleic acid tests for use in clinical laboratories. It is anticipated that these tests will eventually become routine tests to be used in conjunction with antibody tests for detecting infection in blood units.

Test Methodologies, Limitations, and Interpretation of Results

Enzyme-Linked Immunosorbent Assays/Enzyme Immunoassays (ELISA/EIA)

For screening blood, most laboratories use ELISA methodologies based on the indirect or antigen sandwich principles; about 10 FDA-licensed ELISAs are commercially available (6). In the indirect method, antigen is attached to a microtiter plate well or to a bead, and antibody in the sample is allowed to react. Subsequent addition of a conjugate (an anti-human immunoglobulin labeled with an enzyme) reacts with the specific antibody attached to the antigens on the solid phase. Addition of an appropriate substrate results in color development, which is proportional to antibody concentration and is measured in optical density (OD) units by a spectrophotometer.

Alternatively, in the antigen sandwich method, antibody in the sample binds to both an immobilized antigen on the solid phase and to a labeled antigen (antigen conjugate). Both methods possess equivalent degrees of sensitivity for detecting most individuals with established infection; the antigen sandwich method has a slightly higher analytical sensitivity due to its ability to detect all isotypes of antibody (including IgM) (2). The antigen sandwich methods require larger sample volumes (e.g., 150 UL), making repeat testing or the testing of infants more difficult.

These screening tests have limitations due to their propensity for technical and biological false-positive results. Thus, they must be repeated in duplicate and subsequently followed by confirmatory tests. Optical density to cut-off ratios (OD/CO) above 1.0 signal a reactive result, although some laboratories incorporate a 10% to 20% "gray zone" in which a closer examination is considered warranted as a vigilant measure to detect individuals who may be in the seroconversion phase. The lack of a perfect specificity presents a problem when testing low-risk populations, as exemplified by the positive predictive value. For example, when testing a population of 1000 persons, a test having a specificity of 99% produces 10 biological false-positive results. If this population contains one truly infected individual, a positive result will be a correct result only 10% of the time (one true-positive for every 10 false-positive results). These limitations must be realized, and tests and testing algorithms must be selected carefully depending on the testing situation.

FDA-licensed screening tests that use saliva or urine are indirect ELISAs specifically designed for testing these media, and share the same characteristics as those used for testing blood. In general, these tests possess a higher degree of sensitivity to detect lower levels of antibodies as are found in crevicular fluid (saliva) and urine. Details describing the origin of antibodies in these media, the performance characteristics of the assays, and their limitations have been published (23–25).

Rapid HIV Screening Tests

The most widely used of the two FDA-licensed rapid HIV tests is the SUDS HIV-1. In this assay, antibodies react with microparticles coated with viral lysate and synthetic peptide antigens, and the particles are trapped on a membrane where a subsequent conjugate/substrate system produces a color reaction. This assay can be used for all testing purposes and has gained popularity for testing source patients in exposure cases. It possesses equal sensitivity and specificity to the ELISAs.

Although the test is extremely easy to perform, carelessness among users can cause inconsistent results, particularly when the timing of steps is compromised (when there are attempts to use multiple cartridges simultaneously) and when droppers are not held in a vertical position. A reaction grading template is supplied and should always be used to assist in the interpretation of results. One limitation of this assay is that it is designed to detect antibodies to HIV-1 only.

Western Blot Confirmatory Assay

The Western blot technique is based on the separation of a lysate preparation of viral components by SDS electrophoresis and transfer of the antigens to a nitrocellulose membrane. Thus, the viral components are separated based primarily on their molecular weights, and are supplied ready to use. Subsequently, reaction with antibody in serum and the use of an ELISA methodology produces "profiles" depicting reactivity to specific antigens, including gag proteins (p18, p24, p55), pol proteins (p31, p51, p66), and the gp41, gp120, and gp160 envelope gene products (**Fig. 34-2**). The presence of host cell proteins can cause the occurrence of nonspecific reactivity, making interpretation sometimes difficult. The most technically challenging procedural steps involve the elimination of cross contamination from splashing from one trough to another.

Several criteria exist for the classification of a positive Western blot profile (6). The most widely used is that of the CDC/ASTPHLD, which proclaims the presence of reactivity to any two of the following three antigens signaling a positive result: p24, gp41, and gp120/160. The FDA criteria, which include the inclusion of p31 in addition, are based on the kit manufacturer's criteria at the time of submission for approval. It is universally accepted that a negative result is the absence of all reactivity, although some organizations allow this classification with minimal nonspecific reactivity. The classification of "indeterminate" is reserved for those sera that produce reactivity that does not meet the criteria for negative or positive (i.e., inconclusive). The choice of criteria is user dependent for all testing situations except for the purposes of blood donor reentry. In the latter case, a licensed Western blot and the criteria dictated by the kit manufacturer must be used. In addition, for blood donors, the presence of any markings on the strip (i.e., non-

FIGURE 34-2

HIV-1 Western blot profiles: 1. Strong positive control. 2. Weak positive control. 3. Negative control. 4. Indeterminate result. 5. Indeterminate result, suggestive of HIV-2 infection.

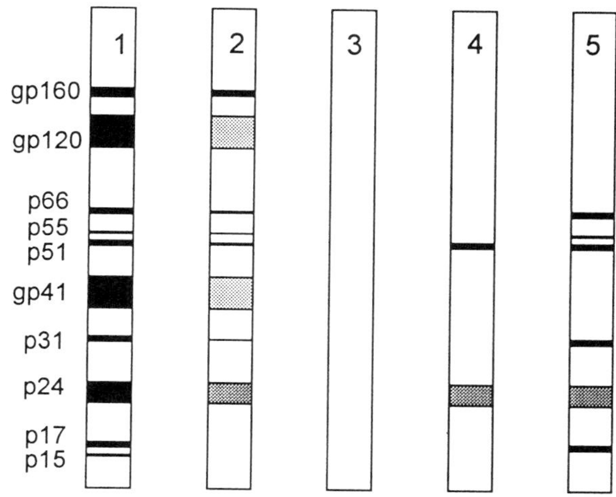

specific reactions, debris) without meeting the criteria for positive must be considered as a classification of indeterminate.

Indeterminate Western blot classifications present substantial concern, and result in a large number of inquiries to the immunology laboratory. This classification can be caused by specific reactivity to several HIV antigens, nonspecific reactivity to host-derived proteins, or weak intensity (+/−) reactions to any component. For the former and latter, reactivity that fails to meet the criteria for positive may signal early infection as during seroconversion, but may also represent nonspecific reactions to HIV antigens in individuals who are subsequently shown to be uninfected.

Indeterminate reactions due to a lack of sufficient numbers of bands (nonqualitative reactivity) can sometimes be suggestive of early infection, depending on the particular profile. For example, reactivity to several gag and pol gene products is much more likely to be from a seroconverting individual than a profile of p24 reactivity only. However, caution much be exercised, because reactivity to any one band can be exhibited during seroconversion. For weak reactivity to antigens (nonquantitative reactivity), some laboratories consider the reactivity as indicating the presence of that antibody when classifying the result as indeterminate, but do not include this reactivity in the criteria for classifying a Western blot profile as positive. For nonspecific reactivity to host proteins, some experts agree that if only nonspecific bands are present by Western blot, an extensively experienced laboratory can consider the sample as negative. However, many recommend that a more conservative approach be taken, with the classification of indeterminate when any reactivity is present. Many initially indeterminate results that subsequently become negative or remain indeterminate are probably a result of nonspecific reactions, hypergammaglobulinemia, the presence of cross-reactive antibodies, infection by HIV-2, or infection by an unknown but related retrovirus.

Some confusion exists in the interpretation of infection status when an individual is classified as negative by Western blot, while having a repeatedly reactive screening test result. In this case, and even with indeterminate Western blot classifications, many laboratory personnel will consider the screening test result to be a false positive. However, it is important to realize that the true status of this individual must remain unknown. Evidence shows that when testing seroconversion panels of sera, there are time points when screening test results are reactive while Western blot results are negative or indeterminate. Although the situation is rare, depending on the population of individuals being tested, negative and indeterminate Western blot results may represent early infection, and those individuals should be subsequently followed or tested by alternative methods (e.g., IFA) for resolution. In this case, the screening test is not producing a false-positive result, but is identifying true early infection.

Biological false-positive Western blot results have been documented. However, these are limited to profiles that meet the positive criteria only minimally (19). There have been several individuals whose sera exhibited reactivity to p24 and one of the envelope antigens only or to only envelope antigens, but who were later shown to be uninfected by HIV. For persons with such reactivity it is now advised to include a statement on the HIV report form: "This person meets the minimum criteria for confirmation of infection by HIV; however, in rare instances persons having this profile have been shown to be uninfected, so we strongly recommend that another sample be submitted for retesting after 1 to 3 months."

In addition, with the institution of vaccine studies, the use of candidate vaccines made from envelope glycoproteins (e.g., subunit gp160) can result in the production of antibodies that may misclassify a person as a confirmed positive when the individual is not truly infected. Conversely, false-negative Western blots also occur. These results can be due to early infection or to testing persons infected with HIV-1 group O variants (26).

Diagnostically, sera from individuals infected by HIV-2 can present problems when using HIV-1 Western blot results. Cross-reactions of antibodies against the heterologous viral antigens may occur, in most cases directed to the core and/or pol antigens because these are highly conserved between the two viruses. But a lack of definitive reactivity with heterologous viruses dictates the need for an extra measure of vigilance to identify infection. By HIV-1 Western blots, the results may be indeterminate with no reactivity to the envelope antigens of HIV-2, or may be completely negative. In the former, characteristic patterns may develop, as illustrated in Figure 34-2. In these instances, testing the serum using HIV-2 specific tests should be considered. Subsequent differentiation of HIV-1 and HIV-2 infections may require the use of highly specific ELISAs (e.g., synthetic-peptide–based), specific HIV-2 Western blots, radioimmunoprecipitation assays, or the polymerase chain reaction. Current algorithms require that negative or indeterminate results by an HIV-1 Western blot be further tested using specific HIV-2 tests. For HIV-2 confirmation, most organizations that have created criteria for positive HIV-2 Western blots agree on the necessity for reactivity to the envelope antigens. The World Health Organization requires reactivity to at least two HIV-2 envelope antigens, while other organizations require reactivity to p26 (gag) and gp34 or gp105 (env). If a specimen is tested by both HIV-1 and HIV-2 Western blots, the blot exhibiting the strongest reactivity to envelope antigens usually indicates which infection is present. Infection by both HIV-1 and HIV-2 viruses simultaneously (dual infection) can occur.

In all instances in which a person's serum exhibits a negative or indeterminate Western blot profile, the individual should be retested in 1 to 3 months for evidence of seroconversion or seroprogression (an increase in the number of antibodies present or in the intensity of reaction to antigens). Because seroconversion occurs in most individuals within several weeks, it is likely that retesting will result in a progression in reactivity over that time. However, because lot-to-lot variations occur in test kits, it is recommended that follow-up samples be tested in parallel with the original (stored) sample to make a direct comparison of profiles and minimize the chances of differences due to kit lots.

It is generally accepted that if a person does not seroconvert or seroprogress within 6 months, he or she can be considered to be noninfected with HIV (18).

Indirect Fluorescent Antibody (IFA) Confirmatory Test

In the IFA technique, immortalized human T lymphocytes infected with HIV are fixed to a microscope slide and allowed to react with specific antibodies. The presence of antibodies is detected using a fluorochrome-labeled conjugate, and is visualized using a fluorescence microscope. Separate wells of uninfected cells act as a control. As with the Western blot, indeterminate results may occur, especially when fluorescent patterns are uncharacteristic and when there is fluorescence in the uninfected cells.

This technique can be used as a confirmatory test or as a screening test in settings where enzyme immunoassays are not practical or available (21). It can also be used to resolve indeterminate Western blot results, with the IFA being definitive if positive or negative. It cannot, however, be used to negate Western blot results for purposes of donor reentry. Because the test is not conducive to handling large numbers of samples, and because the end point interpretation is operator-dependent, the IFA is not recommended for screening of blood.

It is highly recommended that laboratory personnel who perform the IFA be adequately trained and assessed to qualify as a reader. The IFA may not detect all HIV-2 infections, and appropriate algorithms must be used to resolve indeterminate results.

p24 Antigen Tests

The p24 antigen test methodology is a typical ELISA, but with an anti-p24 antibody, rather than antigen, attached to the solid phase. Repeatedly reactive results must be confirmed by a neutralization reaction to increase specificity in which the sample is pre-incubated with a monoclonal anti-p24 (neutralized serum). Subsequently, the p24 antigen test is repeated using both neat serum and neutralized serum, and the OD values are compared. Depending on the assay, at least a 50% reduction in OD of the neutralized serum is required to confirm the presence of true p24 antigen; other requirements may also be needed (e.g., high OD values).

The test can be of value in helping to diagnose infection in newborns (27) (see below) and in monitoring antiviral therapy (28). A major limitation is that the test is insensitive when testing blood, both because low levels of antigen are difficult to detect and because antigenemia is transient (8). Procedures to dissociate antigen-antibody complexes improve the sensitivity of the p24 test, but p24 antigen remains undetectable in most asymptomatic patients (29).

Viral Load Test

Although several varieties of nucleic acid assays are available to detect viral RNA in plasma, all are remarkably similar in sensitivity and reproducibility. However, only the Amplicor HIV-1 Monitor assay (Roche) is licensed for use. In this assay, a specimen-preparation step to purify RNA is followed by a combined reverse transcription and amplification step by PCR using a thermostable polymerase. Biotinylated primers allow the resultant amplicon, after hybridization to oligonucleotide probes bound to a microtiter plate, to be detected through a colorimetric reaction.

The incorporation of a quality standard allows control for inhibitors and the amplification process. The standard is a noninfectious RNA transcript with known copy number, and is subsequently captured by a unique probe. Comparison of the absorbance of the standard to that of the target allows for quantification.

A number of quality control measures are incorporated into the procedure to ensure that the test has performed as expected. In general, these consist of the observation that OD values are of a certain level, have decreased in dilution series, and that the quality standard values have not been abnormally decreased due to the presence of substances that are inhibitory to the amplification process. The ranges provided for the positive controls must be met for acceptability.

The manufacturer recommends that work flow proceed in a unidirectional manner, beginning in the reagent preparation area and moving through the specimen preparation area to the amplification/detection area. Limitations of the procedure include a detection limit of 400 RNA copies/mL, a linear response between 400 and 750,000 RNA copies/mL, and a precision having a coefficient of variation approaching 50%. In addition, there is concern that these assays are not adequate to detect all subgroups of HIV, including HIV-1 group O variants and HIV-2 (30).

Diagnosis of HIV Infection in the Newborn

The early diagnosis of HIV infection in the newborn has long been problematic due to the omnipresence of maternal antibody. However, recent advances in technology, particularly the detection of viral nucleic acid, have allowed better estimates of true infection and have offered prognostic capabilities. The use of either virus isolation or viral DNA detection methods has allowed a greater than 90% prediction of infection after 1 month of age (31) and a 97% prediction by 3 months (32). The detection of p24 antigen in newborns is less sensitive (50% to 80%) but can achieve similar sensitivities by 6 months. At birth, the combined use of p24 antigen, viral culture, and DNA PCR allows a prediction of infection of only 50%, although the specificity is 100% (33). A negative PCR result in the first month of life confirms noninfection with a probability of greater than 90% (34). For prognosis, viral load assays are reported to yield estimates of the risk of newborns to develop severe disease, with median DNA levels peaking about 3 months earlier (at 1 to 2 months) in children who by age 24 months developed severe disease, and can predict death at an early age (35).

The institution of quality assurance measures for amplification techniques (i.e., DNA PCR) is paramount. Because of intra-run, inter-run, inter-laboratory, and inter-lot variations in the assay, it is recommended to obtain at least two similar results by independent laboratories to verify the HIV status in newborns; one result is presumptive (36). Similarly, a negative DNA PCR result should be confirmed. It has been reported that extraordinary measures, such as diluting sera to reduce the presence of inhibitors, can increase the sensitivity of PCR methods (35).

In summary, advances in technology and the combined use of several methodologies allow early detection of HIV infection and offer some prognostic value. However, these techniques are sophisticated and require careful and dedicated quality assurance measures.

Test Algorithms

Test algorithms for the diagnosis of HIV infection are well-established and essentially standardized. Algorithms for the testing of blood donors and for reentry into the donor pool are more complicated, and are described elsewhere (18). For diagnosis, initially reactive screening test results are followed by repeat testing in duplicate to minimize the chance of technical error; at least two reactive results of the three signify a repeatedly reactive result. Reflex testing to the Western blot or IFA is aimed to confirm that the screening test result is correct. A negative result by these tests can be reported as negative (although one should realize that in a high risk population this could represent early infection). Positive confirmatory results indicate infection, while indeterminate results require follow-up testing or testing by other methods. Follow-up testing is the best means to resolve indeterminate results, and should be conducted within 1 to 3 months, but may require longer periods for resolution. As mentioned, the IFA may be used to help resolve indeterminate Western blot results. Alternatively, p24 antigen testing and nucleic acid tests may be of help. The presence of p24 verifies infection, while a negative p24 test does not rule out infection due to its relative lack of sensitivity when testing blood (17). Tests to detect HIV RNA should not be used for diagnosis, but information obtained from these tests may be used to suggest early infection.

Sample Requirements

For all antibody and antigen tests, either serum or plasma may be used; these samples should be processed and stored as for all immunologic assays. Viral load testing requires the use of plasma samples obtained from EDTA or ACD anticoagulated blood; heparinized specimens are unsuitable for use. The whole blood can be stored at 2° to 25°C for no longer than 6 hours without refrigeration. Plasma should be separated from cells within 6 hours of collection; it can be stored at room temperature for up to one day, at 2° to 8°C for up to 5 days, or frozen at −20°C. The use of ACD specimens will yield test results that are about 15% lower than those of EDTA specimens.

Controls, Standards, Available Reference Preparations

A number of preparations that can be used to assist in the monitoring of HIV test performance on a routine basis are available commercially. Alternatively, preparations can be assembled in-house and tailored to the laboratory's needs (e.g., made to contain multiple analytes). These reagents offer a means to estimate precision and can be used to monitor assay systems for random, systematic, and technical errors. Their use allows for the monitoring of the test procedure to provide added confidence that the assay system is performing as expected and that the values assigned to unknowns are correct. These preparations are quality control reagents, and offer a means for identifying inconsistencies and problems that may arise due to small changes, such as variations in temperature, pipetting techniques, and other procedural steps. They can be used to monitor assay performance by targeting intra-run, inter-run, inter-technologist, lot-to-lot variations, trends, shifts, and other biases, and can be used to compare a laboratory's performance to that of others. Importantly, these reagents can be used as a means to detect variations in different test kit lots (e.g., sensitivity); such variations have been documented (37). In summary, controls can be used for training purposes, to verify acceptance of reagents and kits, to evaluate different test kits, to troubleshoot assay systems, and as a means to assess proficiency. These standards must be assayed identically to unknown samples, and resultant values must be evaluated statistically for acceptability.

Commercial preparations are available from several sources, and usually consist of human plasma that has been chemically modified to remove unwanted materials and ensure stability by using preservatives, stabilizers, and antimicrobial agents (38). They are usually configured in 5 or 20 mL sizes, allowing use in multiple run monitoring. Most of these reagents have been prepared from dilutions of several reactive human source materials, but undiluted reagents are available and may be important as it has been reported that the sensitivity of HIV antibody tests with diluted samples does not correlate with their sensitivity with naturally occurring low reactive sera (39). These reagents may not have assigned values (e.g., OD/CO) but are accompanied by charts showing reactivity by several manufacturers' test kits as a means to give representation of typical test procedures; each laboratory must establish its own performance characteristics. A description of the use of these reagents as external controls is presented below.

Seroconversion panels, which are available from several commercial companies, allow for comparison of sensitivities of different test kits. However, it should be emphasized that certain test kits perform excellently with some panels but less well with others (2); therefore, it is important to evaluate a particular test using several seroconversion panels. Low performance panels are also available and offer highly characterized specimens over a wide range of reactivity; these can be efficiently used to monitor technicians' performances or to assess proficiency when training or retraining is needed.

Finally, quality assessment panels of sera are available from several organizations such as the CDC and College of American Pathologists (CAP). These panels are sent to laboratories as an external proficiency program designed to determine the ability of the laboratories to accurately test samples and report results. Most are sent quarterly, with feedback of proficiency provided and comparison to that of other laboratories. Poor proficiency on the CAP proficiency panels can jeopardize a laboratory's accreditation.

The commercial preparations can be obtained from the following partial list of sources: Boston Biomedical, Inc., West Bridgewater, MA; Blackhawk Biosystems, Inc., San Ramon, CA; Serologicals, Inc., Marietta, GA; and North Atlantic Biologicals, Inc., Boca Raton, FL.

Quality Control Guidelines

Quality control (QC) refers to those specific measures that ensure that a test is performing to the degree that it was designed. Such measures include careful inspection to validate internal (kit) control values, monitoring of physical parameters (temperatures, functioning of equipment), validation of new reagents (different kit lots), and using additional measures such as external controls to verify the manufacturer's claims (the use of external controls is recommended but not required). A detailed description of quality control measures and related calculations for monitoring HIV tests has been published (6).

The most important quality control measures for HIV testing are the monitoring of assay performance using internal kit controls and the following of manufacturer's recommendations. Next in importance is the institution of an external control system to monitor all aspects of the test, including the performance of the internal controls. Importantly, quality control is only one part of a quality assurance program aimed at ensuring that a suitable specimen was obtained, the correct specimen was tested, the test was performed accurately, and results were reported correctly.

The monitoring of internal kit controls is most often accomplished automatically by the associated instrumentation. Such calculations will indicate acceptability or rejection. Rejected runs cannot be salvaged, and must be repeated after appropriate troubleshooting to determine the cause. Although acceptable runs allow the reporting of results, the values of the internal controls should be examined in relation to previous runs to determine if trends are occurring. Such trends, signaled by optical density changes in one direction over time, may alert personnel to test systems that are about to fail or that may be "near misses." Although rare, it is possible that low internal control values can cause a weakly reactive sample to react just below the cut-off value. This has been documented in ELISA systems (40), and is most likely due to the artificially stabilized kit controls which will cause a fairly constant cutoff while sample signals vary to a greater degree. In fact, in simulated situations, kit controls indicated an invalid run in 13%, as compared to an external control which warned of a problem in at least 63% of the runs. Because of the ability of external controls to detect minor, but sometimes significant changes, the use of these reagents is highly recommended and is discussed below. To further monitor internal controls, controls from one lot should be tested in parallel with new kit lots to ensure that reactivity is as expected.

Controversy exists concerning the use of external controls (37,41). Many institutions, and organizations such as the ASTPHLD have recommended external controls be used to detect variability in test kits (6,19). On more than one occasion, test kits which have been released for use have been found to be incapable of performing as expected (for detecting low levels of antibodies) by observing performance using external controls (37). Their use may also be important for detecting errors or equipment malfunction in the latter part of a test run (where internal kit controls are not placed), and for detecting pipetting errors by automated equipment (in test systems where the kit controls are not subjected to the same dilution steps). Conversely, the FDA has indicated that the use of external controls can be used as a supplement to kit controls, but they do not consider their use as absolutely necessary to ensure proper kit performance (40). In fact, the FDA will not allow the performance of external controls to invalidate a test run containing a reactive sample (42).

Nevertheless, the author and others strongly recommend that external controls be used in all HIV assays, particularly the ELISA. To be most effective, this control should be tested in each run, on each plate, and in duplicate; this will allow for monitoring of inter-run variability, intra-run variability, and intra-plate variability, respectively. Inter-run variability checks can detect lot to lot (inter-lot) variations or kit-to-kit (inter-kit) variations (one kit could be damaged during shipment). Intra-run variability can be caused by equipment malfunction (e.g., inconsistent washer or dilutor), while intra-plate variability may be due to varying incubation times or equipment malfunction. Consistently divergent values in the same direction between the duplicate external controls, which should be run at the beginning and at the end of each plate, can signal a deteriorating conjugate (personal observation).

The statistical methods used for establishing acceptability of external controls must be determined by each laboratory. Some general guidelines are presented as to the most used methods. To establish target ranges, the external control should be tested in replicate on multiple test runs (at least 20 runs), by multiple test kit lots (usually three), and by several operators. From the resultant values, a mean and standard deviation are determined. For subsequent runs, it is expected that the external control values will fall on both sides of the mean with essentially equal frequency. Also, it is expected that the values should be within 2 standard deviations 95% of the time; 5% of the time the values will be outside this range due to random error (not due to test kit or operator error). Values between 0 to 2 standard deviations indicate that the run is performing as expected, while values above +2 or below −2 standard deviations are an alert that there may be a problem and an investigation should be performed. Values outside of 3 standard deviations should be considered as a failure, and the run rejected; an appropriate investigation should be performed before repeating the run. Results that fall outside of acceptable limits are most often due to pipetting technique, variations in assay conditions (most often temperature), cross contamination, improper instrument operation, deterioration of test kits, or variations in test kit lots. **Figure 34-3** is an example of a Levey-

FIGURE **34-3**

Levey-Jennings chart showing shifts and trends as detected by an external control.

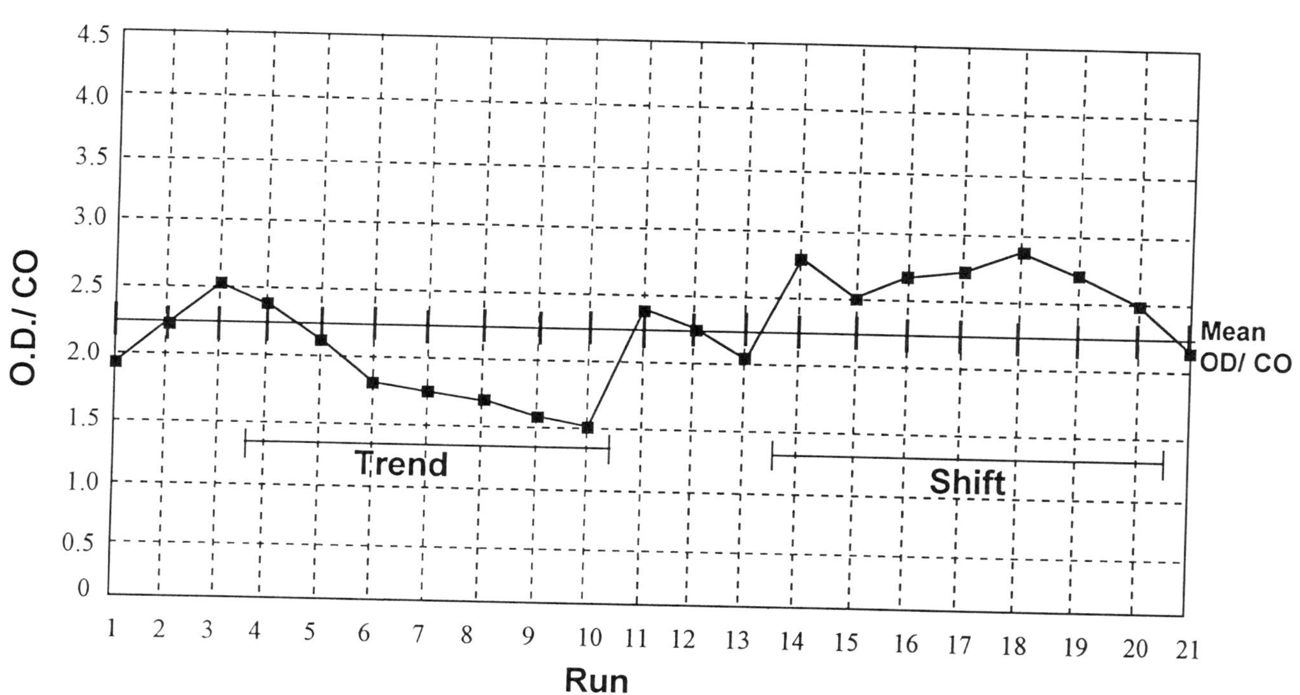

Jennings chart used to monitor external controls; details for setting up such a chart can be found elsewhere (43). Trends occur when at least 6 consecutive points (runs) fall in one direction, and signal slowly deteriorating reagents or a pipet slowly losing its calibration. Shifts are defined as at least 6 consecutive points falling on one side of the mean. This may suggest a major change such as changing to a new kit lot, new reagents, substantial changes in incubation temperatures, changes in equipment, or perhaps even variations in technique by a different technologist (6,44).

Quality Assurance Recommendations

Quality assurance (QA) is an overall program that ensures that correct results are reported on the correct patient. The components of this program for HIV testing do not differ from those of other analytes in any clinical laboratory. CLIA 1988 regulations (in Code of Federal Regulations 42 CFR 493.1701) recommend that each laboratory establish and follow written policies for QA programs. The FDA considers blood as a manufactured product, and this has prompted the AABB to increase emphasis on QA programs by having a written quality plan that includes description of the QA and improvement process, mechanisms for detecting errors, a means to identify and institute suitable corrective action, and the need for reassessment after corrective action has been taken. Other regulatory agencies (e.g., state agencies) may have additional requirements for QA programs.

Laboratory quality assurance includes all aspects from receipt of specimens through final reporting. Specimens must be inspected upon arrival for suitability; logging, processing, and review of all accompanying paperwork must be carefully performed and monitored. Also included are an organized record-keeping system, standard operating procedure manuals to act as references, a continuing education program, supervisory review of results, a system for the evaluation of laboratory personnel, use of the most appropriate tests/strategies, a mechanism for timely reporting, compliance with regulatory requirements, storage of specimens for follow-up testing, appropriate reporting forms, variance reporting for errors/inconsistencies, a good management system, and, of course, a good quality control and quality assessment program. General measures to ensure quality in the clinical immunology laboratory can be found in other chapters of this book and elsewhere (45). It is recommended that all documented quality assurance measures be followed, with continual assessment and improvement.

REFERENCES

1. HL&B proposal. RFP NHLBI-HB-95-09; Refinement of New Assays for National Heart, Lung, and Blood Institute, NIH, July 1996.
2. Constantine NT, van der Groen G, Belsey E, et al. Sensitivity of HIV antibody assays as determined by seroconversion panels. AIDS 1994;8: 1715–1720.
3. Dodd R. Should we do more? Advance 1995; 1:8–9.
4. Salahuddin SZ, Groopman JE, Markham PD, et al. HTLV-III in symptom-free seronegative persons. Lancet 1984;2:1418–1420.
5. Farzadegan H, Polis MA, Wolinsky SM, et al. Loss of human immunodeficiency virus type (HIV-1) antibodies with evidence of viral infection in asymptomatic homosexual men. Ann Intern Med 1988;108:785–790.
6. Constantine NT, Callahan J, Watts DM. Retroviral testing: essentials for quality control and laboratory diagnosis. Boca Raton, FL: CRC Press, 1992.
7. Loussert-Ajaka I, Ly TD, Chaix ML, et al. HIV-1/HIV-2 seronegativity in HIV-1 subtype O infected patients. Lancet 1994;343:1393–1394.
8. Goudsmit J, de Wolf F, Paul DA. Expression of human immunodeficiency virus antigen (HIV-Ag) in serum and cerebrospinal fluid during acute and chronic infection. Lancet 1986; 2:177–180.
9. FDA Memorandum. Recommendations for donor screening with a licensed test for HIV-1 antigen. Washington, DC: August 8, 1995.
10. Dodd R. For safety's sake. Advance 1995;1: 47–50.
11. HIV-1 antigen test implementation guidance. AABB Association Bulletin #96-2: January 5, 1996.
12. Dixon NR. Global goals of today's blood banks. Adv/Lab Med 1996;Oct:20–30.
13. Busch MA. HIV and blood transfusions: focus on seroconversion. Vox Sang 1995;67:13–18.

14. Mellors JW, Rinaldo CR, Gupta P, et al. Prognosis in HIV-1 infection predicted by the quantity of virus in plasma. Science 1996;272:1167–1170.

15. Constantine NT. HIV testing revisited. Adv/Lab Med 1995;May:16–25.

16. Constantine NT. Quantifying viremia: viral load testing offers important information. Clin Lab News 1997;November:8–10.

17. Constantine NT. Serologic tests for the retroviruses: approaching a decade of evolution. AIDS 1993;7:1–13.

18. Revised recommendations for the prevention of human immunodeficiency virus (HIV) transmission by blood and blood products. FDA Memorandum: April 23, 1992.

19. ASTPHLD. Recommendations from the 11th Annual Conferences on Human Retrovirus Testing (Report), Orlando, Florida, March 1996.

20. Centers for Disease Control and Prevention. MMWR Morb Mort Wkly Rep June 7, 1996.

21. Use of fluorognost HIV-1 immunofluorescent assay (IFA). FDA Memorandum: April 23, 1992.

22. Saag, et al. HIV viral load markers in clinical practice. Nat Med 1996;2:625–629.

23. Tamashiro H, Constantine NT. Serologic diagnosis of HIV infection using oral fluids. Bull WHO 1994;72:135–143.

24. Desai S, Bates H, Michalski FJ. Detection of antibody to HIV-1 in urine. Lancet 1991;337:183.

25. Connell JA, Parry JV, Mortimer PP, et al. Preliminary report: accurate assays for anti-HIV in urine. Lancet 1990;335:1366.

26. Gurtler LG, Zekeng L, Simon F, et al. Reactivity of five anti-HIV-1 subtype O specimens in six different anti-HIV screening ELISAs and three immunoblots. J Virol Methodol 1995;51:177–184.

27. Lange JM, Paul DA, Huisman HG, et al. Persistent HIV antigenaemia and decline of HIV core antibodies associated with transition to AIDS. BMJ 1986;293:1459–1462.

28. Spector SA, Kennedy C, McCutchan JA, et al. The antiviral effect of zidovudine and ribavirin in clinical trials and the use of p24 antigen levels as a viral marker. J Infect Dis 1989;159:822–828.

29. Hammer S, Crumpacker C, D'Aquila R, et al. Use of virologic assays for detection of human immunodeficiency virus in clinical trials: Recommendations of the AIDS Clinical Trials Group Virology Committee. J Clin Microbiol 1993;31:2557–2564.

30. Gurtler LG. Difficulties and strategies of HIV diagnosis. Lancet 1996;348:176–179.

31. Scarlatti G. Paediatric HIV infection. Lancet 1996;348:863–868.

32. Bremer JM, Lew JF, Cooper E, et al. Diagnosis of infection with human immunodeficiency virus type 1 by a DNA polymerase chain reaction assay among infants enrolled in the women and infant's transmission study. J Pediatr 1996;129:198–207.

33. Burgard M, Mayaux MJ, Blanche S, et al. The use of viral culture and p24 antigen testing to diagnose human immunodeficiency virus infection in neonates. N Engl J Med 1992;327:1192–1197.

34. Haas J, Geiss M, Bohler T. False-negative polymerase chain reaction-based diagnosis of human immunodeficiency virus (HIV) type 1 in children infected with HIV strains of African origin. J Infect Dis 1996;174:244–245.

35. Brandt CD, Sison AV, Rakusan TA, et al. HIV DNA blood levels in vertically infected pediatric patients: variations with age, association with disease progression, and comparison with blood levels in infected mothers. J Acquir Immune Defic Syndr Hum Retrovirol 1996;13:254–261.

36. Nesheim SR. The diagnosis and management of perinatal HIV infection. Clin Obstet Gynecol 1996;39:396–410.

37. Linden JV, Wethers J, Dressler KP. Controversy in transfusion medicine: use of external controls in transmissible disease testing: pro. Transfusion 1994;34:550–551.

38. Blackhawk BioSystems, Inc. Virotrol I (package insert) San Ramon, CA: 1995.

39. Boston Biomedical. The sensitivity of HIV antibody test kits with diluted samples does not correlate with their sensitivity with naturally occurring low reactive sera. Technical Bulletin #1. West Bridgewater, MA: 1993.

40. Boston Biomedical. Detection of error in infectious disease testing-kit validation criteria versus independent control values. Technical Bulletin #6. West Bridgewater, MA: 1995.

41. Epstein JS. Controversy in transfusion medicine: use of external controls in transmissible disease testing: con. Transfusion 1994;34:552–553.

42. Recommendations for the invalidation of test results when using licensed viral marker assays to screen donors. FDA Memorandum: January 3, 1994.
43. Boston Biomedical. The use of Levey-Jennings charts for run control. Technical Bulletin #3. West Bridgewater, MA: 1993.
44. Boston Biomedical. Troubleshooting EIA assays—what to do when Accurun 1 multi-marker control is out of range. Technical Bulletin #5. West Bridgewater, MA: 1996.
45. Guide to inspections of infectious disease marker testing facilities. FDA: June 1996.

CHAPTER 35

Syphilis

SANDRA A. LARSEN
WILLIAM E. MORRILL

The pathogenic treponemes, *Treponema pallidum*, subspecies *pallidum* (syphilis), *T. pertenue* (yaws), *T. endemicum* (nonvenereal endemic syphilis), and *T. carateum* (pinta) are morphologically, serologically, and chemically indistinguishable (1,2). Moreover, molecular approaches, such as DNA sequencing, DNA probes, and polymerase chain reaction (PCR) techniques have failed to differentiate between the pathogenic treponemes. The diseases are separated based on geographic location of the individual when infected, distinctive lesions, the age of populations infected, mode of disease transmission, and progression of disease (3). In the United States, syphilis is the treponemal disease most frequently encountered.

Test Selection

Untreated syphilis may become a chronic infection with diverse clinical manifestations, occurring in distinct stages. The manifestations of syphilis are easily confused with other diseases and conditions when laboratory tests are not performed. In early syphilis, the skin lesions are frequently mistaken for other dermatoses, whereas the symptoms associated with late syphilis may be mistaken for other neurologic or cardiologic conditions. Unlike agents causing most other bacterial infections, *T. pallidum* cannot be cultured. Therefore, alternative methods for detection of the treponemes or antibodies against *T. pallidum* subspecies have been developed (**Table 35-1**). The use of animal infectivity tests and most DNA-based antigen detection tests are now limited to the research laboratory.

In early syphilis (primary and secondary stages) and congenital syphilis, direct detection of the organism is the most specific and easiest means for diagnosis. A positive result by darkfield examination or by direct fluorescent antibody for *T. pallidum* (DFA-TP) in lesion exudate or in tissue (DFAT-TP) is definitive evidence of syphilis. In addition, preliminary results with the Multiplex PCR test indicate that a reactive PCR test is definitive evidence of syphilis (4). For persons with no previous history of syphilis, diagnosis may be based on the presence of a typical lesion(s); a reactive nontreponemal test such as the Venereal Disease Research Laboratory (VDRL) or rapid plasma reagin (RPR); and a reactive treponemal test, such as the fluorescent treponemal antibody-absorption (FTA-ABS) or microhemagglutination assay for antibodies to *T. pallidum* (MHA-TP). For persons with a previous history of syphilis, a fourfold increase in titer in a quantitative nontreponemal test suggests a recent infection.

In the early latent stage of syphilis, the disease progresses from an acute to a chronic infection. Because lesions are not present in latent syphilis, the diagnosis is based on reactive serologic results for both the nontreponemal and treponemal tests, or a fourfold increase in titer for a person with a history of syphilis.

Late syphilis may occur as benign late syphilis, cardiovascular syphilis, or neurosyphilis. The nontreponemal tests may be nonreactive in late syphilis; therefore, treponemal tests should be performed regardless of non-

TABLE 35-1
Diagnostic Tests for Syphilis

Direct Microscopic Examination
Dark-field
Direct fluorescent antibody for *Treponema pallidum* (DFA-TP)
Direct fluorescent antibody tissue test for *T. pallidum* (DFAT-TP)
Nontreponemal
Venereal Disease Research Laboratory (VDRL) slide
Unheated serum reagin (USR)
Rapid plasma reagin (RPR) 18-mm circle card
Toluidine red unheated serum test (TRUST)
Nontreponemal antibody enzyme-linked immunosorbent assay (ELISA)
Treponemal
Fluorescent treponemal antibody absorption (FTA-ABS)
Fluorescent treponemal antibody absorption 19S IgM (FTA-ABS 19S IgM)
Fluorescent treponemal antibody absorption double-staining (FTA-ABS DS)
Microhemagglutination assay for antibodies to *T. pallidum* (MHA-TP)
Treponemal IgG antibody enzyme-linked immunosorbent assay (ELISA)
Antigen Detection Test
Rabbit infectivity testing (RIT)
Polymerase chain reaction (PCR) for *T. pallidum*

treponemal test results when late stage syphilis is suspected. In benign late syphilis, lesions are present and should be examined for treponemes using DFAT-TP. The diagnosis of cardiovascular syphilis is based on symptoms of aortic insufficiency or aneurysm, reactive serologic test results, and no known history of treatment for syphilis. A definitive diagnosis of neurosyphilis consists of a reactive serum treponemal test, a reactive VDRL-cerebrospinal fluid (CSF) test or identification of *T. pallidum* in tissue or spinal fluid. A presumptive diagnosis of neurosyphilis requires a reactive treponemal test with a serum sample, a CSF cell count of >5 mononuclear cells/cc, and CSF total protein >45 mg/dL.

Congenital syphilis is the result of intrauterine infection of the fetus with *T. pallidum*. The definitive diagnosis of neonatal congenital syphilis is based on the demonstration of *T. pallidum* in umbilical cord, placental, nasal discharge, or skin lesion material. Otherwise, diagnosis is based on reactive nontreponemal and treponemal test results with clinical signs or symptoms of congenital syphilis, an abnormal CSF finding without other cause, or a reactive immunoglobulin M (IgM) antibody test specific for syphilis when the infant's serum is used.

To measure the efficacy of treatment, use quantitative nontreponemal tests. Success or failure of treatment for early syphilis is based on a ≥ fourfold decrease in titer within 8 to 12 months after treatment initiation.

Assay Methods

Dark-Field

Because of their narrow width, treponemes cannot be observed with the ordinary light microscope. Microscopes equipped with a double-reflecting or single-reflecting dark-field condenser are needed to perform the dark-field examination. Illumination for dark-field microscopy is obtained when light rays strike the object in the field at an oblique angle so that no direct light rays enter the objective lens, only the rays that are reflected from the object. Therefore, the treponemes appear to be illuminated against a dark background.

By dark-field examination, *T. pallidum* is distinguished from other spiral organisms by the tightness of the spirals and characteristic corkscrew movement. *T. pallidum* is a delicate, corkscrew-shaped organism with rigid, uniform, tightly wound, deep spirals. The characteristic motion of *T. pallidum* is a deliberate forward and backward movement with rotation along the longitudinal axis.

Dark-field examination is most effective for diagnosis during primary, secondary, infectious relapsing early latent, and early congenital syphilis when moist lesions containing large numbers of treponemes are present. Aspirates from enlarged regional lymph nodes also can serve as a specimen source. The proper specimen for dark-field microscopy is serous fluid containing *T. pallidum* but free of erythrocytes, other organisms, and tissue debris (5). The lesion should be cleansed only if encrusted or obviously contaminated, and only a minimal amount of tap water or physiologic saline (without antibacterial additives) should be used. Because viability (motility) of the treponeme is necessary to distinguish *T. pallidum* from morphologically similar saprophytic spirochetes, dark-field examination must be completed within 20 minutes after the specimen is collected from the patient. Adequate training and experience are necessary to make an accurate diagnosis by dark-field microscopy. Cotton fibers and brownian motion may deceive the untrained observer. Because *T. pallidum* cannot be differentiated from saprophytic spirochetes in oral or intestinal tract lesions, dark-field microscopy should not be used for samples from these areas.

Primary syphilis can be diagnosed by dark-field microscopic examination several days to several weeks before the appearance of reactive serologic tests. According to the Clinical Laboratory Improvement Acts of 1988 (CLIA 1988), dark-field is classified as a high complexity test due to the significant level of expertise required to successfully identify *T. pallidum*. The amount of time required for accurate test reading and interpretation makes this the most expensive syphilis test; the cost of materials and labor is approximately $4.50 per specimen tested.

Direct Fluorescent Antibody Techniques

DFA-TP and DFAT-TP tests detect and distinguish pathogenic treponemes from nonpathogenic treponemes using an antigen-specific conjugate. The direct fluorescent antibody techniques are applicable to samples collected from oral, rectal, or intestinal lesions. Reference monoclonal antibody and controls are available from CDC (Technical Services Branch, National Center for Infectious Diseases [NCID], Centers for Disease Control and Prevention, 1600 Clifton Road, Atlanta, GA 30333).

DFA-TP

Slides for the DFA-TP test may be stained with fluorescein-isothiocyanate (FITC)-labeled anti-*T. pallidum* globulin prepared from the serum (absorbed with Reiter treponemes) of humans or rabbits with syphilis, or with a mouse monoclonal antibody specific for *T. pallidum* (5–8). Sample requirements are identical to those indicated for dark-field microscopy. In addition to lesion exudates, body fluids, suspensions of macerated tissue, or tissue impressions are suitable samples for the DFA-TP as motility is not required. Smears should be air dried and stored at room temperature (23° to 29°C) or refrigerated (4° to 8°C) until they are to be stained. If slides are to be sent to a reference laboratory, the slides should be shipped without fixation. Slides may be stored for a period of months to years at −20°C. If slides have been stored at −20°C, they should be shipped frozen.

Controls slides for each test run include:

1. *T. pallidum* antigen (FTA-ABS test antigen), or human chancre smear from a patient with syphilis, or *T. pallidum*-infected rabbit testicular impression smear.
2. Reiter treponemes or fresh mouth treponemes. *T. pallidum* subspecies *pallidum* in the positive control should show strong (3+ to 4+) fluorescence and typical morphology. Nonpathogenic treponemes in the negative control should show <1+ fluorescence and may have a morphology atypical of *T. pallidum*.

Sources of error in the DFA-TP test procedure are precipitate in the conjugate, improper pH of the mounting medium (mounting media pH must be ≥7.0 for polyclonal conjugate and ≥9.0 for monoclonal conjugate), rinsing control slides in a bulk saline bath so that treponemes may wash onto specimen slides causing a false-positive test result, and talcum powder accidentally deposited on slides from gloves.

Failure to demonstrate treponemes in a sample from a patient with syphilis may be related to the age or condition of the lesion when the sample was collected, treatment of the patient before the specimen was taken, and poor specimen collection technique.

As with all fluorescent antibody techniques, high level technical skill is required. Although not as labor intensive as dark-field microscopy in terms of test interpretation, the cost of the DFA-TP test is still around $3.00 per specimen.

DFAT-TP

A combination of the DFAT-TP test and histologic stains may be used to examine biopsy and autopsy material for the presence of pathogenic *Treponema* (5,8). Generally, tissues for paraffin-embedded sections are collected from the brain, gastrointestinal tract, placenta, umbilical cord, or skin. Approximately, 5 mm to 1 cm of tissue is collected by punch or surgical excision. Regardless of its source, tissue is placed in 10 mL of 10% neutral-buffered formalin (3.7% to 4.0% formaldehyde) at room temperature, then transferred to 70% ethanol for storage if tissue cannot be processed into paraffin blocks within the first 24 hours. (Note: The antigens will tend to degrade in ethanol, but more slowly than if left in formalin.) Sections from the paraffin block are cut at 2 microns, and attached to slides. Slides are deparaffinized, rehydrated, and then treated with either 1% NH_4OH or 0.25% trypsin prior to staining. Slides prepared from sections are stained with a FITC-labeled monoclonal conjugate as for the DFA-TP. A testicular tissue section from a *T. pallidum*-infected rabbit is used as the positive control. Noninfected rabbit testicular tissue is used as the negative control. The condition of the specimen and the thickness of the tissue sections affect the outcome of the test; the thicker the section, the lesser the probability of a positive test result.

Because of its application with tissue samples, the DFAT-TP test procedure requires more specimen preparation time than does the DFA-TP. The additional time and reagents used for specimen preparation increases the cost of the DFAT-TP test to about $4.00 per test.

Serologic Tests

The most common methods for diagnosis of syphilis are serologic tests (5,9). These tests detect either antibodies to lipoidal antigens indicative of an infection (nontreponemal methods) or antibodies against specific treponemal antigens (treponemal methods). Details of the procedure for each of these standard tests and the methods for specimen collection have been previously discussed (5). Reference reagents and control serum samples are available for the nontreponemal and treponemal tests from CDC.

Nontreponemal Tests

The nontreponemal tests are fast, easy to perform, and excellent for screening patient samples. Cardiolipin, when combined with lecithin and cholesterol, forms a serologically active antigen composed of liposomes. This antigen is common to all treponemal tests. Choline chloride and EDTA are added to stabilize the antigen, and sized particles such as charcoal for the RPR card test or paint toner pigment for the toluidine red unheated serum test (TRUST) are used to enhance visualization of the antigen antibody reaction. The nontreponemal tests measure IgM and IgG antibodies to lipoidal material released from damaged host cells, as well as to lipoprotein-like material and possibly cardiolipin released from the treponemes (10,11).

In the macroscopic nontreponemal tests, patient serum is mixed with the antigen on a plastic-coated card. If antibodies are present, antigen-antibody recognition occurs first, followed by aggregation and antigen-antibody lattice formation. The colored particles coagglutinate with the antibodies to produce black or red clumps (depending on the test used) on the white card. If antibodies are not present, the test mixture is uniformly gray or pink.

In the qualitative nontreponemal tests, an undiluted serum specimen from the patient is used to detect the presence or absence of antibodies. In the quantitative nontreponemal tests, serial twofold dilutions of a serum are made until an end point is reached. All serum samples exhibiting any degree of reactivity or roughness in the qualitative test should be diluted because of the possibility of a prozone (antibody excess) reaction.

Serum and plasma are both suitable samples for the qualitative card tests; however, serum is the preferred sample for the quantitative test (5). Serum should be obtained from whole blood collected in a clean, dry tube without an anticoagulant. In contrast, plasma should be obtained from blood collected in a tube containing an anticoagulant. For plasma samples, the collection tube should be filled to capacity.

Plasma samples should be tested within 48 hours after collection or as recommended by the test manufacturer. An acceptable serum or plasma specimen should not contain particulate matter that would interfere with reading test results. Specimens that are excessively hemolyzed, grossly contaminated with bacteria, chylous, or otherwise extremely turbid are unsatisfactory for testing. A specimen is too hemolyzed for testing when printed matter cannot be read through it. (Note: Hemolysis may be caused by transporting blood in freezing or extremely hot weather without proper insulation.) After centrifuging the specimen to sediment cellular elements, the serum specimen may be kept in the original collection tube, if testing is to be performed within a few hours.

Serum should be removed from the clot and stored at refrigerator temperature (2° to 8°C) if testing is to be delayed. If a delay of more than 5 days is anticipated before testing, freeze the serum at ≤ -20°C. Avoid repeated freeze-thawing of specimens. Although unheated serum specimens may be used, serum may be heated at 56°C for 30 minutes without affecting test outcome. Store plasma specimens at refrigerator temperature (2° to 8°C) if testing is to be delayed more than a few hours. Do not heat plasma samples or use plasma samples for confirmatory treponemal tests.

Lyophilized reactive (R), minimally reactive (Rm), and nonreactive (N) control serum specimens on a card, or liquid or lyophilized serum samples of graded reactivity, are used on each test day and whenever a new vial of antigen is placed in service. When performing quantitative tests use a control serum that can be titered to at least a 1:4 dilution. To ensure the delivery of the correct volume of antigen suspension, check the calibrated needle each time a new needle is used, when the needle has been dropped or wiped, or when the control pattern is not met. Errors in test results occur if:

1. The temperatures of the sera, reagents, or testing area are <23°C (73°F) or if temperatures are >29°C (85°F).
2. The speed of the mechanical rotator is too fast or too slow.
3. The time of rotation is too long or too short.
4. The card is excessively rotated and tilted (to-and-fro motions) by hand after removal from the rotator.
5. Lighting produces a glare on the card.
6. The antigen is outdated or not adequately tested for standard reactivity.
7. The serum is spread unevenly in the circle.
8. Hemolyzed, contaminated, or improperly collected serum or plasma samples are tested.
9. The proper humidity is not maintained and test components dry on the card.

Limitations of the card tests include the inability to obtain appropriate results with spinal fluid samples, and the failure of the nontreponemal test titers to decline as expected for persons treated in latent or late stages of syphilis, or if patients have been reinfected.

While the macroscopic tests are easier to interpret and perform than the other nontreponemal tests, the RPR and TRUST are slightly more expensive. The cost of the macroscopic tests, including labor, is about $1.50 per test.

Treponemal Tests

Three treponemal tests are routinely used in the United States: FTA-ABS, FTA-ABS double staining (DS), and the MHA-TP (5). The treponemal tests are not intended for use as screening procedures, but rather to confirm reactivity in nontreponemal tests. In addition, the treponemal tests are technically more difficult and expensive to perform than nontreponemal tests and cannot be used to monitor treatment outcome.

Serum is the specimen of choice for the treponemal tests. Serum samples for the treponemal tests are collected, processed and stored as previously described for the nontreponemal tests. Reference reagents and controls for the FTA-ABS test procedures are available from the CDC.

FTA-ABS and FTA-ABS DS The fluorescent treponemal antibody-absorption tests (5) are indirect fluorescent antibody techniques used as confirmatory tests for syphilis. To perform these tests, the patient's serum is heated at 56°C then diluted 1:5 in sorbent (an extract from cultures of *T. phagedenis*, Reiter treponeme). Next, the serum is layered on a microscope slide to which *T. pallidum* subspecies *pallidum* has been fixed. If the patient's serum contains anti-*T. pallidum* antibodies, the antibodies will coat the treponeme. In the FTA-ABS test, FITC-labeled anti-human immunoglobulin is added; this combines with the patient's IgG and IgM antibodies that are bound to the *T. pallidum* cells, resulting in a visible test reaction when examined by fluorescence microscopy. This test uses only one fluorescent dye and the presence of test antigen must be verified by dark-field microscopy. The FTA-ABS DS test was developed specifically for microscopes with incident illumination.

In the FTA-ABS DS class-specific tetramethylrhodamine isothiocyanate (TMRITC)-labeled antihuman IgG replaces the fluorescein-labeled conjugate in the FTA-ABS test and, if antibodies are present, results in a red test reaction when examined by fluorescence microscopy with the rhodamine filters. A counterstain, FITC-labeled anti-treponemal globulin, is added to locate *T. pallidum* on the slide when it is examined with the FITC filter. Seven controls are performed with each test run as indicated in **Table 35-2**.

Erroneous FTA-ABS or FTA-ABS DS results occur if:

1. Reagent evaluation procedures are not strictly followed.

TABLE 35-2

Control Pattern for the FTA-ABS and FTA-ABS DS Tests

Controls	Dilution	Reading
Reactive serum	a. 1:5 PBS dilution b. 1:5 sorbent dilution	R4+ R (4+ to 3+)
Minimally Reactive	1+ control dilution of reactive serum	R1+
Nonspecific serum	a. 1:5 PBS dilution b. 1:5 sorbent dilution	R (2+ to 4+) N±
Nonspecific staining	a. Antigen, PBS, conjugate b. Antigen, sorbent, conjugate	N N

Note: Test runs in which these control results are not obtained are considered unsatisfactory and should not be reported.

2. Multi-circle slides are used and serum from one well is allowed to run onto another well.
3. Microscope slides are not clean (note: slides may first need to be cleaned by sonic vibration or wiping with alcohol).
4. The FTA-ABS test procedures are used as screening procedures.
5. The microscope is not properly aligned and the control pattern is not obtained.
6. Reagents become contaminated with bacteria.
7. Reagents are not correctly stored.
8. Frozen antigen slides are thawed and refrozen.
9. The patient's serum is contaminated with bacteria or is hemolyzed excessively.
10. Antigen slides are not dried and stored according to the procedure requirements, or too much volume is placed on the slide.
11. Too many smears are fixed in a given volume of acetone.
12. Rehydrated antigen does not adhere to the slide.
13. Precipitate is observed in the conjugate preparation.
14. The atypical staining pattern of beaded fluorescence is not recognized.

The technical difficulties involved in performing the FTA-ABS and FTA-ABS DS tests elevate the cost of these tests into the $3.50 to $4.00 per test range.

MHA-TP The MHA-TP is another confirmatory test for syphilis (5). In the MHA-TP, the patient's serum is diluted in absorbing diluent to remove possible cross-reacting heterophile antibody and to block potentially cross-reacting nonpathogenic treponemal antibodies. Next, sheep red cells sensitized with *T. pallidum* are added. If antibodies to pathogenic treponemes are present, a smooth mat of agglutinated cells form in the microtiter tray. A compact button of nonagglutinated cells forms at the bottom of the tray well if antibodies are not present.

Heat inactivation of specimens is not necessary for MHA-TP testing, but heated specimens may be used. Controls for the MHA-TP include both reactive and nonreactive lyophilized serum samples, as well as unsensitized sheep erythrocytes.

Errors with the MHA-TP test may occur if:

1. Microtitration trays other than those recommended are used for the test.
2. Lint or dirt have contaminated the trays.
3. Inaccurate pipetting of specimens or controls occurs.
4. The plate is tapped too vigorously causing cross-contamination of specimens.
5. Outdated reagents are used.
6. The kits are stored improperly.

The MHA-TP test is simple to perform and, unlike the FTA-ABS, is easily adapted to high-volume testing. Because the MHA-TP is a macroscopic test, interpretation is more objective than with the other treponemal tests. Also, quality control is less complicated than with the FTA-ABS tests. Cost of the test, including labor, is approximately $3.35 per test.

Test Interpretation

How well a test assists in the diagnosis of syphilis is related to the test's sensitivity, specificity, and predictive values. In turn, the test's predictive values are related to the prevalence of the disease in the community. Despite periodic increases in sexually acquired syphilis, overall rates of syphilis have progressively declined since the advent of penicillin therapy. The rates of primary and secondary syphilis for 1994 and 1995 declined to approximately 8 cases per 100,000 population. However, the incidence of syphilis varies widely throughout the United States with the highest rates seen in the rural South.

The nontreponemal tests, while excellent screening tests, are not very sensitive for diagnosing early primary syphilis or late syphilis. Approximately 20% of early primary cases are nonreactive in the nontreponemal tests (**Table 35-3**). Moreover, up to 30% of late, untreated syphilis cases are nonreactive in these tests. All nontreponemal tests are reactive in secondary syphilis, achieving 100% sensitivity in most patient populations. However, antibody excess (prozone phenomenon) may prevent detection of antibodies. The antilipoidal antibodies measured in the nontreponemal tests may also be produced in response to nontreponemal diseases of an acute and chronic nature in which tissue damage occurs (9). Biological false-positive (BFP) results occur occasionally in specimens from persons who abuse drugs; who have diseases such as lupus erythematosus, mononucleosis, malaria, leprosy, or viral pneumonia; or who have recently been vaccinated. Without some other evidence for the diagnosis of syphilis, a reactive nontreponemal test does not indicate an infection with *T. pallidum*. Overall, the sensitivity of the nontreponemal tests is approximately 90% and the specificity 98% (see Table 35-3).

The advantages of the treponemal tests are that they are sensitive in early syphilis, and can distinguish true-positive nontreponemal results from false-positive results (see Table 35-3). Nevertheless, false-positive results do occur in the treponemal tests. These results are often transient and the cause is unknown, but a definite association has been made between false-positive test results and the diagnosis of systemic, discoid, and drug-induced varieties of lupus erythematosus, and aging (9). Unlike nontreponemal tests, the treponemal tests remain reactive for the lifetime of approximately 80% of treated patients and, therefore, cannot be used to monitor the effectiveness of treatment.

TABLE 35-3

Performance Characteristics of the Tests for Untreated Syphilis

Direct Test	Sensitivity	Specificity
Dark-field	76.3%	100%
DFA-TP[a]	88.0%	97%
DFA-TP[b]	87%	100%
DFAT-TP[b]	87%	99%
PCR	91%	99%

[a] Results using polyclonal conjugate.

[b] Results using monoclonal conjugate.

Serologic Tests	Sensitivity by Stage[c]				Specificity
	S10	S20	S30	S40	
VDRL	80	100	95	71	98
USR	80	100	95	—	99
RPR	86	100	98	73	98
TRUST	85	100	98	—	99
VISUWELL-R[d]	93	100	100	—	97
FTA-ABS	84	100	100	96	97
FTA-ABS DS	80	100	100	—	98
MHA-TP	76	100	97	94	99
CAPTIA-G[d]	76	96	92	—	97
VISUWELL-S[d]	93	100	100	—	94

[c] S10 = primary syphilis, S20 = secondary syphilis, S30 = latent syphilis, S40 = late syphilis.

[d] Visuwell-R is a nontreponemal ELISA test. Visuwell-S and Captia-G are treponemal ELISA tests.

Quality Assurance

Quality assurance (QA) in the syphilis serology laboratory ensures the reliability and reproducibility of test results within a laboratory and among different laboratories performing the same tests. An appropriate QA system must address the preanalytical, analytical, and postanalytical phases of diagnostic testing (12). Most technical errors that occur in testing can be eliminated through adherence to recommended techniques and the use of standardized reagents.

Internal QA Procedures

Quality assurance measures that can ensure reliable and reproducible test results for the diagnosis of syphilis include those mandated by CLIA 1988. In addition, internal QA procedures unique to syphilis diagnosis exist (5).

General

1. Each new lot of reagents should be checked in parallel with reference reagents to verify that results are comparable. Testing should be performed on two testing days with at least 10 specimens of graded reactivity (nonreactive, weakly or minimally reactive, and reactive).
2. Periodic intra-laboratory reading comparisons should be performed to maintain

uniform reading levels for all testing personnel.

Nontreponemal Tests

1. All reagents and specimens must be at room temperature (23° to 29°C) for optimal tests results.
2. The mechanical rotator speed must be calibrated to 180 ± 2 rpm for the VDRL, VDRL-CSF, and unheated serum reagin (USR) tests, and 100 ± 2 rpm for the RPR and TRUST each day the tests are performed.
3. Nondisposable, stainless steel, calibrated needles without bevels are used for the VDRL, VDRL-CSF, and USR tests (5). Because these needles are usually prepared by the user, delivery volumes of these needles must be carefully standardized.
4. Disposable glassware may be used for all testing with the following exceptions; VDRL antigen suspension bottles, VDRL slides, and VDRL-CSF Kline concavity slides. Nondisposable glassware should be cleaned according to recommended procedures (5).

Treponemal Tests

1. Every 2 to 3 months, microscopes should be calibrated using an FITC quality control slide to standardize fluorescent staining intensity.
2. For the FTA-ABS tests, precleaned, 1 × 3 inch microscope slides approximately 1-mm thick are recommended.
3. The FTA-ABS tests and MHA-TP results should be monitored for increases in the false-positive rate above 1% (reactive minimals in the FTA-ABS tests and heterophile reactions in the MHA-TP). Abnormal increases may indicate the existence of diseases other than syphilis in a patient population or poor quality of reagents.

Direct Fluorescent Antibody Tests

1. New conjugates for the DFA-TP and DFAT-TP tests are tested in parallel with reference conjugates and characterized control antigens (smears or tissue sections). To determine conjugate specificity, each conjugate dilution is tested with *T. pallidum*, *T. denticola*, *Borellia burgdorferi*, and *Leptospira* sp. control slides.
2. Clean, 1 × 3 inch slides approximately 1-mm thick are suitable for each of the direct microscope tests (dark-field, DFA-TP, and DFAT-TP).

External QA Procedures

The syphilis serology laboratory should participate in an established proficiency testing (PT) program that evaluates the quality of diagnostic testing on a quarterly or semiannual basis. External QA procedures may detect problems within a laboratory by comparing its testing results with those of reference laboratories and peers. Proficiency testing samples should be handled and analyzed as if they were patient specimens, and by personnel who routinely perform the tests. The syphilis serology PT programs are administered by the College of American Pathologists (CAP), several state health departments, and the American Association of Bioanalysts (AAB). All PT records should be retained for a minimum of 2 years.

If a certified PT program is not available for a particular test technique such as the direct microscopic tests for syphilis, an inhouse PT program must be developed using the best available reference materials, or by split-sample analysis with other laboratories, clinical validation by chart review, or other suitable documented means. These alternative programs must be administered at least every 6 months. PT performance results and any documentation of remedial actions taken for PT failure must be kept in a QC manual that is available for review.

Comments and Future Improvements

One recent development is the use of colored gelatin particle carriers sensitized with purified *T. pallidum* to replace the sensitized erythrocytes in the MHA-TP test. This passive particle agglutination test (Serodia-TP PA) has replaced the MHA-TP test in several markets outside the United States. The manufacturer plans to discontinue the production of the MHA-TP test in the near future.

Currently two commercial companies are conducting preliminary evaluations of Western blot test kits. The Western blot offers the advantage of direct visualization of the protein antigens reacting with the patient's antibody. In addition, the Western blot with IgM conjugate appears to be more sensitive and specific than other test techniques for the diagnosis of congenital syphilis (13).

The enzyme-linked immunosorbent assays (ELISA), both nontreponemal and treponemal, were introduced to the clinical laboratories for the serodiagnosis of syphilis in the early 1990s. The advantages of these tests are the capability to run several hundred tests in a day and the elimination of subjective reading because the tests are read spectrophotometrically. The sensitivities and specificities of the ELISAs are comparable to those of the RPR and FTA-ABS tests (see Table 35-3). To date, the number of laboratories using the ELISA techniques is small, but interest in the tests is increasing as reflected by increases in the number of laboratories reporting ELISA test results in PT surveys.

Despite the significant number of treponemal and nontreponemal tests for syphilis, the diagnosis of syphilis remains a problem. PCR could be extremely valuable in diagnosing congenital syphilis (passively transferred antibodies now confuse the diagnosis), neurosyphilis (the only serologic test is only 50% sensitive), early primary syphilis (the only tests available are microscopic), and finally, in distinguishing new infections from old infections (now only a rise in titer can be used). Results from one study comparing DFA-TP with a PCR using a primer encoding for the 47 kd protein found a concordance of 95.5%, when touch preparations of genital lesions were examined (14), and initial studies with the Multiplex PCR (4) indicate that the test is at least as sensitive and specific as the direct methods (see Table 35-3).

REFERENCES

1. Engelkens HJH, Judanarso J, Oranje AP, et al. Endemic treponematoses. I. Yaws. Int J Dermatol 1991;30:77–83.
2. Engelkens HJH, Niemel PLA, van der Sluis JJ, et al. Endemic treponematoses. II. Pinta and endemic syphilis. Int J Dermatol 1991;30:231–238.
3. Benenson AS, ed. Control of communicable diseases in man. 15th ed. Washington, DC: American Public Health Association, 1990: 323–324, 425–426, 483–486.
4. Orle KA, Gates CA, Marten DH, Body BA, Weiss JB. Simultaneous PCR detection of *Hemophilus ducreyi, Treponema pallidum* and herpes simplex virus types 1 and 2 from genital ulcers. J Clin Microbiol 1996;34:49–54.
5. Larsen SA, Hunter EF, Kraus, eds. A manual of tests for syphilis. 8th ed. Washington, DC: American Public Health Association, 1990.
6. Romanowski B, Forsey E, Prasad E, et al. Detection of *Treponema pallidum* by a fluorescent monoclonal antibody test. Sex Transm Dis 1987;22:156–159.
7. Ito F, Hunter EF, George RW, Swisher BL, Larsen SA. Specific immunofluorescence staining of *Treponema pallidum* in smears and tissues. J Clin Microbiol 1991;29:444–448.
8. Ito F, George RW, Hunter EF, et al. Specific immunofluorescent staining of pathogenic treponemes with a monoclonal antibody. J Clin Microbiol 1992;30:831–838.
9. Larsen SA, Steiner BM, Rudolph AH. Laboratory diagnosis and interpretation of tests for syphilis. Clin Micobiol Rev 1995;8:1–21.
10. Matthews HM, Yang TK, Jenkin HM. Unique lipid composition of *Treponema pallidum* (Nichols virulent strain). Infect Immunol 1979; 24:713–719.
11. Belisle JT, Brandt ME, Radolf JD, Norgard MV. Fatty acids of *Treponema pallidum* and *Borrelia burgdorferi* lipoproteins. J Bacterol 1994;176:2151–2157.
12. Department of Health and Human Services. Policies and continuous quality improvement. Atlanta: Centers for Disease Control and Prevention, 1996.
13. Norgard MV. Clinical and diagnostic issues of acquired and congenital syphilis encompassed in the current syphilis epidemic. Curr Opin Infect Dis 1993;6:9–16.
14. Jethwa HS, Schmitz JL, Dallabetta G, et al. Comparison of molecular and microscopic techniques for detection of *Treponema pallidum* in genital ulcers. J Clin Microbiol 1995;33:180–183.

CHAPTER 36

The Laboratory's Role in the Diagnosis of Lyme Disease

NICK S. HARRIS

This chapter has a dual purpose: to inform about the nature of the course of Lyme disease and the difficulty concerning the clinical diagnosis; and to integrate such information into an appreciation of the laboratory tests and decisions regarding their use.

The individual who was responsible for discovering Lyme disease in the United States was Polly Murray, a Lyme, Connecticut, artist and housewife. The following excerpts from her book, *The Widening Circle,* describe the various symptoms exhibited by her family (1):

> Todd [son] . . . had increased swelling of the knee and was hobbling. And he had developed a rash on his chest. Sandy [son] . . . had severe swelling of his knee, and could hardly walk. His flare-up had hit at exactly the same time as Todd's. . . . [Later, Sandy] became dizzy and nauseated and developed a terrible headache. . . . Sandy had another reaction while in the sun. His face became an alarming purple-red and he spiked a fever. His knee was painful again. . . . I [Polly] awoke feeling terrible. It hurt to get out of bed. I could hardly move. My hands were throbbing and swollen, my eyes were gooky, and my lips were sore also. . . . When we had flare-ups we also noticed tiny pinpricklike rashes of blood under the skin; measleslike blotches, butterfly rashes; hot, burning sensations; numbness; and even black-and-blue marks and blisters. . . . I was convinced that a flulike illness, including recurrent sore throat, gastrointestinal problems and fever, was also part of the syndrome. . . . Gil [husband] had knee problems again and I also had strange symptoms, including "lightning pains." I awoke one morning . . . and had trouble hearing out of my left ear. My left eye was blurry and my balance was off. I felt disoriented, and I was running a slight fever. My jaw was cracking again. . . . [Gil] too, was experiencing lightning or stitch-like pains, which affected his neck, shoulder, and lumbar regions . . . he had extreme pain and swelling in right ankle and right mid foot . . . pronounced limp, feverish feeling, general stiffness and slowness in all actions. . . . In our family we had some puzzling eye symptoms. Both David [son] and I found that our pupils were different sizes; he had a wandering eye for awhile; we all had bouts of conjunctivitis; I had subconjunctival hemorrhages; and Sandy and Wendy [daughter], and I had swelling and drooping of the eyelid. We all also had uncontrolled twitching of the eyelid during Lyme disease flare-ups.

This brief section is only a small part of the voluminous records Polly shared with one of her doctors. That interchange started the important studies that led to the recognition of the clinical entity Lyme disease (2–4). In 1909, Afzelius in Sweden first described erythema chronicum migrans (or ECM, now shortened to EM), and its association with a tick bite of *Ixodes ricinus* (5). The first description of EM in the United States was detailed by Rudy Scrimenti in a case study of a physician bitten by a tick in Wisconsin during hunting season (6). From the correlation study by Steere (7), the classic discovery of spirochetes in the midgut and hindgut of *Ixodes dammini* (now *Ixodes scapularis*) by Willie Burgdorfer (8) and the isolation from blood (9) and the initial culture of the organism by Alan Barbour (10) led to the recognition of *Borrelia burgdorferi* (**Fig. 36-1**) with its host ticks, *Ixodes scapularis* and *Ixodes pacificus* (11–13), as the causative agent of Lyme disease.

The Centers for Disease Control and Prevention (CDC) has since established certain epidemiological and clinical criteria (**Table 36-1**) that contribute to the case definition for public health surveillance and reporting of Lyme disease (14). The criteria place great emphasis on the presence of an EM. Although it is generally accepted that a physician's diagnosis of an EM in a patient from an endemic area is extremely useful for ruling in a diagnosis of Lyme disease, more than a third of the patients do not present with an EM (15–17). The variable nature of the EM (18,19)—in its duration, its benign and asymptomatic qualities, and its presentation in obscure areas (axilla and hair regions)—inhibit its use as a consistent diagnostic marker.

FIGURE **36-1**

***Borrelia burgdorferi*, the causative agent of Lyme disease. (Courtesy of Russell C. Johnson. Univ. Minnesota. Minneapolis, MN.)**

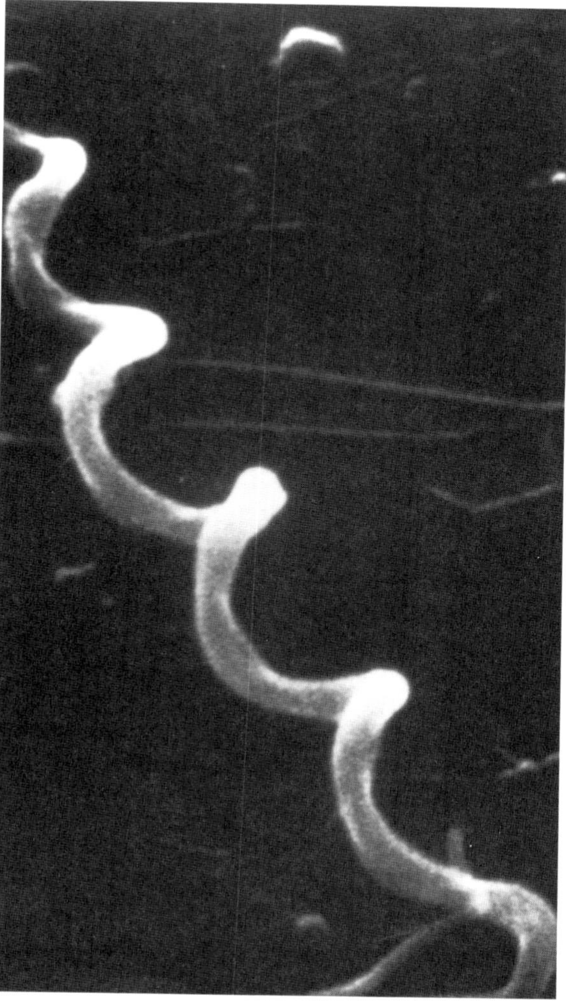

Lyme disease is a problematic diagnosis because it is a complicated clinical entity. Some patients do not make an antibody response large enough to be positive by the currently available ELISA assays. Furthermore, if patients are treated early with antibiotics, their antibody response may be reduced or curtailed (12). The initial symptoms may be overlooked if they were mild and flu-like or mimicked another disease. Later, if the symptoms return, most of the antibody markers have disappeared. The picture is not entirely bleak if we approach Lyme disease for what it is: a complicated clinical entity that cannot be diagnosed at the laboratory level with one test. Thus, if the laboratory assays for Lyme disease using panels of tests instead of a single test, there will be fewer problems with the diagnosis and fewer patients will be missed.

The presence of organisms in infected tissue is rare. In fact, the general sparsity of organisms contributes to the difficulty of trying to get blood or tissue to grow organisms (12,20). Even if one is able to get a positive culture, the patient still may not make an antibody response. Rawlings (21) presented a group of 14 patients in whom she was able to culture *B. burgdorferi*; only 3 of those patients had positive antibody titers. Studies by Aguero-Rosenfeld et al. (18,19) have indicated that only 70% of the patients have a significant antibody response. Interestingly, the degree of antibody response is related to the length of time the EM rash persists. Additionally, in their studies the rate of seroconversion from an IgM response to an IgG response was only 64%.

Several reports have suggested that considerable interlaboratory and intralaboratory variability exists in Lyme disease testing (22–24). That may have been true in 1991, but a review of the 1996 Lyme proficiency results by CAP (College of American Pathologists) and those by New York State demonstrate an agreement between the majority of laboratories, comparable to other bacterial infections or autoimmune conditions.

Table 36-2 presents the tests that are most commonly available for Lyme disease. To provide adequate support for the clinical eval-

TABLE 36-1

Case Definition for Public Health Surveillance of Lyme Disease

Clinical Description

A systematic, tick-borne disease with protean manifestations, including dermatologic, rheumatologic, neurologic, and cardiac abnormalities. The best clinical marker for the disease is the initial skin lesion, erythema migrans, that occurs among 60% to 80% of patients.

Clinical Case Definition

Erythema migrans, or at least one late manifestation, as defined below, and laboratory confirmation of infection.

Laboratory Criteria for Diagnosis

- Isolation of *Borrelia burgdorferi* from clinical specimen, or
- Demonstration of diagnostic levels of IgM and IgG antibodies to the spirochete in serum, or
- CSF, or
- Significant change in IgM or IgG antibody response to *B. burgdorferi* in paired acute, and
- Convalescent-phase serum samples.

Case Classification

Confirmed Case

A *confirmed case* is one that meets one of the clinical case definitions above. This surveillance case definition was developed for national reporting of Lyme disease; it is *not* appropriate for clinical diagnosis.

Erythema Migrans (EM)

For purposes of surveillance, *erythema migrans* (EM) is defined as a skin lesion that typically begins as a red macule or papule and expands over a period of days to weeks to form a large round lesion, often with partial central clearing. A solitary lesion must reach at least 5 cm in size. Secondary lesions may also occur. Annular erythematous lesions occurring within several hours of a tick bite represent hypersensitivity reactions and do not qualify as EM.

For most patients, the expanding EM lesion is accompanied by other acute symptoms, particularly fatigue, fever, headache, mild stiff neck, arthralgia, or myalgia. These symptoms are typically intermittent. The diagnosis of EM must be made by a physician. Laboratory confirmation is recommended for persons with no known exposure.

Late Manifestations

Late manifestations include any of the following when an alternate explanation is not found.

Musculoskeletal System Recurrent, brief attacks (weeks or month) of objective joint swelling in one or a few joints, *sometimes* followed by chronic arthritis in one of a few joints. Manifestations not considered as criteria for diagnosis include chronic progressive arthritis not preceded by brief attacks and chronic symmetrical polyarthritis. Additionally, arthralgia, myalgia, or fibromyalgia syndromes alone are not criteria for musculoskeletal involvement.

Nervous System Any of the following alone or in combination: lymphocytic meningitis; cranial neuritis, particularly facial palsy (may be bilateral); radiculoneuropathy; or rarely, encephalomyelitis. Encephalomyelitis must be confirmed by showing antibody production against *B. burgdorferi* in the cerebrospinal fluid (CSF), demonstrated by a higher titer of antibody in CSF than in serum. Headache, fatigue, paresthesia, or mild stiff neck alone are not criteria for neurologic involvement.

Cardiovascular System Acute onset, high-grade (2° to 3°) atrioventricular conduction defects that resolve in days to weeks and are sometimes associated with myocarditis. Palpitation, bradycardia, bundle branch block, or myocarditis alone are not criteria for cardiovascular involvement.

TABLE 36-1
Continued

Exposure

Exposure is defined as having been in wooded, brushy, or grassy areas (potential tick habitats) in a country in which Lyme disease is endemic not more than 30 days before onset of EM. A history of tick bite is *not* required.

Disease Endemic to County

A county in which Lyme disease is endemic is one in which at least two definite cases have been previously acquired, or in which a known tick vector has been shown to be infected with *B. burgdorferi*.

Laboratory Confirmation

As noted above, *laboratory confirmation* of infection with *B. burgdorferi* is established when a laboratory isolates the spirochete from tissue or body fluid, detects diagnostic levels of IgM and IgG antibodies to the spirochete in serum or CSF, or detects a significant change in antibody levels in paired acute- and convalescent-phase serum samples. States may determine the criteria for laboratory confirmation and diagnostic levels of antibody. Syphilis and other known causes of biologic false-positive serologic tests results should be excluded when laboratory confirmation has been based on serologic testing alone.

MMWR Morb Mortal Wkly Rep 1990;39:19–21.

TABLE 36-2
Laboratory Assays for Lyme Disease

- Direct
  - Biopsy
  - Culture
- Antibody Assays
  - IFA
  - ELISA
  - Western Blot
- Antigen Assays
  - Antigen Capture
  - PCR
- Other
  - Gunderson Borreliacidal Activity Assay
  - Lyme Immune Complex Test
  - Human Granulocytic Ehrlichiosis (HGE)
  - Human Monocytic Ehrlichiosis (HME)
  - *Babesia microti*

uation, multiple tests should be used. Not only is a correct diagnosis advantageous for the patient, but ultimately it is the most cost-effective route. This chapter discusses most of these tests, with the exception of the culture and tissue-section pathology.

Indirect Fluorescent Antibody (IFA)

With the indirect fluorescent antibody (IFA) assay, *B. burgdorferi* spirochetes are affixed to glass slides; usually an isothiocyanate-conjugated goat anti-human immunoglobulin of either IgM or IgG specificity is used (25). Both the conjugate and slides are commercially available. If a laboratory chooses to prepare in-house slides, the ATCC (American Type Culture Collection, Rockville, MD) offers two of the most useful strains of *B. burgdorferi* available, low passage B31 and 297. For laboratories not experienced in growing cultures of *B. burgdorferi,* the ATCC will grow them to whatever density desired for a nominal charge.

Tests for Lyme disease using IFA have received mixed reviews. Some authors feel that the interpretation of IFA assays are overly subjective and that the tests are either functionally insensitive for Lyme-specific antibodies or display considerable cross-reactions for patients with antibodies to other spirochetal organisms (26–27). The studies by Magnarelli et al. (28–29) and the report by Mitchell et al. (25) were favorable to IFA if it is used in conjunction with a clinical evaluation. In fact, Mitchell's study, which used an IgM-IFA, observed no cross-reactivity with the following:

Infectious mononucleosis (n = 20)

Rheumatoid arthritis (n = 19)

Systemic lupus (n = 22)

Syphilis (n = 13)

Streptococcal sequelae (n = 20)

Healthy subjects (n = 16)

Mitchell relates the success of his test to the antigenic and morphologically consistent quality of the substrate slides. Another aspect of primary importance in this study concerns the level of experience of his technologists. He feels that IFA microscopy becomes less subjective with experience. In addition, their observation of heterogeneously stained borrelias proved to be a characteristic pattern in early Lyme disease. This pattern recognition is important to discriminate between specific and nonspecific fluorescence that could lead to false-positive interpretation. As will be discussed in a later section, all positive and borderline IFA assays should be confirmed by Western blot.

The following method for the IgM-IFA detection of *B. burgdorferi* was kindly provided by Paul Mitchell, (Marshfield Laboratories, Marshfield, WI 54449). His method follows the procedure standardized by the CDC (26).

Principle

Intact *B. burgdorferi* spirochetes are used for the antigenic substrate for the detection and titration of antibodies in human serum. Serum is reacted with the antigenic substrate. Antibodies, if present, will bind to the spirochetal antigens forming antigen-antibody complexes. Fluorescein-labeled anti-human IgM is added to the reaction site, which will react (bind) with the antigen-antibody complexes if formed in the first step. This results in a positive reaction of bright apple-green fluorescing spirochetes when viewed with a properly equipped fluorescent microscope. If no antigen-antibody complexes are formed in the first step or if the complexes involve a class of antibody not being tested for, the fluorescent antibody will be washed free with a resultant negative reactivity.

IFA Lyme Test Components

- Lyme disease antigen slides—12-well slides (Bion Enterprises, Chicago, IL)—are ready once they come to room temperature (RT). Store at 4°C.
- Positive control: Serum is selected with a titer of 1:256. Store at −20°C.
- Negative control: Select is selected with a titer of <1:64. Store at −20°C.
- Coplin jars.
- Oxford or MLA pipettor (50 UL and 10 UL) and Oxford microdoser (50 UL).
- Microtitration plates, Autotrays-U.
- Coverslips, 22–60 (Fisher 12-545J).
- Incubation moist chamber.
- Conjugate anti-human IgM immunoglobulin (goat), fluorescein labeled (Kallestad#105). Store at 2 to 8°C. Each lot of conjugate is titered to determine the correct working dilution. Diluted conjugate should be prepared fresh with each run.
- PBS, pH 7.2. Store at 2 to 8°C. (Difco 2314-33, 6 (1 liter)).
- Glycerol mounting media: pH 9.0. Store RT (Difco 3340-57,6 (5 mL)).

IFA Lyme Procedure: IgM

Step 1. Remove the required number of slides and allow them to reach RT (1 slide/6 patients). Divide slide into six sections, two wells for each patient. Prepare a 1:16 dilution of each patient's serum in PBS (0.01 mL serum + 0.15 mL PBS).

Step 2. Using a microtiter plate and 50 UL microdoser, add 50 UL of PBS to wells 1 to 2.

Step 3. Using an MLA pipettor, add 50 UL of the 1:16 dilution to the first well. Mix and transfer 50 UL to the second well. Dilutions are 1:32 and 1:64.

Step 4. Using a dispopipet, add one drop of each serum dilution (1:32 to 1:64) to the appropriate well on each slide, starting with the 1:64 well and working backward to the 1:32 well.

Step 5. Incubate the slides in a moist chamber at 35 to 37°C for 30 minutes.

Step 6. Rinse the slides, then soak slides in a Coplin jar of PBS with an agitating motion for 10 minutes.

Step 7. Rinse slides with distilled water and gently blot.

Step 8. Dilute IgM conjugate to the correct working dilution. Add one drop of the conjugate to each well. Place slides in a moist chamber and incubate at 35 to 37°C for 30 minutes.

Step 9. Repeat steps 7 and 8.

Step 10. Place a small drop of mounting media to each well and coverslip.

Step 11. For best results, the slides should be read immediately at a magnification of 40×.

Quality Control

FITC-conjugated antisera (Kallestad Laboratories) are titered to determine the optimal working dilutions using positive and negative control sera. Each lot number of conjugate is titered prior to use. Positive and negative control sera are tested each time the procedure is performed with patient specimens. Each lot number of antigen substrate slides is tested prior to use with negative and positive control sera and with selected patient sera in parallel, which have been tested with another lot number.

Titration of Conjugate to Determine Working Dilution

Step 1. Prepare the following dilution of conjugate, using diluent recommended by the manufacturer.

IgM 1:40 1:80 1:100

Step 2. Use at least two positive sera of patients with clinically confirmed Lyme borreliosis. For IgM, select two positive sera (>1:64), and one known negative serum (<1:32).

Step 3. Test dilutions of each of the patient sera with each of the three dilutions of the conjugates according to the test procedure.

Step 4. Determine the optimal conjugate dilution. A good working dilution is the highest dilution which will give 3–4+ staining with little background fluorescence when testing positive sera and clearly negative results when testing negative sera. Specific serum titers should compare with results obtained with previously used lot numbers of conjugates.

Reading of Test Results

Fluorescent intensity of homogeneously stained spirochetes may be semiquantitated according to the following guidelines.

4+ Maximal fluorescence; brilliant yellow-green.

3+ Less brilliant yellow-green fluorescence.

2+ Definite, but dull yellow-green fluorescence.

1+ Very dim, subdued fluorescence.

Testing for IgM antibodies, positivity is defined as a heterogeneous (spotty, lumpy, etc.) staining of the spirochetes at a 1:64 dilution. A serum dilution is considered to be negative if the spirochetes exhibit less than a 2+ heterogeneous fluorescence.

Interpretative Criteria

The indirect fluorescent antibody (IFA) assay offers an advantage in that qualitative judgments can be made about patterns of observed fluorescence. As indicated above, IgM reactivity results in a heterogeneously stained substrate spirochete and is easily discernible by the experienced microscopist.

Interpretation of Test Results

Lyme IgM Ab: titers >1:32 are considered presumptive evidence of past or present infection with *Borrelia burgdorferi* in patients with appropriate clinical history. Sera of patients with other infectious diseases or connective tissue disorders may cross-react in these assays. In patients with early disease, antibodies may not be detected for several weeks after exposure, so repeat testing in 2 to 4 weeks may be necessary.

Enzyme-Linked Immunosorbent Assay (ELISA)

Since 1984, testing by ELISA for *B. burgdorferi* has been available (30). Most commercial assays use a sonicate of the whole spirochete of the *B. burgdorferi* organism. Excellent descriptions of "home-brew" methods for a Lyme disease ELISA can be found in the publications by Craft et al. (30), Magnarelli et al. (28), and Russell et al. (26). Standard ELISA techniques have been employed in all these assays (31).

A large number of commercial ELISA tests are available. It is often complicated to evaluate a significant number of them. One technique employed by this author's laboratory is to review past proficiency events by CAP and the New York State Health Department. (Serum controls are available and will be discussed later.)

The problem with most commercially available ELISA is a lack of sensitivity for the more unique and specific *B. burgdorferi* antigens. Therefore, they are poor screening assays for Lyme disease (32). These more unique antigens, which are visualized by Western blot (**Fig. 36-2**), are Osp A (31 kd), Osp B (34 kd), Osp C (23 to 25 kd), 39 kd, and 93 kd (33–38). Initially, some investigators identified 93 kd as 94 kd and Osp C as 22 kd. Most commercial kits do have reactivity to all these antigens, because most are prepared with a sonicate of *B. burgdorferi.* Most also have reactivity against 41 kd, 58 kd, 66 kd, and 73 kd, which are appropriate antigens, but are extremely cross-reactive to other spirochetes, heat-shock proteins, and some viruses.

All borderline and positive ELISA assays (polyvalent, IgG-only, and IgM-only) for Lyme disease must be confirmed by a high quality Western blot for *B. burgdorferi.* Luger and Krause (23) found up to a 56% false-negative rate, depending on the commercial kit used, as compared to their own clinical diagnosis. Golightly et al. (39) encountered a lack of sensitivity (over 70% false-negative rate) with commercial kits in early Lyme disease and from 4% to 46% with late manifestations of Lyme disease. Newer Lyme ELISA assays are often compared in the 510K application to earlier kits, so this lack of true sensitivity has perpetuated itself. For this reason, this chapter author recommends performing both the ELISA and Western blot assays simultaneously.

FIGURE **36-2**

Western blots of *B. burgdorferi* B31 strain. The blots were: (1) stained with amino black, (2) reacted with rabbit antisera, (3) with goat antisera, (4–7) with various monoclonal antibodies, and (8) with pooled patient sera. (Reproduced by permission from Ma B, Christen B, Leung D, Vigo-Pelfrey C. Serodiagnosis of Lyme borreliosis by Western immunoblot: reactivity of various significant antibodies against *B. burgdorferi*. J Clin Microbiol 1992;30: 370–376.)

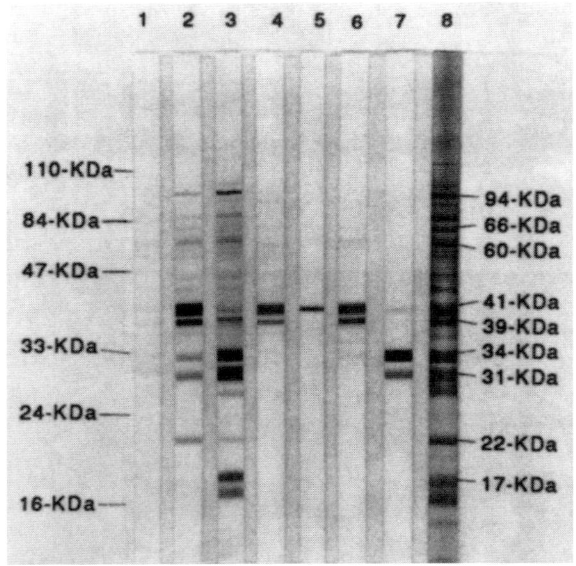

Lyme Western Blots

The Western blot or immunoblot for *B. burgdorferi* is the most useful antibody test available if performed in a quality laboratory by experienced testing personnel. It is performed for the IgG and for the IgM antibodies produced in Lyme disease. Even with the advent of commercially available reagents, the assay takes considerable skill to perform and interpret. Specific and unique quality control for the Western blot is necessary for commercial as well as "home-brew" assays.

The technique for the Western blot in this author's laboratory is essentially covered in a publication of Ma et al. (40). Briefly, either a single or combination of the strains B31, 297, or 2591 of *B. burgdorferi* is sonicated and mixed with lysing buffer, heated in boiling water, and added to sodium dodecyl sulfate-polyacrylamide gel (12.5%). Electrophoresis is carried out at 25 mA at room temperature until a marker dye migrates to a certain predetermined point on the gel. Proteins separated on the gel are transferred to nitrocellulose and then blocked with 5% nonfat dry milk. The nitrocellulose sheets are then cut into strips, and at least four strips from each membrane are used for quality control. If a commercial kit is used, at least four strips from each batch of 20 to 30 strips should be used for quality control.

In the performance of the assay, patient sera, positive control sera, and negative control sera must all be treated in the *exact same manner.* Some commercially available assays do not treat positive and negative controls in the same way as the patient samples, use high dilutions of their controls, or add blocking reagents to their controls. The best control and performance in the assay is achieved using sera from both positive and negative patients. A negative normal serum control, a positive serum control, a low-positive control, and a previously-run positive patient should be used for every run or batch. Our laboratory also includes a previously-run negative patient in addition to the negative normal serum control.

This test is technically difficult and labor intensive, but also very rewarding for a quality effort. Attempts to read it with various densitometric methods have not proved reliable. Appropriately trained technologists can visualize subtle changes with more reliability than instruments have so far demonstrated. As mentioned, it is important to have high and low positive and multiple true serum negative controls on each run. Some commercial assays use very dilute sera to act as a negative, but this approach does not permit the technologist to visually subtract negative background levels from their readings.

Figure 36-3 illustrates a group of IgG-IgM Western blots (lanes 1–48) from clinically confirmed Lyme patients with various levels of antibodies to *B. burgdorferi*. This same figure shows (lanes 48–57) IgM Western blots to *B. burgdorferi.* Even though these patients have different patterns of antibody reactivity, all were confirmed, clinically positive Lyme patients with physician-diagnosed EM. These different patterns of the Western blot demonstrate the variability in immune response so characteristic of other diseases (i.e., Hashimoto's thyroiditis, SLE, Sjögren's syndrome, scleroderma). Our own clinical study of 186 defined patients and 320 negative controls (**Fig. 36-4**) found excellent sensitivity and specificity for IgM using any two of the following bands: 23 to 25 kd (OspC), 31 kd (OspA), 34 kd (OspB), 39 kd, and 41 kd (40). The study also demonstrated good specificity and sensitivity for IgG using any two (also 93 kd) of the above bands.

Admittedly, it is difficult for each laboratory to perform clinical studies and establish its own ranges for normal and disease populations. For this reason, the CDC assembled a group of academic scientists with the assistance of the FDA and the Association of State and Territorial Public Health Laboratory Directors (ASTPHLD) to reach a consensus on certain criteria for the Western blot. After several meetings they arrived at the CDC/ASPHLD consensus criteria presented in **Table 36-3** (41,42). These criteria were based in large part on the work of Dressler et al. (43), using well-defined patients with active Lyme arthritis or neuroborreliosis. Interestingly, in this publication none of the three recommended strains of *B. burgdorferi* (B31, 297, and 2591) was used. Rather, they used

FIGURE 36-3

Western blots to *B. burgdorferi* from various patients with Lyme disease. Lanes 1-48 are IgG/IgM blots from clinically confirmed patients with various levels of antibodies. Lanes 48-57 are IgM-only blots. (Reproduced by permission from Ma B, Christen B, Leung D, Vigo-Pelfrey C. Serodiagnosis of Lyme borreliosis by Western immunoblot: reactivity of various significant antibodies against *B. burgdorferi*. J Clin Microbiol 1992;30:370-376.)

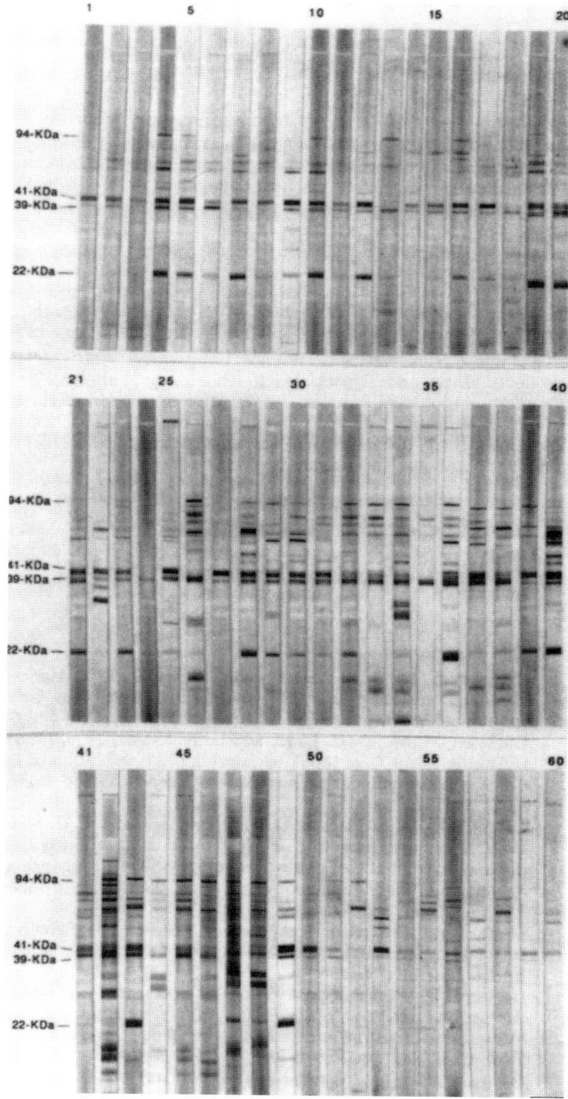

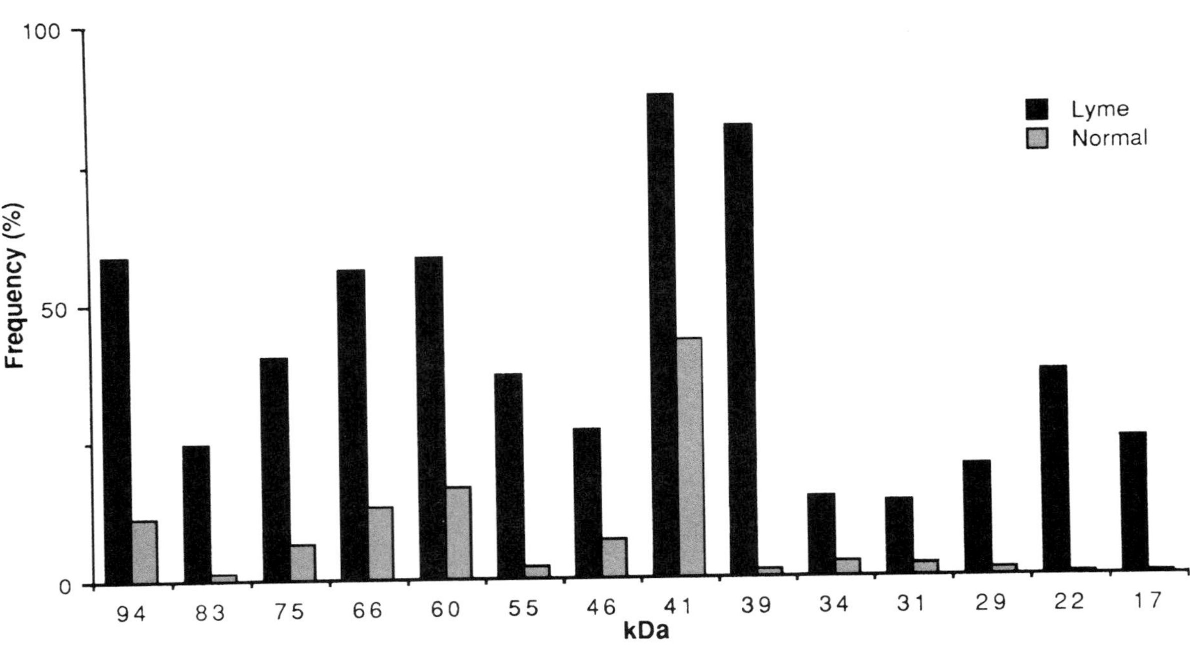

FIGURE 36-4
Comparison of antibody reactivity to various *B. burgdorferi* antigens. The dark bars are from 186 patients with clinically confirmed Lyme disease and the light bars are from 320 normal controls. (Reproduced by permission from Ma B, Christen B, Leung D, Vigo-Pelfrey C. Serodiagnosis of Lyme borreliosis by Western immunoblot: reactivity of various significant antibodies against *B. burgdorferi*. J Clin Microbiol 1992;30:370–376.)

G39/40 and a 10% acrylamide gel. A gel with this low percentage of acrylamide usually does not permit good resolution and definition of all the important antigens of *B. burgdorferi*.

The CDC/ASPHLD criteria for positive Western blots are very conservative and require 5 of 10 antibody bands for IgG positivity; they do not recognize equivocal or borderline results. This cut-off assumes that all Lyme patients, even if they do not have arthritis and neuroborreliosis, have similar immune systems. This criteria makes no adjustment for the length of time which has elapsed since the start of the infection. It also ignores the diversity of immune response seen in other diseases. In addition, the criteria *include* antibodies to 41 kd, a common antigen of most flagella-bearing organisms and *overlook* two of the most important and specific antigens: 31 kd (OspA) and 34 kd (Osp B), which appear later in the response. In reviewing a group of 50 patients with confirmed Lyme disease, Hilton et al. (44) would have missed 4 patients by excluding 31 kd (OspA) and 34 kd (OspB). The author's own laboratory would have missed 2 of 18 proficiency samples by excluding antibodies to these two antigens.

Studies by Engstrom et al. (17) and those of Aguero-Rosenfeld et al. (18,19) confirmed that almost one-third of all Lyme patients are IgG seronegative during the first year. Two years after a physician diagnosed EM, 45% of the patients were negative by ELISA. In another study, Aguero-Rosenfeld et al. (19) showed that the ELISA response declined much more rapidly than the Western blot response. In addition, their study also demonstrated that the CDC/ASPHLD criteria fail to detect some patients with culture-proven EM.

The CDC/ASPHLD criteria (41,42) for a positive IgM Western blot include the 23 to 25 kd (OspC), 39 kd, and the 41 kd, but overlook the 31 kd (OspA) and 34 kd (OspB). During the presentation at the Dearborn meeting (41), the specificity of the IgM Western blot was reported to be greater than 95%, based on several hundred negative controls. Engstrom et al. (17)

TABLE **36-3**

CDC/ASPHLD Criteria for the Serologic Diagnosis of Lyme Disease

Test Performance and Interpretation

Recommendation 1.1. Two-Test Protocol

All serum specimens submitted for Lyme disease testing should be evaluated in a two-step process, in which the first step is a sensitive serological test, such as an enzyme immunoassay (EIA) or immunofluorescent assay (IFA). All specimens found to be positive or equivocal by a sensitive EIA or IFA should be tested by a standardized Western Blot (WB) procedure. Specimens found to be negative by a sensitive EIA or IFA need not be tested further.

Recommendation 1.2. WB Controls

Immunoblotting should be performed using a negative control, a weakly reactive positive control, and a high-titered positive control. The weakly reactive positive control should be used to judge whether a sample band has sufficient intensity to be scored. Monoclonal or polyclonal antibodies to antigens of diagnostic importance should be used to calibrate the blots.

Recommendation 1.3. Testing and Stage of Disease

When Western immunoblot is used in the first 4 weeks after disease onset (early Lyme disease), both IgM and IgG procedures should be performed. Most Lyme disease patients will seroconvert within this 4-week period. In the event that a patient with suspected early Lyme disease has a negative serology, serologic evidence of infection is best obtained by testing of paired acute- and convalescent-phase samples. In late Lyme disease, the predominant antibody response is usually IgG. It is highly unusual that a patient with active Lyme disease has only an IgM response for *Borrelia burgdorferi* after 1 month of infection. A positive IgM result alone is not recommended for use in determining active disease in persons with illness of longer than one month duration, because the likelihood of a false-positive test result is high for these individuals.

Recommendation 1.4. WB Criteria

Use of the criteria of Engstrom et al. (17) is recommended for interpretation of IgM immunoblots. An IgM blot is considered positive if two of the following three bands are present: 24 kd (OspC), 39 kd (BmpA), and 41 kd (Fla). Monoclonal antibodies to these three proteins have been developed and are suitable for calibrating immunoblots (40). Once antibodies are developed to the 37 kd antigen, this protein could be used as an additional band for IgM criteria (>2 of 4 bands). Interim use of the criteria of Dressler et al. (42) are recommended for interpretation of IgG immunoblots. An IgG blot is considered positive if 5 of the following 10 bands are present: 18, 21 (OspC), 28, 30, m 39, (BmpA), 41 (Fla), 45, 58 (not GroEL2), 66, and 93 kd. Monoclonal antibodies have been developed to the OspC, 39 (BmpA), 41 (Fla), 66, and 93 kd antigens and are suitable for calibrating IgG immunoblots (40).

The apparent molecular mass of OspC is recorded above as it was denoted in the published literature. The protein referred to as 24 kd or 21 kd is the same, and should be identified in immunoblots with an appropriate calibration reagent (see 1.6).

Recommendation 1.5. Reporting of Results

An equivocal or positive EIA or IFA result followed by a negative immunoblot result should be reported as negative. An equivocal or positive EIA or IFA result followed by a positive immunoblot result should be reported as positive. An explanation and interpretation of test results should accompany all reports.

Recommendation 1.6. Standardization of WB Nomenclature

The apparent molecular mass of some proteins of *Borrelia burgdorferi* such as OspC will vary depending on the *B. burgdorferi* strain and gel electrophoresis system used. The molecular weights of proteins of diagnostic importance should be identified with monoclonal or polyclonal antibodies (17). When possible, the molecular weight of the protein should be followed by the descriptive name (e.g., OspC).

MMWR Morb Mortal Wkly Rep 1995;44:590–591.

reported specificities of their IgM Western blot to be between 92% and 94%. It has been reported that the IFA and ELISA IgM assays may cross-react with ANA, EBV, and other spirochetal infections (29). However, studies by Mitchell et al. (25) and Ma et al. (40) did not observe this with their IFA and Western blot assays, respectively. However, so as to rule out this possibility, some laboratories suggest that an ANA/DNA/RF screen be included in the differential diagnosis.

The CDC/ASPHLD group seems to have overlooked its reported excellent specificity on the IgM Western blot, defining that it should only be used in the first month after infection with *B. burgdorferi.* Our laboratory (45), as well as some studies by Steere's group (34) and the study by Jain et al. (46), points to the importance of the IgM Western blot in later, recurrent, or persistent disease. In relation to an IgM-only response, an elegant study by Oksi et al. (47) used culture and PCR to confirm Lyme disease reports in patients in whom the specific IgM to *B. burgdorferi* is sometimes the only antibody detected in persistent disease. This strongly suggests that some Lyme patients may have a restricted IgM-only response to *B. burgdorferi.*

The CDC/ASPHLD criteria Table 36-3 (41, 42) make the recommendation that all sera be tested as part of a two-tier (step) process, using a sensitive ELISA (EIA) before doing the Western Blot. This statement causes a major problem in routine diagnosis. Bakken et al. as representatives of the group responsible for the Lyme disease proficiency testing for the College of American Pathologists (CAP) is concerned about the sensitivity of the screening tests. They state ". . . data indicated that the sensitivity and specificity of the currently used tests for Lyme disease are not adequate to meet the two-tier approach being recommended. Ideally, a screening test should have a high degree of sensitivity (>95%). The current methodologies need to be improved to adequately screen serum samples for confirmatory testing (32)".

Specific Aspects of Western Blot Quality Control

Previous proficiency samples are an excellent source of controls for evaluating what antibodies may be seen in the laboratory's Western blot. Laboratories that participate in New York State Department of Health Services (NYDOH, Albany, NY) proficiencies can receive extra samples free of charge by requesting them from the NYDOH. The CDC (Division of Vector Borne Diseases) provides samples that have been characterized by ELISA and Western blot for *B. burgdorferi.* These are provided at no cost to nonprofit organizations and at a nominal fee for commercial laboratories. The CDC sends the samples blinded, the laboratory performs the tests and sends the results back. The laboratory's results are kept confidential and the laboratory receives an analysis of the CDC's results. In addition, Boston Biomedica (West Bridgewater, MA) offers an extensive panel with multiple results from analyses using several commercially available assays. Because of the expense, this panel may be more appropriate for a manufacturing facility than for single laboratory.

In addition to molecular weight markers, monoclonal antibodies to the important antigens must be employed if a laboratory prepares its own blots. These antibodies can also serve as additional quality control for commercial blots. Many monoclonal antibodies to important antigens of *B. burgdorferi* are available, for a nominal charge, from Denee Thomas (University of Texas Health Science Center, San Antonio, TX). Some monoclonal antibodies are also available from the CDC and various research groups (41).

Antigen and Antigen-Capture Assays for Lyme Disease

Many research studies using mice, rats, guinea pigs, and dogs have found *B. burgdorferi* antigen in the urine of naturally occurring and induced Lyme infections (48–51). Dorward et al. (49) and others (48,52) also detected antigen in the urine of patients with Lyme disease. Dorward's study (49) indicated that pieces (**Fig. 36-5**) of *B. burgdorferi* were more common in urine than was the entire organism. Coyle et al. (53) has successfully used antigen-capture with monoclonal antibodies to 31 kd (OspA) and 34 kd (OspB) to detect antigen in cerebral spinal fluid (CSF) of patients with neuroborreliosis.

Our laboratory has published information about the development (54) and use of antigen-capture for the detection of *B. burgdorferi* antigen in urine of Lyme patients (55). **Figure 36-6** illustrates the capture-inhibition method employed. The antibody used is a unique polyclonal antibody that was absorbed and purified to be specific for the 31 kd (OspA), 34 kd

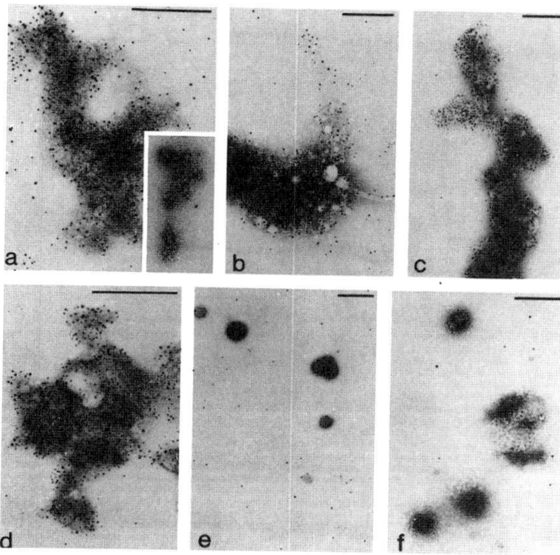

FIGURE 36-5

Immune electron microscopic detection of *B. burgdorferi* antigen in mammalian urine and blood. Pieces of labeled antigen were detected in urine from (**a**) mouse, (**c**) dog, and (**d**) human. Similar material was seen in (**b**) mouse blood. Labeled membrane vesicles were also seen (**a** insert). No specific labeling was seen in (**e**) urine and (**f**) blood from normal mice. (Reproduced by permission from Dorward DW, Schwan TG, Garon CF. Immune capture and detection of *Borrelia burgdorferi* antigens in urine, blood, or tissues from infected ticks, mice, dogs, and humans. J Clin Microbiol 1991;29:1162–1170.)

(OspB), 39kd, and 93kd antigens of *B. burgdorferi.* The assay is very specific for these antigens, and in more than 408 negative controls there was less than a 1% false-positive rate. Blocking and interference studies with human RBCs, WBCs, whole blood, serum, or human serum albumin showed no effect on the urine or CSF antigen-capture assays (55).

Serum and urine from 251 patients with Lyme disease (confirmed after a physician-diagnosed erythema migrans) were evaluated. As seen in **Table 36-4**, 30% of this group of Lyme patients had a positive Lyme Urine Antigen Test (LUAT). Only 8% of this group had a concurrent positive IgG/IgM ELISA. Other studies (56) have suggested that antigenuria may not be a constant daily occurrence. Therefore, multiple sampling days for urine may be more effective for detecting antigenuria (45) than a single collection.

TABLE 36-4

Patients with Physician-Diagnosed EM (n = 251)

History of tick bite	133/251	53%
>3 other symptoms	204/251	81%
History of arthritic symptoms	177/251	71%
Positive concurrent ELISA	19/251	8%
Positive LUAT	75/251	30%

Harris NS, Stephens BG. Detection of *Borrelia burgdorferi* antigen in urine from patients with Lyme borreliosis. J Spirochet Tick-Borne Dis 1995;2:37–41.

Polymerase Chain Reaction (PCR)

Every laboratory that offers Lyme disease testing may not be able to set up a PCR assay for *B. burgdorferi,* but each should be able to understand the assay and have a referral center to which it can send requests. Until proficiency testing is available for Lyme PCR, requests to referral laboratories for general aspects of their methodology, quality control, and validation data are definitely appropriate. Several published articles provide excellent background to this area (57–61). The referring laboratory must also understand and specify what type of PCR for Lyme is requested.

Lyme disease is characterized by a sparsity of organisms, as mentioned earlier (12,20). Some laboratories perform the genomic assay, which requires a minimum of one recoverable bacterium or at least the DNA from one. Our laboratory does dilution assays to validate that we can detect down to the level of 10° organisms/mL (i.e., 1 to 10 organisms).

A plasmid PCR assay is also available from some laboratories. Dorward et al. (49) used an immune electron microscopic technique to detect pieces of antigen rather than intact organisms in urine and other tissues. In an earlier study, Garon, Dorward, and Corvin (62) detected blebs (**Figs 36-7** and **36-8**) or membrane vesicles shed from the surface of *B. burgdorferi.* These blebs contain the same antigen as the intact organism (Dorward, personal communication). These blebs and fragments of *B. burgdorferi* antigen may be the reason for the antigen capture and plasmid PCR having great practical sensitivity. Nocton et al. (59) reported on the use of a plasmid PCR that had excellent sensitivity in the synovial fluid of patients with Lyme arthritis. The specificity of the plasmid PCR assay is still being studied;

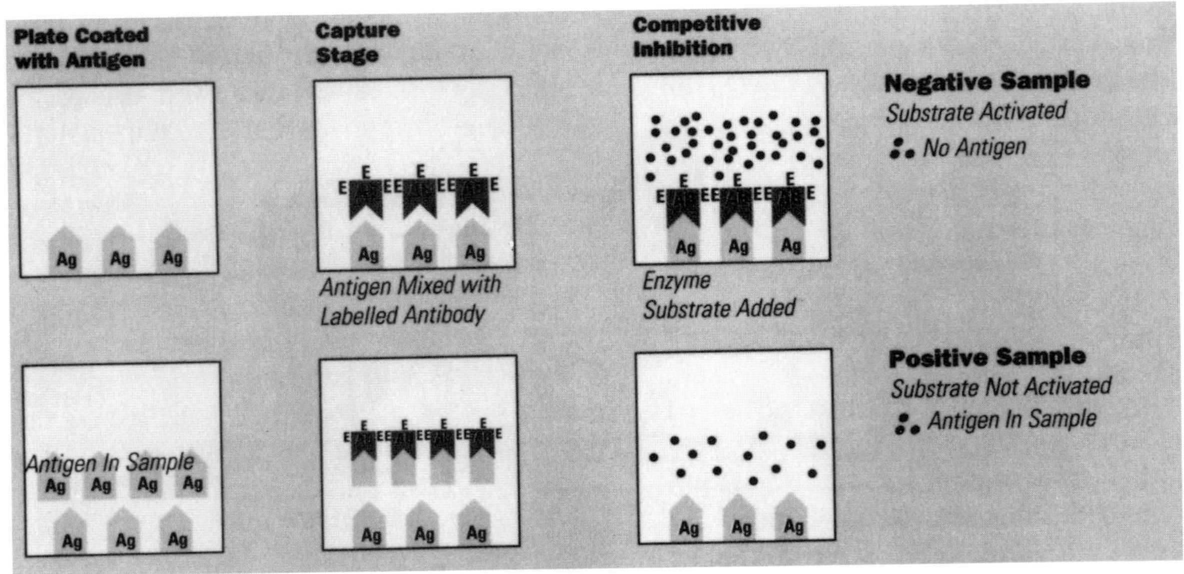

FIGURE 36-6

The Lyme urine antigen-capture inhibition test (LUAT). This test is covered by U.S. Patent 4,888,276. IGeneX, Inc. Reference Laboratory has exclusive license from Bio Whittaker, Inc., Walkersville, MD. (Reproduced by permission from Harris NS, Stephens BG. Detection of Borrelia burgdorferi antigen in urine from patients with Lyme borreliosis. J Spirochet Tick-Borne Dis 1995;2:37–41.)

FIGURE 36-7

Outer membrane blebs of *B. burgdorferi.* The blebs appear as buds coming off the membrane. (Reproduced by permission from Garon CF, Dorward DW, Corwin MD. Structural features of *Borrelia burgdorferi*—the Lyme disease spirochete: silver staining for nucleic acids. Scanning Microscopy 1989(suppl 3):109–115.)

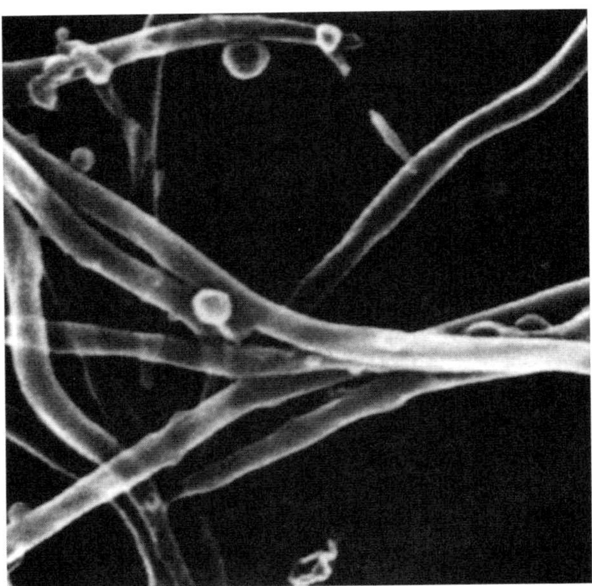

FIGURE 36-8

Membrane vesicles or blebs shed from surface of *B. burgdorferi.* (Reproduced by permission from Garon CF, Dorward DW, Corwin MD. Structural features of *Borrelia burgdorferi*—the Lyme disease spirochete: silver staining for nucleic acids. Scanning Microscopy 1989(suppl 3):109–115.)

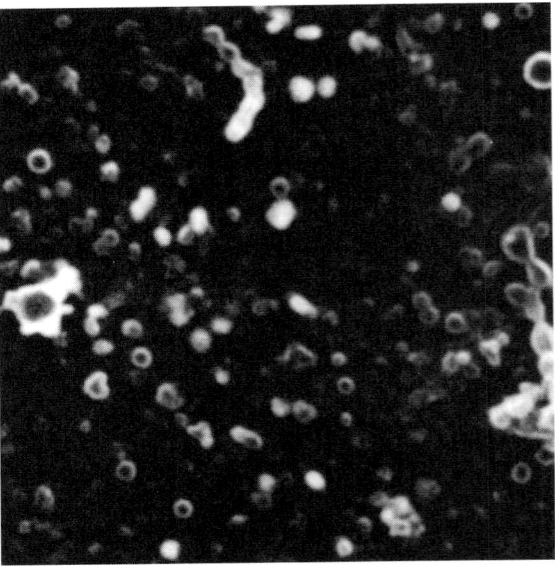

therefore, it is premature to rank it against other methods.

To avoid contamination problems, most laboratories performing PCR use separate facilities for testing by this method. For example, our laboratory uses separate rooms and dedicated UV laminar-flow hoods for assay setup, reagent dispensing, thermal cycling, and gel analysis. Each assay must have multiple negative and positive controls interspersed throughout the assay. Although contamination in the clinical laboratory is much less common than in the research laboratory, a contamination episode can wipe out assays for a considerable period of time. Decontamination may involve the development of new primers and an entirely new validation, which is comparable to a mini-PMA (pre-market approval).

Immune Complex and Borreliacidal Assays

Studies by Schutzer et al. (63,64) have provided preliminary data on a serum immune complex dissociation and subsequent Lyme Western blot. Serum from suspected Lyme patients or the appropriate control is initially precipitated by PEG, then dissociated by various ionic strength buffers, and subsequently assayed by an IgG and IgM Lyme Western blot. The authors suggest this technique can detect specific *B. burgdorferi* antibodies in previously seronegative Lyme patients. The concept is provocative, and in a small study our laboratory was able to detect specific antigen, as well as antibodies after dissociation. Considerable control populations now need to be evaluated before this assay gains wider acceptance.

Calister et al. (65) developed an assay that measures the killing of viable *B. burgdorferi* organisms with the serum from patients with Lyme disease. This borreliacidal activity was increased in convalescent serum of patients with early Lyme disease. Expanded studies by this group demonstrated that this borreliacidal activity caused by immune serum plus complement can easily be detected by flow cytometry (66). Their clinical data shows high specificity, but at the expense of sensitivity. A better use of this assay may be to monitor different antibiotic treatments in some selected patients.

Which Tests to Perform?

There is a logical sequence for laboratory tests to aid in the diagnosis of Lyme disease. Similar to the hepatitis model, antigen is present early after infection. Schmidt et al. (61) detected *B. burgdorferi* antigen in urine by PCR within the first weeks after infection. Our laboratory has found antigen by the LUAT as early as 3 days after a tick bite.

Later there is an antibody response in about 70% of the patients. IgM appears first, followed by IgG. Even in the presence of an IgM response, seen with the Western blot, our laboratory has detected *B. burgdorferi* using a genomic PCR with serum and plasma.

For completeness, both of the two major antibody assays (ELISA and Western blot) should be run, even though the Western blot is more sensitive. The increased sensitivity of the Western blot is analogous to a mountain where the base is a Western blot and the summit is an ELISA. The Western blot has considerably more sensitivity because it provides detection before the peak of the response. As mentioned before, the Western blot is a qualitative assay based upon an individual visualization of a patient's unique antibody against the various *B. burgdorferi* antigens. This type of assay should not be restricted by the same sensitivity and specificity concerns as the ELISA. An ELISA with a quantitative or semiquantitative cut-off, which is not necessarily specific to only the most unique of the *B. burgdorferi* antigens, needs to consider population aspects of false positive (specificity) and false negative (sensitivity).

These relationships can be depicted in the hypothetical model of an "idealized" *B. burgdorferi* infection (**Fig. 36-9**). After the first year or with persistent/recurrent disease, the left side of Figure 36-9 may not be valid. Therefore, multiple tests as used with other disease screening such as for hepatitis, thyroid deficiencies, or autoimmunity give a more complete picture to help with the clinical diagnosis and are ultimately more economical for the patient.

Persistent/recurrent infection offers a unique diagnostic problem, because the IgG response may be absent in more than 50% of the patients (17–19). The IgM Western blot has proved helpful for some patients with persistent/recurrent disease (34,47), but care must be taken to rule out possible cross-reactions due

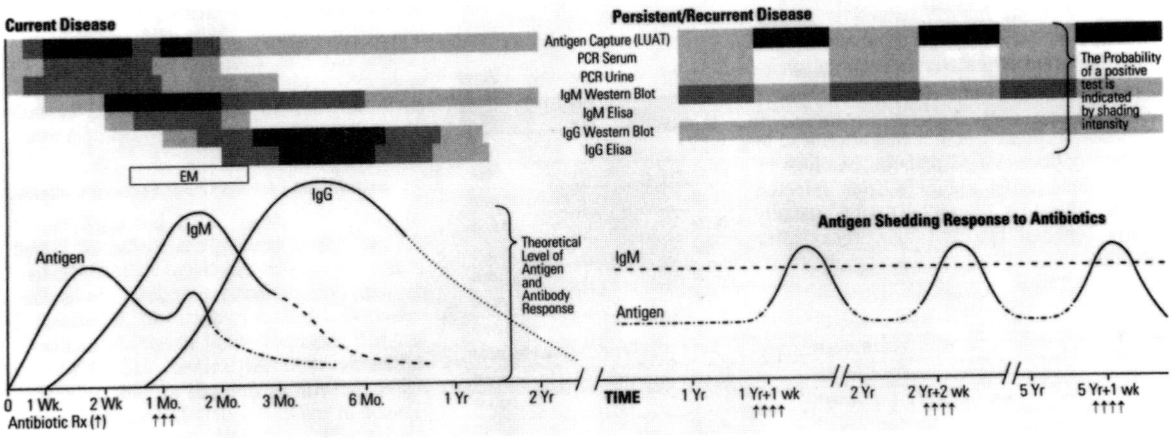

FIGURE 36-9

A model suggesting the tests applicable in different phases of Lyme disease. The left side of the figure indicates a hypothetical patient making antibodies soon after infection. Less than 70% of current patients are in this category. The theoretical responses shown on the right side of Figure 36-9 are typical of many patients with recurrent/persistent disease. (Courtesy of IGeneX, Inc. Reference Laboratory, Palo Alto, CA.)

to rheumatoid factor, other spirochetal disease, and perhaps mononucleosis (23,29).

During persistent/recurrent disease, assays that focus on antigen detection may be particularly useful (55). Antigen capture in urine has been a useful diagnostic assay, especially during the start-up of new antibiotics, which seem to enhance antigenuria (45).

The LUAT and the PCR are often complimentary. The PCR does seem to be more positive when patients are not on antibiotics. The genomic PCR requires at least one recoverable bacterium or at least the DNA from one. Studies at the Rocky Mountain National Laboratory (49) have shown that pieces of antigen are more common in urine than whole or semiwhole *B. burgdorferi*.

Antigen capture or PCR should be considered for studying the synovial fluid of inflamed joints in Lyme disease. In fact, the role of a plasmid PCR as a diagnostic aid in synovial fluid has proven to be very effective (59).

Lyme Neuroborreliosis

Lyme disease has been reported to cause a wide range of neurological symptoms: Bell's palsy, meningitis, meningoencephalitis, radiculoneuritis, encephalopathy, psychiatric syndromes, fatigue, MS-like symptoms, and Parkinson-like symptoms (53,67–74). Appropriate diagnostic assays must evaluate the CSF (75–77). In fact, according to Coyle, the blood of the brain is CSF, and it is impossible to make a diagnosis of neurological Lyme disease without performing a spinal tap and analyzing the CSF for antibodies and antigens to *B. burgdorferi* (personal communication).

One necessary assay is the CNS (central nervous system) or CSF index; it is a combination of immunological tests that measure specific antibodies to *B. burgdorferi* in both serum and spinal fluid. This index shows a relationship between serum and spinal fluid in Lyme disease. Calculations are based on the results of quantitation of both serum and CSF total IgG. This then provides the dilution values for the serum and CSF Lyme IgG ELISA. A CSF/serum ELISA index greater than 1 suggests in situ synthesis of antibody in the CNS. This index is important, because if a test is only performed on the CSF, there would be no control for leakage across the blood-brain barrier. Unfortunately, this series of tests uses the same flawed ELISA assays approved by the FDA for serum. Therefore, sensitivity is always a concern. A positive result, however, is excellent support for CNS Lyme infection.

The Western blot should be considered for ultimate antibody sensitivity in CSF. Our laboratory uses a 1:2 dilution for CSF (serum is 1:100 dilution) with longer incubation times for sensitivity. Because of concerns about leakage across the blood-brain barrier, these Western blots should be compared to those of the patient's serum.

Antigen capture and PCR assays have also been helpful with some patients (52,53,78). Patients with neurological symptoms of Lyme disease often have detectable levels of antigen in the CSF. These patients may be entirely negative for all assays in blood and urine.

Other Tick-Borne Diseases

It is important that the "complete" Lyme laboratory be aware of the connection between Lyme disease, ehrlichiosis, and babesiosis (79–84). Human ehrlichiosis is a disease caused by rickettsial-type organisms, transmitted in part by the same ticks that carry Lyme disease. Human granulocytic ehrlichiosis (HGE) has been closely linked to the bites of *Ixodes scapularis* and *Ixodes pacificus* (85,86). Human monocytic ehrlichiosis has been linked to the bites of *Amblyomma americanum* (Lone Star tick) (85,86). The *Dermacentor variablis* (dog tick) has also been suggested to be involved in transmission of both diseases.

Two forms of the human disease are caused by the *Ehrlichia* species. *E. chaffeensis* and *E. phagocytophilia* cause the human diseases human monocytic ehrlichiosis (HME) and human granulocytic ehrlichiosis (HGE), respectively. Serology by IFA is done using *E. chaffeensis* (87) for HME, and the closely related *E. equii* (88) for HGE. Seroconversion usually occurs between 2 and 4 weeks after infection.

Ehrlichiosis usually presents with high fever, malaise, headache, myalgia, sweats, and nausea. Patients diagnosed with *Ehrlichia* organisms should also be tested for Lyme disease, because the disease is transmitted by the same tick and coinfections have been shown to occur (82,84).

Babesiosis is caused by an intraerythrocytic parasite, *Babesia microti* (81,89), which is similar in effect and appearance to *Plasmodium falciparum*, the causative agent of malaria. In fact, the symptoms and the appearance of ring-shaped intraerythrocytic parasites in red cells stained with Giemsa or Wright's often lead to the wrong diagnosis of malaria. Serology by IFA is done using red cells from infected Syrian hamsters. Seroconversion usually occurs between 2 and 4 weeks after infection.

B. microti is also transmitted by the same ticks that transmit *B. burgdorferi*, the causative agent of Lyme disease (79–81,83). Symptoms of babesiosis are also somewhat similar to some of the symptoms of Lyme disease: fatigue, malaise, myalgia, arthralgia, chills, and fever. Usually the fever is high. This disease is particularly life threatening in splenectomized patients.

The physician may find it helpful to have all these tests performed at the same time. As with all IFA antibody assays for bacterial infections, paired testing of acute and convalescent sera is recommended.

General Aspects of Quality Control and Quality Assurance

Quality control concerns itself with the specifics of a particular assay. For Lyme disease this chapter has stressed the importance of proficiency events and their associated samples, which can provide one level of control. Panel samples from the CDC are available as well as commercial Lyme disease panels. A wide range of specific monoclonal antibodies to unique antigens of *B. burgdorferi* are also available (90–98). These monoclonal antibodies become imperative if a laboratory embarks upon the development of its own Western blot for *B. burgdorferi.*

In addition, a laboratory should send serum samples to various laboratories for comparison purposes of band identification and evaluation of their blot's sensitivity. This type of cross reference is the beginning of test validation. It is, of course, followed by ongoing control testing of each individual test batch. Criteria, independent of the CDC/ASPHLD criteria (even though they have sensitivity problems), require a laboratory to establish an elaborate clinical study. This type of study has tremendous benefits, because it can increase a Western blot's sensitivity with very minimal effect on specificity. However, such a study is expensive and time consuming.

Quality assurance is a much more general and ever-changing program which includes quality control. Our laboratory defines quality assurance as:

> . . . an administrative program for the systematic monitoring of all key management areas including quality control, which impact on the patient. The program must meet prescribed conformance to specific criteria and thresholds: e.g., quality, efficacy, turn-around-time, medical appropriateness, practicality and safety. Results of a quality assurance program should upgrade or downgrade given laboratory management areas, meet overall management objectives: e.g., appropriate patient care, safe working environment, resource utilization, team effectiveness, and strategic planning. This implies that the laboratory has four customers with unique needs:

1. The patient, with satisfactory service toward medical care
2. The physician, with satisfactory state of the art and turnaround-time
3. The employee, with satisfactory state of safety
4. The company, with satisfactory state of fiscal balance

The Future

Improvements will evolve in laboratory diagnostics as recombinant antigens become available to the unique antigens of *B. burgdorferi* (36,95,97,99–101). Individual recombinant antigens will be able to be added, one by one, to construct a series of highly specific ELISA assays. Retrospective clinical studies must be performed to observe what combinations of antigens are needed to approach the needed degree of sensitivity (>95%) and acceptable specificity (>85%) for a screening assay (32). Furthermore, new genetic markers for *B. burgdorferi* will most likely be discovered, and new PCR-like assays will become easier to perform in the laboratory.

However, little additional progress will be made in the scope of new diagnostics until we learn more regarding the biology of *B. burgdorferi.* In the course of disease, long periods of remission are followed by acute symptoms, which may last for weeks or months. Therefore, basic research studies at the animal level are needed to evaluate the cyclical nature of the disease as well as the idiosyncrasies of the organism—for example, where it hides in the body.

Science has progressed to the point where it is enamored with techniques associated with molecular diagnostics and genetics, but some of the traditional techniques may also be appropriate to study this organism. Tissue culture studies provide one level of understanding of how the bug interacts with lymphocytes. Natural infection of mice and dogs by ticks with radiolabeled *B. burgdorferi* will provide information in a homeostatic environment where different types of cells and tissues can be studied. Progress for better diagnostics and treatment will come through better knowledge of the spirochete *B. burgdorferi.*

Acknowledgments

I would like to thank Alana Hansen, Aline Harris, Steven Harris, and Diana Stephens for editorial assistance. I would also like to thank Brenda Shiplett for help with manuscript preparation.

REFERENCES

1. Murray P. The widening circle. New York: St. Martin's Press, 1996.
2. Steere AC, Malawista SE, Snyderman DR, et al. Lyme arthritis: an epidemic of oligoarthritis in children and adults in three Connecticut communities. Arthritis Rheum 1977;20:7–17.
3. Steere AC, Gibofsky A, Patarroyo ME, et al. Chronic Lyme arthritis: clinical and immunogenetic differentiation from rheumatoid arthritis. Ann Intern Med 1979;90:896–901.
4. Steere AC, Hardin JR, Ruddy SM, et al. Lyme arthritis: correlation of serum and cryoglobulin IgM with activity, and serum IgG with remission. Arthritis Rheum 1979;22:471–483.
5. Afzelius A. Erythema chronicum migrans. Derm Venereol (Stockh) 1921;2:120–125.
6. Scrimenti RJ. Erythema chronicum migrans. Arch Dermatol 1970;102:104–105.
7. Steere AC, Malawista SE. Cases of Lyme disease in the United States: locations correlated with distribution of *Ixodes dammini.* Ann Intern Med 1979;91:730–733.
8. Burgdorfer W, Barbour AG, Hayes SF, et al. Lyme disease—a tick borne spirochetosis? Science 1982;216:1317–1319.

9. Benach JL, Boster EM, Hanrahan JP, et al. Spirochetes isolated from the blood of two patients with Lyme disease. N Engl J Med 1983;308:740–742.

10. Barbour AG. Isolation and cultivation of Lyme disease spirochetes. Yale J Biol Med 1984;57:71–75.

11. Barbour AG, Burdorfer W, Grunwaldt E, Steere AC. Antibodies of patients with Lyme disease to components of the *Ixodes dammini* spirochete. J Clin Invest 1983;72:504–515.

12. Steere AC, Grodzicki RL, Kornblatt AN, et al. The spirochetal etiology of Lyme disease. N Engl J Med 1983;308:733–740.

13. Burgdorfer W, Lane RS, Barbour AG, et al. The western black-legged tick, *Ixodes pacificus*: a vector of *Borrelia burgdorferi*. Am J Trop Med Hyg 1985;34:925–930.

14. CDC. Lyme disease: case definitions for public health surveillance. MMWR 1990;39:19–21.

15. Williams CL, Strobino B, Lee A, et al. Lyme disease in childhood: clinical and epidemiologic features of ninety cases. Pediatr Infect Dis J 1990;9:10–14.

16. Berger BW. Dermatologic manifestations of Lyme disease. Rev Infect Dis 1989;11:S1475–1481.

17. Engstrom SM, Shoop E, Johnson RC. Immunoblot interpretation criteria for serodiagnosis of early Lyme disease. J Clin Microbiol 1995;33:419–427.

18. Aguero-Rosenfeld ME, Nowakowski J, McKenna DF, et al. Serodiagnosis in early Lyme disease. J Clin Microbiol 1993;31:3090–3095.

19. Aguero-Rosenfeld ME, Nowakowski J, McKenna DF, et al. Evolution of the serologic response to *Borrelia burgdorferi* in treated patients with culture-confirmed erythema migrans. J Clin Microbiol 1996;34:1–9.

20. Wallach FR, Forni AL, Hariprashad J, et al. Circulating *Borrelia burgdorferi* in patients with acute Lyme disease: results of blood cultures and serum DNA analysis. J Infect Dis 1993;168:1541–1543.

21. Rawlings JA, Fournier PV, Teltow GA. Isolation of Borrelia spirochetes from patients in Texas. J Clin Microbiol 1987;25:1148–1150.

22. Schwartz BS, Goldstein MD, Ribeiro JMC, et al. Antibody testing in Lyme disease: a comparison of results in four laboratories. JAMA 1989;262:3431–3434.

23. Luger SW, Krauss E. Serologic tests for Lyme disease: interlaboratory variability. Arch Intern Med 1990;15:761–763.

24. Bakken LL, Case KL, Callister SM, et al. Performance of 45 laboratories participating in a proficiency testing program for Lyme disease serology. JAMA 1992;268:891–895.

25. Mitchell PD, Reed KD, Aspeslet TL, et al. Comparison of four immunoserologic assays for detection of antibodies to *Borrelia burgdorferi* in patients with culture-positive erythema migrans. J Clin Microbiol 1994;32:1958–1962.

26. Russell H, Sampson JS, Schmid GP, et al. Enzyme-linked immunosorbent assay for Lyme disease. J Infect Dis 1984;149:465–470.

27. Hedberg CW, Osterholm MT, MacDonald KL, White KE. An interlaboratory study of antibody to *Borrelia burgdorferi*. J Infect Dis 1987;155:1325–1327.

28. Magnarelli LA, Meegan JM, Anderson JF, Chappell WA. Comparison of an indirect fluorescent-antibody test with an enzyme-linked immunosorbent assay for serological studies of Lyme disease. J Clin Microbiol 1984;20:181–184.

29. Magnarelli LA, Anderson JF, Johnson RC. Cross-reactivity in serological tests for Lyme disease and other spirochetal infections. J Infect Dis 1987;156:183–188.

30. Craft JE, Grodzicki RL, Steere AC, Antibody response in Lyme disease: evaluation of tests. J Infect Dis 1984;149:789–795.

31. Voller A, Bidwell D. Enzyme-linked immunosorbent assay. In: Manual of clinical immunology. 3rd ed. Washington, DC: ASM, 1986:99–109.

32. Bakken LL, Callister SM, Wand PJ, Shell RF. Inter-laboratory comparison of test results for detection of Lyme disease by 516 participants in the Wisconsin State Laboratory of Hygiene/College of American Pathologists Proficiency Testing Program. J Clin Microbiol 1997;35:537–543.

33. Barbour AG, Tessier SL, Hayes SF. Variation in a major surface protein of Lyme disease spirochetes. Infect Immunol 1984;45:94–100.

34. Craft JE, Fischer DK, Shimamoto GT, Steere AC, Antigens of *Borrelia burgdorferi* recognized during Lyme disease: appearance of a new immunoglobulin M response and expansion of the immunoglobulin G response late in the illness. J Clin Invest 1997;78:934–939.

35. Coleman JL, Benach JL. Isolation of antigenic components from the Lyme disease spirochete: their role in early diagnosis. J Infect Dis 1987; 155:756–765.

36. Simpson WJ, Schrumpf ME, Schwan TG. Reactivity of human Lyme Borreliosis sera with a 39 kilodalton antigen specific to *Borrelia burgdorferi*. J Clin Microbiol 1990;28:1329–1337.

37. Wilske B, Preac-Mursic, Schierz G, et al. Antigenic variability of *Borrelia burgdorferi*. Ann NY Acad Sci 1988;539:126–143.

38. Zoller L, Burkyard S, Schafer H. Validity of Western immunoblot band patterns in the serodiagnosis of Lyme borreliosis. J Clin Microbiol 1991;29:174–182.

39. Golightly MG, Thomas JA, Viciana AL. The laboratory diagnosis of Lyme borreliosis. Lab Med 1990;21:299–304.

40. Ma B, Christen B, Leung D, Vigo-Pelfry C. Serodiagnosis of Lyme Borreliosis by Western immunoblot: reactivity of various significant antibodies against *Borrelia burgdorferi*. J Clin Microbiol 1992;30:370–376.

41. Association of State and Territorial Public Health Laboratory Directors (ASTPHLD). Proceedings of the second national conference on the serological diagnosis of Lyme disease, October 27–29, 1994. Dearborn MI. Washington, DC: ASTPHLD, 1995.

42. CDC. Recommendations for test performance and interpretation from the second national conference on serologic diagnosis of Lyme disease. MMWR Morbid Mortal Wkly Rep 1995;44:590–591.

43. Dressler F, Whalen JA, Reinhardt BN, Steere AC. Western blotting in the serodiagnosis of Lyme disease. J Infect Dis 1993;167:392–400.

44. Hilton E, Devoti J, Soo S. Recommendation to include OspA and OspB in the new immunoblotting criteria for serodiagnosis of Lyme disease. J Clin Microbiol 1996;34:1353–1355.

45. Harris NS, Harris SJ, Joseph JJ, Stephens BG. *Borrelia burgdorferi* antigen levels in urine and other fluids during the course of treatment for Lyme disease: a case study. Presented at the VII International Congress of Lyme Borreliosis meeting, San Francisco, CA, June 16–21, 1996.

46. Jain VK, Hilton E, Maytal J, Dorante G, Ilowite NT, Sood SK. Immunoglobulin M immunoblot for diagnosis of *Borrelia burgdorferi* infection in patients with acute facial palsy. J Clin Microbiol 1996;34:2033–2035.

47. Oski J, Uksila J, Marjamaki M, et al. Antibodies against whole sonicated *Borrelia burgdorferi* spirochetes, 41 kilodalton flagellin and P39 protein in patients with PCR- or culture-proven late Lyme borreliosis. J Clin Microbiol 1995;33: 2260–2264.

48. Hyde FW, Johnson RC, White TJ, Shelburne CE. Detection of antigens in urine of mice and humans infected with *Borrelia burgdorferi*, etiologic agent of Lyme disease. J Clin Microbiol 1989;27:58–61.

49. Dorward DW, Schwan TG, Garon CF. Immune capture and detection of extracellular *B. burgdorferi* antigens in fluids or tissues of ticks, mice, dogs, and humans. J Clin Microbiol 1991; 29:1162–1171.

50. Goodman JL, Jurkovich P, Kodner C, Johnson RC. Persistent cardiac and urinary tract infections with *Borrelia burgdorferi* in experimentally infected Syrian hamsters. J Clin Microbiol 1991;29:894–896.

51. Magnarelli LA, Anderson JF, Stafford KC. Detection of *Borrelia burgdorferi* in urine of *Peromyscus leucopus* by inhibition enzyme-linked immunosorbent assay. J Clin Microbiol 194;32: 777–782.

52. Goodman JL, Jurkovich P, Kramber JM, Johnson RC. Molecular detection of persistent *Borrelia burgdorferi* in the urine of patients with active Lyme disease. Infect Immun 1991;59:3–12.

53. Coyle PK, Deng Z, Schutzer SE, et al. Detection of antigens in cerebrospinal fluid. Neurology 1993;43:1093–1097.

54. Shelburne CE. Method and composition for the diagnosis of Lyme disease. US Patent 4,888,276, 1989.

55. Harris NS, Stephens BG. Detection of *B. burgdorferi* antigen in urine from patients with Lyme Borreliosis. J Spirochetal Tick-Borne Dis 1995;2:37–41.

56. Harris N, Drulle J, Eiras E, Stephens B. Detection of *B. burgdorferi* antigen and antibody in patients presenting with an erythema migrans. Presented at 6th annual Lyme disease scientific conference, Atlantic City, NJ, May 5–6, 1993.

57. Rosa PA, Schwan TG. A specific and sensitive assay for the Lyme disease spirochete *B. burgdorferi* using the polymerase chain reaction. J Infect Dis 1989;160:1018–1029.

58. Persing DH, Telford SR, Spielman A, Barthold SW. Detection of *Borrelia burgdorferi* infection

in *Ixodes dammini* ticks with the polymerase chain reaction. J Clin Microbiol 1990;28:566–572.

59. Nocton JJ, Dressler F, Rutledge BJ, et al. Detection of *Borrelia burgdorferi* DNA by polymerase chain reaction in synovial fluid from patients with Lyme arthritis. N Engl J Med 1994;330:229–234.
60. Goodman JL, Bradley JF, Ross AE, et al. Bloodstream invasion in early Lyme disease: results from a prospective, controlled, blinded study using the polymerase chain reaction. Am J Med 1995;9:6–12.
61. Schmidt B, Muellegger RR, Stochenhuber C, et al. Detection of *Borrelia burgdorferi*—specific DNA in urine specimens from patients with erythema migrans before and after antibiotic therapy. J Clin Microbiol 1996;34:1359–1363.
62. Garon GF, Dorward DW, Corwin MD. Structural features of *Borrelia burgdorferi*—the Lyme disease spirochete: Silver staining for nucleic acids. Scanning Microscopy Suppl 1989;3:109–115.
63. Schutzer SE, Coyle PK, Belman AL, et al. Sequestration of antibody to *Borrelia burgdorferi* in immune complexes in seronegative Lyme disease. Lancet 1990:335:312–315.
64. Schutzer SE. Method and materials for detecting Lyme disease. US Patent 5,187,065, 1993.
65. Callister SM, Schell RF, Lourich SD. Lyme disease assay which detects killed *Borrelia burgdorferi.* J Clin Microbiol 1991;29:1773–1776.
66. Liu YF, Lim LCL, Schell K, et al. Differentiation of Borreliacidal activity caused by immune serum or antimicrobial agents by flow cytometry. Clin Diag Lab Immunol 1994;1:145–149.
67. Finkel MF. Lyme disease and its neurologic complications. Arch Neurol 1988;45:99–104.
68. Pachner AR, Neurologic manifestations of Lyme disease: the new "great imitator." Rev Infect Dis 1989;11(suppl 6):S1483–1486.
69. Halperin JJ. Nervous system manifestations of Lyme disease. Rheum Dis Clin North Am 1989;15:635–647.
70. Pahner AR, Duray P, Steere AC. Central nervous system manifestations of Lyme disease. Arch Neurol 1989;46:790–795.
71. Halperin JJ, Luft BJ, Anand AK, et al. Lyme neuroborreliosis: central nervous system manifestations. Neurology 1989;39:753–759.
72. Logigian EL, Kaplan RF, Steere AC. Chronic neurologic manifestations of Lyme disease. N Engl J Med 1990;323:1438–1444.
73. Fallon BA, Nields JA, Burrascano JJ, et al. The neuropsychiatric manifestations of Lyme borreliosis. Psychiatr Q 1992;63:95–117.
74. Coyle PK, Neurologic complications of Lyme disease. Rheum Dis Clin North Am 1993;19:993–1009.
75. Wilske B, Schierz G, Preac-Mursic V, et al. Intrathecal production of specific antibodies against *Borrelia burgdorferi* in patients with lymphocytic meningoradiculitis. J Infect Dis 1986;153:304–314.
76. Steere AC, Berardi VP, Weeks KE, et al. Evaluation of the intrathecal antibody response to *Borrelia burgdorferi* as a diagnostic test for Lyme neuroborreliosis. J Infect Dis 1990;161:1203–1209.
77. Halperin JJ, Volkman DJ, Wu P. Central nervous system abnormalities in Lyme neuroborreliosis. Neurology 1991;41:1571–1582.
78. Keller TL, Halperin JJ, Whitman M. PCR Detection of *Borrelia burgdorferi* DNA in cerebrospinal fluid of Lyme neuroborreliosis patients. Neurology 1992;42:32–42.
79. Benach JL, Coleman JL, Habicht GS. Serologic evidence for simultaneous occurrences of Lyme disease and babesiosis. J Infect Dis 1981;144:473–477.
80. Grunwaldt E, Barbour AG, Benach JL. Simultaneous occurrence of babesiosis and Lyme disease. N Engl J Med 1983;308:1166.
81. Anderson JF, Mintz ED, Gadbaw JJ, Magnarelli LA. *Babesia microti,* human babesiosis, and *Borrelia burgdorferi* in Connecticut. J Clin Microbiol 1991;29:2779–2783.
82. Magmarelli LA, Dumler SJ, Anderson JF, et al. Coexistence of antibodies to tick-borne pathogens of babesiosis, ehrlichiosis, and Lyme borreliosis in human sera. J Clin Microbiol 1995;33:3054–3057.
83. Krause PJ, Telford SR, Spielman A, et al. Concurrent Lyme disease and babesiosis: evidence for increased severity and duration of illness. JAMA 1996;275:1657–1660.
84. Mitchell PD, Reed KD, Hofkes JM. Immunoserologic evidence of coinfection with *Borrelia burgdorferi, Babesia microti,* and human granulocytic Ehrlichia species in residents of Wisconsin and Minnesota. J Clin Microbiol 1996;34:724–727.
85. Fishbein DB, Dawson JE, Robinson LE. Human ehrlichiosis in the United States, 1985 to 1990. Ann Intern Med 1994;120:736–743.

86. Dumler JS, Bakken JS. Ehrlichial diseases of humans: emerging tick-borne infections. Clin Infect Dis 1995;20:1102–1110.

87. Anderson BE, Dawson JE, Jones DC, Wilson KH. *Ehrlichia chaffeensis*, a new species associated with human ehrlichiosis. J Clin Microbiol 1991;29:2838–2842.

88. Goodman JL, Nelson C, Vitale B, et al. Direct cultivation of the causative agent of human granulocytic ehrlichiosis. N Engl J Med 1996; 334:209–215.

89. Persing DH, Mathiesen D, Marshall WF, et al. Detection of *Babesia microti* by polymerase chain reaction. J Clin Microbiol 1992;30:2097–2103.

90. Barbour AG, Tessier SL, Todd WJ. Lyme disease spirochetes and ixodid tick spirochetes share a common surface antigenic determinant defined by a monoclonal antibody. Infect Immun 1986; 41:795–804.

91. Barbour AG, Hayes SF, Heiland RA, Schrumpf ME, Tessier SL. A borrelia-specific monoclonal antibody binds to a flagellar epitope. Infect Immun 1986;52:549–554.

92. Luft BJ, Gorevic PD, Jiang W, et al. Immunologic and structural characterization of the dominant 66–73 kDa antigens of *Borrelia burgdorferi*. J Immunol 1991;146:2776–2782.

93. Coleman JL, Benach JL, Characterization of antigenic determinants of *Borrelia burgdorferi* shared by other bacteria. J Infect Dis 1992;165: 658–666.

94. Sadzeine A, Rosa PA, Thompson PA, et al. Antibody-resistant mutants of *Borrelia burgdorferi*: in vitro selection and characterization. J Exp Med 1992;176:799–809.

95. Luft BJ, Mudri S, Jiang W, et al. The 93-kilodalton protein of *Borrelia burgdorferi*: an immunodominant protoplasmic cylinder antigen. Infect Immun 1992;60:4309–4321.

96. Comstock LE, Fikrig E, Shoberg RJ, et al. A monoclonal antibody to OspA inhibits association of *Borrelia burgdorferi* with human endothelial cells. Infect Immun 1993;61:423–431.

97. Padula SJ, Sampieri A, Dias F, et al. Molecular characterization and expression of p23 (OspC) from a North American Strain of *Borrelia burgdorferi*. Infect Immun 1993;61:5097–5105.

98. Schwan TG, Schrumpf ME, Karstens RH, et al. Distribution and molecular analysis of Lyme disease spirochetes, *Borrelia burgdorferi*, isolated from ticks throughout California. J Clin Microbiol 1993;31:3096–3108.

99. LeFebvre RB, Perng GC, Johnson RC. The 83-kilodalton antigen of *Borrelia burgdorferi* which stimulates Immunoglobulin (IgM) and IgG responses in infected hosts is expressed by a chromosomal gene. J Clin Microbiol 1990;28: 1673–1675.

100. Magnarelli LA, Fikrig E, Berland R, et al. Comparison of whole-cell antibodies and an antigenic flagellar epitope *of Borrelia burgdorferi* in serologic tests for diagnosis of Lyme borreliosis. J Clin Microbiol 1992;30:3158–3162.

101. Probert WS, Allsup KM, LeFebvre RB. Identification and characterization of a surface-exposed 66-kilodalton protein from *Borrelia burgdorferi*. Infect Immun 1995;63:1933–1939.

CHAPTER 37

Pneumococcal Serotype Assays

JØRGEN HENRICHSEN

Streptococcus pneumoniae is a gram-positive, lanceolate capsulated diplococcus that also appears in short chains. Based on differences in the capsular polysaccharides recognized by the immune system of both rabbits and humans, it is divided into 90 capsular types (1), each of which introduces type-specific protective antibodies that are necessary for opsonophagocytosis.

The pneumococcus causes sinusitis, otitis media, pneumonia, and severe invasive diseases such as bacteremia and meningitis. Pneumococcal otitis media is common in children all over the world. Annual hospital admissions for all pneumococcal pneumonias in the elderly in western Europe were estimated to amount to as many as 175,000 to 275,000 in 1995 (David Fedson, personal communication), and the overall annual mortality from pneumococcal infections lies in the range of 75,000 deaths. Of course many more patients who suffer from pneumococcal pneumonia are being treated in their homes.

In Denmark the incidence of invasive pneumococcal infections in 1995 was found to be 18 cases per 100,000 inhabitants and the highest rates were seen in the very young (23/100,000) and in the elderly (55/100,000) (2). In 1996, the overall incidence had risen to 27 cases per 400,000 inhabitants. In the United States, the annual incidence of pneumococcal bacteremia in Ohio was 83 per 100,000 in the elderly (3), and in Australia it was found to be as high as 1025 per 100,000 in aboriginal children under 5 years of age (4). When one adds to this that the number of pneumococcal disease isolates that are resistant to penicillin and other antibiotics seems to be increasing worldwide, it is not surprising that pneumococcal vaccination is receiving increasing attention as a preventive measure, especially in the US and Europe.

The laboratory diagnosis of pneumococcal disease is still mainly based on culture (5). Attempts to detect pneumococcal capsular polysaccharide in urine and serum may be a useful diagnostic supplement in the search for the etiologic agent in blood culture–negative cases of pneumonia (6). Determination of type-specific pneumococcal antibodies in serum seems to be of little or no diagnostic value, whereas some have claimed the merit of determination of antipneumolysin antibodies in paired serum samples (7). Knowledge about pneumococcal antibody levels, which today are usually measured by enzyme-linked immunosorbent assay (ELISA), is, on the other hand, necessary in order to assess susceptibility to pneumococcal infections, especially in risk groups.

Finally, surveillance of types of pneumococcal isolates and of their antibiotic sensitivity is highly important for the formulation of vaccination policy.

Culture

As *Streptococcus pneumoniae* is a fastidious microorganism with growth requirements, it is essential to use enriched media to obtain good growth. These are described in bacteriologic textbooks such as *Manual of Clinical Microbiology* (8). Media should always be tested for their ability to sustain growth of pneumococci by the use of a few known pneumococcal strains. Blood and chocolate agar culture plates of good quality represent standard media but are not of sufficient quality everywhere in the world (9). The most widely used liquid media are Todd-Hewitt, serum, and brain-heart infusion broths.

The species diagnosis is easily secured by testing for ethylhydrocupreine (Optochin) sensitivity and bile solubility. Also, omniserum (see below) can be used.

If not cultured immediately specimens should be collected and transported in a proper transport medium such as Amies.

An excellent manual on all aspects of laboratory procedures has been published by the World Health Organization (10).

Typing of Pneumococci

To facilitate the typing procedure, those of the altogether 90 types that cross-react most extensively are grouped together. From **Table 37-1** it can be seen that 65 of the 90 types belong to 21 groups that contain from 2 to 5 types.

Typing Antisera

Statens Serum Institut (Copenhagen, Denmark) manufactures diagnostic pneumococcal antisera, primarily intended for typing of pneumococci by means of the capsular reactions test. These antisera are:

1. *Omniserum,* which gives a positive capsular reaction with all 90 types. It is primarily intended as a quick diagnostic tool for use directly on clinical specimens, especially cerebrospinal fluid (CSF). It was originally described by Lund and Rasmussen in 1966 (11).
2. *Nine pooled sera* labeled from A to I. Each of the 90 types will give positive capsular reaction with one of these sera. Types with strong cross-reactions are grouped in the pooled sera, thereby reducing the need for absorption of antibodies that react with types not included in a pool. The pooled sera consist of the following types or groups:

TABLE **37-1**

Pneumococcal Types and Groups[a,b,c]

Type	Group	Types Within Groups
1		
2		
3		
4		
5		
	6	6A, *6B*
	7	*7F*, 7A, 7B, 7C
8		
	9	9A, 9L, *9N*, *9V*
	10	10F, *10A*, 10B, 10C
	11	11F, *11A*, 11B, 11C, 11D
	12	*12F*, 12A, 12B
13		
14		
	15	15F, 15A, *15B*, 15C
	16	16F, 16A
	17	*17F*, 17A
	18	18F, 18A, 18B, *18C*
	19	*19F*, *19A*, 19B, 19C
20		
21		
	22	*22F*, 22A
	23	*23F*, 23A, 23B
	24	24F, 24A, 24B
	25	25F, 25A
27		
	28	28F, 28A
29		
31		
	32	32F, 32A
	33	*33F*, 33A, 33B, 33C, 33D
34		
	35	35F, 35A, 35B, 35C
36		
37		
38		
39		
40		
	41	41F, 41A
42		
43		
44		
45		
46		
	47	47F, 47A
48		
25	21	65

[a] 25 + 65 = 90 types altogether (nos. 26 and 30 not in use). 25 + 21 = 46 types or groups.

[b] To distinguish between types within groups, factor sera are needed.

[c] Types present in the currently available pneumococcal polysaccharide vaccines are underlined.

Pool	Types or Groups
A	1, 2, 4, 5, 18
B	3, 6, 8, 19
C	7, 20, 24, 31, 40
D	9, 11, 16, 36, 37
E	10, 12, 21, 33, 39
F	17, 22, 27, 32, 41
G	29, 34, 35, 42, 47
H	13, 14, 15, 23, 28
I	25, 38, 43, 44, 45, 46, 48

3. *Forty-six type or group sera* that react with single types or groups numbered from 1 to 48. Numbers 26 and 30 are not in use because they were shown to be types 6B and 15A, respectively. Heterologous reactions have been absorbed out. These sera are used for the diagnosis of both individual types and groups of closely related types (see Table 37-1).
4. *Factor sera* that are rather heavily absorbed and thereby usually rendered monospecific (12). These sera are necessary for the differentiation of types within groups.

Complete Typing Procedure

Typing of pneumococci, the diagnosis as to species level having been verified by Optochin sensitivity or bile solubility, or both, and/or a positive reaction with omniserum, by means of the capsular reaction test using successively pooled sera A-I, the relevant type or group sera, and, whenever necessary, factor sera, has been described in detail elsewhere (12,13).

Typing with PNEUMOTEST

An alternative, and much simpler, typing procedure has been described recently (14). It is based on the combined use of 12 pooled sera. Seven of the above mentioned A-I, that is, A, B, C, D, E, F, and H, plus five new pools, designated P-T, are available together from Statens Serum Institut as the PNEUMOTEST kit. The formulation of these 12 pooled sera is seen in **Table 37-2**. The typing strategy is shown diagrammatically in **Figure 37-1**. Using this procedure more than 90% of strains isolated from blood or CSF can be typed or grouped; however, it does not allow differentiation of types within groups.

TABLE 37-2

A Chessboard System for Typing/Grouping of most Pneumococci Isolated from Blood or Cerebrospinal Fluid[a]

Pool	P	Q	R	S	T	Nonvaccine Types/Groups
A	1[b]	18[c]	4	5	2	
B	19[c]	6[c]	3	8		
C	7[c]				20	24[c]; 31; 40
D			9[c]		11[c]	16[c]; 36; 37
E			12[c]	10[c]	33[c]	21; 39
F				17[c]	22[c]	27; 32[c]; 41[c]
H	14	23[c]		15[c]		13; 28[c]
G[d]						29; 34; 35[c]; 42; 47[c]
I						25[c]; 38; 43; 44; 45; 46; 48

A-I, existing pooled sera; P-T, new pooled sera.

[a] The five pooled sera P-T are composed in such a way that each of the 21 vaccine-related types/groups reacts both in one of these sera and in one of the seven pooled sera A-F plus H.

[b] All 46 types or groups are shown in the table (nos. 26 and 30 are not in use).

[c] Groups containing the following types; **6**: 6A and **6B**; **7**: **7F**, 7A, 7B, and 7C; **9**: 9A, 9L, **9N**, and **9V; 10**: 10F, **10A**, 10B, and 10C**; 11**: 11F, **11A**, 11B, 11C, and 11D; **12**: **12F**, 12A, and 12B; **15**: 15F, 15A, **15B**, and 15C; 16: 16F and 16A; **17**: **17F** and 17A; **18**: 18F, 18A, 18B, and **18C; 19**: **19F**, **19A**, 19B, and 19C; **22**: **22F** and 22A; **23**: **23F**, 23A, and 23B; 24: 24F, 24A, and 24B; 25: 25F and 25A; 28: 28F and 28A; 32: 32F and 32A; **33**: **33F**, 33A, 33B, 33C, and 33D; 35: 35F, 35A, 35B, and 35C; 41: 41F and 41A; 47: 47F and 47A. Types/groups present in the currently available 23 valent pneumococcal vaccine are entered in boldface.

[d] Pools G and I do not react with vaccine types and are, therefore, not included in the chessboard system.

SOURCE: Reprinted by permission from Sørensen UBS. Typing of pneumococci by using 12 pooled antisera. J Clin Microbiol 1993;31:2097–2100. (The six newly described types have been added.)

Capsular Reaction Test

Although first described in 1902 by Neufeld, capsular reactions were not used for typing of pneumococci until 1931, when Neufeld and Tulczynska reported on the application of the reaction for this purpose [see (13) for a review of this reaction]. It has therefore also been referred to as the Neufeld reaction and, because under the microscope it appears as a swelling of the capsule, as the quellung reaction.

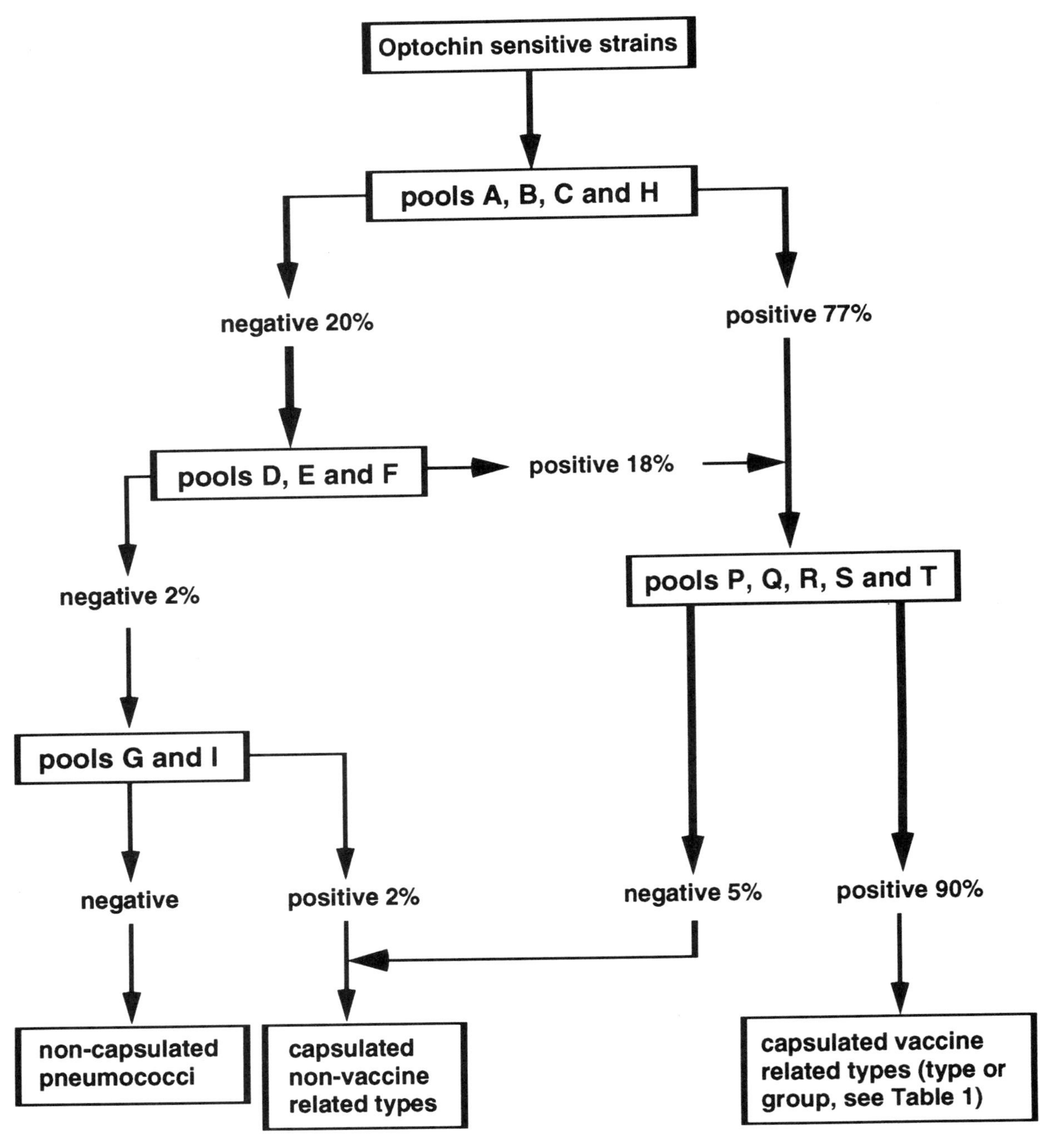

FIGURE 37-1

Typing strategy of pooled sera. (Reprinted by permission from Sørensen UBS. Typing of pneumococci using 12 pooled antisera. J Clin Microbiol 1993;31:2097–2100.)

A loopful (a few microliters) of a young (preferably 5–7hr) broth culture or a suspension of bacteria in, for example, saline, is mixed thoroughly with a loopful of antiserum on a microscope slide. A coverslip is placed over the mixture and the preparation is examined under the microscope with an oil immersion lens (magnification, ×100). It is preferable to use phase contrast but if this is not available a drop of methylene blue added to the mixture makes the examination easier by coloring the body of the bacteria. If the reaction is positive, the

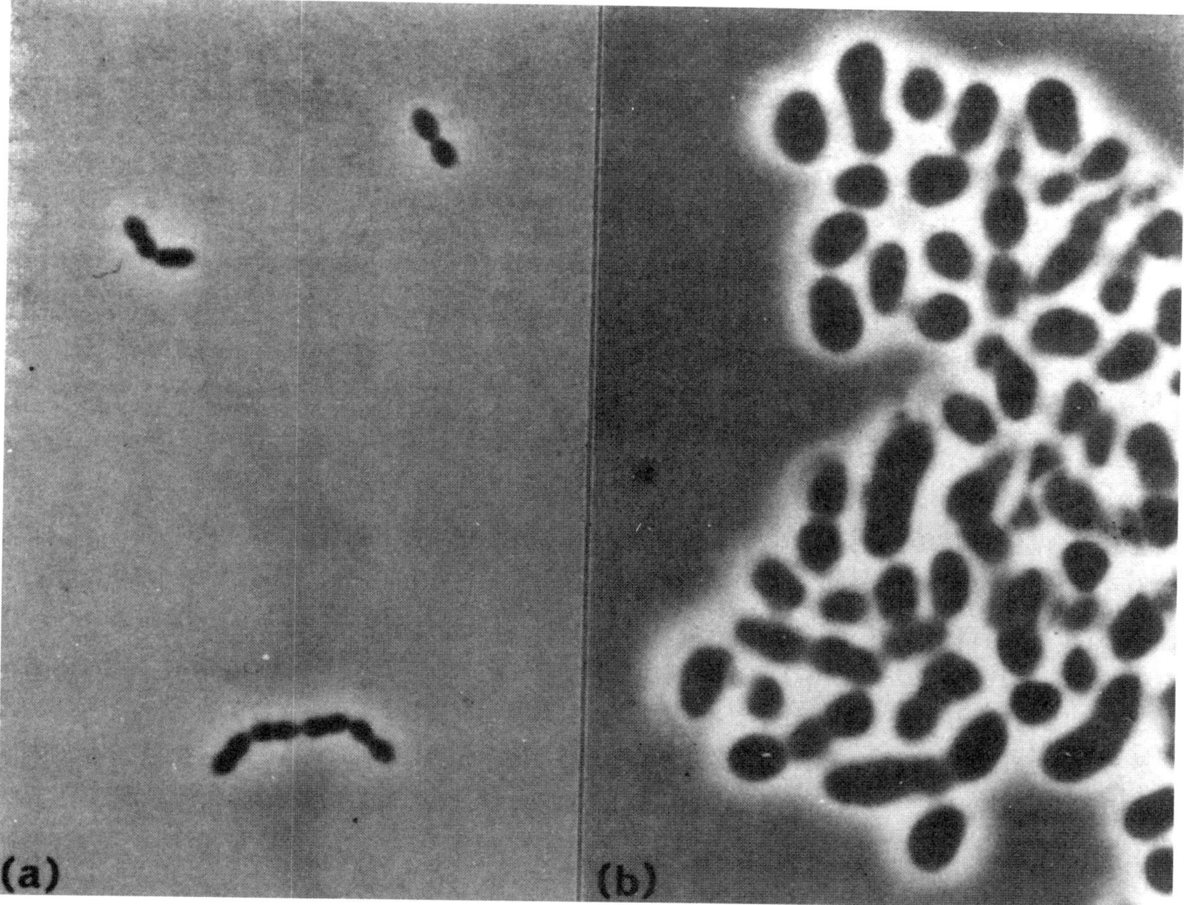

FIGURE 37-2

Preparations of a type 17F pneumococcal strain with saline (a) and the group 17 antiserum (b), the latter showing both a positive quellung reaction and agglutination (approximately ×1000). (Reprinted by permission from Henrichsen J. The pneumococcal typing system and pneumococcal surveillance. J Infect Dis 1979;1(suppl 2):31–37.)

capsules become visible because of an in situ immunoprecipitation leading to a change in their refractile index; in addition, the bacteria agglutinate. A typical positive reaction is shown in **Figure 37-2B**. Both a pronounced capsular reaction and an agglutination are evident when compared with the negative control in Figure 37-2A (15).

A strain that grows in broth with a sediment and shows agglutination in all pools (A-I) is likely to be noncapsulated, that is, rough. Such strains as well as those that give equivocal capsular reactions should, however, be subjected to serial passages in broth before finally being labeled noncapsulated. A well-suited preincubated broth is inoculated in the morning and incubated at 37°C. After 5 to 7 hours of incubation when growth has just become visible, it must be transferred to a refrigerator, where it is left overnight. The next morning 10 drops are used to inoculate a fresh preincubated broth and the procedure is repeated for 3 to 5 days. In this way poorly capsulated strains will usually have regained their full capacity to produce well-defined capsules and, therefore, have become easy to type.

Alternative Typing Methods

Although the diagnostic pneumococcal antisera are manufactured for use in the capsular reaction test, and their specificity is controlled by this test, they are also being used for typing utilizing various other techniques, notably coagglutination, capillary precipitation, and counterimmunoelectrophoresis. In general, it should be noticed that because the specificity of the typing antisera is being controlled by the capsular reaction test any other test that is more sensitive may theoretically reveal cross reactions that are not detected by the capsular reaction.

Coagglutination

The typing antisera can be adsorbed to protein A that contains staphylococci as described by Kronvall (16) and used for typing by slide agglutination. Such reagents are actually being manufactured by a number of producers of diagnostic reagents using omniserum for coating the staphylococci or latex particles. Such agglutination reagents are intended for diagnosis of, for example, the causative agent of bacterial meningitis, by mixing them directly with cerebrospinal fluid. They perform well if used according to the directions of the manufacturers.

Capillary Precipitation

Capillary precipitation using the supernatant of an overnight broth culture and the various diagnostic antisera in the same sequence as in the capsular reaction test is, as far as I know, a procedure employed successfully by the Centers for Disease Control and Prevention in Atlanta.

Immunoelectrophoresis

Immunoelectrophoresis is also used, although it is both more tedious and expensive than the capsular reactions test (17). Its limitations have been described elsewhere (18,19).

Quality Assurance Measures

The performance of the diagnostic pneumococcal antisera is guaranteed for at least 2 years from the date of delivery when stored in the dark at 2° to 6°C. Statens Serum Institut possesses typing antisera, produced almost 50 years ago, that still perform very well.

When starting to type pneumococci, the most important thing to control is the ability of the growth media in use to support optimal capsulation of the pneumococci. This is done by examining the growth of, for instance, a type 1 strain after 5 to 7 hours of incubation at 37°C in Todd-Hewitt broth (or any other similarly enriched broth) or a suspension of bacteria made from an overnight blood agar culture plate with the homologous antitype 1 antiserum. All the bacteria should exhibit distinct capsules when viewed under the microscope, as described under Capsular Reaction Test. The media and the growth conditions have to be evaluated carefully if the test results are not positive. For the purpose of being able to carry out this kind of control the PNEUMOTEST kit in addition to the 12 pooled antisera contains a type 1 strain and its homologous antiserum.

Determination of Antigen

The etiologic diagnosis of pneumococcal pneumonia is difficult to establish; blood cultures are only positive in approximately 20% of cases. Examinations of sputa should give reliable findings, but proper samples are often difficult to obtain. Because they demand an invasive procedure examination of direct lung aspirate, these tests are used only by very few.

Countercurrent Immunoelectrophoresis

Detection of pneumococcal capsular polysaccharide antigens in urine by means of countercurrent immunoelectrophoresis (CIE) has been used in a number of studies during the last 20 years [see (6) for review]. Most workers have found this method to be of low sensitivity in nonbacteremic patients. However, we found a dose correlation of the sensitivities in both bacteremic and nonbacteremic patients, probably because the diagnosis, pneumococcal pneumonia, was based on rather strict diagnostic criteria. In about one third of the patients with pneumococcal disease we could not demonstrate antigenuria by CIE. Our conclusion was that this method is valuable as a diagnostic supplement in adults hospitalized with pneumonia (6).

Polymerase Chain Reaction (PCR)

Considering the sensitivity of CIE, that is, less than 0.1 μg/mL (19), it does not seem likely that PCR can be more useful in the demonstration of gene fragments in urine. However, recently a PCR assay based on the amplification of pneumolysin gene fragments in patient sera for the diagnosis of acute pneumococcal pneumonia was described (20). In a very limited number (20) of blood culture–positive patients, the sensitivity was shown to be 100% and the specificity 94%. The authors did not show whether their laborious method also is useful in detecting cases of blood culture–negative pneumococcal pneumonia.

Determination of Antibody

In recent years only two methods have been used: radioimmunoassay (RIA) and ELISA. For a number of reasons, ELISA has become the method of choice: It is cheaper; it does not involve handling of radioactive material; and, perhaps most importantly, it is easy to avoid measuring anti–C-polysaccharide (C-ps) antibodies in addition to the type-specific antibodies by simply adding C-ps to the serum samples before the assay proper (21). Although measurement of type-specific antibodies, even in paired serum samples, has little or no value in the diagnosis of pneumococcal infections, some claim that measurement of antipneumolysin antibodies in paired samples is of potential value (22).

Surveillance of Disease Susceptibility and Response to Vaccination

It is in this context that ELISA for measuring type-specific anti-pneumococcal antibodies becomes indispensable. For instance, it has been shown that certain ethnic groups, such as Alaskan Eskimos, Navajo Indians, and Australian aboriginals have substantially lower levels of anti-pneumococcal antibodies than do whites. Even Colombian preschool children have lower levels than American children of the same age. Further, elderly individuals have lower levels than younger adults and adolescents.

With the increasing use of pneumococcal polysaccharide vaccines and also with the introduction of polysaccharide-protein conjugate vaccines, it is of definite importance to be able to accurately measure antibody responses with a good reproducibility. This is done with the ELISA.

ELISA

This method has been described in detail elsewhere (21). Briefly, microtiter plates are coated with purified pneumococcal capsular polysaccharides. (We originally used phenylated polysaccharides but this later was shown to be unnecessary.) The serum to be tested is then added after having been incubated overnight with C-ps. Next, enzyme-conjugated rabbit anti-human immunoglobulin (total Ig, class- or IgG-subclass specific) is added, and finally the substrate of the enzyme employed (horseradish peroxidase or alkaline phosphatase) goes into the wells. The plates are washed thoroughly between each step. After the enzyme-substrate reactions have been stopped, the optical density values of each well are read in an ELISA reader; the data are transferred to a computer with a program that leads to a calculation of the antibody level expressed in units relative to an international standard. Usually an inhouse standard serum, which has been calibrated by the use of the international standard 89SF, is tested on all plates to allow for correction of intra- and interassay variations.

Two workshops on pneumococcal ELISA standardization, one in 1994 and the other in May 1996, have been held at the Centers for Disease Control and Prevention in Atlanta under the auspices of the World Health Organization. As a result, a revised standard ELISA protocol has been agreed on concerning all aspects of the ELISA, including all reagents, steps, and computing. It has recently been tested in a number of laboratories using 25 pairs of quality control sera as well as 10 blinded pairs and six duplicates for consistency and, of course, the international standard but the results have not been published yet. Hopefully, in the near future, a full and detailed description of the entire procedure as well as the international standard serum will be made available to the scientific community.

REFERENCES

1. Henrichsen J. Six newly recognized types of *Streptococcus pneumoniae.* J Clin Microbiol 1995;33:2759–2762.

2. Nielsen SV, Henrichsen J. Incidence of invasive pneumococcal disease and distribution of capsular types of pneumococci in Denmark 1989–1994. Epidemiol Infect 1996;117:411–416.

3. Plouffe JF, Breiman RF, Facklam RR. Bacteremia with *Streptococcus pneumoniae*: implications for

therapy and prevention. JAMA 1996;275:194–198.

4. Trotman J, Hughes B, Mollison L. Invasive pneumococcal disease in central Australia. Clin Infect Dis 1995;20:1553–1556.
5. Kalin M, Lindberg AA. Diagnosis of pneumococcal pneumonia: a comparison between microscopic examination of expectorate, antigen detection and cultural procedures. Scand J Infect Dis 1983;15:247–255.
6. Nielsen SV, Henrichsen J. Detection of pneumococcal polysaccharide antigens in the urine of patients with bacteraemic and non-bacteraemic pneumococcal pneumonia. Zbl Bakt 1994;281: 451–456.
7. Kettula Y, Leinonen M, Mäkelä PH. The aetiology of pneumonia. Application of bacterial serology and basic laboratory methods. J Infect Dis 1987;14:21–30.
8. Murray PR, Baron EJ, Pfalser MA, et al. Manual of clinical microbiology. Washington, DC: ASM Press, 1995.
9. Grahen M, Bahistutta D, Torzillo P, et al. Comparison of goat and horse blood in culture medium supplements for isolation and identification of *Haemophilus influenzae* and *Streptococcus pneumoniae* from upper respiratory tract secretions. J Clin Microbiol 1994;32: 2871–2872.
10. Acute respiratory infections. Laboratory manual of bacteriological procedure. Manila: World Health Organization, Regional Office for the Western Pacific, 1986.
11. Lund E, Rasmussen P. Omni-serum, a diagnostic pneumococcus serum reacting with the 82 known types of pneumococcus. Acta Pathol Microbiol Scand 1966;68:458–460.
12. Lund, E, Henrichsen J. Laboratory diagnosis, serology and epidemiology of *Streptococcus pneumoniae*. In: Bergan T, Norris JR, eds. Methods in microbiology. vol. 12. New York: Academic Press, 1978:241–262.
13. Austrian R. The quellung reaction, a neglected microbiologic technique. Mount Sinai J Med 1976;43:699–709.
14. Sørensen UBS. Typing of pneumococci by using 12 pooled antisera. J Clin Microbiol 1993;31: 2097–2100.
15. Henrichsen J. The pneumococcal typing system and pneumococcal surveillance. J Infect Dis 1979;1(suppl 2):31–37.
16. Kronvall G. A rapid slide-agglutination method for typing pneumococci by means of specific antibody adsorbed to protein A containing staphylococci. J Med Microbiol 1973;6:187–190.
17. Colding H, Lind I. Counterimmunoelectrophoresis in the diagnosis of bacterial meningitis. J Clin Microbiol 1977;5:405–409.
18. Coonrad JD, Rytel MW. Detection of type specific pneumococcal antigens by counterimmunoelectrophoresis. I. Methodology and immunologic properties of pneumococcal antigens. J Lab Clin Med 1973;81:770–777.
19. Henrichsen J, Berntson E, Kaijser B. Comparison of counterimmunoelectrophoresis and the capsular reaction test for typing of pneumococci. J Clin Microbiol 1980;11:589–592.
20. Salo P, Örtqvist Å, Leinonen M. Diagnosis of bacteremic pneumococcal pneumonia by amplification of pneumolysin gene fragment in serum. J Infect Dis 1995;171:479–482.
21. Konradsen HB, Sørensen UBS, Henrichsen J. A modified enzyme-linked immunosorbent assay for measuring type-specific anti-pneumococcal capsular polysaccharide antibodies. J Immunol Methods 1993;164:13–20.
22. Jalonen E, Paton JC, Koskela M, et al. Measurements of antibody responses to pneumolysin: a promising method for the presumptive aetiological diagnosis of pneumococcal pneumonia. J Infect Dis 1989;19:127–134.

CHAPTER 38

Hepatitis A, B, and C

STEPHEN B. LAMBERT
HOWARD A. FIELDS

Hepatitis

Liver disease can be brought about by a number of microorganisms, pharmaceuticals and industrial chemicals. The pathogenic effects of these agents are similar in that they damage hepatocytes, which leads to inflammation and impaired liver function. Certain factors that are produced by the liver, such as the components of the clotting cascade, may be reduced as a result of liver damage. Bilirubin, which is principally composed of the porphyrin ring of degraded hemoglobin, is normally processed in the liver and expelled as bile through the gallbladder and pancreas into the duodenum. When the microcanaliculi of the liver are closed off by inflammation, bilirubin is redirected, to be excreted in the urine and deposited in the skin. **Table 38-1** lists some of the agents that are capable of bringing about clinical hepatitis.

Table 38-2 lists the most common clinical symptoms of hepatitis. Jaundice is the hallmark of liver disease, but actually is present in a minority of cases. Otherwise the symptomatology is rather generic, which is why the milder cases frequently go unrecognized, even in the presence of considerable histopathology. Although the liver has a remarkable ability to regenerate itself, degradation may progress irreversibly after a certain level of damage is reached.

Viral Hepatitis

Most clinical hepatitis is viral in etiology. **Table 38-3** compares the known human hepatitis viruses. Most of these organisms have little in common other than hepatic tropism. Hepatitis viruses A, B, and C collectively comprise about 98% of the viral hepatitis infections in the United States.

Hepatitis A virus (HAV) is most often transmitted by way of contaminated food or water. In some less developed countries, practically the entire population is infected in early childhood. In the United States about 11% of the population has acquired the serologic markers of HAV infection by age 5, which increases linearly to about 74% by age 50.

The probability of a patient with hepatitis A being symptomatic increases with age. The disease is rarely life threatening, with a case fatality rate of 0.3%, and is usually resolved without sequelae.

Hepatitis A infection typically elicits a very high antibody titer, which is protective against subsequent infection. Hepatitis A vaccines have been in use in much of the world for several years. The first HAV vaccine licensure in the United States was granted to Smith Kline Beecham Pharmaceuticals in 1995. The HAV vaccines are 94% to 100% effective and induce a negligible incidence of adverse reactions.

Hepatitis B virus (HBV) is transmitted through blood products, sexually and perinatally. About 300,000 new cases of HBV infection occur in the US each year. Many of these cases are asymptomatic and most resolve spontaneously. However, some HBV-infected persons go on to carry the virus chronically for life. The probability of a case progressing to chronicity is dependent upon the age at which the infection is acquired. Up to 90% of infants who are infected perinatally, 25% to 50% of children who are infected between 1 and 5

TABLE **38-1**

Some of the Agents that Are Capable of Bringing About Clinical Hepatitis

Hepatitis viruses
- Hepatitis A virus
- Hepatitis B virus
- Hepatitis C virus
- Hepatitis D virus
- Hepatitis E virus
- Hepatitis G virus(?)

Bacteria
- *Salmonella typhi*
- *Clostridium perfringens*
- *Leptospira* spp

Parasites
- *Entamoeba histolytica*
- *Plasmodium* spp
- *Leishmania donovani*
- *Faciola hepatica*

Viruses other than hepatitis viruses
- Cytomegalovirus
- Epstein-Barr virus
- Adenovirus
- Yellow fever virus

Chlamydia
- *Chlamydia psittaci*

Drugs/Chemicals
- Acetaminophen
- Tetracycline
- Ethanol
- Carbon tetrachloride
- Trinitrotoluene
- Vinyl chloride
- Tannic acid
- *Amanita* spp mushroom toxin

years of age, and 6% to 10% of HBV-infected older children and adults will become chronic HBV carriers. The effects of chronicity vary greatly from negligible to cirrhosis or hepatocellular carcinoma. Hepatitis B virus vaccines have been available since the 1970s. The ones that are in use in the US are recombinant in nature, induce minimal side effects, and are up to 95% effective. HBV vaccines that are produced from hepatitis B surface antigen (HBsAg) purified from the plasma of carriers are still in use in many regions of the world.

For many years HAV and HBV were the only characterized hepatitis viruses, and were referred to as "infectious" and "serum" hepatitis, respectively. However, there were other entities causing clinical hepatitis that were believed to be viral in nature. These were collectively referred to as non-A, non-B, or NANB.

TABLE **38-2**

Major Symptoms of Clinical Hepatitis

Jaundice/icterus
Lassitude
Loss of appetite
Nausea
Weakness
Fever
Vomiting
Headache
Abdominal pain

In 1989, Choo and colleagues at Chiron Corporation in collaboration with Bradley and colleagues at the Centers for Disease Control and Prevention described certain genomic regions and corresponding immunoreactive recombinant proteins specific to hepatitis C virus (HCV). Like HBV, HCV transmission is blood borne. Hepatitis C virus can also be transmitted sexually, although less efficiently than HBV. Detection in semen by the polymerase chain reaction (PCR) has been problematic. The nature of perinatal transmission is currently under study by a number of investigators.

Before the introduction in 1990 of screening tests to identify HCV contamination in the blood supply, the incidence of HCV infection in the US was believed to be approximately 15,000 cases per year. That number decreased by about 50% in the 2 years thereafter, partially due to blood screening for HCV and partially due to a general increase in awareness of blood-borne infections brought about by the HIV epidemic. The probability that an HCV infection will become chronic is very high. Since most of these cases are asymptomatic or subclinical, many of the individuals who are chronic carriers are unaware of it.

The hepatitis D virus (HDV) is a satellite virus of hepatitis B. It is dependent upon the presence of HBV to provide HBsAg, which is used to encapsulate the HDV genome. HDV can be transmitted to a susceptible individual at the same time as HBV, resulting in a coinfection, or to an individual who is already chronically infected with HBV, producing a superinfection. The symptoms in either case are similar to those brought about by HBV infection alone, but tend to be more severe. Hepatitis D virus is most frequently seen in the tropical regions of South America, Africa, and Asia, and is very rare in the US.

TABLE 38-3

Hepatitis Virology at a Glance

Attribute	HAV	HBV	HCV	HDV	HEV	HGV
Virus group	Picornavirus	Hepadnavirus	Flavivirus	Satellite	Calicivirus	Flavivirus
Virion size	30 nm	42 nm	45 nm	36 nm	30 nm	45 nm
Nucleic acid	ss+RNA	ssDNA	SS+RNA	SSRNA	SS+RNA	SS+RNA
Genome size	7.5 Kb	6.4 Kb	9.4 Kb	1.7 Kb	7.5 Kb	9.4 Kb
Envelope?	No	Yes	Yes	Yes	No	Yes
Transmission	Enteric	Blood/STD	Blood/STD	Blood/STD	Enteric	Blood/STD?
Incubation	15–40 days	60–160 days	40–80 days	60–160 days	35–45 days	?
Chronicity?	No	Sometimes	Usually	Frequently	No	Probably
Incidence, US	0.01%	0.01%	0.001%	Rare	Very rare	TBD

HAV, hepatitis A virus; HBV, hepatitis B virus; HCV, hepatitis C virus; HDV, hepatitis D virus; HEV, hepatitis E virus; HGV, hepatitis G virus; STD, sexually transmitted disease; TBD, to be determined.

TABLE 38-4

Generic Markers that Have Value in the Diagnosis of Liver Disease

Analyte	Specimen of Choice	Storage
Bilirubin	Serum, most plasma*	4°C <24 hr or freeze
Albumin	Serum, most plasma*	4°C <24 hr or freeze
ALT (SGPT)	Serum, most plasma*	4°C <48 hr or freeze**
AST (SGOT)	Serum, most plasma*	4°C <48 hr or freeze**
Alkaline phosphatase	Serum, most plasma*	4°C <24 hr or freeze
γ-Glutamyl transferase	Serum, most plasma*	4°C <24 hr or freeze
Fibrinogen	Citrate plasma	4°C <72 hr or freeze
Plasminogen	Citrate plasma	4°C <8 hr or freeze
Antithrombin III	Citrate plasma	Test fresh or freeze

SGPT, serum glutamic pyruvic transaminase; SGOT, serum glutamic oxaloacetic transaminase.

*i.e., plasma collected, into most anticoagulants; Consult test manufacturer's instructional literature for specific exclusions.

**It is preferred that ACT and AST testing be done on fresh samples. When frozen storage prior to testing is unavoidable, the sample should be stored at −70°C immediately after collection.

The epidemiology of hepatitis E is similar to that of hepatitis A. It is enterically transmitted usually via fecally contaminated drinking water. Most cases resolve without complications. A notable exception is in pregnant women in whom the mortality is 15% to 25%, the biology of which is not known. Hepatitis E virus does not induce a chronic carrier state. Epidemics that comprise thousands of cases of HEV infection have been reported in India and China. Infections reported in the US are almost exclusively in recent travelers to endemic regions of the world.

Hepatitis G and hepatitis virus GB-C have recently been demonstrated to be independent isolates of the same virus. It is classified as a member of the flavivirus family, as is HCV. It appears to be blood borne and to be capable of inducing acute and persistent infections without strong evidence of chronic disease. Immunoassay and PCR methods are being used to study this virus, but no diagnostic methods are commercially available.

Hepatitis Diagnostics

The clinical chemistry of hepatitis diagnostics includes nonspecific and specific markers with respect to the etiology of the disease. **Table 38-4** lists some of the markers of liver disease that are independent of the cause. These and others are routinely included in patient profiles. Deviation of some of these analytes from normal ranges is unique to liver dysfunction while others may indicate a problem in other organs as well.

Table 38-5 lists the serologic markers of viral hepatitis that are commonly tested for as part of diagnostic protocols. For the viral agents that do not induce a chronic state of infection (i.e., HAV and HEV), serologic differentiation of the status of disease is straightforward. Acute infection is characterized by the presence of the immunoglobulin M (IgM) class of antibodies directed against the viral proteins. Both acute and resolved cases will have total (primarily IgG) antibody. Total anti-HAV antibodies may persist at high titer for decades while total anti-HEV antibody titers decline over time.

The diagnostic algorithms for viral agents that cause chronic infections are much more complex. For hepatitis B three antigens are used as diagnostic determinants: HBsAg, the nucleocapsid or hepatitis B core antigen (HBcAg), and the hepatitis B e antigen (HBeAg). Immunoassays are readily available that detect these antigens or antibodies directed against them, or both.

Immunoglobulin M anti-HBc is the primary marker of acute infection. With rare exceptions, it is not detectable after the acute phase. HBsAg is the earliest serologic marker of acute disease, but may persist into the chronic phase. HBsAg is not present in resolved cases. Along with PCR, HBsAg and HBeAg quantitation can be used for tracking the effectiveness of treatment, which most often consists of some form of interferon therapy. Total antibody directed against HBcAg (T-anti-HBc) appears later in the acute phase and persists for many years in both resolved and chronic cases. Anti-HBs antibody appears near the end of the acute phase and usually persists for many years. The HBV vaccine is derived from HBsAg, and therefore anti-HBs is a marker of immunity in vaccinees.

Hepatitis B e antigen is synthesized at about the same time as HBsAg. It is generally used as evidence of the presence of infectious virus and is associated with the ability of the infected individual to transmit the disease. HBeAg testing is frequently used, along with HBsAg subtyping, as a tool for epidemiologic tracking. Although anti-HBe is often associated with

TABLE **38-5**

Specific Serologic Markers of Viral Hepatitis

Serologic Marker	**Acute**	**Resolved**	**Chronic**	**Vaccinee**
Hepatitis A				
Total anti-HAV antibody	×	×		×
IgM anti-HAV antibody	×			
Hepatitis B				
HB surface antigen	×		×	
Anti-HBsAg antibody		×	×	×
Total anti-HB core antibody	Probably	×	×	
IgM anti-HB core antibody	×			
HBe antigen	×		×	
Anti-HBe antibody	Unlikely	×	×	
Hepatitis C				
Total anti-HCV antibody	×	×[a]	×	
Hepatitis D				
Total anti-HDV antibody	Probably	×	×	
IgM anti-HDV antibody[b]	×			
HD antigen[b]	×		×	
Hepatitis E				
Total anti-HEV antibody[b]	×	×		
IgM anti-HEV antibody[b]	×			
Hepatitis G				
Anti-HG E2 antibody[b]	Unlikely	Maybe	Maybe	

[a] If any HCV infection is actually resolved.

[b] Not licensed for clinical applications in the US.

resolved disease, it may also be found in chronic infections.

Hepatitis C virus progresses to chronicity in more that 80% of cases. The only conventional specific serologic test of value is for total anti-HCV antibody, which is a marker of both acute and chronic infection. Immunoglobulin M is produced sporadically over the course of HCV infection and thus is of no value in discriminating between acute and chronic cases. There are reports of IgM anti-HCV being of value for monitoring therapy. Like HBV, interferon is the treatment of choice for chronic HCV infections. PCR is the principal method for monitoring its efficacy.

In the US, the only licensed immunoassays for HDV are for total anti-HDV antibody. Due to the infrequent occurrence of HDV infection and its exclusive association with hepatitis B infection, additional testing is rarely justifiable. However, assays for IgM anti-HDV and HDV antigen are available in some locations.

Clinical laboratories frequently group hepatitis diagnostics into panels of tests. The panel of hepatitis tests that is ordered by a physician is based upon the condition and history of the patient. For example, an individual who presents with acute clinical hepatitis will generally be tested using an acute marker panel. An HBV panel can be used near the time of delivery for pregnant women who are known to be HBV carriers. The Food and Drug Administration (FDA) regulates the panel of hepatitis tests that are used to screen blood products. The responsibility of the laboratory is to receive and process the specimen, assure that the requested testing is carried out, and report results as quickly and accurately as possible. The laboratory may also be asked to help interpret the data or to recommend follow-up testing for difficult cases.

Assay Methodology

Immunoassays for the viral markers listed in Table 38-4 are conventional, commercially available methodologies, except as noted. They tend to be available as direct or competition format heterogeneous radioimmunoassay (RIA) or enzyme immunoassay (EIA) kits that use polystyrene beads or microtiter plates as the solid-phase. Positive and negative controls are included with each group of samples tested and the control data are used to validate the testing and to calculate the cutoff value for that group. They tend to require one to three reagent incubation steps and a similar number of manual or semiautomated wash steps between incubations. However, the diagnostics industry is in the process of undergoing major changes with respect to many of the viral markers. Technologic advances in reagent, instrument, and software engineering have led to the development of several stand-alone instruments that will accommodate infectious disease testing. This has been further driven by a market demand for faster tests that require less technician time. Such instrumentation has been available for some time for routine clinical chemistry such as the tests for bilirubin, enzymes, and clotting factors. However, underestimation of the complexity of making the research and development transition from small, highly defined molecules to viral antigens and antibodies has been a source of great discouragement for many commercial test manufacturers. The upcoming generation of diagnostic instruments will mostly utilize microparticle beads as the solid-phase because of their greatly increased surface area per reagent volume and their ease of handling.

Specimens

Specimen handling is a very important factor in maximizing the confidence in the data that are generated from it. Most hepatitis immunoassays are licensed for the use of plasma that contains any of the conventional anticoagulants or serum. However, this should not be assumed. The manufacturer's instructional literature will always include a section that describes the type of samples that are acceptable or not acceptable, or both. Hemolysis, autoimmune factors, preservatives, and certain anticoagulants may be a problem for some tests.

The serum or plasma should be separated from the cells within a few hours of being drawn. Safe, aseptic technique should always be used. Samples that will be tested for hepatitis antigens or antibodies within 3 days can be refrigerated for that period of time. Samples that are to be tested using PCR methods should be frozen immediately, as should those that will be held for more than 3 days before conventional testing. Additional sample handling requirements specific to the generic markers are included in Table 38-4. Multiple freeze-thaw cycles are severely damaging to diagnostic specimens, and therefore dividing a sample into several individually labeled aliquots while it is fresh may be beneficial. No specimen should ever be stored or shipped at ambient temperature or as whole blood.

Many infectious disease markers can be detected to clinically relevant levels of sensitivity in saliva specimens or in dried blood spot eluants. The principal advantage of dried blood spots is that, when sealed in airtight containers with desiccant, they can be shipped or stored for relatively long periods of time at ambient temperature. Their actual stability is dependent on the analyte that is to be assayed. Saliva is a very convenient sample to collect, but tends to be subject to enzymatic degradation of its components. Saliva specimens should be refrigerated immediately upon collection and frozen if testing is to be delayed for more than a few hours.

Validation and Quality Control of Reagents

Very few clinical laboratories manufacture their own reagents for routine hepatitis testing. Manufacturers take responsibility by virtue of kit licensure for assuring that the individual reagents contained within those kits are sufficient to satisfy the performance claims of the product. The responsibility of the laboratory is to assure the fidelity of those performance claims.

For most commercial test kits, certain quality assurance and reagent validation procedures are described in detail in the manufacturer's instructional literature. It is critical that these procedures be followed and documented without exception. In addition to the controls and standards that are included as part of diagnostic test kits, additional laboratory standards are of great value. The manufacturer's controls tend to be optimized within the context of individual kit lots and may not be close to the assay cutoff. An independent laboratory standard can be used to define the variability between assay kit lots and to monitor the performance of the assay from the perspective of a point near the cutoff. Laboratory standards can be prepared according to internal procedures or obtained commercially. In either case, there must be some assurance that they are truly standards (i.e., exactly the same over periods of storage and between preparations). Highly defined protocols are important for the manufacture and validation of new preparations of standards.

Most clinical analytes are reported in quantitative values. Many of the viral hepatitis markers can be quantitated as well. Anti-HAV, anti-HBs, and anti-HEV can be expressed as milli-international units per milliliter (mIU/mL, also seen as IU/liter); total anti-HBc, IgM anti-HBc, HBeAg, and anti-HBe as Paul-Ehrlich Institute units (PEIU) per milliliter; and HBsAg as PEIU/mL or ng/mL. Except for the ng/mL designation, these units are somewhat arbitrary in nature, but are nonetheless internationally recognized standards. The quantitated standards that are available through various institutions tend to be rather expensive and available only in small quantities. They can be used, however, as calibrators for the preparation of inhouse standards for individual laboratories.

The most valuable laboratory standard for a given test must have defined characteristics. First, it must be manufactured according to a highly defined protocol and narrow acceptance criteria. This will minimize lot-to-lot variability between preparations. Standards are by definition nonvariable. Second, it must be prepared using a diluent that conforms to the specimen limitations of the assay and is nonreactive for the analyte that is detected by the assay. If the assay requires serum as a clinical specimen, then the diluent that is used to prepare the standard must also be serum. Moreover, the diluent will be most accurately representative of the mean value of negative specimens if it is a pool of several sera that have been demonstrated to be negative for that analyte both as individual samples and as the pooled reagent. It is important to note, however, that elevation of background values can occur if too many serum or plasma samples are used to formulate a pool. Third, it must contain a known unit per volume quantity, based upon a recognized calibrator. Fourth, it must generate a value that is just to the positive side of the assay cutoff. Inhouse controls are typically targeted to a signal cutoff value of 1.1 to 1.4 for direct immunoassays or 0.7 to 0.9 for competition immunoassays. An exception to this is a standard that is used as a marker of vaccine-induced immune protection, which may be of a considerably higher value than the assay cutoff. Fifth, it must be stored frozen in single-use aliquots that are clearly labeled with the identity, concentration, preparation date, and expiration date of the reagent.

A test run comprises specified controls and a number of clinical specimens, all tested together under identical conditions. When the kit controls or laboratory standards of a test run do not conform to acceptance criteria, the run is disqualified and the data are invalid. Under no circumstances shall control data be manipulated or exchanged for other control data, even with similar test runs that are performed at the same time.

There are as many possible reasons for a defective test run as there are reagents and protocol steps in the assay. However, by far the most common source of difficulty is the detection phase reagent or conjugate. The conjugate is usually an antigen or antibody that is chemically bound with a reporting agent such as an enzyme, radioisotope, fluorescent dye, or visible particle. It is frequently the most difficult reagent to manufacture and the one that dictates the shelf life of the test kit because of its instability. Depending on their nature, conjugates may be inhibited or degraded by temperature, light, preservatives, contamination with other kit reagents or specimens, detergents, pH, chelating and reducing agents, and disinfectants, including the vapors of household bleach. Assay failures can be minimized by handling conjugates with great respect.

Laboratories that do have the research and development resources to manufacture their own diagnostic test methods must do so with the same level of precision and documentation that a commercial manufacturer would, although generally on a smaller scale. Every reagent, whether produced in the laboratory or purchased from an outside source, must be thoroughly validated to standard operating procedure specifications. No assumptions can be made regarding any reagent, from raw materials to utility and stability of the final product.

Practicability

Routine hepatitis serology tends not to be prohibitively difficult to carry out. Standard methods and technologies are generally used and the protocols of commercial test kits are highly defined. However, a certain level of technical precision, customer focus, and dedication to quality is required to process a large number of specimens with a high degree of efficiency and accuracy. In many cases, people's lives and families are profoundly affected as a result of the data that are generated in clinical laboratories. Even in laboratories that have become testing factories as a result of automation, assay performance specifications are inconsequential compared with the value of employees carrying an extended vision for the significance of their work. A responsible employee relations policy is a critical component of any quality management plan.

Sensitivity and Specificity

Sensitivity is the measure of a test to correctly identify samples that contain the analyte in question. Specificity is the measure of a test to correctly identify samples that do not contain the analyte in question. The sensitivity and specificity of the commercially available tests for the markers listed in Table 38-5 are typically 97% to 100%, depending on the test methodology, manufacturer, and population under study. Exceptions to this are the "rapid" methods such as lateral flow immunochromatography and latex agglutination assays. These methods are designed to be instrument independent, inexpensive, fast, simple, and compatible with field use. Although these attributes provide a means of taking immediate action, they frequently come at the expense of sensitivity. These tests are generally excellent for population-based studies in which a decline in sensitivity can result in an underestimation of the overall seroprevalence. For clinical diagnosis, however, more sensitive assays should be considered.

The dynamics of immunochemistry within the context of tests that are reasonably simple and inexpensive to perform dictate that sensitivity and specificity will be in competition with each other near their respective limits. The art of optimizing an immunoassay for maximum performance involves balancing the available reagents so as to achieve levels of sensitivity and specificity that are compatible with the intended use of the test.

Immunoassays for HBsAg, total anti-HBc, and anti-HCV serve a dual purpose: screening of blood donors and clinical diagnosis of disease. For screening of blood donors, maximum sensitivity is the more desirable parameter. In this environment the negative samples vastly outnumber the positive samples and those that are demonstrated to be negative will be transfused into individuals who presumably are also negative. False-positive test results will contribute to waste of blood products, but false-negative results will cause infection in a susceptible transfusion recipient. For the clinical diagnosis of disease, maximum specificity is the more desirable characteristic. Symptomatic patients for whom clinical evidence suggests the presence of a particular infectious agent generally produce relatively substantial amounts of the identifying analytes associated with that agent. Borderline true positive results in the absence of other supporting data are uncommon. In the clinical laboratory, false-negative results will be unlikely but false-positive results will lead to incorrect diagnosis and treatment. Tests that serve a dual purpose must have the best combination of performance characteristics that can be engineered.

Immunoassays for anti-HAV and anti-HBs serve a dual purpose of a different sort: clinical diagnosis of disease and assessment of immune status, particularly as related to vaccine-induced antibody. For anti-HBs, the assay cutoff value that is calculated from the kit controls has relevance in identifying the outcome of HBV infections. This cutoff value is 2.1 SRU (signal/$\bar{x}$NC) by RIA or approximately 1.7 mIU/mL when a standard curve is used in an EIA format. The threshold of immune protection according to Centers for Disease Control (CDC) recommendations is 10 SRU or 10 mIU/mL.* Therefore, specimens with anti-HBs SRU or mIU values between the assay cutoff and 10 are technically positive, but may not provide immunologic protection from infection. Five percent to 10% of healthy HBV vaccinees do not attain protective levels of circulating antibody, although there is some question as to the level of protection afforded by immune response to challenge other than antibody production. At any rate, a carefully calibrated 10-mIU/mL anti-HBs in-house standard is of great value for all anti-HBs test runs.

Similarly, the threshold of protection against HAV infection is believed to be 10–20 mIU/mL, although this value has yet to be firmly established. Antibody titers generated in response to natural HAV infections tend to be very high, while the average antibody response to HAV vaccine is significantly lower. Therefore, prior to the recent licensure of the HAV vaccines, there was little demand for tests with thresholds of sensitivity below 75–100 mIU/mL. Consequently, vaccinees who generate antibody titers within the range of 20–75 mIU/mL are protected from infection, but are nonreactive in most commercial assays. When more sensitive anti-HAV assays become available, an anti-HAV laboratory standard calibrated to 20 mIU/mL (or whatever the recommended threshold level of protection is determined to be) will be of value.

Laboratory Quality Assurance Programs

Most laboratories that carry out diagnostic testing are required by law to operate under a comprehensive quality assurance program. For laboratory environments that are not under such legal mandates, it is equally advisable that a similar program be undertaken voluntarily. Implementation of a comprehensive quality assurance program can be quite strenuous and is often met with significant opposition from technicians and management alike who are not used to the level of documentation that is required. However, it is only when quality is a fully standardized and integrated way of life that the laboratory can expect to have confidence in the value of the data that it generates.

There is no reason for every laboratory to reinvent its own quality assurance program. There are many established programs that are highly defined and applicable to a diversity of laboratory functions. Most medical diagnostic laboratories in the US fall under the requirements of the Clinical Laboratory Improvement Act of 1988 (CLIA '88) and are regulated and inspected under state or federal statutes, or both. Many laboratories that are part of manufacturing facilities are certified under one of the ISO 9000 management system standards. Research and development laboratories can choose to conform to the provisions of good laboratory practices. There are numerous publications and training opportunities that are helpful in determining which program is suitable for a given laboratory environment and in implementing the one that is chosen.

Under a given quality assurance program, there are certain packaged components that are also helpful in keeping each individual laboratory from having to reinvent them. For example, the blood-borne pathogen panel of the

* Around the value of 10, SRU and mIU of anti-HBs activity are considered to be equivalent. In one determination, however, 10 +/− 1 mIU was demonstrated to be equal to 8.4 +/− 1 SRU (unpublished data).

American College of Pathologists is an excellent source of intralaboratory proficiency assessment and interlaboratory comparison of hepatitis and retrovirus test performance. Certain commercially available hepatitis standards may serve as inhouse control reagents or standardized starting materials from which inhouse control reagents may be manufactured. A partial list of sources of various hepatitis standards is shown in **Table 38-6**.

Highly detailed standard operating procedures (SOPs) for every imaginable laboratory function comprise the central dogma of the regulated laboratory. Some diagnostic test kit manufacturers provide their instructional literature as electronic files that can be converted into SOPs. Material safety data sheets (MSDS) for thousands of laboratory chemicals are also available as electronic files. Several computer-based data management systems are available frequently referred to as laboratory information management systems (LIMS) or laboratory information tracking systems (LITS). In addition to routine data processing, these software packages provide a number of quality summary functions, such as plotting Levey-Jennings charts to monitor method variability.

A comprehensive quality assurance plan and a genuine, long-term dedication at every level of the organization to making it work are the keys to having confidence in the data that are generated. Broadly distributing the responsibility for the elements of the plan gives every employee a stake in its success; however, this is difficult to manage. There should be one person who holds primary responsibility for assuring that the plan is adhered to. One of the functions of the quality assurance manager should be to visit as many similar laboratory operations as possible to study how other organizations handle similar programs. In this way, quality assurance and quality control can be an integral component rather than an inconvenience in any laboratory environment.

TABLE **38-6**

Some Sources of Hepatitis Standards

Central Laboratory of the Netherlands Red Cross Transfusion Service
Plesmaniaan 125
PO Box 9190
1006 AD Amsterdam
The Netherlands

College of American Pathologists
325 Waukegan Road
Northfield, IL 60093

National Institute for Biological Standards and Controls
PO Box 1193
Potters Bar
Hertfordshire EN6 3QH
United Kingdom

Paul-Ehrlich Institut
Paul-Ehrlich Straςςe 51–59
D-63207 Langen
Germany

BIBLIOGRAPHY

Alter MJ. Epidemiology of hepatitis C in the West. Semin Liver Dis 1995;15:5–14.

Alter MJ, Mast EE. The epidemiology of viral hepatitis in the United States. Gastroenterol Clin North Am 1994;23:437–455.

Choo QL, Kuo G, Weiner AJ, Overby LR, Bradley DW, Houghton M. Isolation of a cDNA clone derived from a blood-borne non-A, non-B viral hepatitis genome. Science 1989;244:359–62.

Clements RB. Quality manager's complete guide to ISO 9000. Englewood Cliffs, NJ: Prentice Hall, 1993.

Gunter EW, Lewis BL, Koncikowski SM. Laboratory methods used for the Third National Health and Nutrition Examination Survey (NHANES III), 1988–1994. Hyattsville, MD: Centers for Disease Control and Prevention, 1996.

Linnen J, et al. Molecular cloning and disease association of hepatitis G virus: a transfusion-transmissible agent. Science 1996;271:505–508.

Mahoney FJ, Burkholder BT, Matson CC. Prevention of hepatitis B virus infection. Am Fam Physician 1993;47:865–872.

Mast EE, Krawczynski K. Hepatitis E: an overview. Ann Rev Med 1996;47:257–266.

Moyer LA, Warwich M, Mahoney FJ. Prevention of hepatitis A. Am Fam Physician 1996;54:107–114.

Nilsen CL. Managing the analytical laboratory: plain and simple. Buffalo Grove, IL: Interpharm Press, 1996.

Ratliff TA Jr. The laboratory quality assurance system. New York: Van Nostrand Reinhold, 1993.

Schiff L, Schiff ER (eds). Diseases of the liver. Philadelphia: Lippincott, 1987.

Tietz NW (ed). Clinical guide of laboratory tests. Philadelphia: Saunders, 1995.

CHAPTER 39

Rubella

TERYL K. FREY

The Agent and its Associated Diseases

Rubella virus occurs solely in humans and infects systemically during primary infection. The associated disease is known as rubella, German measles, or three-day measles. The primary symptom is a rash, although it is estimated that up to 50% of primary infections are asymptomatic. The disease is generally benign and serious complications rarely develop. However, when infection occurs during early pregnancy (most significantly during the first trimester), virus penetration of the placenta and infection of the fetus can lead to abortion or a constellation of severe birth defects known collectively as congenital rubella syndrome [CRS; there are many excellent reviews on rubella, including chapters in standard medical microbiology textbooks; a selected review is Wolinsky (1)].

Before the institution of a vaccination program in the United States in 1969, rubella was primarily a disease of childhood with a peak incidence in late winter and early spring. Epidemics typically occurred every 5 to 7 years. The virus was not isolated until 1962. Spurred by an epidemic in 1964 that resulted in over 20,000 CRS cases, live attenuated vaccines were rapidly developed. Since the inception of the vaccination program, the vaccination strategy in the US has included both universal vaccination at 15 to 18 months and selective vaccination of at-risk adults, primarily seronegative women who are planning pregnancy and seronegative health care workers. Aggressive implementation of this strategy after 1980 resulted in a precipitous drop in rubella and CRS through 1988. However, a resurgence occurred between 1989 and 1991, concentrated among foci of unvaccinated individuals. Since these persons were largely past childhood, the ratio of CRS to rubella cases was much higher than in prevaccination epidemics. Since the resurgence, vaccination policy has become even more aggressive, and the vaccination strategy has been augmented with both institution of an additional vaccination before adolescence and enforcement of vaccination requirements, particularly for school enrollment. Since 1991, both rubella and CRS have plummeted to all-time low levels (2). The outbreaks that do occur are localized and are thought to be initiated primarily by imported cases.

Rubella and the Clinical Immunology Laboratory

Although acute rubella is currently rarely encountered in the US, extensive serologic testing is done. Most of the testing is for immunologic screening to identify seronegative individuals who are subsequently vaccinated. Serologic testing is a standard part of prenatal health care (seronegative women who are vaccinated are advised not to become pregnant for 3 months postvaccination; if a patient found to be seronegative is already pregnant, vaccination is contraindicated and is deferred to the postpartum period). To avoid nosocomial infections, some states and many health care facilities require serologic testing of prospective health care workers. Some states mandate rubella testing for marriage licenses. With increasing frequency, serologic testing is also being done on school students who do not have proof of vaccination. Such students have the option of receiving the vaccine without testing; however, many choose testing to ascertain whether vaccination is necessary.

Serologic testing is also used to diagnose rubella. Rubella is a reportable disease in all 50 states and initial diagnosis is based on symptomatology. However, the symptoms can be confused with those of other diseases. Additionally, with the general disappearance of rubella in the US, many physicians are unfamiliar with the symptomatology of the disease. Furthermore, the National Immunization Program as well as state public health departments are interested in tracking and containing rubella outbreaks. Therefore, the US Public Health Service recommends that diagnosis be confirmed by virus isolation or by serologic testing. Although well-established virus isolation methods exist, they are lengthy and expensive and are not generally available, and therefore serologic testing is the sole method currently used to diagnose acute rubella. Serodiagnosis of rubella requires either the detection of an immunoglobulin M (IgM) response or demonstration of a significant rise in titer between paired acute and convalescent specimens. Likewise, CRS is also a reportable disease and is diagnosed at birth by the presence of symptoms. However, confirmation requires virus isolation (which is detectable in most CRS patients up to 6 months to a year after birth), the presence of IgM antibodies, or the persistence of an IgG titer above and beyond that expected for maternal antibody.

Outside of epidemiologic tracking and containment, the only other health care situation that requires diagnosis of acute rubella is one in which a woman in early pregnancy develops rubella-like symptoms or comes in contact with someone suspected of having rubella (3). Unfortunately, if rubella is diagnosed the only recourse possible is termination of the pregnancy, as prophylactic treatment with immunoglobulin has proved to be ineffective. However, even during the first trimester of pregnancy, there is a chance that fetal infection will not occur. Fetal infection can be confirmed by serologic testing of fetal blood to detect the presence of IgM antibodies to rubella virus; however, this procedure is encumbered by the fact that fetal IgM antibodies are not detectable until the 22nd week of gestation and at this time titers may be very low. Virus isolation and detection of virus nucleic acid by polymerase chain reaction in fetal blood, chorionic villous, and amniotic fluid specimens have been reported, although these techniques are not available in the US (4,5).

Rationale for Rubella Test Selection by the Clinical Immunology Laboratory

Historical Background on Rubella Serologic Testing

The initial serologic test employed to detect antirubella antibodies was hemagglutination inhibition (HAI or HI). This assay is sensitive to lipoprotein substances in serum, which causes false positives, and specimens initially had to be diluted 1:8 to overcome this problem. Most of the studies in the literature on detection of antibody levels induced by natural infection and determination of the level that conferred a protective response to natural infection employed the HAI assay. Therefore, the 1:8 dilution became fixed in the literature. Studies indicate that natural infection generally induces an HAI titer in excess of 1:8, that HAI titer correlates with neutralizing titer, and that individuals with a titer in excess of 1:8 rarely suffer reinfection. Therefore, an HAI titer of 1:8 was standardized as 15 international units (IU)/mL by the World Health Organization and the WHO recommends this as the cutoff value for immunity [a concise review on the history of rubella serologic testing is presented in Skendzel (6)].

Subsequently, a number of rubella serologic tests were developed using techniques such as complement fixation, radial hemolysis, passive hemagglutination, immunofluorescence, latex agglutination, and enzyme immunoassay. These tests do not suffer from interference by serum components to the extent that HAI does and thus are capable of detecting an antibody response at serum dilutions of less than 1:8. Studies in the literature indicate that antibody titers of less than 1:8 are generally protective. Furthermore, vaccination induces lower titers than does natural infection and thus the percentage of individuals with low-range titers has increased since the vaccination program was initiated. Considering these factors, the US Public Health Service at one time considered that a rubella titer above the cutoff level of any standard test was indicative of immunity (7). However, as discussed below, this recommendation has been revised and the recommended cutoff value is now 10 IU/mL.

Due to the size of the rubella serodiagnostic market, commercial test kits were developed and have been available and in widespread use for many years. The passage of the Clinical Laboratory Improvement Act of 1988 mandated extensive validation of all tests used in clinical laboratories from which results would be reported to patients. This requirement made inhouse tests impractical and shifted rubella test kits completely to the commercial arena. In response to requests from the American Society for Microbiology, the Food and Drug Administration (FDA) Center for Devices and Radiological Health, and several manufacturers, the National Committee on Clinical Laboratory Standards (NCCLS) undertook a review of rubella serologic tests and issued guidelines. At the time of this writing, these guidelines are tentative (8); however, approved guidelines were issued in 1997 (9). Among the guidelines were recommendations that all rubella tests used in clinical laboratories be cleared by the FDA and that the cutoff value for immunity be standardized at 10 IU/mL. Standardization is done using reference sera available from both the Centers for Disease Control (CDC) and WHO. The 10 IU/mL cutoff was originally proposed by the manufacturers of the Abbott Laboratories (Abbott Park, IL) IMx rubella test, who standardized their test to IU/mL and published data that a 10-IU/mL titer was protective. Since issuance of the NCCLS guidelines, both CDC and the FDA have embraced the 10 IU/mL cutoff value. However, test kits cleared before these guidelines are not required to be standardized to the 10 IU/mL value and many commercially available kits make no mention of it.

Currently Available Tests

Rubella tests based on methods such as hemagglutination inhibition, passive hemagglutination, radial hemolysis, complement fixation, and neutralization are described in most current clinical immunology manuals and were commercially available 10 years ago (10). However, commercial tests using these methods have since been discontinued and all tests currently available in the US are based on either latex agglutination (LA), enzyme immunoassay (EIA), immunochromatography (IC), or immunofluorescent assay (IFA). A list of commercial tests is given in **Table 39-1**.

Latex Agglutination

Latex agglutination tests employ latex spheres that have been coated with rubella antigen. In the absence of antibody, the spheres will settle from solution in a uniform pattern. However, in the presence of antibody, the spheres clump or agglutinate. The test is entirely manual; agglutination is determined by visual inspection. Positive and negative control sera are run concurrently with test sera to aid in interpretation. Total antibody (IgM plus IgG) is measured and the test is not quantitative unless serum dilutions are assayed to determine reciprocal titer. Latex agglutination tests are much more sensitive than HAI; some LA tests on undiluted serum can measure titers equivalent to 1 to 2 IU/mL. However, some manufacturers have adjusted the sensitivity of the test so that the positive/negative border corresponds to the 10 IU/mL cutoff and other manufacturers recommend that the sera be diluted 1:10 for the test to mimic the HAI assay.

Enzyme Immunoassay

In standard EIA, microtiter wells or plastic beads coated with rubella antigen are incubated with a serum specimen with the result that antirubella antibodies in the serum will bind to the surface of the well or bead. Subsequently, antihuman IgG antibodies (usually goat) conjugated with horseradish peroxidase (HRP) or alkaline phosphatase (AP) are added that will bind to the antirubella antibodies forming an antigen-antibody-antibody sandwich. The sandwich is exposed to a substrate (*o*-phenylenediamine or tetramethylbenzidine for use with HRP; *p*-nitrophenyl phosphate for use with AP), which is catalyzed into a product of a different color by the enzyme. The reaction is stopped by the addition of acid or base and color development is determined spectrophotometrically using a microtiter plate reader or spectrophotometer. The intensity of color is proportional to antibody titer. Enzyme immunoassay tests thus require instrumentation, minimally a plate reader or spectrophotometer. Manufacturers also market equipment to carry out the washes required by the assay, which increases the efficiency and convenience of the assay. The standard EIA used for immunologic screening measures IgG; however, many manufacturers

TABLE 39-1

Commercial Rubella Serodiagnostic Tests

Test Commercial Kit (supplier, location)	IU/mL Standardization* (10 IU/mL cutoff)
Latex agglutination	
Impact Rubella Slide Test (Wampole Laboratories, Cranbury, NJ)	Yes (yes)
Rubagen (Biokit USA, Lexington, MA)	Yes (no)
Rubalex (Orion Diagnostics, Somerset, NJ)	Yes (no)
Ruba-Test (Murex Diagnostics, Norcross, GA)	Yes (yes)
Rubascan (Becton Dickinson, Cockeysville, MD)	No
Seratest Rubella (Seradyn, Indianapolis, IN)	Yes (yes)
Enzyme immunoassay	
Access Rubella IgG (IgG only) (Sanofi Diagnostics Pasteur, Chaska, MN)	Yes (15 IU/mL)
Captia Rubella-G and Rubella-M (Sanofi Diagnostics Pasteur, Chaska, MN)	Yes (15 IU/mL)
Diamedix Rubella Microassay (IgG only) (Diamedix Corp, Miami, FL)	Yes (no)
Gull Laboratories Rubella IgG and IgM ELISA (Gull Laboratories, Salt Lake City, UT)	No
IMx System Rubella IgG 2.0 (IgG only) (Abbott Laboratories, Abbott Park, IL)	Yes (yes)
INCSTAR Rubella IgG ELISA and "fast" ELISA (IgG only) (INCSTAR Corp., Stillwater, MN)	Yes (yes)
Microstar Rubella IgG and Rubella IgM (Kenstar Corp, North Miami, FL)	No
Rubazyme and Rubazyme-M (Abbott Laboratories, Abbott Park, IL)	No
Sigma Rubella IgG and IgM (Sigma Diagnostics, St. Louis, MO)	No
Vidas Rubella IgG (IgG only) (BioMerieux Vitek, Hazelwood, MO)	No
Wampole Rubella IgG and IgM ELISA (Wampole Laboratories, Cranbury, NJ)	No
Zeus Rubella IgG and IgM ELISA Test System (Zeus Scientific, Raritan, NJ)	No
Immunochromatography	
BioSign Rubella IgG (Princeton BioMeditech, Princeton, NJ)	No
Rubella Plus (Wampole Laboratories, Cranbury, NJ)	Yes (yes)
Immunofluorescence	
Virgo Rubella IgG IFA (Hemagen Diagnostics, Columbia, MD)	No

*Yes/no refers to whether the assay results can be converted or correlated to titers in IU/mL. (Yes/no) refers to whether the recommended cutoff value is 10 IU/mL. Two assays for which the recommended cutoff value is 15 IU/mL are so indicated.

SOURCE: Compiled from the 1996 Medical Devices Register and 1996–97 Clinical Laboratory Reference. Current availability of all tests was confirmed by phone; this list is current as of February 1997. All suppliers provided product inserts, which were used in preparation of this manuscript.

have EIA tests that are specific for IgM as well. The IgM assays are based on the same principle as the IgG assays; however, enzyme-conjugated antihuman IgM is used as the secondary antibody.

Enzyme immunoassay tests yield a numeric measure of antibody titer that is determined by calibration against low-positive ("calibrator") control sera and must be run each time the test is performed. Each test has a predetermined cutoff value for immunity, which is either equivalent to the reading obtained with the calibrator serum or a factor multiplied by the calibrator serum reading. The reading for some specimens will be below the cutoff value, but above the negative control. Many EIA tests consider the range just below the cutoff value as "indeterminant" and it is recommended that the test be done on a second serum specimen before vaccination is performed. Enzyme immunoassay is more sensitive than is HAI. Although it would be relatively easy for manufacturers to standardize EIA tests to IU/mL titers, many do not do so.

Two variations on standard EIA have been developed based on the ability of HRP and AP to cleave novel substrates. The first, known as enzyme-linked fluorescent immunoassay (ELFA), is based on the ability of HRP to cleave 4-methylumbelliferyl phosphate (MUP) to 4-methylumbelliferone (MU). When excited by light with a wavelength of 365 nm, MU emits at wavelengths of 387 and 448 nm. Using the proper emission filters, emission at the longer wavelength can be measured spectrophotometrically. Two commercially available tests employ ELFA; both tests are completely automated and require specific instruments. The BioMerieux Vitek (Hazelwood, MO) Vidas rubella IgG test employs a pipet tip coated with antigen into which are drawn sequentially the specimen, the conjugated antibody, and the MUP substrate. Total fluorescence is measured after a standard reaction time. The Abbott Laboratories IMx rubella IgG test uses microparticle beads coated with antigen that are captured on a glass filter following incubation with the serum specimen. After incubation with the conjugated second antibody, the glass filter is immersed in the MUP substrate solution and the initial rate of the reaction is measured. Since the fluorometers used in both assays are computerized, calibration can be entered into the computer and stored for up to 2 weeks. Calibration of the Vidas test is based on a single calibrator sample provided with each pack of tests while with the IMx test, a calibration curve is generated using a standard series of six sera specimens whose titer has been determined in IU/mL. With both tests, positive and negative control specimens are assayed with each run.

The second EIA variant is based on the ability of AP to cleave dioxetane phosphate to dioxetane, a chemiluminescent reaction that generates light and is measured in a luminometer. As with the ELFA tests, the commercially available enzyme-linked chemiluminescent assay (ELCA), the Sanofi Diagnostics Pasteur (Chaska, MN) Access Rubella Immunoassay System, requires specific instrumentation. A second novel innovation of this test is that it employs paramagnetic particles coated with rubella antigen and thus a magnetic field is used to effect washing. A calibration curve is generated using a series of five sera whose titers have been determined in IU/mL. Although the calibration curve can be stored for up to 4 weeks, positive and negative quality control sera are assayed with each run.

Immunochromatography

Immunochromatography (IC) is based on the same general principle as is EIA. A serum or plasma specimen is spotted on a chromatographic membrane in which has been embedded successive bands of rubella antigen and antimouse IgG antibody. As the specimen migrates up the membrane by capillary action, human antirubella IgG antibody is captured by the rubella antigen band. Developer (phosphate-buffered saline) is added on a pad below the chromatographic membrane that contains mouse antihuman IgG conjugated to a dye. As the developer migrates up the chromatographic membrane carrying the antibody-dye conjugate with it, the conjugate binds to human antirubella IgG that has bound to the rubella antigen band, resulting in development of a colored band (if no antirubella IgG is present, a colored band does not appear). The remaining conjugate is captured by the antimouse IgG antibody band, resulting in a second colored band that serves as a control. Although the currently available IC tests detect only IgG, by using an antihuman IgM antibody-dye conjugate, the test could be adapted for detecting IgM. IC tests are entirely manual and are read by visual inspection. The currently available tests may or may not include control positive and negative sera. Though the test is qualitative, the manufacturers claim that since the intensity of the rubella-specific band is related to antibody titer, increases in titer between paired sera can be detected. The sensitivity of the currently available IC tests is equivalent to that of HAI.

Source of Rubella Antigen Used in LA, EIA, and IC Tests

In all of the currently available LA and EIA kits, the rubella antigen consists of highly purified rubella virus that has been chemically disrupted and thus inactivated. In Europe, one EIA test has been developed that utilizes noninfectious, subviral particles produced in cell cultures transfected with the rubella virion protein genes (11). It has also been shown that the rubella proteins produced in *Escherichia coli*, yeast, and baculovirus are immunoreactive (12–14) and such bioengineered antigens could be used in test kits developed in the future.

Immunofluorescence

In IFA, the serum specimen is pipetted onto a well on a microscope slide that contains acetone-fixed, rubella-infected culture cells. Antibody in the serum binds to rubella antigen in the infected cells. After removal of the specimen, a secondary antihuman IgG antibody (usually goat) conjugated with fluorescein isothiocyanate (FITC) is added, which binds to the human antibody bound to the infected cells. The slide is then examined under a fluorescence microscope for apple-green FITC-specific fluorescence (FITC absorbs at 490 nm and emits at 520 nm) in the cytoplasm of the infected cells. Interpretation of IFA is subjective since the fluorescence intensity varies (qualitatively graded from 1+ through 4+). While intense (3+ to 4+) fluorescence is readily apparent, borderline fluorescence (1+) is difficult to distinguish. The presence of autoimmune antibodies can also cause false positives (to overcome this problem, manufacturers mix infected and uninfected cells in the slide well; antirubella antibodies will not bind to all cells and thus nonfluorescing cells will be present whereas autoimmune antibodies will bind to all of the cells). Although the intensity of fluorescence is roughly proportional to the antibody titer, IFA is only quantitative if dilutions are made to determine reciprocal titer. Immunofluorescence could be adapted to detect IgM if FITC-conjugated anti-human IgM antibodies were used as the secondary antibody; however, the only IFA test currently available is only specific for IgG. The sensitivity of IFA is equivalent to that of HAI.

Criteria for Test Selection

Functionally, the main criterion for test selection is the availability of instrumentation. The instruments that are necessary for ELFA and ELCA are expensive (in excess of $25,000); once purchased, the automated nature of the instrumentation dictates dedication of the laboratory to the corresponding test. Interestingly, however, the automation also allows for classification of ELFA tests as only moderately complex under Clinical Laboratory Improvement Act (CLIA) guidelines and thus highly trained personnel are not required to run the tests. The manufacturers of these tests offer courses for training personnel. The instrumentation required for EIA tests are less expensive (in the neighborhood of $10,000 for washing equipment and a microplate reader or spectrophotometer). However, the frequent manual intervention required results in EIA tests being classifed as highly complex under CLIA guidelines and thus technically trained personnel are required for operation. (Once the equipment has been procured for the ELFA, ELCA, and EIA tests, it can, of course, be used for a broad spectrum of tests and assays other than rubella.) Both LA and IC tests require minimal equipment (LA requires a rotator that costs less than $500) and are classified as moderately complex under CLIA guidelines. Immunofluoresence assay tests require both expensive equipment (a fluorescence microscope) and personnel who are skilled in performing the assay. Once instrumentation has been factored out, the cost per assay of all of these tests is roughly equivalent (in the $3–$6 range per specimen). All of these tests can be done on individual specimens or in batches. In terms of time required to perform the assay, the LA and IC tests are the shortest, taking less than 15 minutes. The ELFA tests require 45 minutes, while the EIA tests take 2.5 to 3 hours.

A second criterion is the need for the laboratory to diagnose acute infection (a rare occurrence in the US). Practically, this requires EIA capability since the ability to detect IgM or an increase in overall titer is necessary. Neither of the ELFA tests has been modified for IgM and neither has been validated for detecting and interpreting significant increases in titer. The LA tests detect total IgG plus IgM antibody and none has been modified to detect only IgM. By doing serial dilution, LA tests can be used to determine and compare reciprocal titers; the extent to which this is actually practiced is not known. Practically, a laboratory without EIA capability does not necessarily need to acquire it since there is always the option of referring a specimen from a potential acute infection to a laboratory with EIA capability, particularly county and state health laboratories that are responsible for tracking rubella outbreaks. In most or many instances, these laboratories take the initiative to obtain specimens from reported rubella cases.

Practical Considerations for Rubella Testing in the Clinical Immunology Laboratory

NCCLS has published proposed guidelines for specimen handling and use of rubella serology tests in the clinical laboratory (15). These guidelines were included in the approved overall guidelines on rubella testing that were issued in 1997 (9). Additionally, all of the commercially available tests contain instructions in the package insert.

Specimen Collection and Handling

Most rubella tests based on LA and EIA require serum; only the Abbott IMx rubella test and the IC tests have been validated for either serum or plasma. Most tests recommend specimen analysis within 48 hours of collection (specimens are stored refrigerated in the interim). If specimens must be stored longer than this (particularly when paired serum specimens are being collected), they should be stored frozen. The chance of contracting rubella through specimen handling is remote, particularly since most specimens are collected for immunologic screening. However, standard safety procedures employed for handling and processing blood specimens eliminate all possibility of laboratory infection.

In terms of the test kits themselves, all control sera contained in such kits are screened for common blood-borne pathogens such as human immunodeficiency virus (HIV) and hepatitis B. However, standard safety procedures should still be employed in handling these sera. Although the antigen in the test kits is derived from rubella virus, the virus has been inactivated and does not impose a safety hazard.

Internal and External Quality Control

The NCCLS tentative guideline for rubella tests (8) recommends that test kits contain negative, low-positive, and high-positive sera as controls and that these controls be included with every run. "Calibrator" serum is also to be included for calibrating quantitative tests and determining cutoff values. In practice, the low-positive control serum and calibrator serum are often the same. With the exception of the IC tests, all of the commercially available kits require that negative and positive serum controls be included with every run (or minimally every 8–24 hr for high-usage automated testing). Some of the tests that utilize computerized instrumentation (particularly the ELFA and ELCA tests) only require periodic calibration using the calibrator serum. For proficiency testing as mandated by CLIA '88, most laboratories subscribe to services provided by individual state health laboratories, the College of American Pathologists, or both.

Interpretation of Test Results

For immunologic screening, the presence of a positive titer as determined by the test employed is evidence of immunity to rubella. Conversely, the absence of titer is indicative of lack of immunity and vaccination is recommended. Some of the quantitative EIA and ELFA tests have an intermediate "equivocal" outcome. In such cases, it is recommended that an independent specimen be assayed for determination of immunity.

For diagnosis of acute infection, a serum specimen taken less than 7 days after onset of symptoms is required. Convalescent specimens are collected 1 to 2 weeks later, but not earlier than 10 days after onset of symptoms. The presence of IgM antibody in any specimen collected within 2 weeks of onset of symptoms is evidence of acute infection. Alternately, a significant rise in titer between the acute and convalescent specimens is also evidence of acute infection. Interpretation of significance in rises in titers is addressed in each test kit.

When a pregnant woman is suspected of having been exposed to rubella, determination of susceptibility is most expeditiously done using a specimen collected within 10 days of exposure. The presence of titer is evidence of immunity due to previous exposure to rubella. When such a recent specimen is not available, specimens must be processed as for acute specimens. Follow-up specimen collection is advisable until the danger period has passed.

Current and Future Issues in Rubella Serodiagnostic Testing

Test Standardization

The most visible current issue in rubella serodiagnostic testing is the effort to standardize available tests to the 10 IU/mL cutoff value for immunity. The only enforcement of this cutoff value is at the time of application for clearance by the FDA. Many of the currently available tests were granted clearance before implementation of the 10 IU/mL cutoff value, and the manufacturers of these tests do not need to resubmit for FDA clearance unless the test or its production is changed. The expense involved in changing tests is a deterrent to manufacturers that adopt the 10 IU/mL cutoff [ironically, some of the European tests that are standardized on the old 1:8 HAI (15 IU/mL) cutoff value also have to be changed]. Thus, it may be a number of years before the FDA clearance process effects universal standardization to the 10 IU/mL value.

Adoption of the 10 IU/mL cutoff value would also address the standardization of rubella test kits. Currently, no standardization exists. All manufacturers present comparative data on the sensitivity (ability to detect positive sera), specificity (ability to discriminate negative sera), and reproducibility of their assays. Some of the kits use panels of sera that were titered by HAI (the old "gold standard," which is no longer routinely available in the US); others use a panel of 100 serum specimens (82 positive, 18 negative) available from CDC, while still others use serum panels that were titered by other commercially available kits. The tentative NCCLS guidelines recommend that both sensitivity and specificity be greater than 95% on panels of 200 positive and negative sera [of the 200 positive sera, 40 must be in the low range (10–20 IU/mL)](8). At one time, CDC compared commercially available rubella tests and reported the results of the tests that were judged acceptable, but this service was discontinued in 1985. Adopting the 10 IU/mL cutoff as well as collecting sensitivity and selectivity data on panels of sera that were titered in IU/mL would serve to standardize rubella test kits. Troublingly, however, a recent study that compared commercial tests that reported IU/mL found that while the individual tests were internally consistent and reproducible, the international units expressed were inconsistent among the tests (16).

Although rubella test standardization is a highly worthwhile goal, it needs to be kept in perspective that the rubella vaccination effort in the US, with its indispensable immunologic screening component, has been overwhelmingly successful. Reinfection of individuals with low titers has neither been a medical problem nor a source of virus spread.

Diagnosis of Acute Infection

Although acute infection can be diagnosed either by the presence of IgM antibody or a significant rise in titer between paired sera, in practice diagnosis is more generally done on the basis of IgM antibody. This is due to the convenience of testing a single specimen for IgM as well as the difficulty of collecting the second specimen.

Two problems have been encountered with IgM tests: 1) competition for antigen by IgG that is also present in the specimen, which can lead to false negatives, and 2) the presence of rheumatoid IgM factor, which can bind to IgG bound to the specific antigen in the EIA, leading to a false positive since the secondary enzyme–anti-IgM conjugate will bind to the rheumatoid IgM. One means of overcoming these problems is by designing an EIA that utilizes "IgM capture": The EIA microtiter well or bead is coated with antihuman IgM antibody that binds (or "captures") IgM present in the serum specimen. Antigen (rubella virions) is then added, which binds to antirubella IgM. Finally, enzyme-conjugated antirubella antibody is added, which binds to rubella antigen (forming an antibody-antibody-antigenantibody sandwich). The IgM capture approach is standard in rubella IgM tests marketed in Europe, but not in tests available in the US. In the US, most rubella IgM assays include antihuman IgG antibodies in the preliminary dilution solutions, which bind to and complex IgG, thus removing it from the test. NCCLS has not issued guidelines that cover IgM tests and thus there are no standard criteria for the formulation of such tests.

Despite reliance on IgM testing for diagnosis of acute infection, the presence of IgM is not always indicative of acute infection. While IgM usually wanes over the month following development of symptoms, it can persist beyond this time period and cases of persistence of IgM over long periods without evidence for recent infection have been reported (17). Immunoglobulin M is also occasionally induced following reinfection (which is usually subclinical). Although reinfection occurs in individuals with naturally induced immunity, it appears to be more common in vaccinees whose antibody levels are lower. In vaccinated populations in which natural virus still circulates, a situation encountered in several countries in central and southern Europe as well as Japan (due to differences in vaccination strategy from the US), reinfection is viewed as a significant problem. Reinfection during pregnancy is not considered a danger to the fetus, although rare cases of CRS following reinfection have been reported [S Katow, as cited in (18)]. A more significant problem is that reinfection can mimic acute infection in that both induction of IgM antibodies and elevation of IgG titers can occur. In the case of a pregnant woman, a recommendation for termination of the pregnancy can result. It has been pointed out that the presence of low-avidity antibodies is a more consistent indicator of acute infection, and modifications of standard EIA kits to test for low-avidity antibodies have been described (19). However, in the US, which has little circulating wild rubella, reinfection rarely occurs and development of tests to specifically diagnose reinfection would not seem to be necessary.

Vaccine-Related Arthralgia and Arthritis

Transient arthralgia and arthritis are common manifestations of rubella infection, particularly in adult women. Not surprisingly, transient arthritis and arthralgia also follow vaccination of adult women, with an expected incidence of 10% to 20%. Chronic arthritis following natural infection or vaccination has also been reported. The HPV-77 vaccine, which was used in the US vaccination program between 1969 and 1979, was associated with chronic arthritis as well as neurologic symptoms in children. This was a major factor in the withdrawal of this vaccine in 1979. The RA 27/3 vaccine, which replaced it, was associated with a lower incidence of overall arthritic complications. Nevertheless, chronic arthralgia, arthritis, and neurologic symptomatology have been reported following RA 27/3 vaccination in adult women (20).

The phenomenon of chronic complications associated with the RA 27/3 vaccine is surrounded by controversy. The US Public Health Service (USPHS) through the Advisory Committee on Immunization Practices has generally taken the position in its publications that vaccine-related chronic complications are extremely rare, if not nonexistent (7). An initial study by one group in British Columbia indicated that the incidence may be as high as 5% (although the population sizes used in this study were not large enough that this incidence was statistically significant) (21). However, three recently completed studies using much larger sample sizes (including one by the British Columbia group) failed to find a statistically significant incidence of chronic arthritis following rubella vaccination (22, 23, 24). A complicating factor in such studies is the general background incidence of arthritis in adult populations, which can approach 5% to 10%. The pathogenesis of vaccine-associated chronic symptoms is also not understood; studies by the British Columbia group have indicated that both long-term virus persistence and immunologic dysfunction may be involved (20), although individuals who suffer from chronic symptoms exhibit immunity to rubella that is not consistently different from that of unaffected immune individuals. Other groups have failed to reproduce the virus persistence findings (25).

The issue of rubella vaccine–associated chronic complications was publicized on an ABC News "20/20" program in 1990. Subsequently, the Institute of Medicine undertook a review of available data and concluded that chronic symptomatology was consistent with that of natural rubella pathogenesis, but no accurate evaluation of incidence could be made (26). Rubella was included in the Vaccine Compensable Injuries Act, given that a temporal series of complications following rubella vaccination could be documented.

Unfortunately, there are no predictive parameters (such as ethnic background or major histocompatibility haplotype) or tests that can be employed on seronegative adults to identify individuals who are potentially more likely to suffer chronic complications. In that regard, recent data from the British Columbia group indicate that both transient and chronic arthritic complications are most likely to occur in "true seronegatives" who have no antibody titer by any available commercial test or sensitive immunodiagnostic tests developed by that group [LA Mitchell, as reported in (18)]. This reverses an earlier report by the same group that stated that chronic complications were usually encountered in individuals who were "borderline negative" or "equivocal" on commercial EIA assays (27). Therefore, until more research on the phenomenon is forthcoming, there is no recourse except to require vaccination for adults who test seronegative. In this regard, it needs to be emphasized that all parties who have studied chronic complications, including the British Columbia group, recommend that rubella vaccination programs not be interrupted.

Serodiagnosis in Conjunction with Worldwide Eradication Efforts

Efforts are currently being considered to eradicate rubella both regionally and worldwide, and serodiagnosis will play an important role in the surveillance and containment required in these efforts. Until recently, rubella was not seriously considered for eradication, even though a highly effective vaccine exists that could be employed in mass vaccination efforts, as have been undertaken successfully against both polio and measles. Ironically, mass measles vaccination campaigns in Latin America have focused attention on rubella. In these campaigns, all reported rash illnesses require investigation and the majority turn out to be rubella. Additionally, recent epidemiologic studies that have underscored the presence of both rubella and CRS in underdeveloped countries have served to emphasize the societal load imposed by these diseases and the benefit of eradication. Finally, the USPHS has a goal of elimination of endemic rubella by the year 2000 and this goal is well under way toward being met. However, as long as rubella is endemic in other regions of the world, the US vaccination program will have to be maintained. Therefore, eradication is in the best interests of the US. Rubella elimination efforts are currently being discussed by the Pan American Health Organization. Rubella elimination will also soon be considered by the World Health Organization, although at the time of this writing rubella is not included in the WHO's Expanded Programme for Immunization.

In virus elimination programs, diagnosis is necessary not only for epidemiologic surveillance, but also for containment. Containment is generally accomplished by mass vaccination in the locality where case reports are made. As in the US, diagnosis of acute rubella is done serologically, primarily by testing for the presence of IgM antibodies. A current diagnostic issue specifically regarding measles elimination programs that will also affect similar efforts against rubella is discrimination among the "rash illnesses" (rubella, measles, and dengue fever) so that the correct vaccine can be employed for containment (as discussed above, the measles programs in Latin America have focused attention on rubella). Rubella tests employed in the US and Europe are currently available worldwide. However, the development of rapid, inexpensive "field" tests utilizing blood from finger or ear pricks that can diagnose and discriminate rash illnesses will greatly facilitate eradication efforts for both measles and rubella. The IC tests modified for IgM might possibly be applicable in this regard.

Acknowledgments

I would like to thank Kyung-ah Kim, Mark Kopnitsky, Denise Lynch, Paul Rota, Jeanette Stringer, David Schwartz, Bob Studholme, and John Stewart, all of whom provided essential information for this manuscript. I would also like to thank the technical service representatives at a number of companies for answering my questions and faxing me product inserts.

REFERENCES

1. Wolinsky JS. Rubella virus. In: Fields BN, Knipe DM, Howley PM, eds. Virology. 3rd ed. Philadelphia: Lippincott-Raven, 1996:899–930.
2. Centers for Disease Control. Rubella and congenital rubella syndrome–United States, January 1, 1991–May 7, 1994. MMWR 1994;43:391 and 397–401.
3. Tanemura M, Suzumori K, Yagami Y, Katow S. Diagnosis of fetal rubella infection with reverse transcription and nested polymerase chain reaction: a study of 34 cases diagnosed in fetuses. Am J Obstet Gynecol 1996;174:578–582.
4. American College of Obstetricians and Gynecologists, Committee on Technical Bulletins.

Rubella and pregnancy; ACOG Technical Bulletin No. 171–August 1992. Int J Gynecol Obstet 1992;42:60–66.

5. Bosma TJ, Corbett KM, Eckstein MB, et al. Use of PCR for prenatal and postnatal diagnosis of congenital rubella. J Clin Microbiol 1995;33: 2881–2887.
6. Skendzel LP. Rubella immunity: defining the level of protective antibody. Am J Clin Pathol 1996;106:170–174.
7. Centers for Disease Control. Rubella prevention. Recommendations of the Immunization Practices Advisory Committee (ACIP). MMWR 1990;39, No. RR-15, 1–18.
8. National Committee for Clinical Laboratory Standards. Evaluation and performance criteria for multiple component test products intended for the detection and quantitation of rubella IgG antibody; tentative guideline. NCCLS document I/LA6-T (ISBN 1-56238-158-X). Villanova, PA: NCCLS, 1992.
9. National Committee for Clinical Laboratory Standards. Detection and quantitation of rubella IgG antibody: evaluation of performance criteria for multiple component test products and specimen handling and use of test products in the clinical laboratory; approved guideline. NCCLS document I/LA6-A. Villanova, PA: NCCLS. *In Press.*
10. Herrmann KL. Available rubella serologic tests. Rev Infect Dis 1985;7:S108–S112.
11. Grangeot-Keros L, Pustowoit B, Hobman T. Evaluation of cobas core rubella IgG EIA recomb, a new enzyme immunoassay based on recombinant rubella-like particles. J Clin Microbiol 1995; 33:2392–2394.
12. Seppanen H, Huhtala M-L, Vaheri A, et al. Diagnostic potential of baculolvirus-expressed rubella virus envelope proteins. J Clin Microbiol 1991;29:1877–1882.
13. Lindquist C, Schmidt M, Heinola J, et al. Immunoaffinity purification of baculovirus-expressed rubella virus E1 for diagnostic purposes. J Clin Microbiol 1994;32:2192–2196.
14. Starkey WG, Newcombe S, Corbett M, et al. Use of rubella virus E1 fusion proteins for detection of rubella virus antibodies. J Clin Microbiol 1995; 33:270–274.
15. National Committee for Clinical Laboratory Standards. Specimen handling and use of rubella serology tests in the clinical laboratory; proposed guideline. NCCLS document I/LA7-P (ISSN 0273-3099). Villanova, PA: NCCLS, 1984.
16. Dimech W, Bettoll A, Eckert D, et al. Multicenter evaluation of five commercial rubella virus immunoglobulin G kits which report in international units per milliliter. J Clin Microbiol 1992; 30:633–641.
17. Thomas HIJ, Morgan-Capner P, Roberts A, Hesketh L. Persistent rubella-specific IgM reactivity in the absence of recent primary rubella and rubella reinfection. J Med Virol 1992;36:188–192.
18. Frey TK. Report of an international meeting on rubella vaccines and vaccination, 9 August 1993, Glasgow, United Kingdom. J Infect Dis 1994;170:507–509.
19. Thomas HIJ, Morgan-Capner P, Connor NS. Adaptation of a commercial rubella-specific IgG kit to assess specific IgG avidity. Serodiagn Immunother Infect Dis 1993;1:13–16.
20. Tingle AJ, Chantler JK, Kettyls GD, et al. Failed rubella immunization in adults: association with immunologic and virological abnormalities. J Infect Dis 1985;151:330–336.
21. Tingle AJ, Allen M, Petty RE, et al. Rubella-associated arthritis. I. Comparative studies of joint manifestations associated with natural rubella infection and RA 27/3 rubella immunisation. Ann Rheum Dis 1986;45:110–114.
22. Slater PE, Ben-Zvi T, Fogel A, et al. Absence of an association between rubella vaccination and arthritis in underimmune postpartum women. Vaccine 1995;13:1529–1532.
23. Tingle AJ, Mitchell LA, Grace M, et al. Randomised double-blind placebo-controlled study on adverse effects of rubella immunization in seronegative women. The Lancet 1997;349: 1277–1281.
24. Ray P, Black S, Shinefield IT, et al. Risk of chronic arthropathy among women after rubella vaccination. JAMA 1997;278:551–556.
25. Frenkel LM, Nielsen K, Garakian A, et al. A search for persistent rubella virus infection in persons with chronic symptoms after rubella and rubella immunization and in patients with juvenile rheumatoid arthritis. Clin Infect Dis 1996; 22:287–294.
26. Howson CP, Fineberg HV. Adverse events following pertussis and rubella vaccines. Summary of a report of the Institute of Medicine. JAMA 1992;267:392–396.
27. Tingle AJ, Yang T, Allen M, et al. Prospective immunological assessment of arthritis induced by rubella vaccine. Infect Immunol 1983;40: 22–28.

CHAPTER 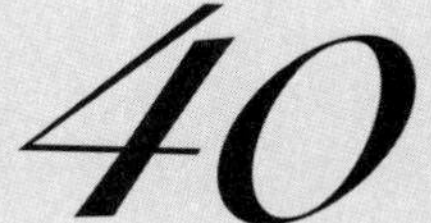

Epstein-Barr Virus and Mononucleosis-like Illnesses

CHARLES A. HORWITZ
THERESA A. STEEPER

Whereas classic infectious mononucleosis (IM) refers to an illness dominated by pharyngitis, cervical lymphadenopathy, and heterophil-antibody positivity (Het-Pos IM), its clinical features often overlap with other illnesses, including other viral processes and malignant lymphoma. Mononucleosis-like illnesses (IM-like) with negative heterophil antibody studies (Het-Neg) can be caused by Epstein-Barr virus (EBV), cytomegalovirus (CMV), *Toxoplasma gondii*, human immunodeficiency virus (HIV), or human herpesvirus-6 (HHV-6) (1–3). Rarely, drugs such as dapsone, halothane, hydantoin, and sulfasalazine (Azulfidine) produce similar findings. As a group these illnesses are only held together by the presence of blood smears, meeting the minimal morphologic criteria for the diagnosis of IM, that is, reactive lymphocytoses with over 50% lymphocytes, including at least 10 atypical lymphocytes of Downey type per 100 white blood cells (WBCs). Such smears demonstrate considerable morphologic heterogeneity within the lymphoid cells. Clinically, the heterophil-negative, IM-like syndromes must be separated from more serious conditions such as malignant lymphoma and acute leukemia. Because some cases of EBV-induced IM and most cases of CMV-induced mononucleosis (CMV-mono) lack significant lymphadenopathy, suspicion of an IM-like illness often occurs only after evaluation of peripheral blood smear data that show a significant atypical lymphocytosis.

The laboratory diagnosis of either Het-Pos IM or a heterophil-negative mononucleosis-like (Het-Neg, IM-like) illness is based on a combination of morphologic and immunoserologic data including heterophil or virus-specific antibody profiles. Our algorithm to diagnosis is summarized in **Figure 40-1** (3). This cost-effective approach begins with a careful analysis of the peripheral blood smear and can be performed in the physician's office as well as in large hospital laboratories. Once the presence of an atypical lymphocytosis is confirmed, a test for heterophil antibodies is indicated if the clinical presentation is dominated by pharyngitis and peripheral lymphadenopathy. If the clinical symptoms are dominated by persistent fevers, and splenomegaly without lymphadenopathy, virus-specific tests for CMV should be considered. The age of the patient is often important, as a differential diagnostic consideration, for example, CMV mononucleosis, is rarely encountered in children below the age of 10 years whereas primary EBV infections occur frequently in patients less than 48 months of age as heterophil-negative illnesses.

Selection and Accuracy of Confirmatory Heterophil Antibody Tests

A variety of techniques have been developed for the detection of heterophil antibody responses utilizing sheep, horse, or beef erythrocytes (RBCs). The most widely used heterophil tests require differential absorption of the patient's sera before titration to retain

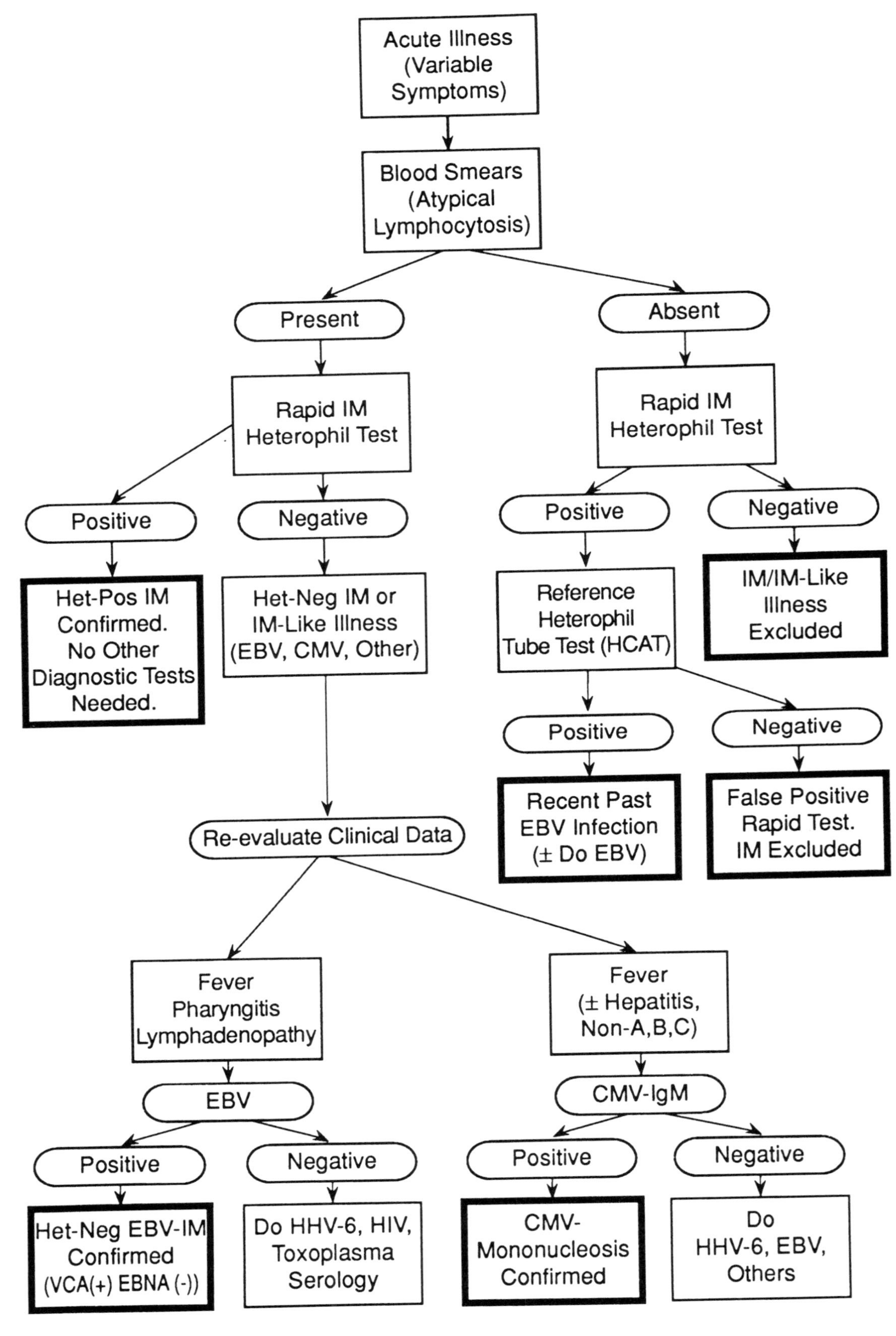

Acute Illness (Variable Symptoms)
Blood Smears (Atypical Lymphocytosis)
Present
Absent
Rapid IM Heterophil Test
Rapid IM Heterophil Test
Positive
Negative
Positive
Negative
Het-Pos IM Confirmed. No Other Diagnostic Tests Needed.
Het-Neg IM or IM-Like Illness (EBV, CMV, Other)
Reference Heterophil Tube Test (HCAT)
IM/IM-Like Illness Excluded
Positive
Negative
Recent Past EBV Infection (± Do EBV)
False Positive Rapid Test. IM Excluded
Re-evaluate Clinical Data
Fever Pharyngitis Lymphadenopathy
Fever (± Hepatitis, Non-A,B,C)
EBV
CMV-IgM
Positive
Negative
Positive
Negative
Het-Neg EBV-IM Confirmed (VCA(+) EBNA (-))
Do HHV-6, HIV, Toxoplasma Serology
CMV-Mononucleosis Confirmed
Do HHV-6, EBV, Others

specificity for EBV-IM. The standard reference heterophil differential absorption test is referred to as the Paul-Bunnell-Davidsohn or sheep cell differential absorption test (SDAT) (4). It is a 2-hour tube test that measures sheep RBC agglutinin titers before and after differential absorption of the test serum with both Forssman antigen [guinea pig kidney (GPK) suspensions] and beef RBCs. Antisheep agglutinins of IM type are minimally absorbed by GPK but mainly removed by beef cells. The SDAT test is highly specific for EBV-IM but it is relatively insensitive compared to similar test methods that utilize horse cells. Only rare false-positive SDAT reactions are reported. The sensitivity of the SDAT test depends in part on the time after onset of illness that the test is performed since peak heterophil titers are encountered during the second or third weeks of illness. Similar test principles are utilized in the Lee-Davidsohn modification of the SDAT test wherein horse erythrocytes are substituted for sheep cells following differential absorption of the patient's serum as described above (HDAT) (5,6). The use of horse erythrocytes in the HDAT results in greater sensitivity for detection of IM-type heterophil antibodies. The retention of differential absorption in the procedure retains test specificity EBV-IM; that is, Forssman-specific heterophil antibodies are separated from IM-specific heterophil antibodies. If the GPK-absorbed horse agglutinin titers exceed simultaneously performed beef-absorbed titers, the HDAT is interpreted as positive. When this result is accompanied by an atypical lymphocytosis, the diagnosis of EBV-IM is confirmed and no further diagnostic testing is indicated. If the beef cell absorbed titers are equal to or greater than the GPK-absorbed titers, the test is interpreted as negative. Negative results do not rule out an active EBV infection (i.e., Het-Neg, EBV-IM) or a mononucleosis-like illness due to other causes such as CMV. With primary EBV infections heterophil antibody responses are age dependent; that is, they are detectable in up to 98% of young adults, in only 16% of infants 7 to 24 months of age, in 50% of children 25 to 48 months of age, and in 81% of children between 5 and 10 years of age. Clearly, many more cases of Het-Neg EBV-IM will be encountered in children's hospitals versus cases from college health services.

Whereas heterophil antibody data are useful for qualitative diagnostic purposes, they cannot be used to monitor the patient's clinical course. Thus, EBV-IM patients with negative or very low peak heterophil titers can have very severe protracted illnesses whereas other patients with very high heterophil antibody responses may have short illnesses and very few clinical signs of mononucleosis. Delayed heterophil antibody responses where the initial testing is negative occur in 2.7% of Het-Pos cases of EBV-IM. As mentioned earlier, peak heterophil antibody titers occur 2 to 3 weeks after onset of EBV-IM, after which they may still be detectable at 12 months and can take as long as 2 to 3 years before becoming negative. The persistence of IM-type heterophil antibodies does not correlate with persistence of a particular patient's clinical illness. Because of their labor-intensive nature and a requirement for 2-hour test incubation, the reference heterophil tests, including the sensitive HDAT test, have largely been replaced in routine laboratories by 1- to 2-minute rapid heterophil IM slide tests.

Rapid Heterophil Infectious Mononucleosis Tests

Most confirmatory slide tests for EBV-IM utilize fine suspensions of GPK and beef RBC stroma for rapid differential absorption of serum followed by the use of horse RBC stroma to detect circulating IM-heterophil antibodies. Because of

FIGURE **40-1**

Algorithmic approach to the diagnosis of infectious mononucleosis and related heterophil-negative, mononucleosis-like syndromes. IM, infectious mononucleosis; Het-Pos, heterophil-antibody positive; Het-Neg, heterophil-antibody negative; HCAT, horse cell differential absorption tube test; CMV, cytomegalovirus; CMV-IgM, CMV macroglobulins; EBV, Epstein-Barr virus; HHV-6, human herpesvirus-6; HIV, human immunodeficiency virus; EBNA, EBV nuclear antigen; VCA, viral capsid antigen. (Modified by permission from Steeper TA, Horwitz CA, Henle W, Henle G. Selected aspects of acute and chronic infectious mononucleosis and mononucleosis-like illnesses for the practicing allergist. Ann Allergy 1987;59:243–250.)

their overall simplicity and convenience, these slide tests are the screening tests of choice for EBV-IM. They demonstrate reasonable sensitivity compared to the 2-hour HDAT test; that is, they are generally positive if the GPK-absorbed horse agglutinin titer in the HDAT is 1:224 or greater. Such levels (i.e., GPK titers of ≦1:224) are noted in approximately 91% of initial samples from Het-Pos EBV-IM. In 551 Het-Pos cases recently analyzed by us, 8.2% had peak initial GPK-absorbed titers of ≤1:112, and false-negative rapid IM were often encountered. Thus the rapid IM tests are not quite as sensitive as the more time-consuming HDAT. In the 2.7% of EBV-IM cases with delayed IM-heterophil antibody responses, true negative results initially occur with both rapid slide and HDAT heterophil tests. The aforementioned data are derived from cases in which 4.4% of EBV-IM patients were children aged 7 to 48 months of age.

Recently, rapid heterophil enzyme immunoassay tests (EIA) have been developed in which "IM-specific antigen" derived from either sheep or bovine erythrocytes is coated onto solid-phase surfaces that are then incubated between washing steps with patient serum that contains IM-specific heterophil antibodies. Enzymes labeled with antihuman IgM are added to the mixture, after which a substrate for a particular linking enzyme is added, yielding a colorimetric end point that determines the heterophil test result. These tests have been marketed heavily because of their longer shelf life, distinctive visual end points, and lack of a requirement for differential absorption. As a group they are much more expensive than the simpler agglutination tests and have not been extensively evaluated in the medical literature. In College of American Pathologists (CAP) proficiency testing studies from 1991 to 1995, heterophil EIA tests have done no better and at times have done worse than more traditional IM heterophil slide agglutination tests.

Immunoserologic Diagnosis of Heterophil-Negative, Mononucleosis-like Illnesses

In the 1970s and 1980s, the majority of baseline serologic data in primary EBV infections were acquired by immunofluorescence assay (IFA) methods (7–11). These techniques are limited by their tedious and time-consuming nature and the fact that subjective visual end points limit cellular detail and make ultrastructural localization impossible. In addition, a variety of interfering substances that induce circulating rheumatoid factors (RhFs) can significantly limit interpretation or produce erroneous results, or both, especially in immunoglobulin M (IgM)-specific tests (12–15) (**Table 40-1**). Some of these interferences that are capable of yielding falsely positive IgM responses can be eliminated by separating IgM class antibodies from IgG or IgA antibodies before IgM testing. This is optimally accomplished by pretreatment of the patient's serum with an antihuman IgG antiserum, after which the IgM-specific test is performed on the adsorbed supernate. Such separation decreases the likelihood of false-positive reactions due to rheumatoid factors and, in addition, eliminates false negatives due to quenching phenomena where small high-affinity IgG molecules compete with IgM molecules for antigen binding sites. The latter phenomenon is more commonly encountered in solid-based techniques such as EIA.

Other methods for separation of IgG and IgM include the use of commercially available sucrose density gradient columns or preabsorption of test serum with staphylococcus protein A and streptococci to remove IgG_3, the subtype that is notably increased in viral infections. Both of the latter methods appear to be limited because of false negatives due to loss of virus-specific IgM during the separation process.

It is also important to recognize that heterotypic cross reactivity can significantly affect test accuracy; for example, acute EBV-IM sera interfere significantly with accuracy in CMV-IgM tests, and this interference is not entirely eliminated by IgG/IgM serum separation (13,16,17). Circulating antinuclear antibody (ANA) interference can produce invalid test data with some viral IgG-specific tests, and appropriate negative controls are required for detection. Such ANA interference limits interpretation of anti-EBV nuclear antigen-IgG (EBNA-IgG) data by anticomplement immunofluorescence methods (ACIF) in approximately 3% of sera submitted for EBV-specific testing.

Overall, IFA is more sensitive for viral diagnosis than are older methods such as complement fixation (CF), but it is less sensitive than solid-phase immunoassays such as EIA. Enzyme immunoassays combine high precision and sensitivity with objective end points that are read in a spectrophotometer or enzyme rate analyzer.

TABLE **40-1**

Selected Serologic Problems and Interferences in Diagnosis of Heterophil-Negative Mononucleosis-like Illnesses in Healthy Individuals

Type of Test	Problem/Interference	Result	Solution
IgM	Rheumatoid factors (RF)	FP	1. Pretesting separation of IgM/IgG (e.g., goat antihuman IgG) 2. ±viral capture assays 3. ±absorption of serum by Fc fragments
IgM	Quenching phenomenon (high IgG levels compete with IgM for antigen sites)	FN	1. Usually seen in solid-based assays at low serum dilutions 2. Overcome by IgM/IgG separation methods
IgM	Heterotypic cross-reactions	FP	Careful evaluation of CMV/EBV data (shared virus effect vs reactivation of latent virus by present illness); R/O dual infections
IgM	Persistence of CMV-IgM	FP	History, usually low titer, evaluate other viral data
IgG	ANA	Invalid test data	Need negative controls for ANA recognition
IgG	Nonspecific IgG reactivity with Fc receptor of virus-infected cells	Nonspecific end point in CMV IgG IFA test	Generally separable visually from true positive

FP, false positive; FN, false negative; IFA, indirect immunofluorescence assay; Ig, immunoglobulin; CMV, cytomegalovirus; EBV, Epstein-Barr virus; ANA, antinuclear antibodies.

The reagents for EIA are inexpensive and have long shelf lives. Antibody titers in EIA tests can be calculated from standard curves in an objective fashion. Despite the advantages of EIA, IFA remains the gold standard immunoserologic test for the diagnosis of active EBV infections.

Whereas standard serologic techniques (IFA or EIA) remain the methods of choice in diagnosing EBV- or CMV-induced illnesses in immunocompetent individuals, serology plays only a limited role in immunocompromised patients who are undergoing active EBV or CMV infection, or both. With significant immunosuppression such as is seen in patients with acquired immunodeficiency syndrome (AIDS) or bone marrow transplants, CMV infections are best diagnosed by direct methods such as shell vial or deoxyribonucleic acid (DNA) hybridization assays, or conventional cultures. These methods are clearly preferred over standard serologic methods since the humoral responses are often very limited in immunosuppressed states. Also, detection of CMV antigens in buffy coat preparations correlates well with active infection in immunosuppressed patients.

Serologic Confirmation of Primary Epstein-Barr Virus Infections

Several distinctive groups of EBV-related antigens have been differentiated in human sera by serologic methods. These groups include EBV-specific viral capsid antigens (VCA), EBV-induced early antigens (EA), diffuse (D) and restricted (R) types, and EBV-induced nuclear antigens (EBNA). Detection of antibodies to VCA and EA are classically detected by IFA methods and anti-EBNA by ACIF (7,9,10). The lymphoblast cells used in these tests include smears from producer and nonproducer lines for respective detection of anti-VCA and anti-EBNA. Abortively infected nonproducer lines are used for detection of anti-EA of either D or R types. The differentiation is made following cell line fixation with methanol. Anti-D of the EA complex results in diffuse staining of target nuclei and is detected in most acute EBV-IM sera and in nasopharyngeal carcinoma in high titers. Anti-R (EA) staining is confined to cytoplasmic aggregates and is found at low titer in some patients with old EBV infections and in high titer in patients with Burkitt's lymphoma. The appearance of different EBV-specific antibodies at different time frames during the course of primary EBV infection is utilized for diagnostic purposes. Thus, evidence for an ongoing primary EBV infection is obtained when an initial serum sample shows the presence of VCA-specific IgM antibodies (over 1:10), high titers of IgG anti-VCA (over 1:320), some anti-D, and the initial absence (<1:2) of anti-EBNA. Sequential samples usually demonstrate the disappearance of IgM antibodies to VCA and of anti-D and, eventually, the evolution of anti-EBNA. Anti-EBNA may not be detectable for up to 6 months after onset of illness, and when it is present in acute sera (10% of EBV-IM cases) it usually is detected at low titers (1:2 or 1:5). Because IgM responses are found by IFA in only 85% of patients with primary EBV infections, the full panel of EBV-specific tests is often required (i.e., at least IgM and IgG anti-VCA and anti-EBNA). Primary EBV infections are documented in patients without VCA-IgM responses by demonstrating the serial evolution of anti-EBNA along with positive IgG responses on serial samples. The presence of constant VCA-specific IgG and anti-EBNA titers in the absence of VCA-specific IgM and anti-D in serial samples indicates a long-past EBV infection. Anti-VCA IgG titers show fourfold titer rises in only 20% of cases of EBV-IM and thus, must always be considered along with other data (anti-VCA-IgM and EBNA). The absence of all antibodies in serial samples excludes past as well as recent primary EBV infections. **Table 40-2** summarizes the diagnostic aspects of the various antibodies to EBV-related antigens. Anti-EA data are not necessary in most primary EBV infections but are helpful when the question of a chronic active EBV infection arises many years after onset of EBV-IM.

As was mentioned earlier, the vast majority of reference quantitative EBV serologic data were acquired by standard IFA methods. These studies include data on sequential serial samples that were drawn many months or years after the onset of a primary EBV infection (18,19). These data showed that both VCA-IgG and anti-EA may take several years to reach baseline levels in immunocompetent individuals following the onset of EBV-IM. Thus, even at 40 to 104 months after onset of illness, low levels (1:10–1:40) of anti-D (39%) or anti-R (12%) may persist and only anti-EA levels above 1:40 can be used serologically to support a clinical diagnosis of a chronic EBV infection. Similar follow-up studies demonstrate that caution should be used in interpreting high titers of anti-VCA-IgG within 2 to 3 years after onset of EBV-IM. Presently, EIA methods for EBV testing are commercially available; however, IFA is the only test method in which EBV data have been correlated with clinical disease (20,21). The latter authors and others have found no correlation between IFA titers and EIA absorbances, EIA indices, and enzyme-linked immunosorbent assay (ELISA) values. Poor correlation between IFA and EIA data is especially noted for VCA-IgG and VCA-EA, making it very hard to utilize EIA results when a chronic active EBV state is a diagnostic consideration. It is also unclear from EIA data just when anti-EBNA evolves during a primary EBV infection and what increased sensitivity levels can be expected in EBV-IM for VCA-IgM detection (vs 85% by IFA). In a recent study of VCA-IgM detection in EBV-IM with numerous EIA kits, sensitivity varied from 52.8% to 93.5% and specificity from 70.1% to 100% (21).

Standard IgG viral serology by itself is of limited usefulness in viral diagnosis, and this is especially true for herpesviruses that regularly establish lifelong latency states. Recently the differential use of high- and low-affinity IgG antibodies has been noted to be of value in the diagnosis of various infectious diseases (22–24). Such studies have shown that IgG affinity is initially low after primary antigenic challenge and then increases over the next several months. Presently a variety of methods are available for affinity/avidity measurements, with the dissociating effects of urea, quinidine, and diethylamine (DEA) being applied to solid-phase systems and IFA with much success. Such methods hold considerable promise diagnostically in heterophil-negative EBV-IM when IgM responses are negative. Their use can potentially eliminate the requirement for anti-EBNA testing in EBV profiles (22,24,25). Such differential avidity testing also has the ability to differentiate primary from secondary immune responses where the latter are associated with secondary IgM response, as has been seen in secondary CMV and HHV-6 infections (26,27).

TABLE **40-2**

Representative EBV/CMV Profiles in Acute Heterophil-Negative Mononucleosis-like Illnesses

	VCA IgM (<1:10)[a]	**VCA IgG (<40)[a]**	**EBNA IgG (<1:2)[b]**	**EA-IgG Diffuse (<1:10)[a]**	**EA-IgG Restricted (<1:10)[a]**	**CMV IgM (<1:32)[a]**	**CMV-CF or IgG**	**Comments/ Interpretation**
I[c]	Pos	Pos	Neg	Pos	Neg	Neg	±Stable (low titer, usually)	Current primary EBV infection; seen in 85% of cases; EA-IgG data are unnecessary
II[c,d]	Neg	Pos	Neg	Pos	Neg	Neg	±Stable (low titer, usually)	Suggestive, not diagnostic of recent primary EBV infection; definitive if anti-EBNA evolves on convalescent samples
III[c]	Pos	Pos	Neg	Pos	Neg	Pos	Stable (low titer, usually)	Current primary EBV infection; also ± heterotypic serologic cross reaction in CMV-IgM test; dual EBV/CMV infection less likely
IV	Neg	Pos	Pos	Neg	Neg	Neg	Stable (low)	Remote EBV infection; CMV also unlikely cause of present acute illness
V[c]	Neg	Pos	Pos	Neg	Neg (±)	Pos	±Rising (±high)	Consistent with CMV-mononucleosis; old EBV infection
VI	Neg	Neg	Neg	Neg	Neg	Neg	(±)	Still susceptible to EBV; CMV also unlikely

IFA, indirect immunofluorescence assays; EA, early antigens, D or R types; EBNA, EBV-associated nuclear antigens; CMV-IgM, CMV-macroglobulins; IgG-CMV by complement fixation (CF) or IFA.

[a] IFA.

[b] Anticomplement immunofluorescence.

[c] Associated reactive IM-type blood smear.

[d] Pattern II above also seen in severely immunosuppressed patients (e.g., bone marrow transplants or AIDS).

Further evaluations on the specificity of such avidity studies for acute viral illnesses are needed (24).

Serologic Confirmation of Cytomegalovirus-Induced Mononucleosis

The original laboratory studies on CMV mononucleosis (CMV-Mono) in healthy individuals included the technically complex CF method (26). These studies and others showed that many cases had entirely negative (<1:8) or very low (1:8–1:16) anti-CMV CF levels on initial samples and that peak anti–CMV-CF levels (1:128) were found in only 65% of cases (16). Also, studies with paired serum samples showed fourfold titer changes by CF in only 50% of cases. Because of technical limitations, the need for follow-up convalescent samples, and the large number of cases without fourfold titer changes, CF methods are of limited usefulness in CMV mononucleosis. Furthermore, fourfold titer rises by CF or other IgG methods only imply the presence of an active CMV infection and do not firmly establish CMV as the cause of the patient's current illness. For example, 20% of patients with primary EBV infections will also demonstrate fourfold anti–CMV-CF titer rises, indicative of secondary reactivation of the CMV latency state by an active EBV infection. Other less complex methods such as hemagglutination inhibition (HAI), EIA, and passive latex agglutination offer greater sensitivity than CF for detection of CMV-IgG antibodies but are limited by many of the same considerations as is CMV-CF testing. These more sensitive IgG tests are the methods of choice for determination of CMV viral immunity.

The detection of anti-CMV IgM antibodies (1:32) by IFA methods is seen during the acute phase of most CMV-Mono cases (99%), with 91% of positive results occurring on the initial serum sample (16). Thus, only occasionally is a second sample required. Because of heterotypic cross-reactivity of acute EBV-IM sera in CMV-IgM tests, EBV panel results must always be evaluated along with those from CMV tests when the principal pathogen of a Het-Neg IM-like illness is determined. Approximately 30% of acute EBV sera react positively (1:16) in IFA tests for CMV-IgM. Similar cross-reactivity is seen in solid-based EIAs. With IFA methods, this cross-reactivity is generally noted at low levels (1:16–1:32) although on occasion higher levels can be seen. Sera from the acute phase of CMV-Mono much less commonly (<2%) interfere in EBV-IgM–specific tests. Also, most serial samples from confirmed cases of CMV-Mono with significantly increased EBV levels of VCA-IgG and IgG-EA are reflective of EBV carrier state reactivation by the active CMV infections rather than true dual infections. If clinically indicated, complex tests such as DNA hybridization assays, tissue biopsies, and/or assays for EBV in throat washings may be necessary to differentiate dual EBV/CMV viral infections from cases with serologic overlap or secondary carrier state reactivation. The use of EIA for detection of IgG- and IgM-specific CMV antibodies is common today in large commercial laboratories, and such EIA-generated CMV data are generally more easily comparable to IFA data than for EBV.

General Comments

The above discussion summarizes the diagnostic aspects and technical limitations of the various assays utilized for the diagnosis of a heterophil-negative mononucleosis-like illness in previously healthy individuals. Many but not all of the problems for IgM assays can be circumvented by IgM/IgG separation before viral testing. While this generally eliminates interference from rheumatoid factors, quenching phenomena, and so forth, it does not eliminate serologic cross-reactions that result from shared viral antigens between CMV and EBV that are noted by EBV sera in IgM-specific CMV tests. The diagnostic situation is complicated by the occasional occurrence of dual infections that must be differentiated from serologic cross-reactions and others. The herpesvirus latency state can be reactivated by a variety of stimuli including other viral infections that complicate the interpretation of various viral-specific tests, particularly IgG-specific tests. This is especially seen with HHV-6 infections that are capable of producing heterophil-negative IM-like illnesses with high anti–HHV-6 IgG titers (19,27). Since IgG anti–HHV-6 titers are often increased by other viral infections, HHV-6 should only be considered as the causative agent in a Het-Neg IM-like illness after exclusion of both active EBV and CMV infections by appropriate serologic methods. When this is done, the demonstration of anti–HHV-6 IgM by either IFA or EIA favors HHV-6 as the cause of the patient's present acute illness. Finally, in previously healthy individuals with clinical signs that are suggestive of an IM-like illness, viral testing should be limited to Het-Neg cases with significant numbers of atypical lymphocytes in the peripheral smear since the diagnostic yield from EBV or CMV viral testing of healthy adults without many Downey cells is very low (16).

REFERENCES

1. Horwitz CA, Steeper TA. Immunoserology of infectious mononucleosis and related heterophil-negative mononucleosis-like illnesses. In: McClatchey KD, ed. Clinical laboratory medicine. Baltimore: Williams & Wilkins, 1994:1535–1542.
2. Penman HG. The problem of seronegative IM. In: Carter RL, Penman HG, eds. Infectious

mononucleosis. Oxford: Blackwell Scientific, 1969:201–224.

3. Steeper TA, Horwitz CA, Henle W, Henle G. Selected aspects of acute and chronic infectious mononucleosis and mononucleosis-like illnesses for the practicing allergist. Ann Allergy 1987;59: 243–250.
4. Davidsohn I, Nelson DA. The blood. In: Davidsohn I, Henry JB, eds. Todd-Sanford's clinical diagnosis by laboratory methods. 14th ed. Philadelphia: Saunders, 1968:280–292.
5. Lee CL, Zandrew F, Davidsohn I. Horse agglutinins in infectious mononucleosis. III. Criterion for differential diagnosis. J Clin Pathol 1968;21: 631–634.
6. Evans AS, Niederman JC, Cenabre LC, et al. A prospective evaluation of heterophile and Epstein-Barr virus-specific IgM antibody tests in clinical and subclinical infectious mononucleosis. Specificity and sensitivity of the tests and persistence of antibody. J Infect Dis 1975;132: 546–554.
7. Henle W, Henle G, Horwitz CA. Epstein-Barr virus-specific diagnostic tests in infectious mononucleosis. Hum Pathol 1974;5:551–565.
8. Sumaya CV. Endogenous reactivation of Epstein-Barr virus infection. J Infect Dis 1977;135:374–379.
9. Reedman BM, Klein G. Cellular localization of an Epstein-Barr virus–associated complement-fixing antigen in producer and non-producer lymphoblastoid cell lines. Int J Cancer 1973;11:499–520.
10. Henle W, Henle G, Horwitz CA. Infectious mononucleosis and Epstein-Barr virus–associated malignancies. In: Lennette EH, Schmidt NJ, eds. Diagnostic procedures for viral, rickettsial and chlamydial infections. Washington, DC: American Public Health Association, 1979:441–470.
11. Schmitz H, Voltz D, Krainick-Reichert C. Acute Epstein-Barr virus infections in children. Med Microbiol Immunol 1972;158:58–70.
12. Smith TF, Shelley CD. Detection of IgM antibodies to CMV and rapid diagnosis by shell vial assay. J Virol Methods 1988;21:87–96.
13. Schmidt NJ. Update on class-specific viral antibody assay. Clin Immunol Newsletter 1984;5:81–85.
14. Henle G, Lennette ET, Alspaugh A, Henle W. Rheumatoid factor as a cause of positive reactions in tests for EBV-specific IgM antibodies. Clin Exp Immunol 1979;36:415–422.
15. Smith TF. Viral serology in clinical medicine. In: Homburger H, Batsaikis J, eds. Clinical laboratory annual. Norwalk, CT: Appleton-Century-Crofts, 1983;31–56.
16. Horwitz C, Henle W, Henle G, et al. Clinical and laboratory evaluation of CMV-induced mononucleosis in previously healthy individuals. Report of 82 cases. Medicine 1986;65:124–134.
17. Hanshaw J, Niederman JC, Chessen LN. CMV macroglobulin in cell-associated herpesvirus infection. J Infect Dis 1972;125:304–306.
18. Horwitz CA, Henle W, Henle G, et al. Long term serologic follow up of patients for Epstein-Barr virus after recovery from infectious mononucleosis. J Infect Dis 1985;151:1150–1153.
19. Linde A, Fridell E, Dahl H, et al. Effect of primary EBV infection on herpesvirus-6, CMV, measles virus immunoglobulin G titers. J Clin Microbiol 1990;28:211–215.
20. Strauss SE, Cohen JI, Tosato G, Meier J. Epstein-Barr virus infections: biology, pathogenesis, and management. Ann Intern Med 1993;118:45–58.
21. Wiedbrauk DL, Bassin S. Evaluation of five immunoassays for detection of immunoglobulin M antibodies to Epstein-Barr virus viral capsid antigens. J Clin Microbiol 1993;31:1339–1341.
22. DeOry F, Antomaya J, Fernandez MV, Echevarria JM. Application of low-avidity immunoglobulin-G studies to diagnosis of Epstein-Barr virus infectious mononucleosis. J Clin Microbiol 1993;31:1669–1671.
23. Andersson A, Vetter V, Kreutzer L, Bauer G. Avidities of IgG directed against viral capsid antigen or early antigen: Useful markers for significant Epstein-Barr virus serology. J Med Virol 1994;43:238–244.
24. Hedman K, Lappalainen M, Soderlund M, Hedman L. Avidity of IgG in serodiagnosis of infectious diseases. Rev Med Microbiol 1993;4: 123–129.
25. Horwitz CA, Henle W, Henle G, et al. Heterophil-negative IM and mononucleosis-like illness. Laboratory confirmation of 43 cases. Am J Med 1977;63:947–957.
26. Klemola E, Kaariainem L, von Essen R, et al. Further studies on cytomegalovirus mononucleosis in previously healthy individuals. Acta Intern Med 1967;182:311–322.
27. Fox JD, Ward P, Brigs M, et al. Production of IgM antibody to HHV6 in reactivation and primary infection. Epidemiol Infect 1990;104:289–296.

CHAPTER 41

Herpes, Varicella, and Cytomegalovirus

JOHN L. SEVER

There are now eight human herpesviruses: herpes simplex viruses (HSV-1 and HSV-2), varicella-zoster virus (VZV), cytomegalovirus (CMV), Epstein-Barr virus (EBV), and the human herpesviruses (HHV)-6, -7, and -8. Infections with these viruses may be asymptomatic, mild, moderately symptomatic, or sometimes fatal. Severe disease is more likely to occur with infections in infants and immunocompromised patients. This chapter reviews the clinical findings, treatment, and laboratory tests that are of value in diagnosing, evaluating, and monitoring patients who are infected with HSV-1, HSV-2, VZV, and CMV.

Herpes Simplex Virus (HSV-1 and HSV-2)

Clinical Findings

Infections with HSV-1 and HSV-2 are common and result in primary and recurrent disease. By adulthood 80% of the US population are seropositive for HSV-1 and 15% to 50% are seropositive for HSV-2. Many infections are subclinical; however, mild to severe or fatal disease can occur. Herpes infections are generally self-limited and the severity of disease depends on the location of the infection, age, immunologic status of the patient, and whether the infection is primary, initial, or recurrent. Both HSV-1 and -2 can infect the lips and oral cavity, genital area, eyes, and skin, and can persist in the sensory ganglia of the nervous system. HSV-1 infections, however, occur more frequently "above the belt" whereas HSV-2 infections are more often seen "below the belt." HSV-1 is most frequently transmitted between children by oral contact while HSV-2 is usually transmitted sexually as a venereal disease or congenitally from mother to infant at birth. Severe HSV infections are seen in patients with cancer, organ transplants, and immunosuppression due to disease, drugs, or infections such as human immunodeficiency virus (HIV). Severe ocular and neurologic disease can be caused by these viruses.

Oral-Labial Herpes and Skin Infections

HSV-1 is a frequent cause of cold sores or fever blisters and gingivostomatitis. Most primary infections are subclinical and occur in children between 1 and 5 years of age. Oral ulcers, pharyngotonsillitis, or severe gingivostomatitis may occur in some patients. Recurrent lesions are unusually due to reactivation of virus, which persists in a latent form. Stimuli for reactivation can include sunlight, trauma, stress, fever, menstruation, and other factors. Infections of the skin can occur by autoinoculation or by close contact. Severe skin infections are seen in patients with eczema, chronic dermatosis, or immunosuppression.

Genital Herpes

Most genital herpes infections are due to HSV-2. The infections can be asymptomatic or symptomatic and can involve the external genitalia as well as the vagina and cervix in women. Primary infections are more likely to be more severe, with multiple lesions. Recurrent infections are usually more limited and of shorter duration. In men, lesions appear as vesicles or ulcers on the penis and sometimes on the scrotum. Anal sex can result in anorectal lesions. Genital lesions can also be spread to the buttocks and thighs and by autoinoculation. In children genital infections can occur by sexual abuse or autoinoculation from HSV infection of the mouth. In adults, genital infections with HSV-1 can be transmitted by oral sex.

Central Nervous System Involvement

The encephalitic form of HSV is usually due to HSV-1 while benign meningitis associated with HSV is generally caused by HSV-2. Herpes simplex virus encephalitis can be very severe, and, if it is untreated, mortality is over 70%.

Ocular Herpes

Herpes simplex virus of the cornea is usually due to HSV-1 and is an important cause of blindness. Primary infection is usually limited to conjunctivitis, occasionally with keratitis. Recurrences of keratitis are painful and can cause severe scarring of the cornea.

Disseminated Herpes

Patients with cancer, organ transplants, or immunosuppression can have severe forms of primary herpes or reactivation of latent herpes with chronic or recurrent extensive lesions. Skin lesions can become massive in these patients and the infection can involve organs such as the liver, lungs, and central nervous system (CNS).

Congenital Herpes

Newborns can become infected at birth or just before birth when the mother has genital herpes at the time of delivery. The mother's infection is usually due to HSV-2 and may be clinically evident or subclinical. Infection of the newborn is reported in 1 in every 1000 to 10,000 births. The infection of the child can be localized to the skin or disseminated with or without involvement of the central nervous system. Untreated infected neonates have a fatality rate of over 50%. Early diagnosis is important for treatment but often difficult since symptoms usually do not appear until about one week after birth and only about 50% of infants have skin lesions.

Treatment

Acyclovir (Zovirax) can be used for the treatment of HSV infections and the prevention of recurrences. The drug can be given orally in a suspension, capsules, or tablets for severe genital and skin infections and to prevent recurrent disease. An ointment that contains acyclovir can be used topically to treat genital HSV or can be given at the onset of the recurrence of symptoms. The intravenous form of the drug is used for the most severely affected patients and for HSV encephalitis. Other drugs that can be considered include valacyclovir (Valtrex), a drug related to acyclovir, and foscarnet (Foscavir) for acyclovir-resistant HSV.

Cesarean section delivery is used for women who have active genital HSV infection at the time of the birth. This reduces the risk of infection of the newborn.

Laboratory Tests

The availability of drugs and procedures for the prevention and treatment of HSV infections and the prevention of recurrences has increased the importance of laboratory tests to detect HSV infection in asymptomatic individuals and to confirm the diagnosis of HSV when the clinical findings are not clear (**Table 41-1**).

Serology

Tests for antibody to HSV-1 and -2 are used to document prior infections with specific herpesviruses and for epidemiologic studies. Enzyme-linked immunosorbent assays (ELISA) and immunofluorescent assay (IFA) assays are generally used; however, these tests frequently give cross-reactions between antibody to HSV-1 and HSV-2 (1). The tests may be labeled as being specific for HSV-1 or -2, but they are not.

The College of American Pathologists (CAP) proficiency program provides survey kits to evaluate performance with these tests (**Table 41-2**).

Newer tests using Western blot or a specially absorbed HSV antigen have been reported to be type specific. Investigators at the University of Washington have developed a Western blot test that is specific for HSV-1 and HSV-2

TABLE **41-1**

Laboratory Tests for Herpes Simplex Viruses, Varicella, and Cytomegalovirus

Virus	Serology	Detection of Virus/Antigens
Herpes simplex *(HSV-1, HSV-2)*: Serious infections of genital area and skin, congenital infections, and disease in immunosuppressed patients	ELISA and IFA tests frequently have cross-reactions between antibody to HSV-1 and -2; newer Western blot and purified glycoprotein G tests appear to be specific for antibody to HSV-1 and -2 and should be useful for documenting past infections	Virus isolation with tissue culture and fluorescent labeled antibody to identify HSV-2; shell vial assay more rapid; ELVIS culture system available ELISA antigen tests generally less sensitive than cultures; PCR of spinal fluid best for CNS HSV
Varicella: Severe disease with congenital infection in immunosuppressed patients and elderly	ELISA or FAMA tests for IgG antibody are used for identifying patients at risk for infection; other tests are also available	Varicella-specific immunofluorescent stain (DFA) of scrapings can be used to confirm the diagnosis Culture available but slow (5–10 days) PCR of spinal fluid best for CNS syndrome and unusual lesions
Cytomegalovirus: Fetal disease and death with congenital infection; immunosuppressed and organ transplant patients at high risk for severe disease	ELISA and IFA tests for IgG for identifying past infection IgM antibody indicates recent infection but 10%–20% false negatives make test somewhat unreliable	Virus isolation with cultures best; shell vial cultures more rapid Antigen labeling used to detect virus in PBLs PCR is best for confirming infections in CNS and other organs and to identify resistant virus

ELISA, enzyme-linked immunosorbent assay; IFA, indirect fluorescent antibody; PCR, polymerase chain reaction; CNS, central nervous system; IgG, immunoglobulin G; DFA, direct fluorescent antibody; FAMA, fluorescent antibody to membrane antigen; PBLs perepheral blood leukocytes.

TABLE **41-2**

Quality Assurance for Herpes Simplex Viruses, Varicella, and Cytomegalovirus: College of American Pathologists (CAP) Survey Kits

		CAP Survey Kits[a]		
Virus		**Antibody**	**Virus Isolation**	**Antigen**
Herpes simplex (HSV-1 and -2)	VR-3	HC-4[b] or VR-1	HC-2[b] or VR-2	VR-4
Varicella	VR-3	VR-1	VR-2	VR-4
Cytomegalovirus	VR-3	VR-1	VR-2	VR-4

[a] Survey kits are provided three times each year. Herpesvirus challenges are included in certain kits each year. For further information call 1-800-323-4040.

[b] HC-4, HC-2 survey kits provide challenges for HSV-1 and -2 only.

(2). Also, a new ELISA test that uses an absorbed, purified glycoprotein G in the COBAS COR HSV-2 IgG test has been reported to be type specific (3). If further evaluation of these methods confirms that they are type specific, they should replace the present cross-reacting ELISA test methods.

Detection of Herpesviruses/Antigens

Tests for the detection of herpesvirus are used to detect or document HSV infections so that appropriate management or treatment can be instituted. Virus isolation in tissue culture has been considered the most sensitive and specific method for detecting herpesviruses in vesicle fluid, ulcerating lesions, nasopharynx, conjunctiva, and urine. Cultures usually become positive in a few days. The presence of the virus is recognized by the cytopathic effect on the culture, and the type of virus can be determined with the use of type-specific fluorescent labeled antibodies. Some laboratories now use a rapid shell vial assay that combines tissue culture on a coverslip in a one-dram shell vial, low-speed centrifugation (700 × g for 60 min), incubation, and indirect immunoperoxidase staining (4). A new tissue culture method called ELVIS (BioWhitaker, Walkersville, MD) uses a genetically engineered baby hamster kidney cell line that, in the presence of HSV, activates the enzyme beta-galactosidase, and this can be detected by a color change in the cells.

ELISA and direct fluorescent antibody (DFA) tests for HSV antigens are commercially available (HERPCHEK, Dupont, and others) but are not as sensitive as cultures, particularly when used for asymptomatic patients. Some laboratories test specimens with both culture and antigen tests. The antigen test is rapid and the culture identifies infections that are missed by the antigen test. In a small percent of cases the antigen test may be positive while the culture is negative. Positive tests can be confirmed by blocking with HSV antibody.

College of American Pathologists survey kits are available for proficiency testing of laboratories that perform virology cultures, antigen determinations, and also specifically HSV cultures (Table 41-2).

Polymerase chain reaction (PCR) is the method of choice for the early diagnosis of herpes encephalitis (5). The tests of spinal fluid are usually positive at the time of onset of clinical symptoms and remain positive for at least 5 days after the initiation of therapy with acyclovir. The sensitivity of the method is about 95%. Since about 90% to 95% of the cases of herpes encephalitis are due to HSV-1 and the remainder are caused by HSV-2, the primers used for the PCR must be able to detect both viruses.

Varicella

Clinical Findings

Primary infection with varicella-zoster virus is almost always symptomatic and is characterized by a generalized vesicular rash. VZV is highly contagious and is spread from the lesions through the air. The recent licensing of a vaccine for varicella for use in children in the United States should change the frequency of occurrence of this illness in the future. Herpes zoster (shingles) usually occurs in adults and is caused by the reactivation of latent VZV along sensory nerves; it results in painful areas of the skin and vesicles.

Varicella (Chickenpox)

The vesicular lesions of varicella usually appear about 14 days (10–20 days) after exposure to a case of varicella. About 24 hours before the onset of rash, the patient may have fever, headache, anorexia, and malaise. The rash usually begins on the scalp or trunk as red macules, which progress to papules and then vesicles. The lesions appear in crops, predominantly on the trunk, but also on the face and extremities over a period of 1 to 5 days. Itching is frequently quite pronounced. Within 1 to 3 days, the lesions develop into brown scabs. The active period of the disease usually lasts for 7 to 10 days.

Congenital Varicella

The occurrence of varicella early in pregnancy can result in severe malformations of the fetus, while chickenpox at the time of delivery can be transmitted to the fetus and cause disseminated infection and death. To reduce the risk of severe varicella in the mother and to protect the infant, varicella-zoster immune globulin (VZIG) should be used (see Treatment).

Herpes Zoster (Shingles)

Pain usually precedes the onset of the skin lesions of herpes zoster. The latent VZV in the sensory ganglia becomes activated and travels down the sensory nerve. The lesions then develop along the distribution of the nerve and are usually larger than for varicella. Various nerves of the face (trigeminal), neck, thorax, and lumbar area may be involved. Pain and headache are frequent complaints. Patients under 60 years usually have spontaneous resolution of the lesions within 4 weeks. Chronic or disseminated zoster, or both, are more common in immunocompromised and elderly patients. In these cases the infection may spread to the brain, lungs, and liver and can result in death.

Treatment

Varicella

Normal Individuals Treatment of chickenpox in healthy children is symptomatic. Antihistamines and calamine lotion are used for itching. Fever can be treated with acetaminophen or ibuprofen. Aspirin should not be used because of the association with Reye's syndrome.

Antiviral therapy is possible with acyclovir. If the drug is started within 24 hours of the onset of rash the number of lesions is decreased and the duration of lesions is shortened. The value of this treatment for children under 13 years of age is limited and chemotherapy is not generally recommended for young children. Acyclovir is recommended for adolescents and adults because of their increased risk for severe disease.

High-Risk Individuals Immunocompromised individuals with chickenpox or patients with varicella pneumonia should be treated with acyclovir intravenously (6). Individuals who must take large doses of steroids may also require acyclovir.

Congenital Varicella

Pregnant women who are exposed to varicella in the first 20 weeks of gestation are at risk for becoming infected and transmitting the infection to the fetus (7). Under these circumstances there is about a 2% risk of severe fetal damage. Approximately 95% of women have experienced varicella in childhood and are immune. To determine if a specific pregnant woman is immune she should be tested for varicella antibody with the ELISA or FAMA (fluorescent antibody to membrane antigen) methods. If no varicella antibody is present, she can be given VZIG to reduce the severity or prevent varicella and to lessen the risk of congenital varicella.

Varicella that is present 5 days before delivery to 2 days after delivery can be transmitted to the infant and cause severe generalized infection that can be fatal. These children should be given VZIG as soon as possible after birth to reduce the risk of this serious infection.

Herpes Zoster

Normal Individuals In normal children and adults under 60 years of age, herpes zoster is usually a painful but limited disease. Acyclovir can be used if the nerves near the eye are involved. The drug has also been shown to shorten the duration of lesions and pain and to reduce the prevalence of other neurologic symptoms, particularly for patients over 60 years of age.

High-Risk Individuals Acyclovir should be used to treat immunocompromised patients with herpes zoster. Two other antiviral agents, famciclovir (Famvir) and valacyclovir, are also used for the treatment of herpes zoster in adults. Acyclovir is started intravenously and later changed to oral administration.

Prevention Varicella vaccine is now available to be given to children 12 months of age and older. Adolescents and adults 13 years of age and older should receive a second dose of vaccine 4 to 8 weeks after the first dose.

Varicella zoster immune globulin can be used for susceptible pregnant women who are exposed to varicella, infants born to women who have varicella near term, and high-risk individuals such as immunocompromised patients who are exposed to varicella.

Laboratory Tests (See Table 41-1.)

Serology

Tests for antibody to varicella are used to identify susceptible patients, for epidemiologic studies, and, in rare instances, to document infections. ELISA and FAMA tests for varicella immunoglobulin G (IgG) antibody are most useful for this purpose (Table 41-1). IFA and latex agglutination tests may be quite sensitive. Other tests are available but are not generally used. The complement fixation test is not sensitive and should not be used to determine susceptibility. Varicella IgM antibody tests using ELISA and FAMA can be utilized to identify recent infections. The CAP proficiency program for serology provides survey kits for varicella.

Detection of Varicella-Zoster Virus

(See Table 41-2.)

The diagnosis of chickenpox and shingles is usually based on the characteristic rash and the clinical syndrome. If confirmation is needed, scrapings of the lesions can be stained with Giemsa's or Wright's stain. The presence of multinucleated giant cells indicates the detection of herpesvirus but does not distinguish varicella from herpes simplex. The use of varicella-specific immunofluorescent antibody staining of the scrapings (DFA) provides a better test. The lesions can be cultured for virus; however, this test takes 5 to 10 days to complete. The CAP proficiency program issues survey kits for culture of varicella.

Polymerase chain reaction tests are available for varicella and are recommended for the diagnosis of unusual varicella or herpes zoster–like lesions, CNS syndromes, infected body fluids, and vesicle fluid specimens that are negative for VZV by culture or direct fluorescence, or both, where the identification of an etiologic agent is important.

Cytomegalovirus

Infections with cytomegalovirus (CMV) are very common and are usually asymptomatic in normal individuals. Some patients experience an infectious mononucleosis-like syndrome. Infants can be infected in utero and severe disease and death may occur. Patients with acquired immunodeficiency syndrome (AIDS), those who are immunocompromised, and those who have undergone organ transplants are also at risk for severe disease due to CMV.

Clinical Findings

Congenital Cytomegalovirus

About 1% of newborns are infected with CMV at birth and are excreting this virus. Approximately 10% of these children have some evidence of damage due to CMV. The full severe syndrome occurs infrequently but can include hepatosplenomegaly, chorioretinitis, thrombocytopenia, encephalitis, pneumonitis, nephritis, microcephaly, mental-motor retardation, and blindness.

Organ Transplant Patients

About 20% of patients who have undergone a renal organ transplant may have symptoms related to CMV, including fever, malaise, hepatosplenomegaly, hepatic dysfunction, and pneumonia. There is some evidence of increased graft rejection if CMV infection is present. In bone marrow organ transplant patients pneumonia due to CMV may be a problem.

Posttransfusion Syndrome

About 1 to 8 weeks after multiple transfusions, particularly after open heart surgery, a syndrome similar to CMV mononucleosis may be seen. Pharyngitis and lymphadenopathy may not be present but a hemolytic anemia can occur. In premature infants ($<1500\,g$) who are infected by transfusion, poor respiratory function, hepatosplenomegaly, gray pallor, thrombocytopenia, and anemia may develop.

Immunocompromised Patients

Progressive pneumonia with cough, fever, shortness of breath, rapid breathing, and rapid heart rate can be due to CMV. Ulcerative lesions in the gastrointestinal tract may occur and CMV myocarditis has been reported. Patients may experience CMV retinitis with loss of vision and infection of the central nervous system. Patients with AIDS are at high risk for complications due to disseminated infection with CMV. Among these patients, 20% to 40% have involvement of the brain with CMV at autopsy.

Treatment

Ganciclovir (Cytovene) can be used for the treatment of CMV retinitis in immunocompromised patients, including patients with AIDS. It is also used to prevent CMV disease in organ transplant recipients who are at risk for CMV disease. Foscarnet and cidofovir (Vistide) are also indicated for the treatment of patients with AIDS who have CMV retinitis.

Laboratory Tests (See Table 41-1.)

Serology

About 60% to 80% of adults are seropositive for CMV. ELISA and IFA tests for CMV-IgG antibody can be used to confirm past infections, to screen blood or donors before selection for transfusion or organ transplant, and for epidemiologic studies (Table 41-1). ELISA and IFA tests for CMV-IgM–specific antibody are positive in about 90% of primary infections and the antibody persists for several months. With reactivation of CMV, CMV-IgM tests may again become positive. In children infected with CMV in utero, ELISA CMV-IgM antibody develops in about 80% of cases and the antibody persists for several months. The frequency of false-negative IgM antibody tests makes serology less valuable for identifying recent infections. The CAP proficiency program for serology provides survey kits for CMV (Table 41-2).

Detection of Cytomegalovirus/Antigens

In most cases infections with CMV are best identified by detection of the virus. Conventional tube cultures have been used for more than 30 years for detecting CMV. These cultures become positive in a few days with urine samples from infected newborns but can require 14 days or more for samples from other tissues and patients. In recent years, many laboratories have switched to shell vial cultures with tissue culture monolayers on coverslips (8). The cultures are centrifuged and stained with a CMV-specific immunofluorescent antibody. This method reduces the time for detection of CMV infection and is more sensitive than the conventional tube cell cultures. The CAP proficiency panel survey kits can be used for CMV viral cultures.

Antigenemia assays to detect pp65 antigen in peripheral blood leukocytes after centrifugation use either immunofluorescence or enzyme-labeled monoclonal antibodies (CMV Brite, Biotest Diagnostics, Denvill, NJ; CMV Light, Chemicon International, Temecular, CA; CMV-Vue, INCSTAR Corp, Stillwater, MN). A chemiluminescent hybrid capture method is available for the detection of CMV DNA in white blood cells using a modified sandwich ELISA (Digene, Beltsville, MD). Similar tests for quantitation of CMV in leukocytes are being evaluated using flow cytometry that utilizes DNA probes (9). These tests are used to monitor CMV infections in immunosuppressed patients.

The PCR technique is the method of choice for the identification of CMV in the spinal fluid of patients with AIDS (10). It can also be used to identify CMV in the plasma to document CMV resistance to antiretroviral chemotherapy (11).

REFERENCES

1. Ashley RA, Cent A, Maggs V, et al. Inability of enzyme immunoassays to discriminate between infections with herpes simplex virus types 1 and 2. Ann Intern Med 1991;115:520–526.
2. Ashley RA, et al. Comparison of Western blot (immunoassay) and glycoprotein G–specific immunodot enzyme assay for detecting antibodies to herpes simplex virus type 1 and 2 in human sera. J Clin Microbiol 1988;26:662–667.
3. Johnson AM, Buckley L. Evaluation of a new herpes simplex type 2, glycoprotein G, IgG-specific EIA. ALM Interactions Newsletter Winter 1996;2:2–3.
4. Salmon VC, Turner RB, Speranza MJ, Overall JC. Rapid detection of herpes simplex virus in clinical specimens by centrifugation and immunoperoxidase staining. J Clin Microbiol 1986;23: 683–686.
5. Lakeman FD, Whitley RJ, et al. Diagnosis of herpes simplex encephalitis: application of polymerase chain reaction to cerebrospinal fluid from brain-biopsied patients and correlation with disease. J Infect Dis 1995;171:857–863.
6. Broussard RC, Payne DK, George RB. Treatment with acyclovir of varicella pneumonia in pregnancy. Chest 1991;99:1045–1047.
7. Pastuszak AL, Levy M, Schick B, et al. Outcome after maternal varicella infection in the first 20

weeks of pregnancy. N Engl J Med 1994;330: 901–905.

8. Gleaves CA, Smith TF, Schuster EA, Pearson GR. Comparison of standard tube and shell vial cell culture techniques for the detection of cytomegalovirus in clinical specimens. J Clin Microbiol 1985;21:217–221.
9. Link H, Battmer K, Kleine HD. Detection of cytomegalovirus-infected cells by flow cytometry and fluorescence in suspension hybridization (FLASH) using DNA probes labeled with biotin by polymerase chain reaction. J Med Virol 1992; 37:143–148.
10. Gozlan J, et al. A prospective evaluation of clinical criteria and polymerase chain reaction assay of cerebrospinal fluid for the diagnosis of cytomegalovirus-related neurological diseases during AIDS. AIDS 1995;9:253–260.
11. Spector SA, et al. Molecular detection of human cytomegalovirus and determination of genotypic ganciclovir resistance in clinical specimens. Clin Infect Dis 1995;21:S170–S173.

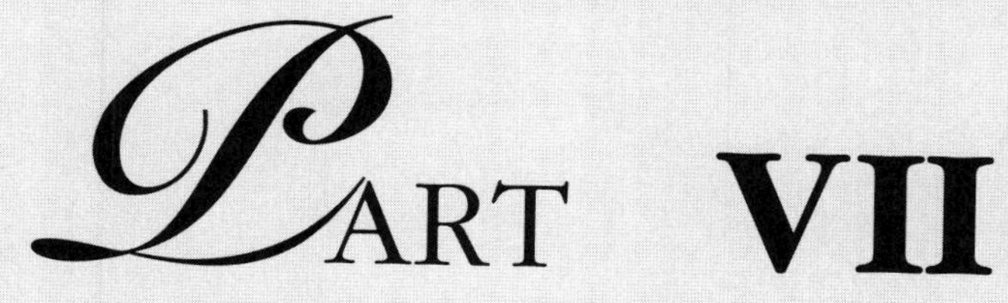

PART VII

Quality Assurance, Quality Control, and Standardization of Molecular Nucleotide Assays

JAMES D. FOLDS, ROBERT M. NAKAMURA, EDITORS

CHAPTER 42

Organization and Structure of a Modern Molecular Diagnostic Laboratory

YIPING CHEN
GARTH D. EHRLICH

The performance of clinical polymerase chain reaction (PCR)-based diagnostic assays requires a specially designed facility. The design objective is to minimize false-positive results due to carry-over contamination of amplified products from one specimen to another.

A suitable laboratory facility can be established either by new multiroom construction or retrofitting of an existing area. The installation of a new heating, ventilation, and air conditioning (HVAC) system is necessary to minimize false-positive results. The laboratory should be staffed with capable professional and technical personnel who have received specialized training. For functional efficiency, the laboratory should be equipped with automated state-of-the-art instrumentation.

The cost to set up such a PCR laboratory is substantial, but improvements in technology that are currently on the horizon may render some of the current physical and procedural safeguards obsolete in the near future. At this time, only a few PCR facilities exist, mostly in tertiary care medical centers associated with universities and at specialty diagnostic laboratories that provide clinical testing for one or several pathogens.

The greatest challenge with PCR technology is to avoid foreign deoxyribonucleic acid (DNA) contamination and the resulting false positives. Future PCR improvements must focus on this problem. The ability to exponentially amplify a small DNA target sequence a billionfold permits the development of assays with exquisite sensitivity, but also allows any contaminating DNA to be amplified as well. Because of this unparalleled sensitivity, a single molecule of target DNA can be amplified and detected using any one of several hybridization formats. The avoidance of contaminating DNA is most critical for achieving reliable results.

The chief source of DNA contamination has been found to be previously amplified DNA that corresponds to the region of current interest. The term *carry-over* is used to designate the vexing problem of PCR end-product contamination in distinction to other possible sources of contamination. The low-molecular-weight amplified DNA can be aerosolized readily during pipetting or opening of test tubes and, hence, may rapidly contaminate everything—all instrumentation, reagents, and even personnel with which it comes in contact. Clearly, molecular isolation of pre- and postamplification procedures is a daunting challenge that requires stringent physical and procedural containment safeguards.

Procedural Safeguards and Policies

Pipets and Pipetting

One of the most important means to avoid contamination of the amplification reaction is use of the proper pipets. During normal pipetting operations a certain amount of microaerosolization occurs, resulting in the deposition of a molecular residue on the tip of the shaft of conventional air displacement micropipettors. This can be avoided by using cotton-plugged disposable pipet tips in all pipetting operations. The cotton in the base of these tips produces a barrier between the liquid and the pipet shaft, thus providing a safeguard against microaerosol contamination. An alternative is to use positive displacement pipets for the transfer of fluids that contain DNA. These pipets are designed with a disposable piston/plunger that moves within a disposable molded capillary tip, physically isolating the pipet shaft from direct contact with the solution, thereby minimizing aerosolization.

Measures to Detect and Reduce False-Positive PCR Results

Inadequate care in conducting experiments can easily lead to false-positive results. All potential sources of DNA contamination must be eliminated including plasmid DNAs and other nucleic acids of small size and low sequence complexity such as purified restriction fragments that contain sequences that have previously been used as target sequences for amplifications. Personnel, equipment, or instruments that have been exposed to DNA preparations should not be used in the pre-amplification processing of clinical specimens for PCR diagnostics.

Besides using great care regarding physical practices, several biochemical methods may be useful in reducing carry-over contamination. Most of these methods aim to either produce metastable DNA that cannot be reamplified or are concerned with destroying template DNA present in the PCR master mix. The former method does nothing to eliminate nonamplified DNA template and the latter method does not prevent carry-over that occurs in the specimen aliquot itself. Hence, the use of both methods together is possible to achieve the greatest degree of protection.

Metastable DNA can be produced in one of several ways. One method is to modify the PCR setup to replace deoxynucleoside thymidine triphosphate (dTTP) with deoxynucleoside uridine triphosphate (dUTP). This results in the generation of amplified DNA that contains uracil residues in place of thymidine residues. Such uracil-containing DNA can be degraded by the addition of the uracil N-glycosylase (*UNG*), which enzymatically modifies the U-containing DNA template. *UNG* is produced by the *Escherichia coli-UNG* gene and functions by removing uracil residues from either single-stranded (ss) or double-stranded (ds) DNA without destroying the DNA sugar-phosphodiester backbone. Since the resulting abasic sites are susceptible to hydrolytic cleavage at elevated temperatures, *UNG*-treated DNA becomes fragmented during the PCR denaturation step and cannot serve as a template for further amplification by the thermostable DNA polymerase. A second way to produce metastable DNA involves the construction of oligonucleotide primers, which support the reaction, so that they contain a ribonucleoside moiety at their 3′ terminus. Therefore, the elongation amplification product contains a cleavage site that can be exploited to destroy only those DNA molecules that are the products of previous amplification reactions.

Ultraviolet (UV) radiation can be used to inactivate template DNA, which may have been accidentally introduced into one of the reagents that make up the PCR master mix. The UV light creates thymidine dimers in the DNA that destroy its ability to serve as an amplification template. However, the nucleoside triphosphates cannot be treated this way since they absorb UV and thereby shield any contaminating DNA.

Each PCR setup must be accompanied by proper controls for establishing the presence or absence of possible contaminating DNA. The selection of appropriate positive and negative controls to be run with each set of PCR reactions is a vital safeguard. The controls should include the following: 1) a reagent that contains all components of the reaction except template DNA, 2) a negative DNA control that does not contain target sequences, and 3) a positive control dilution series of DNA that is known to contain the target sequence.

Reagent contamination is easy to detect since all or almost all reactions will result in amplification. However, random contamination of individual samples that is attributable to aerosolized amplimers is more difficult to control. Therefore, multiple reagent controls and negative DNA controls should be included in each run so as to enhance the chance of detecting contaminations.

Algorithms for Interpreting PCR-Based Results

Means for detecting carry-over are important since carry-over will occasionally occur regardless of all the precautions that are taken to prevent it. The development and utilization of multiple sets of primer pairs and probes for each test organism are the best way to detect spurious carry-over. It is preferable to have at least three sets of primer probes for each organism. Ideally, all the sets should be compatible so they can be used together in a multiplex assay that simultaneously supports amplification of all the targets. To accomplish this, each primer pair should target a unique region so that all products can be resolved in a single lane of an electrophoretic gel. This implies that the products should differ by a minimum of 30 bp in length and, even better, by 40 or 50 base pair (bp). To keep amplification efficiency high, it is best to utilize primer pairs in which all amplimers are between 100 and 300 bp in length.

It is very unlikely that a given sample will sustain two carry-over events that correspond to two amplimers for the same organism since each carry-over event is independent of all other carry-over events. Hence, each specimen to be tested for a given agent should be subjected to a multiplex assay that uses two sets of primer pairs. Then, upon hybridization, if both products are visualized, the specimen is considered positive. On the other hand, if only one of the two primer pairs supported amplification, the sample should be rerun with all three primer pairs. If the second run yields a positive result for two of the three or all three target regions, then the sample can be deemed positive. If it produces a positive result for only one of the three target regions, however, the sample must be considered negative or indeterminate. Clearly, if all three amplification attempts are negative on the second rerun, the sample is also considered negative.

Methods to Detect and Avoid False-Negative PCR Results

Although false positives are the bane of PCR, false-negative results can also be a problem. Inhibitory factors that reduce the efficiency of the PCR process can be introduced from certain specimens as well as from specimen handling procedures and instruments. The heme molecule and, therefore, whole blood samples or fractionated blood samples from hemolyzed blood can inhibit the action of the *Thermus aquaticus* (*Taq*) DNA polymerase if only a quick lysis technique, that is, detergent or sonication, is used to prepare the sample. Another inhibitor that can be introduced into specimens is heparin. It is used as an anticoagulant in some blood collection tubes. Heparin binds the *Taq* polymerase and incidentally is used in *Taq* purification schemes.

These inhibitors can be removed by organic extraction and ethanol precipitation. A faster alternative, however, is to boil the lysate for 10 minutes or longer, which destroys these and many other inhibitors by denaturation. Heparin can be entirely avoided by using blood-collecting tubes that utilize other anticoagulants. Acid citrate dextran (yellow-top Vacutainer) tubes and neutral citrate (blue-top Vacutainer) tubes perform best for PCR studies. In addition, ethylenediaminetetra-acetic acid (EDTA) tubes (purple-top Vacutainer) can be used, but the EDTA if not removed will bind magnesium in the PCR mixture and thus interfere with the PCR process.

A further precaution is to remove the denatured macromolecular aggregates, which may act as inhibitors, by taking the boiled lysate and spinning for 5 minutes in a microcentrifuge. The supernatant is then transferred to a clean tube.

The lysate can be stored frozen at −80°C for weeks. Simple refrigeration is unsuitable for such specimens, as the DNA will rapidly degrade. However, extracted DNA preparations can be stored at 4°C for years so long as precautions are used to avoid contamination with fungal spores.

False negatives are also reduced by use of the multiplex assay format described above. With some highly variable viral species, a given primer pair will not support amplification because of mutations within the primer binding site that prevent annealing or elongation by the polymerase. The sample would be deemed negative if that were the only primer pair being used. However, if two regions are being coamplified, one comes up positive, and, upon repeat, the third primer pair is also positive, the sample that would have been called negative under a single primer pair amplification system can be regarded as a true positive.

The ability of a given clinical specimen preparation to support amplification can be determined by coamplifying for a single-copy human gene such as beta-globin or DR-beta. This process is typically done as a separate amplification reaction due to concerns that in a multiplex format runaway amplification of a high-copy gene will reduce the efficiency of amplifying a very low-copy number sequence. In a usual PCR, 1 μg or the equivalent of DNA is typically used. This translates to about 150,000 cells worth of DNA. Therefore, an infectious agent that is present in 1 of 10,000 cells would have 15 genomes versus 150,000 genomes of competing target sequences if the amplification were performed in a multiplex format.

A negative result and the absence of an amplification product when a single-copy gene is used may not be a correct result. The target infectious agent may actually be present. The ability to amplify a single-copy gene does not always indicate that the specimen preparation will support amplification of a low-copy number sequence such as a retroviral sequence found in 1 of 10,000 cells or less. To circumvent this problem, one method is to spike a low-copy number (less than 100) of a unique sequence into the reaction and then to coamplify for it. For example, DNA can be spiked into the master mix and then, in a multiplex format, amplified and detected with the actual test sequences. This approach will show whether the specimen contains inhibitors that can prevent amplification of very low-copy number sequences.

Construction Specifics

General Construction Specifics

Fundamental to the operation of a successful PCR facility is the segregation of space into physically and functionally discrete laboratories. Ideally, a facility that was built expressly for PCR would encompass at least five separate laboratories (**Fig. 42-1**). However, if existing space is being modified to incorporate PCR technology, the number of additional rooms required will depend on whether or not the PCR facility is attached to a clinical microbiology laboratory and whether darkroom facilities are already available. Each laboratory should be specified for the execution of a given set of procedures, outlined below. As a precaution against carry-over, amplified DNA should never be taken into a laboratory where patient specimen processing is performed or where PCRs are set up. Processing of specimens, preparation and storage of PCR stock reagents, and synthesis of oligonucleotide primers are all considered preamplification procedures and are therefore referred to as "clean." The laboratories that are used for these functions and for PCR setup should be located as far as is practically possible from the area where postamplification product analysis and manipulations will be performed. The PCR amplification process and subsequent procedures involved in the analysis of the reaction products (hybridization, electrophoresis, restriction analysis, and cloning and sequencing of amplified DNA) are considered "dirty" and must not be performed in sample processing or setup laboratories.

Ideally, the PCR facility should be designed as a suite of five laboratories, including 1) the tissue culture laboratory, for receiving and processing patient specimens (this function can be performed in an existing microbiology laboratory equipped with laminar flow biocontaminant hoods); 2) the PCR setup laboratory; 3) the amplification and analysis laboratory; 4) the DNA sequencing and mutation analysis laboratory; and 5) an image analysis laboratory/darkroom, wherein each is used for a particular purpose with respect to the overall goal of obtaining quality PCR results. Once such a facility is built, an accompanying policy must be established for the orderly, unidirectional flow of samples through the system and individual investigators must adhere to this policy. Certain procedures are carried out in each laboratory and the sample is then transferred to the next.

Each laboratory should have its own ventilation system that maintains 100% air exchange with outside air and no exchange between rooms. To accomplish this goal an HVAC system should be designed and built specifically for the PCR facility to bring to an absolute minimum the probability of obtaining false-positive results due to molecular carry-over caused by aerosolization of PCR-amplified DNAs. To further minimize the chance of molecular carry-over, each of these laboratories should be designed so that individuals who enter and leave must go through a two-door airlock system or anteroom when entering any of the laboratories. All outer and inner doors of the

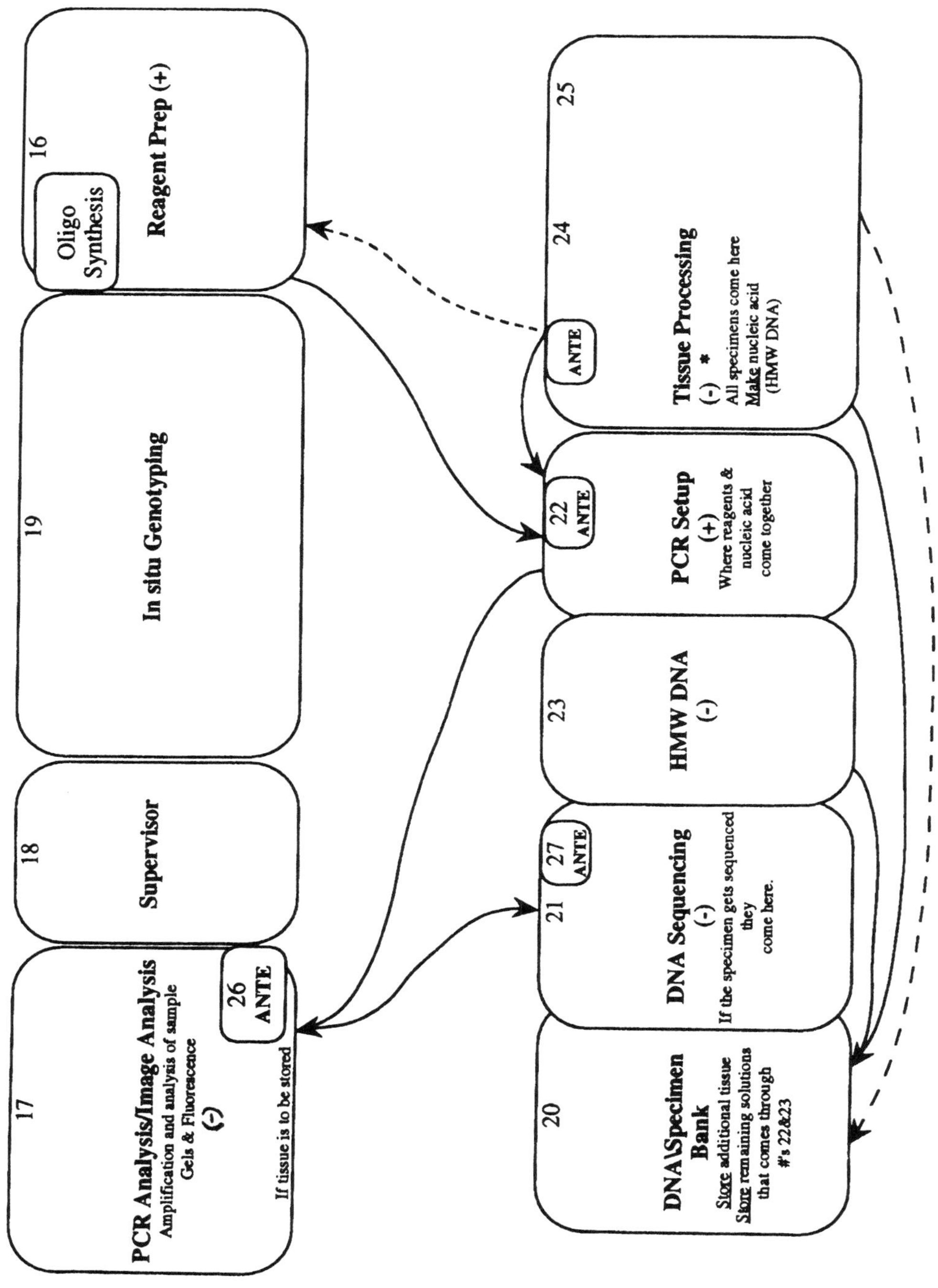

FIGURE 42-1
Diagrammatic representation of the University of Pittsburgh Medical Center's core PCR facility.

laboratories should be fitted with weather stripping to ensure a tight seal. Laboratory policy should mandate that individuals entering and leaving any of the laboratories shut the first door before opening the second.

Tissue Culture/Sample Receiving Laboratory and Signal Amplification Detector System Laboratory

This laboratory is for sample processing, aliquotting, and storage. It should have an anteroom to control air flow and as a site for donning protective clothing. This will also serve to make this laboratory a P2 biocontaminant facility that is suitable for the handling of infectious human pathogens such as retroviruses and tuberculosis. This laboratory should be located as far as is practically possible from the amplification and analysis laboratory in order to avoid contamination, and, because of biohazard concerns, should always be under negative air pressure to the hallways. All aliquots of a given patient specimen, except for the one used for the initial assessment, should be stored in this room at −80°C. This is considered a superclean room and, as such, no plasmid or amplified DNA of any kind should be allowed in this laboratory under any circumstances. No individual who has handled amplified DNA without having showered, shampooed, and changed clothing should be allowed in this laboratory at any time.

If there is sufficient space in this laboratory, the instrumentation for nucleic acid signal amplification systems (i,e., branched-chain DNA) can be installed. Otherwise, a separate facility will be necessary for such nontemplate amplification systems.

PCR Setup Laboratory

The setup laboratory, which is used for DNA and ribonucleic acid (RNA) purification, storage, and preparation of the amplification reactions, is considered a clean laboratory and should have positive air pressure with respect to the hall and to the amplification and analysis laboratory so that the net movement of uncontrolled air flow is from this laboratory to the amplification laboratory. Lysed samples from the tissue culture laboratory should be brought into this laboratory and further processed if DNA extraction is necessary, or used "as is" to support amplification. In some cases individual aliquots of patient specimens prepared in the tissue culture room can be brought into this laboratory for lysis, particularly if the samples are to be processed using a robotic workstation.

No amplified DNA should ever be allowed in this room. Individuals who have handled amplified DNA should not be permitted to enter the setup laboratory unless they have worn protective clothing in the PCR amplification laboratory and have then donned a second set of protective clothing before entering this laboratory. Ideally, individuals should shower and shampoo before entering this laboratory when coming from the amplification laboratory, but this may not be practical in all circumstances. DNA synthesis and oligonucleotide purification instrumentation can also be located in the PCR setup laboratory.

PCR Amplification Laboratory

The amplification laboratory, the "dirty laboratory," should be under negative air pressure with respect to the hall and to the tissue culture and setup laboratories so that the net flow of air is into this laboratory and out of the hall as people pass through the airlock. This laboratory should never be connected directly with either of the clean laboratories in the PCR facility by either doorways or HVAC ducting. All amplifications and analyses of amplified DNA other than sequencing and mutational analyses should be done in this room. In addition, amplified DNAs must be stored within this laboratory, with the exception of wrapped gels; photographic films for imaging or development, or both, in the image analysis laboratory; and PCR products for DNA sequencing and mapping. Nothing should ever go from the "dirty laboratory" into any of the clean laboratories. Any items and/or contaminated materials from the "dirty laboratory" should not be allowed to remain in the hallways outside the other laboratories. Items from this laboratory for autoclaving should have their own schedule and should not be mixed with items from the other laboratories.

DNA Sequencing and Gene-Mapping Laboratory

This laboratory is considered a dirty laboratory. The amplified materials for sequencing or mutational analysis can be transferred between the PCR amplification laboratory and this laboratory. However, any material from this laboratory cannot go to the clean laboratory. The personnel who work in this laboratory should not go to the clean laboratory on the same day unless they change protective clothing and shower.

Imaging Analysis Laboratory and Darkroom

The fifth laboratory serves as an image analysis laboratory or photographic darkroom, or both, for radiometric/fluorometric imaging and development of autoradiograms, and can be built into either of the dirty laboratories or be a stand-alone facility. There is no special air condition requirement, but this laboratory should be considered a dirty laboratory. If possible, the imaging equipment should be separated from the darkroom so that it can be used more effectively.

Equipping of Facilities

Tissue Culture/Sample Receiving Laboratory

At least two laminar flow hoods are needed in this room to permit the processing of all clinical specimens using universal biohazard precautions: one for processing specimens and one for maintaining control cell lines and viral cultures. This arrangement minimizes the chance of specimen-generated mycoplasmal contamination of the type cultures, which can greatly reduce viral production. Each hood should have its own associated humidified carbon dioxide incubator that is connected to a temperature monitor system.

In addition, this laboratory should possess a high-capacity clinical centrifuge; a microcentrifuge; a Coulter counter for determining cell number; a heat block; a water bath; an inverted phase contrast microscope; sufficient −80°C freezer space for storage of patient specimens, preferably with a liquid nitrogen backup system; a liquid nitrogen storage system; a refrigerator; all necessary pipetting devices, including pipet aids, pipetmen, and repeater pipettors; and a fully equipped "kitchen area," including stir plates, pH meters, vortexes, and balances for the preparation of buffers and reagents. All the freezers and refrigerators should be connected to an alarm monitor system that will contact someone who is responsible for these instruments if a failure occurs.

PCR Setup Laboratory

The reaction setup laboratory should contain a sufficient number of PCR setup spaces. If it is possible, this laboratory should have workstations such as Template Tamers (Coy Corp, Grass Lake, MI), which are enclosed, clear Plexiglas boxes with UV light bulbs. These units can provide protection against carry-over by further reducing the probability of aerosol contamination and by producing UV light–induced dimerization of thymidine residues in contaminating DNA, making such DNA an unsuitable template for enzymatic amplification. These workstations provide space for the storage of pipettors and a supply of tips so that the devices used to set up reactions are never exposed to potential contaminants that may escape other control mechanisms.

This laboratory should also contain the following: 1) a controlled-temperature shaking incubator for DNA extractions and bacterial cultures; 2) controlled-temperature water baths with covers for enzymatic reactions; 3) a controlled-temperature convection incubator for bacterial cultures; 4) a refrigerated superspeed or clinical centrifuge; 5) a microcentrifuge; 6) a large sliding-glass-door refrigerator equipped with a variable-speed microcentrifuge; 7) a −20°C, a −50°C, and a −80°C freezer for storage of oligonucleotides, enzymes, aliquotted reagents for PCR setups, and DNA and RNA samples, respectively; 8) vertical and horizontal gel electrophoresis apparatuses and power supplies for running analytic acrylamide and agarose gels to assess the integrity of purified nucleic acids; 9) a UV-Vis spectrophotometer for quantitating DNA and RNA yields; 10) a kitchen area with a microwave oven; and 11) a fume hood for purifying oligonucleotides and further extracting DNA or RNA. All nonambient-temperature equipment should be connected to the alarm monitor system.

If the laboratory is not equipped with an ultrapure water source, it is advisable to install either a glass distillation system or a deionizer/reverse osmosis water purification system. Several laboratory-sized water purification systems are available commercially that will provide type I water (18M resistance). However, any system must be constantly monitored to ensure that bacterial growth does not occur in the holding tanks or lines. Bacterial growth here can result in the generation of false-positive results, particularly if the target amplification sequence is part of a highly conserved gene family. An alternative is to use bottled sterile surgical water for PCR setups and the making of reagents.

A PCR facility that plans to utilize a robotic workstation for lysis of specimens and setup of PCR reactions (1), and/or that will make its own oligonucleotides, can place the appropriate instrumentation in the setup laboratory if additional space is not available elsewhere. The oligo work space should have its own dedicated set of pipettors that are not to be used for any other operations in the setup laboratory. Because the quality and reliability of the oligonucleotides are critical for the successful amplification and detection of amplimers, we recommend that PCR facilities that generate their own "oligos" purchase a proven reliable instrument. The other major piece of instrumentation necessary for oligo preparation is a vacuum centrifuge for drying down the oligonucleotides after purification.

PCR and Amplification Analysis Laboratory

The PCR and analysis laboratory should house all of the thermal cyclers. It is recommended that 96-well thermal cyclers be utilized, as they are compatible with instrumentation designed to work with 96-well microtiter plates (see below for further discussion). Any facility that intends to offer PCR-based clinical diagnostics should possess at least two thermal cyclers or two thermal cycler blocks. The 96-well system employs 0.2-mL, thin-walled, polypropylene reaction tubes, which are designed to fit snugly into wells machined to extremely tight tolerances for the promotion of very rapid and accurate heat transfer without filling the wells with oil. The rapid heat transfer provides the added benefit of substantially reducing cycling times.

Other required equipment includes 1) a fume hood and sink certified for the handling and disposal of radioactive isotopes, 2) Plexiglas shields and waste disposal containers to protect technicians from exposure to radiation, 3) Geiger-Mueller counters for monitoring radiation and a Bioscan (QC-2000) for getting probe counts, 4) an enzyme-linked immunosorbent assay (ELISA) plate reader and washer if enzymatic assays are to be employed, 5) a large glass-door refrigerator for storage of amplified DNAs, 6) a −20°C flammable storage freezer (with temperature monitoring alarm system), 7) controlled-temperature water baths for enzymatic reactions and hybridizations, 8) numerous vertical and horizontal gel electrophoresis apparatuses and power supplies for running analytic and preparative acrylamide and agarose gels, 9) a table-top centrifuge with available fixed-angle and swinging bucket rotors for spin column probe purification and centrifugal filtration operations, 10) a variable-speed microcentrifuge and a shaker/incubator for bacterial culture, 11) a UV transilluminator and Polaroid camera with an isolation hood for benchtop photography of ethidium bromide–stained gels, and 12) all necessary pipetting devices.

DNA Sequencing and Mutation Analysis Laboratory

This laboratory should be equipped with an automated DNA sequencer that is networked with one or more sequence analysis computer workstations. Multiple workstations will be needed to analyze the data generated from a single automated instrument that is running full time.

The additional instrumentation required for this laboratory includes 1) a large sliding-glass-door refrigerator equipped with a variable-speed microcentrifuge; 2) a −20°C freezer for storage of reagents; 3) a refrigerated superspeed or clinical centrifuge; 4) vertical and horizontal gel electrophoresis apparatuses and power supplies for running analytic acrylamide and agarose gels; 5) if possible, a stand alone water purification system; and 6) the PCR products can be brought to this laboratory from the dirty laboratory. However, it is desirable to have a separate thermal cycler for cycle-sequencing reactions.

Image Analysis and Darkroom

A darkroom for developing autoradiographic exposures of gel and filter hybridization should be equipped with a safe light illumination system and outside warning light. An x-ray film developer can be installed in this room. Ideally, this laboratory should also include a Polaroid MP4 camera system (Cambridge, MA) with UV transilluminator to provide a means for producing record quality photographs, and wall mount white light illuminators for displaying autoradiograms. If the facility is to contain phosphor- or fluorescent-image analysis equipment, this is the logical place for its inclusion.

Laboratory Personnel

Laboratory workers must be fastidious in their procedures so as to minimize the possibility of aerosolization from pipetting, opening tubes, and so forth. This strict, careful behavior cannot be overemphasized for all laboratory personnel in order to avoid contamination and erroneous results.

Aerosolized PCR products (amplifiers) can be deposited on skin, hair, and clothing and then later shed into the clean areas (setup or tissue labs) resulting in carry-over. A single molecule of amplified DNA landing on an otherwise negative sample provides a sufficient template for amplification to give a positive detectable signal following 30 cycles of PCR.

Personnel should be separated by duties to avoid carry-over of amplified material from one laboratory area to another. Ideally, both the tissue culture laboratory and the setup laboratory should be staffed with personnel who have minimal contact with the amplification laboratory or the analysis laboratory, thereby minimizing any contact with the PCR amplification products. However, the unidirectional movement of workers from the setup laboratory to the amplification and analysis laboratory is permissible.

Workers must wear disposable gloves in all laboratory areas to minimize contamination and to prevent RNase from destroying RNA templates. If anything is transferred from the amplification or analysis laboratory to one of the other laboratories, it should be washed in 10% bleach or 1 mole/liter HCl before one leaves the laboratory.

Personnel in the amplification laboratory and the analysis laboratory must take special precautions regarding carry-over contamination. Disposable gowns and head coverings should be donned in the airlock area before one enters the laboratory and removed again in the airlock area prior to leaving. Anyone who goes from the amplification and analysis laboratories to either the tissue culture laboratory or setup laboratory should do so on a different day and only after showering to ensure removal of any amplified DNA. One should never go from the laboratories that contain amplified DNA into the tissue culture laboratory, and, if one really must go to the setup laboratory on the same day, one must wear protective clothes that are removed on leaving the amplification laboratory and then put on a second set of protective clothing before entering the setup laboratory.

Stock Reagent Preparation

Each laboratory must have its own instrumentation and kitchen area to prepare reagent stocks. A single senior technical person should be responsible for preparing, quality controlling, aliquotting, storing, and dispensing all of the stock reagents that are necessary for carrying out the PCR. These stock reagents should be 1) prepared in large batches, using sterile solutions and type 1 water or sterile bottled water; 2) aliquotted into volumes that are small enough for a single average setup; and 3) stored at −20°C in the laboratory in which they will be used. All lots of reagents should be subjected to quality control measures and should not be released for clinical setups until these requirements have been met. Each lot of reagents, after passing quality control, should be assigned a lot number that is recorded in a master log that contains the details of preparation. The individual aliquots should each receive a distinguishing character in addition to the lot number. This provides a means to rapidly trace any reagent problem or contamination to its source. Quality control is best achieved by actually determining a reagent's ability to support the PCR. This can be accomplished by performing a setup in which all reagents except the one to be tested have previously passed quality assurance (**Fig. 42-2**). The evaluation of each reagent should include a test of its ability to amplify a dilution series of a known positive control DNA or RNA.

During the preparation of all reagents used in the processing and evaluation of clinical specimens, the following guidelines should be observed:

1. All the chemicals for preparing the reagents should be of molecular grade.
2. Never return any dispensed reagent to the original stock bottle.
3. When preparing any buffer or solution that requires pH measurement, be sure to calibrate the pH meter with standard buffers of known pH before measuring or adjusting the reagent in question.

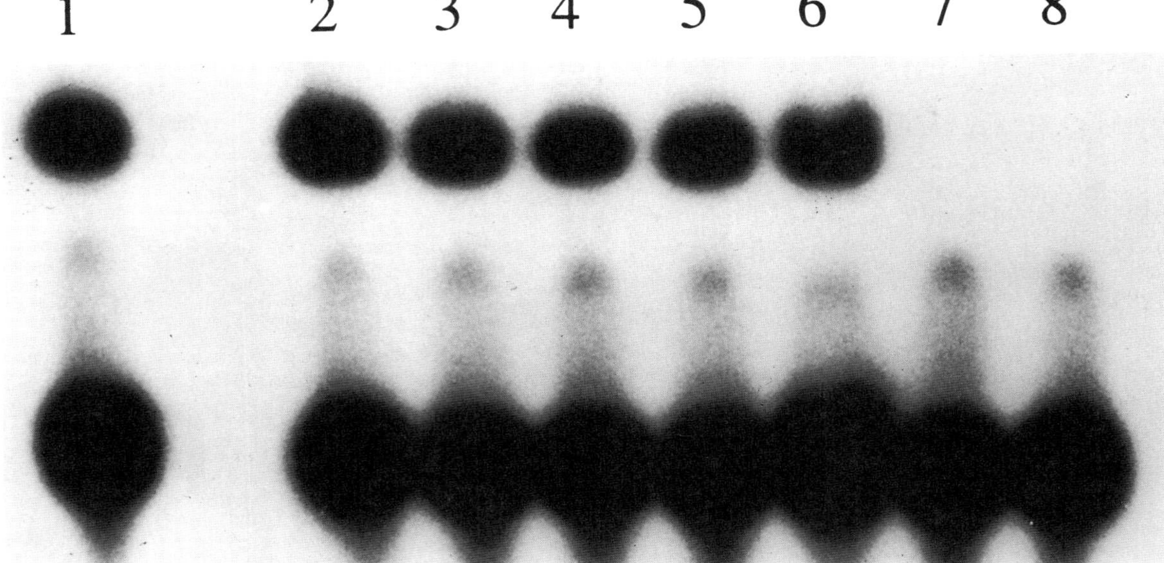

FIGURE 42-2

Positive quality control assay for PCR reagents. Quality control can be accomplished by performing a setup in which all reagents except the one to be tested have previously passed quality assurance. PCR products were hybridized with ^{32}P-labeled internal probes and separated by polyacrylamide gel electrophoresis. Line 1: positive control; line 2: quality control (QC) for $MgCl_2$ lot 11; line 3: QC for dNTPs lot 28; line 4: QC for *Taq* buffer lot 9; line 5: QC for *Taq* lot 40; line 6: QC for H_2O lot 18; lines 7 and 8: negative control.

4. Utilize a balance that has been calibrated using NIST weight standards.
5. Utilize a spectrophotometer that has been calibrated for wavelength, absorbence and photometric linearity, and stray light.
6. Utilize micropipettors that have been calibrated using a NIST-calibrated balance.

The following reagents have been demonstrated over the last several years to provide amplification for almost all DNA templates.

Taq buffer (10×)—500 mmole/liter KCl, 100 mmole/liter Tris-HCl (pH 8.3)

One should prepare 1.2-mL aliquots and store at −20°C in 1.5-mL snap-top tubes. (Some investigators add 0.1–0.2% gelatin or bovine serum albumin to stabilize the enzyme; however, we have not found that this is necessary except in cases in which one is trying to amplify from single cells or very few cells.)

$MgCl_2$ (20×)—50 mmole/liter

One should prepare 1.2 mL and store at −20°C in 1.5-mL snap-top tubes. ($MgCl_2$ should not be added to the *Taq* buffer, as, with time, it becomes unavailable to the enzyme when stored at low concentrations.)

Deoxynucleoside Triphosphates (20×)

These include adenosine 5′-triphosphate (dATP), deoxynucleoside cytadine 5′-triphosphate (dCTP), deoxynucleoside guanosine 5′-triphosphate (dGTP), and 5′-dTTP or 5′-dUTP, which replaces dTTP in reactions in which *ung* is employed to eliminate contamination from amplified DNA (see below). They are supplied by the manufacturer (Amersham Pharmacia Biotech, Piscataway, NJ) as 100-mmole/liter solutions and should be purchased with the specification that they be shipped on dry ice. It is preferable to buy nucleoside triphosphates in solution, as in powder form they are subject to a disproportionation reaction that yields dinucleotides and tetranucleotides.

The dNTP stock solution should consist of 4 mmole/liter each of dNTP (dATP, dCTP, dGTP, and either dTTP or dUTP) in 600-μL aliquots stored in 1.5-mL snap-top tubes at −20°C.

Sterile Ultrapure Water

Sterile water in 1.2-mL aliquots is used for irrigation, USP (Baxter Healthcare Corporation, Deerfield, IL), at −20°C. This is preferable to autoclaved type I water (18M), which can contain bacterial DNA.

Primers (20–100×)

The concentration of each oligonucleotide primer stock is dependent on the yield of its particular synthesis. Concentrated primers should be stored in 2.0-mL screw-cap tubes at −20°C. Working dilutions of 10 pmole/μL (approximately equal to 100 ng/μL for primer length oligonucleotide) should be stored in 100- to 200-μL aliquots at −20°C. All primers should undergo a quality control (QC) test before use in a PCR setup in order to make sure that they will support amplification. The QC results should be filed in a QC file. The pipets for aliquots should be separated from the other pipets, which are used for the other purposes.

UNG

When utilizing the *UNG* strategy, 1 unit of *UNG* should be included as a normal constituent of the reaction mixture. A 10-minute incubation at 37°C immediately before cycling will enable the enzyme to remove uracil residues from potentially contaminating DNA. Because *UNG* is inactivated at high temperature, increasing the initial denaturation step of the first PCR cycle to 94°C for 10 minutes will largely inactivate the enzyme prior to cycling. At this temperature the uracil-free contaminating DNA will be fragmented and thus will be unavailable to act as a hybridization target. The *UNG* enzyme may, however, not be completely irreversibly denatured and some activity may persist after amplification if the reaction is stored at ambient or refrigerator temperatures. Therefore, maintaining the *UNG* in an inactivated state once cycling is complete is necessary to preclude the removal of uracil residues from the desired PCR product. This is accomplished by setting the soak temperature at 72°C rather than the usual 4° or 0°C. Otherwise, amplified DNAs can be stored at −20°C before analysis.

Master Mixes

A master mix that contains all of the PCR components except template DNA should be prepared immediately before use. This minimizes the number of pipetting operations and ensures intrarun uniformity while providing a reagent control to test for carry-over. Because use of a master mix ensures that all of the reactions contain identical chemistry, any inconsistency in expected results can be attributed to reasons other than the chemistry of the stock reagents. One should prepare enough master mix to accommodate the number of reactions to be set up in a single experiment, plus at least two extras to allow for pipetting error, and distribute it among the total number of reaction tubes. The master mix can be dispensed using a motorized multialiquot pipettor for distribution into the reaction tubes. DNA is added to the reaction tubes last, to minimize the possibility of its inadvertent transfer to the wrong reaction; then the tube is immediately capped. As a further precaution against contamination it is recommended that positive control DNAs be pipetted last. Each PCR experiment should include multiple "no DNA" reactions to control for possible aerosol contamination.

Preparation and storage of master mixes for later use have revealed a substantial decrease in the ability to support amplification in as little as a week unless the Mg^{2+} is stored separately.

For assessing the functionality of commercially prepared reagents for the reverse transcriptase (RT) reaction, we suggest the use of QC in order to exclude the possibility of any mishandling during delivery of the reagent from the company to the laboratory.

Laboratory Automation and Efficiency

Robotic Design and Programming for PCR Setup

Numerous vendors currently make robotic instruments for the setup of PCR amplifications. Some instruments are simply designed to deliver simultaneously 96 uniform aliquots (e.g., see Hydra) while others can make multiple master mixes and perform various setups from scratch simultaneously.

Laboratory Efficiency and Coordination with Existing Facilities

In most cases the PCR diagnostic facilities will be installed in preexisting clinical immunology, microbiology, or virology laboratories. This arrangement permits the sharing of the facilities. Usually the "tissue culture laboratory" already exists as part of a clinical laboratory facility. This approach reduces the number of rooms that must be outfitted while providing front-end specimen collection and processing on a 24 hours a day, 7 days a week basis. It is recommended that one technologist trained in molecular biologic techniques be responsible for the organizational structure and procedural aspects concerning handling of specimens for PCR-based diagnostic testing. All personnel in the facility need to be instructed about the entire PCR process so that they can perform their part of the task with the appropriate understanding base to guard against inadvertent contamination.

A networked computer database should be established that permits technicians in each laboratory to access data for incoming samples, to plan their experiments, and to enter the results from the testing respectively. This arrangement will avoid the contamination caused by personnel movement between laboratories and will ensure efficient reporting without compromising the established facility guidelines.

Laboratory Protocols

Clinical Specimen Collection and Handling

All samples should be received and processed by the tissue culture laboratory in as timely a manner as possible following collection to guard against cell lysis and nucleic acid degradation. This is particularly important for those samples from which RNA will be extracted for reverse transcriptase PCR analyses, such as gene expression assays, or for RNA viruses.

Tissue samples will generally need to be lysed by sodium dodecyl sulfate (SDS) and digested with Proteinase K (PK) followed by sequential organic extractions and ethanol precipitation. The advantage of this method is that it is possible to determine by UV absorption spectrophotometry the amount of DNA recovered. Quick lysis procedures are not recommended for most tissue samples; however, in some instances it is possible to sufficiently disrupt, by mechanical means, small pieces of parenchymal tissues that do not contain a lot of stroma. When using a quick lysis approach, it is very difficult to ascertain the quantity of input DNA unless the number of cells can be determined before lysis.

How whole blood samples are handled depends on the test required. The whole blood should not be frozen until the processing of noncoagulated blood is finished. This includes pipetting off and saving the plasma fraction after centrifugation of the cellular material, and, if necessary, either washing the buffy coats or purifying the mononuclear cell population over a Ficoll step gradient. The blood components to be saved and tested will depend on the assay that will be performed. In some instances only plasma will be needed and in some cases white blood cells or mononuclear cells will be required. All plasma and cell samples should be aliquotted before freezing. This provides a very important procedural control by banking material that can be reanalyzed if the first sample through the system is lost, destroyed, or contaminated. Only one aliquot at a time of a clinical specimen should be utilized for testing purposes unless it is necessary that the material be differentially prepared for two different tests; that is, both DNA and RNA are needed from one sample. If it is important to know the number of cells to be analyzed, the buffy coats or mononuclear cells can be counted by hemocytometer or Coulter counter prior to freezing or lysis, or both. By keeping track of the amount of lysate used, it is possible to determine the cell equivalents in the sample to be tested.

Samples obtained by swabbing of mucosal membranes should be collected using devices with plastic shafts instead of aluminum shafts, which can inhibit the PCR process. Because of their viscous nature, many mucosal samples, that is, sputum, otitis media, and wound exudates, need to be clarified before lysis. This can be accomplished by adding *N*′-acetyl-L-cysteine to the specimen before centrifugation and lysis [see (1), Chaps 28 and 29, for protocol].

In analyzing whole blood, cerebrospinal fluid (CSF), or other body fluid samples for viral or bacterial DNA, we suggest the use of the

QIAgen kit. We use 200 μL specimen for extracting DNA. After extraction, the DNA volume is reconstituted in a volume of 50 μL. In general, 1 μL of this is used for PCR.

Quick lysis protocols are becoming increasingly popular for rapid preparation of specimens for PCR. Historically these have utilized some combination of nonionic detergents, such as trition X-100 and NP40. While these agents are less inhibitory to the *Taq* polymerase than are ionic detergents, such as SDS, they can still reduce amplification yield. Recently, we have found that sonication can serve as an effective mechanical lysis procedure with no concern about the introduction of inhibitory agents. Plasma, cerebrospinal fluid, clarified sputum, or almost any other fluid specimen (or palette material from the same) can in most cases be sonicated. The diluted specimens are placed in microfuge tubes and treated in bulk using a water bath–type sonicator for 1 hour. As a general rule specimen lysates should be stored frozen, boiled before use, and centrifuged to remove inhibitory aggregates prior to use for PCR-based analyses.

Setting Up a PCR

Several basic parameters should be kept in mind while performing the PCR setup. First and foremost is to organize the work and employ proper instrumentation to reduce the chance of introducing material from one specimen to another or from a control tube to a specimen. As described above, setup should be performed in a laboratory where amplified DNA is never handled and should ideally be done in an isolation box using specially designated pipettors that are not used for handling anything else, particularly plasmid DNAs. All reagents and the master mix should be held on ice until needed and then should be pipetted using cotton-plugged pipet tips. A standardized log sheet should be prepared for each setup. The setup sheet should have space for indicating the lot number of each reagent used and the calculations utilized to prepare the master mix, as well as space to indicate cycling parameters and probe and hybridization conditions. Copies of the setup sheet should 1) accompany the setup to the amplification and analysis laboratory, 2) be stored in a master log, 3) be kept by the individual technicians in their notebooks, and 4) be placed with the autoradiographic exposure (or other final result media) in a test-specific binder, for example, "Lyme disease."

One of the objects of the setup is to denature the DNA and allow primer annealing, but to prevent template reannealing. Hot Start-PCR is becoming more popular as a means to ensure uniform amplifications by reducing or eliminating false priming events, which occur when the primers anneal to near homologous sequences during the heating up of the thermal cycler before it gets to the programmed annealing temperature. This false annealing in the initial round can produce spurious products that will compete for reagents and result in substantial amplification of nonspecific sequences in some cases. The occurrence of this phenomenon cannot be predicted and must be determined empirically by running the reaction products out on an ethidium bromide–agarose gel. If nonspecific band production is a problem with the primer set of choice and it is not possible or practical to switch primer pairs then one of the following approaches may reduce the accumulation of this artifactual amplification. The most facile is the use of a *Taq* DNA polymerase that is not activated until the temperature of the reaction reaches 95°C. This can be accomplished by utilizing a modified *Taq*, or by using anti-*Taq* antibodies.

PCR Protocol

The PCR process is the first fully automated part of the PCR-based diagnostics process. Once the thermal cycler is programmed and the samples are loaded, the operator can walk away from the instrument and be confident that the thermal cycling will occur automatically [(1), Chap 6].

Most amplification schemes are programmed into the thermal cycler by linking together four or five individual programs or files that provide for the temporal control of the thermal parameters required for each PCR. In general, only one file is used for inputting cycling parameters and the others are soak files designed to hold the temperature constant for specific reasons. Because the files are all linked together, it is sufficient to just call up the first file and initiate the start process. When the thermal cycler has completed the operations contained in the first file it automatically transfers to the next linked file and so on.

The first file is usually used to bring the instrument up to a denaturing temperature, that is, 94°C, and to hold that temperature for 3 to 10 minutes to ensure good separation of the target DNA strands and to activate the dormant *Taq* polymerase. The second file is used to program the actual cycling parameters, including the number of steps, the temperature of each step, the speed of change of temperature between steps, the length of time the temperature should be held at each step, and the number of cycles. PCR cycling for most agents employs a three-step process of denaturation (92–95°C, most commonly 94°C), primer annealing (50–65°C), and DNA synthesis or primer elongation (68–74°C, most commonly 72°C); however, some GC-rich target DNA sequences such as those from cytomegalovirus (CMV) can be amplified using a two-step (65–94°C) cycle.

The time for each step varies widely among individual protocols, but it is safe to say that most protocols provide more than sufficient holding time at each step. Denaturing can usually be accomplished in 30 seconds or less, and often 15 seconds is enough; annealing is essentially instantaneous at the appropriate temperature, and holding for more than a few seconds just means that most of the elongation will also occur at the annealing temperature, as the *Taq* polymerase can function over a very wide temperature range. The elongation step rarely needs to be longer than 30 seconds, as the *Taq* DNA polymerase copies somewhere between 100 and 400 bases per second at its optimum temperature.

The third file in the linked series is usually a soak file to hold the cycler at the elongation temperature for 7 to 10 minutes after cycling to ensure that all bound primers are fully extended. This is because in the later cycles it is the polymerase that becomes limiting in the reaction, and the cost of sufficient *Taq* polymerase to overcome this problem is prohibitive.

Finally, the fourth file is to hold the sample at 4°C until it can be removed by the operator. Some practitioners also include a warm-up file that holds the temperature of the cycler at 68°C to 72°C before and during loading. If such a file is used, it is linked to the prolonged denaturation file, which becomes number two.

If *UNG* is used it is important that the samples be immediately removed from the cycler and that they are analyzed, extracted, or frozen, as *UNG* is not completely destroyed by conditions in the thermal cycler and will, over time, digest the newly amplified DNA if left at ambient or refrigerated temperatures. This problem can also be overcome by making the third file a 72°C soak file and not linking it to a 4°C file, where the *UNG* may maintain activity.

Analysis of the PCR Products

This discussion is limited to a comparison of the various techniques that are available to specifically identify the products of the PCR reaction. For purposes of discussion, all assay formats can be divided into two generic types: direct incorporation assays and hybridization assays. The latter are preferable, as they provide an additional degree of specificity to the assay, which is very important, particularly when making a diagnosis that involves the identification of a potentially life-threatening pathogen. For purposes of clinical diagnostics for infectious diseases, however, filter hybridizations (e.g., Southern blot and dot/slot/spot blot) should be avoided for several reasons. First and foremost, these methods are too time consuming; not only do these assays take 2 or 3 days to complete, but they are also labor intensive, requiring multiple preparative steps for the filter and numerous exchanges of hybridization and wash solutions. Secondly, filter hybridizations often generate a high level of background noise, making it difficult to distinguish between a low-intensity positive signal and a negative result. Both of these shortcomings can be overcome by the use of a liquid hybridization/gel retardation (LH/PAGE) assay [(1), Chaps 20 and 22]. The hybridization is carried out in liquid phase between the amplified DNA and an end-labeled internal oligonucleotide probe, and the reaction products are separated by electrophoresis through an 8% polyacrylamide gel. The gels can be prepared in bulk the night before use, or the first thing in the morning using premixed acrylamide (National Diagnostics, Manville, NJ).

This assay, while still not ideal for routine clinical testing laboratories, provides a rapid, high-resolution format that is well suited for simultaneously analyzing the products of a multiplex PCR. Until fully automated detection systems are commercially available LH/PAGE provides the best alternative. Further, there is no problem with background noise so that the signal-noise ratio is very high and results can be interpreted relatively easily. The entire procedure, starting with amplified material, requires about 2 hours of laboratory time to completely process 50 samples. This is followed by an autoradiographic step with routine exposure times of 2 to 12 hours. We have found this technique to be highly reproducible, trouble free, and one that is readily learned by medical laboratory technicians.

Summary

PCR-based clinical diagnostics require dedicated facilities, equipment, and personnel. These strict requirements are chiefly due to the risk of false-positive results caused by amplified DNA contamination of the clinical specimens.

REFERENCE

1. Ehrlich GD, Greenberg SJ. PCR-based diagnostics in infectious disease. Boston: Blackwell Scientific, 1994.

BIBLIOGRAPHY

Ehrlich GD. Caveats of PCR. Clin Micro News 1991; 13:149–151.

Ehrlich GD, Glaser JB, Maese J. Multiple sclerosis, retroviruses and PCR. Neurology 1991;41:335–345.

Kitchin PA, Szotyori Z, Fromholc C, Almond N. Avoidance of false positives. Nature 1990;344: 201.

Kwok S. Procedures to minimize PCR-product carry-over. In: Innis MA, Gelfand D, Sninsky JJ, White TJ, eds. PCR protocols: a guide to methods and applications. San Diego: Academic Press, 1990: 142–145.

Kwok S, Higuchi R. Avoiding false positives with PCR. Nature 1989;339:237–238.

Sarkar G, Sommer SS. Shedding light on PCR contamination. Nature 1990;342:27.

CHAPTER 43

Molecular Oncology

KEVIN L. NELLIS
W. EDWARD HIGHSMITH
JULIE LEANA-COX
DANIEL C. EDELMAN
SANFORD A. STASS

Cancer is defined as an autonomous proliferation of cells with metastatic potential. Within the last decade, using tools of the new science of molecular biology, a picture of the exquisite interplay of genes and gene products that serve to regulate cell growth and proliferation has begun to emerge. As the number of genes identified and implicated in cancer, carcinogenesis, and metastasis grows, the clinical laboratory faces new challenges. The laboratory now uses the techniques and technology of molecular biology to identify and characterize specific gene mutations associated with cancer.

Several core technologies are central to the practice of molecular biology. The first takes advantage of the ability of complementary strands of DNA to find each other in complex solutions and bind together (anneal) to form double stranded DNA. The specific binding is termed hybridization (or annealing), and forms the basis for almost all types of DNA detection methods. The use of enzymes forms the second set of techniques. The enzymes that are involved in DNA metabolism, repair, or bacterial host defense in vivo include polymerases, ligases, restriction endonucleases, and others; they provide the molecular tools with which nucleic acids can be manipulated with extraordinary specificity. The third set of core techniques of modern molecular biology are the detection methods. These methods are required to possess extreme specificity, not for the chemical structure of DNA, which is identical for all genes, but for the sequence of the bases, which determines the information that a particular piece of DNA is carrying. Further, because specific gene sequences form only a tiny fraction of the whole human genome, and DNA is typically available only in microgram amounts, these methods must posses extreme sensitivity. The first of these methods to be widely adopted is the Southern transfer (1). The second is the polymerase chain reaction (PCR) (2). Fluorescence in situ hybridization (FISH) is another method that has been established as a valuable adjunct to conventional cytogenetic techniques, because of its unique ability to directly couple cytological and molecular information (3,4,5). This chapter will focus on analytical molecular oncology and the quality control and quality assurance and standardization of procedures needed to ensure consistent production of reliable information that can be used for patient care.

Sample Requirements and Nucleic Acid Isolation

As with all testing, the quality of the analysis depends on the quality of the specimen. Nucleic acids can be isolated from just about any source of tissue, usually peripheral blood or marrow that is collected in either ACD-A or EDTA. All cellular material should be processed as soon as possible to prevent DNA degradation. Fresh tissue should be processed or frozen immediately. It is recommended that tissue specimens be snap frozen in OCT and thin-sectioned for hematoxylin and eosin staining to determine adequacy of sample before performing the molecular analysis. A pathologist can determine whether the sample contains the cells of interest, precluding tissue sampling error.

Many commercial research nucleic acid isolation reagents and kits are available that may be well suited for clinical use, once they have been validated by the laboratory. The nonorganic methods are usually easier, safer, faster, and less expensive than organic methods. Once isolated, nucleic acid may be quantitated and its quality assessed by UV spectrophotometric methodology. Nucleic acid is measured at an absorbance of 260 nanometers (nm) to determine concentration. Reviewing absorbance ratios will indicate the quality of the DNA, as a 260 nm/280 nm ratio of less than 1.8 indicates protein contamination. A ratio of greater than 2 indicates the presence of RNA. In the case that the isolated DNA is shown to be contaminated with protein or RNA (6), procedures should be in place for sample clean up. Typically these procedures involve the repeat purification of the sample using the primary method of isolation, or the addition of a proteinase K or RNAse to digest the contaminants.

Southern Transfer

In the Southern transfer procedure, DNA is first cleaved into smaller fragments using an appropriate restriction endonuclease(s) which cleaves DNA at specific base pair sequences. The fragments are separated electrophoretically by size through an agarose gel matrix, and then depurinated, denatured, and transferred onto a nylon or nitrocellulose membrane. The position of the fragments is preserved throughout the transfer. The transfer step may be done either by capillary action or by vacuum techniques. The DNA fragments are fixed to the blot by UV cross-linking or baking at 80°C. The blot is blocked with compounds designed to bind nonspecifically to areas on the blot that do not contain any of the transferred DNA. A probe may be either labeled with an isotope (^{32}P or ^{35}S), biotin, or a hapten. The probe is denatured and then hybridized to the fragments on the blot. The blot, now containing the specific fragment-probe complex, is washed to remove excess and nonspecifically bound probe. The signal detection method depends on the probe labeling system. For radioactive methods, the blot is exposed to x-ray film. Nonisotopic detection methods include bioluminescence, chemiluminescence, colorimetry, electrochemiluminescence, fluorescence, and phosphorescence (7). Procedures employing the use of haptens and binding proteins have been developed which improve the sensitivity of nonisotopic methods. Discrete bands will appear in the area where probe has hybridized to specific fragment targets.

Several quality control steps are taken at each step of the procedure to ensure standardized results. After electrophoresis the gel is stained with ethidium bromide and viewed under UV light. A photograph of the gel is taken for visual evaluation and saved as a permanent record. Each lane of DNA is viewed to check for quality and enzyme digestion patterns. The quantity of DNA in each lane is assessed by comparing the fluorescent intensity relative to that of the normal control. Underloading may yield false negatives, while overloading may affect migration patterns, making interpretation difficult. Partial digestion yields inappropriate results and may be a result of protein or salt contamination of the sample, inactive enzyme, or other improper digestion conditions. Each restriction endonuclease yields a typical pattern of digestion. For example, the *Bam*HI digest yields a typical onion bulb appearance. Other enzymes yield characteristic satellite bands visible with ethidium bromide fluorescence. A partial digest is often evidenced by jagged edges of the DNA at the origin of the lane and missing or light satellite bands.

Inspection of the gel photograph will also provide a confirmation of the presence of high-molecular-weight DNA (>23 kb) in each lane. Absence of high-molecular-weight DNA may be an indication of degradation, resulting in either false-negative or false-positive results. RNA contamination may appear as an intensely stained bulbous area in an area around 300 bp. The pattern of the molecular weight marker should also be checked to ensure proper electrophoresis, and the quantity of sensitivity control DNA should be checked to ensure that an adequate volume was loaded. Abnormal migration patterns may indicate that the gel or electrophoresis buffer was made improperly.

Several controls must be used in the Southern blot procedure. A negative (germ line) control should be used for each restriction endonuclease and a positive control should be used for each hybridization probe. Size markers serve as a reference standard to determine the molecular weight of migrating bands. A sensitivity control should be established that is relative to the analysis of the particular assay. A 5% sensitivity control is generally accepted as the limit of detectability in oncology applications by Southern transfer (**Fig. 43-1**) (8).

Each restriction enzyme/probe combination will, under certain circumstances, yield characteristic cross-hybridization bands and partial restriction digestion bands (9,10). These expected band patterns should be documented for each probe used, and one must be careful not to interpret these as positive rearrangements. Other bands may be present due to polymorphism or pseudogenes. Interpretation must be carried out by an experienced individual.

FIGURE **43-1**

Photograph of a Southern transfer using a probe for the T-cell receptor. Lane 1 contains a γ/*Hin*dIII molecular weight marker. Lane 2 contains a germ line (negative) control digested with *Eco*RI. Lanes 3 and 5 contain normal patient DNA digested with *Eco*RI. Lane 4 contains DNA from a patient demonstrating rearrangement with *Eco*RI. Lane 6 contains 50% germ line and 50% rearranged (positive) control. Lanes 7 and 9 contain normal patient DNA digested with *Hin*dIII. Lane 8 contains DNA from a patient demonstrating rearrangement with *Hin*dIII. Lane 10 contains a 5% sensitivity control.

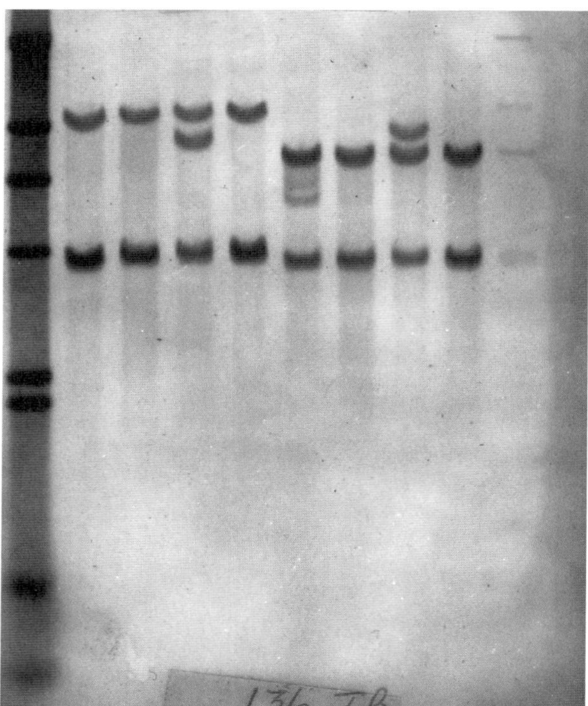

Molecular procedures are labor-intensive, multistep techniques. A problem may develop anywhere throughout the process of each procedure. Problems may be associated with reagent degradation, poor transfer, degraded probe, improperly made reagents, uncontrolled temperature variation of instrumentation, and technologist error. For example, high background in membrane-based systems may be due to problems associated with blocking solution, hybridization reagents, or incorrect washing procedures. Low signal or poor band resolution may be associated with poor transfer. Each step or parameter must be controlled by establishing valid quality control procedures for reagents and instrumentation and maintaining an up-to-date personnel training program and continuing education records.

The multistep procedure carried out in the molecular diagnostics laboratory includes the manual generation of patient worksheets, work lists, patient folders, and computer data entry, all of which are subject to clerical errors. All personnel are responsible for continuously monitoring the work generated for clerical errors, and such errors are to be taken seriously.

Errors may be caused by uncontrollable fluctuations in the temperature, small variations in volumetric apparatus, or minute differences in wavelength measurements. Temperature variations can affect hybridizing and the washing procedures. Improperly calibrated volumetric pipettes may influence the digestion procedure. Wavelength variations would affect the calculation of DNA concentration. Serious variations may be detected by observing trends in the wavelength absorbance ratios and/or recovery rates. Other errors may originate from incorrect operations, instrument malfunction, poor quality of materials, or technologist error. The quality control features of a procedure and the parameters established should address errors of this nature (8).

Interferences can occur during several stages in the procedure, such as during extraction, digestion, transfer, hybridization, and detection. Interferences may possibly be demonstrated as partial digest, cross-hybridization bands, or nonspecific non-germ-line bands. In general, these interferences may not be readily discernible to the technologist until the detection step.

Polymerase Chain Reaction

Polymerase chain reaction (PCR) is a gene amplification process that generates multiple copies of a specific gene target. Detection is possible because of the large amounts of amplified material available when compared to extraneous nuclear material. Specificity is determined by careful design of primers specific to the area of interest so that they recognize targets of identical homology of the nucleic acid. Amplification of target occurs in the presence of a DNA polymerase, Mg++, and nucleotide triphosphates via controlled temperature cycling.

The reaction mixture is first denatured at just below 100°C to separate the strands of the target, and then cooled at a temperature just below the melting temperature of the primers (at which point they anneal to the target sequence). The polymerase extends the primer in the 5′ to 3′ direction of the target strand, thus generating a new strand that contains a binding site for the other primer. Multiple heating and cooling cycles with a polymerase result in multiple copies of the target. Exponential expansion results in a millionfold increase in target copy number.

Reverse transcriptase polymerase chain reaction (RT-PCR) is a method for detection of RNA targets. A reverse transcriptase enzyme is first used to convert the RNA to DNA. The DNA is then amplified as described. Several recent books are available that cover the PCR process and its applications in detail (11–14).

Detection of the amplified target may be done by separating the product by agarose gel electrophoresis, staining with ethidium bromide or Sybr Green I, and photographing under UV light. The target will migrate at a known molecular weight (**Fig. 43-2**). Sensitivity may be improved by using transfer techniques followed by probe detection. Alternatively, a capture probe may be fixed to nylon membranes or the wells in microtiter plates in which an amplified target may hybridize followed by a colorimetric reaction.

A positive control, a sensitivity control, and an amplification or negative control must be employed with each assay to ensure accurate results. As quality control material is not commercially available for many of the assays typically done in the molecular diagnostics laboratory, each lab will have to prepare and validate its own controls. A specimen that yields a proven positive result by at least two trials with a concurrent positive control may be used as a new positive control. A positive specimen that has been diluted to approximate the sensitivity limit of the assay is useful as a sensitivity control. An amplification or negative control is a reaction that contains all reagents, but no template. It is advisable to place amplification controls both at the beginning and the end of the run, as they will assist in troubleshooting for reagent, disposables, or equipment contamination.

Depending on the application, processing, internal, or inhibitor controls may also be used

FIGURE 43-2

Photograph of amplified RT-PCR products electrophoresed on a 3% Nusieve 3 : 1 agarose gel, post stained in Sybr Green I, and photographed under UV light. Lane 1 is a negative patient specimen. Lane 2 is a 100 base pair ladder. Lane 3 is a positive control. Lane 4 is a sensitivity control. Lane 5 is an amplification (negative) control.

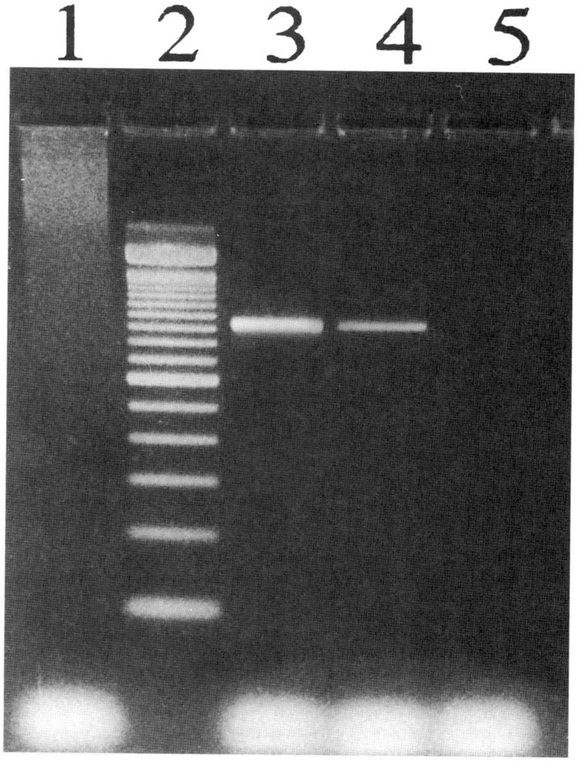

1 2 3 4 5

to enhance the quality control system of a particular assay. A processing control is a sensitivity control prepared from a positive specimen that is processed exactly as a patient specimen. This type of control may be helpful when commercial controls are treated differently than patient samples (for example, stored in a different sample matrix). An internal control may be an additional target that is added to each sample to amplify a different product than the test target. Demonstration of this target indicates that the test system was adequate for the specimen. A negative sample may also be spiked with a weak positive control to rule out the presence of endogenous inhibitors. Demonstration of PCR amplification of products using primers to ubiquitous targets such as the β-globin gene may be used as indicators of adequate amplifiable nucleic acid (8).

PCR techniques are very sensitive and one must guard against carryover of amplified product (amplicon) (15). Poor technique or sloppy conditions will create a contamination problem. The risk of contamination with amplified products is a frustrating possibility in the absence of strict PCR containment policies. The technologist must be trained to be constantly aware of the possibility of contamination. These policies should be emphasized throughout the training period until the practices become habitual.

The technologist should organize the work area before performing a procedure. All reagents and supplies should be available during the procedure to restrict unnecessary movement around the room, thus lessening the risk of contamination. All worksheets should be completed before doing a procedure. All reagents except enzymes should be divided into aliquots. All lot numbers and aliquot numbers should be recorded for each procedure.

The workflow should be unidirectional, from "clean" to "dirty." Each of the pre- and postamplification work areas should be separate and have dedicated supplies, reagents, equipment, pipettors, lab coats, gloves, manuals, pens, and cleaning supplies. Ideally, the work areas should be in separate rooms without air exchange. Air may leave the pre-PCR area and enter the post-PCR area, but air currents from post- to pre-PCR areas must be avoided. Post-PCR products must never enter the pre-PCR work area. Lab coats and gloves must also be changed when changing work areas. Supplies must never be taken from the post- to the pre-PCR area. Amplification of contaminating amplicons could be disastrous, as well as difficult to identify and eliminate.

PCR reactions may be set up in a dead-air box. Supplies, reagents, pipettes, and work surfaces may be wiped down with 70% ethanol or 10% bleach before use. With the exception of nucleic acids (target/primers) and enzymes, reagents may be UV irradiated for about 10 minutes in the dead-air box to inactivate possible contaminating template. The technologist should move his or her hands slowly and deliberately when working in the PCR preparation area to avoid causing extreme air currents within the dead-air box. Tubes should be opened with a tube opener and never left open longer than necessary. The tubes are closed immediately after transferring the aliquot. An aliquot is never returned to an original container.

Filter barrier tips are used to prevent aerosol contamination within the barrel of pipettes. It is preferable to use positive displacement pipettes with capillaries and pistons; however, these are usually more expensive. Tips should never be overfilled. Tips and capillaries/pistons may only be used once, and must be changed after each reagent or specimen addition. Once a box of tips is opened within the dead-air box, it should remain in the box until discarded.

Microcentrifuge tubes and PCR tubes should be autoclaved. When RT-PCR is used, the interior of containers should be wiped down with RNAse decontaminate before use. Tube racks and trays should be autoclaved frequently.

Chemical safeguards may also be employed to reduce the risk of PCR contamination. Isopsoralen may be included in a PCR reaction; it intercalates with DNA and is cross-linked by exposure to UV light, rendering it an unsuitable substrate for PCR amplification. Alternatively, deoxyuridine is used in the place of thymidine in the PCR reaction. The enzyme uracil-N-glycosylase (*UNG*) is added prior to the PCR reaction to destroy amplified products containing the deoxyuridine without effecting authentic target DNA (16).

Fluorescence In Situ Hybridization

A successful technique for fluorescence in situ hybridization (FISH) using biotinylated probes was first described in 1986 and has since been extensively employed (17). Chromosome-specific probe DNA is chemically modified by incorporation of biotin-dUTP via nick translation, followed by its hybridization to metaphase chromosomes or interphase nuclei. For hybridization to occur, both the DNA of the target cells and the labeled probe must be denatured. Incubation at the appropriate temperature allows the probe to bind to complementary sequences in the target DNA. The bound, chemically modified DNA is then rendered fluorescent by successive treatments with fluorescein-labeled avidin and biotinylated anti-avidin antibody. The chromosomes are counterstained with a DNA-specific fluorescent dye, such as propidium iodide, and are visualized under fluorescence microscopy. A modification of this technique, known as chromosomal in situ suppression (CISS), was developed to suppress the repetitive elements distributed throughout the karyotype to allow for the specific hybridization of single-copy DNA sequences or whole-chromosome DNA probes containing such elements (18).

FISH is becoming a widely used method to detect genetic rearrangements or amplifications in cancer cells. For example, the juxtaposition of the *bcr* and *abl* genes (located on chromosomes 9 and 22, respectively) that occurs in chronic myelogenous leukemia (CML) can be identified in either metaphase or interphase cells when the probes for each gene are labeled with different fluorophores (19). Clinical tests for other gene rearrangements, including the *PML/RARA* fusion seen in acute promyelogenous leukemia, are currently being established.

FISH may be performed with DNA probes that are commercially available, or with probes developed within the testing laboratory. Most clinical laboratories rely on commercially available probes, which undergo quality control testing by the manufacturer. In such cases, it is important to test each new lot to ensure that the probe hybridizes to the correct location under the appropriate conditions. Non-commercially-prepared DNA probes must undergo a quality control procedure established within the laboratory, which should include the analysis of several positive and negative control samples to establish the sensitivity, specificity, and reliability of the probe.

To perform FISH, a microscope equipped with fluorescence capability must be available; a mercury light source (100 watt) is preferred over xenon by most laboratories because it provides a more intense signal for the majority of fluorophores used. The microscope filters should match the wavelength of the fluorophores used to allow for optimum visualization of probe signal. In addition, the system must be capable of providing photographic documentation of hybridization results; most laboratories use either a photomicroscope to record images on 35-mm slide film, or a computer-based system that records digitized images.

Often, a control probe is hybridized simultaneously with the test probe to ensure that hybridization conditions are optimum. For metaphase analysis, a control probe may also serve to mark the chromosome pair of interest. A positive and/or negative control specimen should be run with each sample when interphase nuclei are analyzed. Calculation of the mean value of percent abnormal or normal cells within 2 standard deviations can be used for a control range following a sufficient number of independent hybridizations for each probe. For metaphase analysis, a control probe may also serve to mark the chromosome pair of interest. However, for most such assays, an internal control is provided by the normal chromosome homolog(s) present in each metaphase, so a control specimen may be unnecessary.

Hybridization conditions may vary among different probes, and must be carefully optimized; then they are monitored and recorded for each assay. Cross-hybridization, high background signal, or inadequate hybridization should be evident by analysis of the control probe or specimen. Scoring criteria are established to determine which metaphase spreads or interphase nuclei will be included in the analysis. For example, if probes for the *bcr* and *abl* loci are simultaneously hybridized to interphase nuclei, each labeled with a different fluorophore, only cells with four signals—or three signals, with one clearly representing a fusion of the two colors—should be scored. The number of cells analyzed varies; most laboratories score 10 to 50 cells for a metaphase analysis, although 50 to 500 interphase nuclei may be scored.

Validation of Test Methodology and Performance Specifications

Optimal PCR and Southern transfer parameters must be determined for each assay. Southern transfer parameters may include: choice of restriction endonuclease and digestion conditions, or hybridization, washing, and detection conditions. Salt concentration of wash reagents and wash temperatures must be determined for each Southern assay. PCR parameters could include: concentrations of Mg++, dNTP, primers, template, and added enhancers; or pH, primer design, melting temperature (T_m) of primer sequence, annealing temperature, and number of amplification cycles. The empirical determination of optimum parameters can be a labor, resource, and time intensive activity. The laboratory must be willing to make the investment to achieve optimal sensitivity. Literature should also be reviewed prior to establishing a new test methodology.

All new tests must be validated for clinical use under the direction of the laboratory director(s) or their designee. A number of samples must be analyzed and reviewed before the lab begins offering a new test. The specimens tested must represent the full spectrum of possible values. Blind studies from a College of American Pathologists (CAP) accredited laboratory should be used to test the laboratory's proficiency with a new methodology. Sensitivity of the assay should also be determined and maintained. This may be done with the use of a sensitivity control specific for each assay.

CAP requires that sufficient information must be documented regarding the nature of probe(s) or primer(s) used in an assay to permit interpretation and troubleshooting of the test (20). Items of importance include the type and origin of the probe or sequence; oligonucleotide sequence and complementary sequence or gene region recognized; an appropriate restriction enzyme map of the DNA; known polymorphism sites resistant to endonuclease digestion and cross-hybridizing bands; and labeling methods used and standards for adequacy of hybridization or amplification. Documentation of the validation shall be available for the period during which the procedure is used in the laboratory or for the number of years specified by local and national regulatory agencies, whichever is longer.

The laboratory must verify or establish and document each of the following specifications, as appropriate to and applicable for a particular method: analytic accuracy and precision claimed for each method in use and for which the laboratory reports results; analytic sensitivity and specificity claimed for each method in use and for which the laboratory reports results; linear reportable range of patient test results. A reference range shall be established for each method before reporting patient test results. In the case of qualitative and screening tests, the laboratory must determine and document the basis for specifying reportable results as positive, negative, or degree of reactivity. The laboratory must follow these established limits in reporting test results (21).

Periodic evaluation of the appropriateness of reference ranges, and corrective actions if necessary, must be undertaken and documented. A list of current test methods, including performance specifications, must be available to clients upon request. If the laboratory changes its analytic methodology so that test results in their interpretations may be significantly different, the change must be explained to clients. Notification may vary but could include direct mailing, laboratory newsletters, or inclusion as part of the test report. When a laboratory performs the same test using different methodologies or instruments, or performs the same test at multiple test sites, it must have a system in place for evaluation and definition of the relationship between test results at least 3 times a year to meet CAP requirements (21).

Instrumentation

In general, quality control procedures and preventive maintenance on equipment should be done as indicated by the manufacturer. Additional quality control should be performed as indicated by CAP standards. Some procedures that are unique for molecular laboratories (8) include:

- Inhouse DNA absorbance controls for a UV spectrophotometer may be established using calf thymus DNA.
- Linearity studies for these instruments may be established using λ phage DNA.
- Individual wells of the thermal cyclers should be checked using a NIST traceable thermistor.
- UV lamps inside dead-air boxes and safety hoods should be changed at least every 6 months or as indicated by inability to inactivate a biological control.

- Water quality control procedures should be established to ensure quality of type 1 water.
- Autoclave cycles should be spore tested.
- A pipet verification program should be established to ensure accuracy and precision of these instruments.
- Balances should be checked for accuracy and precision in accordance to the frequency of use.
- Temperature-dependent equipment should be checked daily.
- Timer and instrumentation accuracy of timers should be checked against a NIST stopwatch.
- Relative humidity and temperature should be checked daily.

Reagent Quality and Safety

Ensuring the quality of reagents in the molecular lab is imperative. Procedures should be established to ensure biochemical reactivity of reagents. Enzymes in particular should be tested with concurrent lots. A reagent lot log should be established, including the date the reagent was tested, the gel number used for quality control, and the date it was placed in service. Reagent lot numbers should be recorded on appropriate worksheets when they are used. A lot log and worksheets are very useful when troubleshooting procedures. All reagents (with the exception of enzymes) should be divided into aliquots to reduce the risk of contamination with amplified products. Lot numbers of kit components should not be interchanged unless approved by the manufacturer of the kit.

All reagents must be labeled consistently in accordance with CAP standards, with name, lot number, date prepared or opened, and expiration date. Reagent labeling of very small vials is sometimes impossible; it is helpful to use an abbreviated label and put these vials in a single box labeled with all the pertinent information.

All reagents should be stored in accordance with the manufacturer's instructions or as reported in the literature. Frost-free freezers, which maintain cycles of warm and cool temperatures, will destroy the biological activity of enzymes. Therefore, enzymes such as restriction endonuclease and polymerases should be stored in non-frost-free freezers. Enzymes should never be held at the base of the tube as this will warm the small volume of reagent and may speed degradation. When not in the freezer, enzymes should be kept on ice or stored in a cold rack, but not on dry ice.

Few procedures for molecular oncology testing are approved by the Food and Drug Administration (FDA). The majority of procedures are being developed within reference or academic laboratories and regulated through other mechanisms including the Clinical Laboratory Improvement Act of 1988. In 1996, the FDA proposed a classification of analytic-specific reagents (ASRs) for inhouse developed or "home brew" assays, which would subject them to FDA rules and make them available only to those laboratories certified to perform high complex testing. However, this proposition is under review and has been challenged as too destructive to the rapidly evolving field of molecular testing (22,23).

Material Safety Data Sheets (MSDS) must be available for all reagents. It is recommended that a thorough review of information contained in material safety data sheets (MSDS) via OSHA Subpart Z, the International Agency for Research on Cancer (IARC), or the National Toxicology Program (NTP) should be done to assess the chemical toxicity and carcinogenicity of each reagent used in the molecular lab. A summary of this information should be shared with all employees working with the reagents as a part of their continuing education and training program.

Working with isotopes requires obtaining a radiation license, and performing radioactive safety monitoring and radiation safety training for all employees working in the area of use. Personnel protection gear such as eye shields, fluid-proof lab coats, and adequate gloves should be used by all personnel. Universal precautions should be followed for all procedures.

The hepatitis B vaccine should also be offered to all employees. Employees should be safety trained in UV radiation, shock hazards of electrophoresis, fire hazards, burn prevention, and cryogenic and chemical hazards. Each employee should know how to use the eyewash, fire extinguishers, and safety showers. Written procedures should be in place for disposal of chemical, biohazard, and radioactive waste. Emergency chemical spill kits with posted instructions must be available in the laboratory. Certain signs must also be posted as required by the institution and laboratory safety office for general safety and radiation procedures.

Quality Assurance

The CAP general checklist and molecular pathology checklist serve as excellent guides for establishing quality in a molecular laboratory (20,21). CAP has a relationship with the Health Care Finance Administration (HCFA) and the Joint Commission of Accreditation of Health Care Organizations (JCAHO). CAP has deemed status as a private accrediting agency under the Clinical Laboratory Improvement Act of 1988 (CLIA '88). Participation in the CAP accreditation process enables the laboratory to satisfy CLIA '88 regulations. The National Committee for Clinical Laboratory Science (NCCLS) publishes standards that are essential for the molecular laboratory (24,25). NCCLS has published standards for gene rearrangement assays, water quality control, and standardized written procedure format (26). The NCCLS guidelines for infectious disease amplification applications may also be applicable for molecular oncology testing (27).

The molecular diagnostics laboratory should participate in the pathology department's quality assurance plan. Evaluation and corrective action are taken whenever the thresholds exceed the monitors outlined in the plan. Examples of such monitors may include: turnaround-time monitoring, verification that failed hybridization reactions were documented, necessary corrective actions, the number of repeat tests, and the number of failed controls. Comparative studies and statistical analysis should also be done when appropriate. For example, comparisons of molecular studies with cytogenetics, immunophenotype, bone marrow biopsy and smear, and anatomic pathology results should be performed as appropriate. All records and reports shall be well maintained in the laboratory.

The CAP-accredited laboratory will participate in all CAP proficiency surveys appropriate for the testing performed in the laboratory. When a CAP survey is not available for a particular test, an intra-laboratory exchange of blind samples with another CAP-accredited laboratory should be attempted. Testing of survey samples should be rotated among all trained laboratory technical personnel when possible.

Employee Qualifications, Training, and Competency Assessment

Personnel employed in labor-intensive molecular techniques require more training time on new procedures than those performing routine clinical testing. In even the most standardized molecular procedure, troubleshooting will inevitably be required, regardless of the laboratory's level of control. The molecular laboratory is subject to its own particular technical problems, and it is imperative that the technologist understand the entire theory behind each assay, so that he or she may troubleshoot when necessary. A thorough understanding of theory also helps alleviate potential problems and technologist error.

Because of the nature of molecular techniques, it is often beneficial to have a skill mix of both certified medical technologists and molecular biologists or other research scientists. It may be cost effective to have less skilled laboratory technicians who can be adequately trained for routine maintenance and reagent preparation. Additional safety training may be required for molecular technologists because they will be exposed to toxic, carcinogenic, and radiation hazards not associated with other clinical or research laboratories.

CLIA '88 requires that competency be documented when an employee is trained, and again at 6 months after training, and yearly thereafter. Documentation may be in the form of oral review of a training checklist or a written exam. Examples of actual problems should be reviewed in the competency evaluation to determine an employee's ability to troubleshoot various situations. Personnel records must be maintained as required by CAP and CLIA '88 regulations.

Continuing education of each employee should be maintained and documented through attendance at continuing education classes or reading appropriate journal articles. The title of the training, a brief synopsis of the topics covered, and the total time spent on the event should be recorded.

The CAP and state regulatory agencies have qualification standards for supervisory and directoral positions. A supervisor must have 6 to 7 years of molecular biology experience. A director must be a physician or doctoral scientist qualified to judge the medical significance of the data generated by the molecular assay and to ensure standards of performance and quality. It is preferable that the director be board-certified in human molecular genetics. Currently, the only organization that is offering AMA-recognized board examinations is the American Board of Medical Genetics. However, other organizations, including the American Board of Pathology and the American Board of Clinical Chemistry, are debating whether to offer certifying examinations. It is ideal to have both a medical director with expertise in molecular biology and a technical director to guide daily operations, test development, troubleshooting, and monitoring of quality control.

Interpretation and Reporting of Test Results

The individual signing out the test results, typically the laboratory director or pathologist, should have access to such results as generated by cytogenetics, electron microscopy, and immunology for comparison with the molecular diagnostic results. The director will determine if unusual results are obtained, and make recommendations for any follow-up work. Physician notification may be made by the director when appropriate. The director or designate interpreting the results has the final responsibility for determining the validity of the results.

Two qualified people, as determined by the director, must interpret the results of each test. Both designates assigned by the director must initial or sign drafts or report worksheets. The written report should be reviewed and signed by the director or designee for results and interpretation. Reports must indicate the testing methodology used and the limitations and sensitivity of each assay. Reports of the results of tests are submitted only to a physician or the physician's agent. Reports are not issued to the patients concerned except with the written consent of the physician or other authorized person. Copies of reports should be maintained in the molecular diagnostic lab.

Summary

The identification of new genes is increasing our understanding of cancer. Further, the identification of mutations in disease genes leads to new molecular laboratory procedures and a better ability to diagnose affected individuals, monitor therapeutic interventions, make prognostic projections, and offer presymptomatic or carrier testing to family members. The explosion of molecular testing offers the clinical laboratory new challenges. The clinical laboratory has a long history of translating research advances into clinical practice. The clinical laboratory has the ultimate responsibility of ensuring that results are accurate, precise, and of clinical value.

The need to maintain quality is of fundamental importance in the molecular diagnostics laboratory. The introduction of new test protocols brings the requirement for the development of adequate quality control and quality assurance techniques. The majority of molecular test protocols are labor intensive, multistep procedures. The need to maintain control at each step is crucial for the delivery of meaningful results. Techniques and procedure for the monitoring of all steps of molecular test protocols, from sample preparation to result interpretation, are now available. By rigorous adherence to quality control procedures and quality assurance indicators, the clinical laboratory will continue its venerable history of delivering test results that guide and improve patient care.

REFERENCES

1. Southern EM. Detection of specific sequences among DNA fragments separated by gel electrophoresis. J Mol Biol 1975;98:503–517.
2. Saiki RK, Scharf S, Faloong F, et al. Enzymatic amplification of β-globulin genomic sequences and restriction site analysis for diagnosis of sickle-cell anemia. Science 1985;230:1350–1354.
3. Trask NJ. Fluorescence in situ hybridization: applications in cytogenetics and gene mapping. Trends Genet 1991;1:149.
4. Lichter P, Chang Tang C-J, Call K, et al. High-resolution mapping of human chromosome 11 by in situ hybridization with cosmid clones. Science 1990;247:64–69.
5. McNeil JA, Johnson CV, Carter KC, et al. Localizing DNA and RNA within nuclei and chromosomes by fluorescence in situ hybridization. Genet Anal Tech Appl 1991;8:41–58.
6. Manchester, Keith L. Use of UV methods for measurement of protein and nucleic acid concentrations. Biotechniques 1996;20:968–970.

7. Kricka, Larry J. Nonisotopic probing, blotting and sequencing. 2nd ed. Philadelphia: Academic Press, 1995.
8. Farkas DH. Molecular biology and pathology: a guidebook for quality control. San Diego, CA: Academic Press, 1993.
9. Oncor manual for the B/T Blue gene rearrangement test system for the in vitro diagnosis of leukemia and lymphoma: procedure and interpretation guide. Gaithersburg, MD: Oncor, 1992.
10. Sklar J. Antigen receptor genes: Structure, function, and techniques for analysis of their rearrangements. In: Knowles DM, ed. Neoplastic hematopathology. Baltimore: Williams & Wilkins, 1992:215–244.
11. Mullis KB, Ferré F, Gibbs RA, Watson JD. The polymerase chain reaction. Boston: Birkhäuser, 1994.
12. Erlich HA. PCR technology: principles and applications for DNA amplification. New York: WH Freeman, 1991.
13. White BA. Methods in molecular biology. PCR protocols: current methods and applications. Vol 15. Totowa, NJ: Human Press, 1993.
14. McPherson MJ, Quirke P, Taylor GR. PCR: a practical approach. New York: IRL Press/Oxford University Press, 1993.
15. Kwok S, Higuchi R. Avoiding false positives with PCR. Nature 1989;339:237–238.
16. Longo MC, Beringer MS, Hartley JL. Use of uracil DNA glycosylase to control carry-over contamination in polymerase chain reactions. Gene 1990;93:125–128.
17. Pinkel D, Straume T, Gray JW. Cytogenetic analysis using quantitative, high-sensitivity, fluorescence hybridization. Proc Natl Acad Sci USA 1986;83:2934–2938.
18. Schad CR, Dewald GW. Building a new clinical test for fluorescence in situ hybridization. Appl Cytogenet 1995;21:1–4.
19. Dewald GW, Schad CR, Christensen ER, et al. The application of fluorescent in situ hybridization to detect *Mbcr/abl* fusion in variant Ph chromosomes in CML and ALL. Cancer Genet Cytogenet 1993;71:7–14.
20. College of American Pathologists. Inspection checklist. Section XII: Molecular pathology. Northfield, IL: CAP, 1996.
21. College of American Pathologists. Inspection checklist. Section I: Laboratory general checklist. Northfield, IL: CAP, 1996.
22. Department of Health and Human Services. Proposed Rules: Medical Devices; Classification/Reclassification; Restricted Devices; Analyte Specific Reagents. Federal Register (21 CFR 809, 864) March 14, 1996;61(51):10484–10489.
23. Leonard DGB. Clinical news update: FDA proposal for classification of "analyte-specific reagents." Mol Diag 1996;1:153–154.
24. National Committee for Clinical Laboratory Standards. Preparation and testing of reagent water in the clinical laboratory. 2nd ed. Villanova, PA: NCCLS, 1991.
25. National Committee for Clinical Laboratory Standards. Clinical laboratory technical procedure manuals. 2nd ed. Villanova, PA: NCCLS, 1992.
26. National Committee for Clinical Laboratory Standards. Immunoglobulin and T-cell gene rearrangement assays: proposed guideline. Villanova, PA: NCCLS, 1994.
27. National Committee for Clinical Laboratory Standards. Molecular diagnostic methods for infectious disease: proposed guideline. Villanova, PA: NCCLS, 1994.

CHAPTER 44

In Situ Hybridization

ELIZABETH R. UNGER
DAISY R. LEE

There are many variations of in situ hybridization (ISH) assays in the literature. The goal of all of these assays is to demonstrate specific genetic information within the morphologic context of tissues, cells, or chromosomes. These assays have been widely used in such diverse research applications as mapping genes to particular chromosomes, enumerating chromosomes in interphase cells or chromosome spreads, detecting cells that contain infectious or altered gene sequences, and demonstrating cellular subpopulations expressing particular genes. However, ISH has been only tentatively incorporated into the clinical laboratory. Reasons for this delay in technology transfer include the relative lack of automation and limited commercial availability of optimized standardized reagents. This chapter is based upon our laboratory's experience with incorporation of ISH into a diagnostic setting. We will present our recommendations for clinical applications of colorimetric ISH to formalin-fixed paraffin-embedded tissue sections from the surgical pathology laboratory.

Principles of In Situ Hybridization Assay

The basic steps of tissue ISH are shown in **Figure 44-1**. The similarities to immunohistochemistry (IHC) are obvious. Both techniques start with a tissue sample immobilized to a microscope slide and end with identical methods of detection and interpretation. Because of the familiarity of the format, ISH is the molecular technique that has the greatest attraction for diagnostic histopathology laboratories.

Difficulty can arise when laboratories fail to appreciate the differences between ISH and IHC. In both assays, the specificity of the reaction occurs because of the many weak noncovalent bonds that occur between the interacting macromolecules. For ISH, nucleic acid chemistry rather than protein chemistry determines the optimal assay conditions that maintain the desired specificity.

Because ISH is a molecular biologic technique, adherence to the CAP checklist for molecular pathology laboratories is required. Each step of the ISH assay will be briefly considered to emphasize features important in standardization.

Sample Fixation and Processing

Like immunohistochemistry, diagnostic in situ hybridization is used as a supplemental technique following routine histopathologic study of the tissue sample. Therefore, the starting material has been fixed and processed "routinely" for light microscopic examination and ISH must use recut sections of these formalin-fixed paraffin-embedded blocks. The advantage of this approach is that light microscopic examination allows the correct assay to be performed on tissue that is representative of the lesion. The disadvantage is that routine tissue processing is far from reproducible.

Preservation of nucleic acids requires that the tissues are rapidly and evenly fixed. The sample must be cut thin enough to allow for even penetration of fixative, and it must be

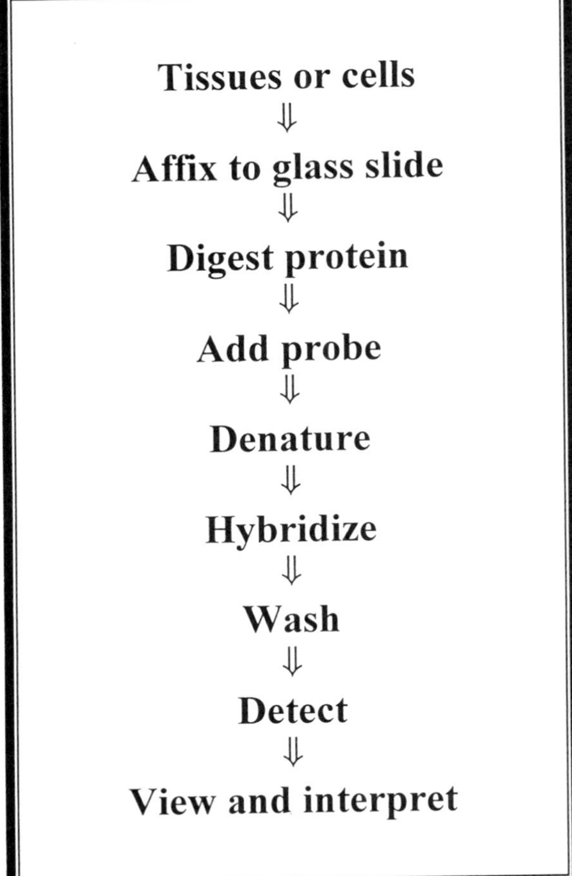

FIGURE 44-1

Outline of the basic steps of an in situ hybridization assay. (Reprinted by permission from Unger ER, Lee DR. In situ hybridization: principles and diagnostic applications in infection. J Histotechnol 1995;18:203–209.)

quickly placed in an adequate volume of fresh formalin. Ideally, the time and temperature of fixation should be standardized, and processing to the paraffin block should use fresh reagents. These ideal conditions are seldom met. Significant variations in fixation and processing that dramatically influence nucleic acid preservation may go unnoticed by standard light microscopic examination. Until histology laboratories develop methods to ensure standardization of fixation and processing, ISH assays on diagnostic samples must include controls that will detect and adjust for variations in tissue preservation (see the discussion on controls).

Although noncrosslinking fixatives may be used, the crosslinks help maintain morphology and increase tissue retention of small nucleic acids during all the steps of the assay. Crosslinking also limits permeation of probe into the tissue, so final probe size, denaturation conditions, and protease treatment must all be adjusted to maximize the balance between target accessibility and retention of morphology.

Histologic Sectioning

The importance of good histologic sectioning is often overlooked. Standard 5-micron sections are adequate, but thickness may be adjusted as desired. Sections must be of uniform thickness without folds or tears, and the thickness must be uniform from section to section to allow for even and reproducible penetration of reagents.

Tissue adherence to glass is also crucial. Conditions for the hybridization assay are drastic and loss of tissue may occur during the assay if steps are not taken to improve tissue adherence. Treatment of the glass slides with 3-aminopropyltriethoxysilane has largely replaced other techniques, such as coating glass with poly-L-lysine or glue. When tissue sections are cut and floated in a protein-free tapwater bath, the silane-treated glass will form a covalent bond with the tissue section. This "silanized glass" is available commercially and greatly minimizes the problem of tissue adherence. Quality of silanization may be monitored by the behavior of tissue sections during cutting. If the glass is properly treated, the tissue will not be able to be "refloated" or moved around on the slide once it has been lifted from the surface of the water. Difficulties with the procedure can be attributed to poorly treated glass, dirty glass, or protein in the water bath. Once the section is picked up on the microscope slide, the slide is placed vertically and allowed to air dry. The paraffin should be retained on the section (i.e., section not melted) until just before the assay is started.

Tissue Pretreatment

Slides are stored air dried at room temperature prior to starting the assay. The first step of tissue pretreatment is removal of paraffin. Tissue adherence is helped by melting paraffin section onto the glass. The paraffin must be completely removed for efficient reagent penetration. Xylene is the most efficient clearing agent, but xylene substitutes may be used if care is taken to ensure dewaxing steps are efficient. Several changes of dewaxing agents are recommended.

Deparaffinization conditions that are satisfactory for routine staining may not be adequate for ISH; overtreatment with dewaxing agents has not been observed. Tissues are prepared for protease treatment by solvent removal with alcohol, followed by hydration to a water-based buffer.

Protease treatment is required for all cross-linked samples. Digestion removes proteins and makes the target more accessible to the probe. Acid conditions also contribute to tissue permeabilization, protein removal, and improved accessibility of target. Conditions are empirically determined and depend on the type of sample and degree of crosslinking. Proteinase K, pronase, pepsin, and other proteases have all been used. For DNA targets, we vary the pepsin concentration and acid concentration depending on results with the control hybridization (see below), and we keep the time and temperature of the protease step constant. Reproducibility of protease performance is ensured by storing the enzyme in aliquots, verifying lot-to-lot performance, and preparing enzyme solutions on the day of use.

Probe and Hybridization Cocktail

In a hybridization assay, the probe is analogous in role and importance to the primary antibody in an immunoassay. Probes may be produced and labeled inhouse, but in most diagnostic settings laboratories rely on commercial sources of these crucial reagents. Probes may be available in purified form or already prepared in a hybridization cocktail. The nature of the probe will influence the assay conditions, selection of controls, and methods of troubleshooting the assay. Even when the probe is provided in a "kit" form with manufacturer-specified conditions for all portions of the assay, it is useful to have some basic technical information about the probe.

Chemical Nature of Probe

The chemical nature of the probe must be known. Probes may be DNA or RNA, single-stranded or double-stranded. They may be prepared from purified genomic material, recombinant (cloned) fragments, or chemically synthesized oligonucleotides. If cloned probes are used, the specific insert may be purified from the plasmid or cosmid vector, or total recombinant plasmid/cosmid used.

Probe Label

Nonradioactive methods for probe labeling provide the required stability for this key reagent of the in situ hybridization assay. Although some probes are labeled with a fluorescent tag allowing direct visualization following hybridization, for most applications in formalin-fixed paraffin-embedded tissue sections, affinity labels are used. The technical information required includes the type of label, method of incorporation, and final size of the labeled probe.

The type of label is needed to match the appropriate detection reagents. The commercially available affinity labels include biotin, digoxigenin, fluorescein, and sulfone. These labels are detected indirectly using the label as a hapten for antibody-based detection or using biotin-avidin specificity. Because of this, the extent of affinity-label incorporation is less crucial to assay sensitivity than the availability of the label to the detection reagents. The extent of affinity-label incorporation is therefore not a required piece of technical information. If desired, lot-to-lot variation in label incorporation can be monitored by dilution dot series of probe followed by detection with the appropriate reagents. This step is most essential when labeling is done inhouse.

The method of incorporation provides information about the nature of the chemical linkage between label and probe, which in turn determines the stability of the crucial linkage. In addition, the method of incorporation will determine how uniformly the label is distributed over the length of the probe and whether both strands of a double-stranded probe will be labeled.

The final size of the probe after labeling is particularly crucial information for in situ hybridization because of the problem of tissue penetration. Optimal results require that the labeled probe fragments be under 500 bases. Larger fragments contribute to background and add little to sensitivity because of steric hindrance to target accessibility. Reproducibility of results requires that lot-to-lot variation in probe size be minimized.

Biologic Nature of Probe

The manufacturer should be able to provide information about what region(s) of the target will hybridize with the probe and whether probe is directed against repetitive or unique sequences. In many instances genetic maps of the probe and target can be provided. This information about the genetic complexity of the probe and nature of the target will provide a guide to the final sensitivity and specificity of the hybridization assay.

Oligonucleotides can be designed to be very specific for a particular target, yet unless the oligo is directed against a highly repetitive target, the sensitivity will be reduced compared to that achieved with a genetically complex recombinant probe. If the target consists of 10 kb of nonrepetitive genetic information, only one copy of a probe 20 to 40 bases in length will hybridize to each target compared to the 5 to 7 kb of genetic information that could be included in a recombinant DNA or RNA probe.

Hybridization Cocktail

Components of the hybridization cocktail vary considerably and are empirically determined to optimize specific hybridization and minimize background. The hybridization cocktail is used to control the chemical environment of probe and tissue during the hybridization reaction. It includes a buffer to control pH, salt to control ionic strength, and in most instances formamide to lower the melting temperature of the nucleic acids. Other components of the mixture may include high-molecular-weight polymers such as dextran sulfate, added to reduce evaporation and favor kinetics of hybridization. A myriad of other reagents such as protein, carrier DNA or RNA, detergent, and Ficoll, may be included to reduce nonspecific probe tissue interactions. It is not necessary to know the exact formulation of the hybridization cocktail, but the final concentrations of probe and formamide should be provided by the manufacturer to assist the laboratory in evaluating assay conditions.

Careful adherence to the manufacturer's guidelines for storage of probe and cocktail is required for reproducible results. Some components of the cocktail may precipitate in the freezer. Just prior to use, the cocktail and probe should be warmed and thoroughly mixed to ensure even distribution of probe and resolubilize all components of the cocktail. Repetitive freeze-thaw cycles are damaging to probe, so storage of probe and cocktail in single-use aliquots helps to ensure reagent stability and reproducibility of assay sensitivity.

Denaturation

Almost all assays use heat to denature the probe and/or target. Efficient denaturation is especially important when both species are double-stranded. The time and temperature of denaturation are empirically determined depending on the nature of the probe and target. For adequate denaturation of crosslinked double-stranded DNA targets in formalin-fixed paraffin-embedded tissue sections, the temperature is much higher and the time longer than that required for DNA in solution. Optimal conditions for denaturation are also influenced by the extent of tissue pretreatment and crosslinking.

In practice, we have found it most practical to keep the conditions of denaturation constant for each assay and to vary protease digestion to reach an optimal combination. If conditions of denaturation are not adequate, accessibility of target and probe are compromised, and sensitivity will in turn be compromised. If conditions of denaturation are too drastic, morphology will be lost and eventually sensitivity will be reduced. Once optimal conditions are established, careful monitoring of temperature and time of denaturation for each assay and for each slide in each assay is required.

Hybridization and Washing

The stringency of the hybridization reaction is determined by conditions of hybridization and posthybridization washes. Stringency refers to the degree of base pair mismatching that will be tolerated in the final probe-target hybrid. At high stringency, nearly all stable hybrids will be an exact base pair match. As stringency is lowered, hybrids with greater numbers of mismatches will be stable. Optimal stringency is once again empirically determined. Temperature, ionic strength, formamide, and base pair composition all are variables that must be controlled.

In practice, the hybridization cocktail that controls the ionic strength, pH, and formamide is kept constant and the temperature of the hybridization is varied to adjust the stringency of the reaction. Higher temperatures increase stringency and lower temperatures reduce stringency. Because the hybrid molecules are dynamic structures, conditions following hybridization will also influence the stringency.

Posthybridization washes are used to remove nonspecifically bound probe so that all label detected can be attributed to a specific probe target interaction. Reducing the salt concentration in the wash and raising the temperature allow the final stringency of the hybridization to be raised. In practice, it is convenient to perform the hybridization at a slightly lower level of stringency to maximize the probe-target interaction and then to raise the stringency to the final desired level with the posthybridization washes. Thus, it follows that temperature, hybridization cocktail, and salt concentration of washing buffers are all essential assay parameters that must be controlled.

The time of the hybridization reaction is another empirically determined variable. The kinetics of a solid phase hybridization assay are complex, but are generally most dependent on the probe concentration. With affinity labels, probe concentration can be increased to allow for shortened hybridization times, 2 hours or less, which can be important for clinical assays. At high probe concentrations with double-stranded probes, solution phase self-hybridization limits the usefulness of further increases in time. High probe concentration can also result in increased nonspecific interaction (background) between probe and tissue. If probe is a limiting reagent, reducing the concentration and increasing the time of hybridization may be used to maintain sensitivity.

Detection

The detection system is matched to the type of affinity label on the probe. Whether the affinity label is detection with an antibody or through biotin-avidin interaction, the subsequent color development depends on enzyme-linked histochemistry. Increased sensitivity will result when detection reagents are optimized to minimize nonspecific tissue interactions and maximize the intensity and localization of the colored product.

The contribution of optimal detection reagents to the final sensitivity and specificity of the ISH assay is frequently overlooked. Alkaline phosphatase-linked systems with color development with BCIP/NBT are generally considered to result in the highest sensitivity. The blue-colored product requires a red counterstain.

The efficacy of detection reagents, even when based on the same histochemical principles, vary considerably among manufacturers and in some cases among lots. Enzyme substrates are also key reagents in colorimetric assays. Buffer composition, temperature, and time of enzyme reaction must be optimized and monitored for optimal results.

Assay Controls

Because so many variables exist in the ISH assay, controls are of paramount importance to monitor the validity of each reaction. The purpose of controls is to provide assurance that tissues without signal are devoid of the target nucleic acid and that tissues with signal do contain the target. Interpretation of a precipitated product as evidence of a particular nucleic acid sequence requires that all other explanations be eliminated. Controls also allow problems in any assay to be detected so that appropriate corrective measures can be instituted. Many different kinds of controls can be included; the three essential controls are listed in **Table 44-1**. These three are the minimum required by the CAP laboratory checklist for molecular pathology.

Positive Tissue Control

With each assay, a sample known to contain the target nucleic acid must be run to demonstrate that all components of the assay are working. The positive tissue control must be fixed and processed using conditions as close as possible to those used for the patient samples. The positive tissue control is then handled as an additional sample in each assay. Use of a positive tissue control near the lower limit of assay sensitivity verifies the lower limit of detection and allows small variations between runs to be noticed and corrected. Cell lines are quite useful positive controls as they can be reproducibly obtained and may contain known quantity of target. Preparation of formalin-fixed paraffin-embedded cell blocks results in a preparation quite similar to tissue, although not tissue per se.

Positive Probe Control

Because of unavoidable variations in tissue fixation and processing, the use of an endogenous positive control probe on each sample is absolutely essential. This probe is selected to be

TABLE 44-1

Controls for In Situ Hybridization

Control	Requirement	Purpose
Positive tissue control (handle as additional tissue sample)	1. Processed in manner identical to test tissue. 2. Contains known amount of target.	Positive results verify reaction of probe and detection reagents.
Positive probe control (use on each tissue)	1. Hybridizes with a target present in all tissues. 2. Labeled in similar manner to test probe and used at similar concentration.	Positive result verifies preservation of nucleic acid and availability to probe.
Negative probe control (use on each tissue)	1. Probe of similar base pair composition to test probe; should not hybridize to test and control tissues. 2. Labeled in similar manner to test probe and used at similar concentration.	Negative results monitor specificity of hybridization and detection.

Adapted with permission from Unger ER, Lee DR. In situ hybridization: principles and diagnostic applications in infection. J Histotechnol 1995;18:203–209.

positive on all tissues if the target nucleic acid has been adequately preserved and made available. This probe should be similar to the test probe in base pair composition, type of nucleic acid (i.e., oligonucleotide, double-stranded DNA, RNA, etc.), labeling, and final concentration. The positive control probe is designed to detect endogenous nucleic acid within the sample. An additional section of the patient tissue is hybridized with the positive control probe under conditions identical to those used for the test probe. If the positive control probe does not give positive results, a negative result for the test probe cannot be interpreted.

Adjustment of digestion conditions will often allow positive results to be obtained, but at times preservation is poor or tissues are so overfixed that the assay must be termed unsatisfactory. A positive result for the test probe under conditions that yielded negative results with the positive control probe can be interpreted with caution if all other components of the assay are valid and the negative control probe gives acceptable results.

Negative Probe Control

Because each patient sample is unique, unanticipated nonspecific interactions may occur with probe, detection reagents, or both. The negative control probe is used to monitor each patient sample for these potential problems. It is selected to be absent from all patient samples. Like the positive control probe, the negative control probe should be similar to the test probe in base pair composition, type of nucleic acid (i.e., oligonucleotide, double-stranded DNA, RNA, etc.), labeling, and final concentration. An additional section of the patient tissue is hybridized with the negative control probe under conditions identical to those used for the test probe.

Results of the assay cannot be interpreted unequivocally if there is color development with the negative control probe. A negative result does not ensure the specificity of the assay, which must be determined by validation studies, but serves as a guide to monitoring results in each run.

General Quality Control

The probe is central to the ISH assay, and clearly, accurate reproducible results will be obtained only when all reagents used during the assay are prepared and stored under controlled conditions. Dewaxing agents, buffers, protease, detection reagents, and substrates all will affect the quality of the final product. Changes in buffers and dewaxing agents should be noted in case variable results are seen, but testing prior to introducing new lots is not required.

Change in all other reagents requires comparison of new lot and old lot results to ensure reproducibility.

Assay Validation

Final responsibility for the validity of the ISH assay must be assumed by the laboratory performing the test. However, when significant components of the assay are supplied by a commercial vendor, especially in a kit format, good laboratory practice dictates that the majority of the potential problems of the assay have been addressed by the manufacturer. Nonetheless, some degree of individual laboratory validation of the assay is required, which can be addressed to some extent by the use of control tissues.

Ideally, results of the ISH assay should be validated by comparison to results obtained with different technology. In the example of an infectious agent, results of culture, immunohistochemistry, or polymerase chain reaction performed on a replicate sample could be compared to those obtained by ISH. Complete concordance between methods can never be expected, but this approach will allow the laboratory to demonstrate sensitivity and specificity of ISH relative to another currently used method. Participation in interlaboratory comparison programs is also recommended to allow the laboratory to see how its results compare with those of other laboratories using the same starting material.

Troubleshooting

Despite careful quality control, problems may occur in any assay. Appropriate controls will allow the laboratory to recognize that a problem exists with a particular assay, run, or tissue. Recognition is the key first step to solving the problem; troubleshooting can be thought of as comprising the subsequent steps to specifically identify and correct the problem.

Lack of Signal in Positive Control

Probably the simplest and most frustrating error is omission of one step or use of incorrect reagents in one step. This type of error is reduced with experience and may be almost eliminated with the introduction of automated methods. In most instances the problem will affect more than one sample in the run.

When an assay that has been working at an acceptable level suddenly no longer works, or works with reduced signal, the probe and detection reagents should be first suspected. Out-of-date reagents cannot be used reliably. Change of lot can alter results. New lots of any crucial reagent should be carefully introduced with side by side comparison to old lots. This will allow the laboratory to pinpoint the problem prior to introduction of the faulty reagent. This not only eliminates errors on patient material, it also presents cogent evidence to the manufacturer when the problem occurs with commercial reagents. Buffers and dewaxing agents are less likely sources of error, but should not be overlooked.

No Signal with Endogenous Positive Control Probe

No signal with an endogenous positive control probe is the most frequently observed problem in ISH assays performed on diagnostic tissue samples. Assuming control tissues give the expected results with the positive control probe, the lack of signal in a test sample reflects either inadequate preservation of target or inadequate pretreatment to make the target available. Obviously if the target is degraded, nothing can be done. Increasing concentration of protease, time, and temperature of digestion may all be attempted to improve detection.

For optimal sensitivity, each test tissue should be assayed initially using only the endogenous control probe to verify and optimize the conditions of pretreatment. The endogenous positive control probe is repeated in subsequent assays, including test probes, to validate the conditions of that assay.

Signal in Negative Controls

Signal in the negative control tissue or in patient tissue with negative probe control prevents unequivocal interpretation of the hybridization result. This problem could result from endogenous histochemical enzyme, nonspecific binding of detection reagent, or nonspecific binding of probe. Repeating the assay with hybridization cocktail only (no probe) on one slide and omission of detection reagent on another slide will pinpoint which of these problems is present. If the slide with no detection reagent generates signal, the problem must be due to endogenous histochemical enzyme. If the slide hybridized with cocktail only generates signal, the problem is attributable to nonspecific sticking of detection reagents. If the problem is eliminated by omission of probe, then nonspecific sticking of probe is the cause.

Nonspecific Binding of Probe

Nonspecific binding of probe is the most frequently encountered explanation for signal in negative controls. Nonspecific binding of probe in most instances reflects low stringency conditions in hybridization and/or wash. The probe may be used at a concentration that is too high, or the time of hybridization may be too long. Drying of tissue during the hybridization reaction will result in very high nonspecific sticking of probe. Adjusting these conditions and repeating the assay will generally solve the problem.

Nonspecific Binding of Detection Reagents

Nonspecific binding of detection reagents, resulting in spurious signal, can occur as the result of interaction between charged cellular components and the antibody or avidin molecules directing localization of the histochemical enzyme. An isolated instance of this problem can be attributed to inefficient washing or elevated time or temperature of incubation with detection reagents. Eliminating a more systematic problem may require trying alternative suppliers of reagents, increasing the salt or protein block during the incubation, or switching to a different approach for detection.

Endogenous Enzyme Activity

When the signal is generated by histochemical enzymes, any enzyme activity remaining in the tissues will contribute to the signal. Endogenous enzyme activity is not commonly encountered in the paraffin-embedded tissues used for hybridization because of the harsh conditions of tissue fixation, processing, and hybridization. However, tissue with very high levels of enzymes, such as the alkaline phosphatase in placenta, may retain enough activity to be detectable in the negative control. Increasing acid treatment may eliminate the problem, but in some instances switching to a different histochemical enzyme may be required.

Tissue Loss

Overdigestion of tissues will cause poor morphology and result in increased tissue loss. Digestion conditions should be adjusted to the minimum required for probe penetrance.

CHAPTER 45

Parentage and HLA Testing Using DNA Polymorphisms

HERBERT F. POLESKY

Tests for DNA polymorphism make it possible to establish relatedness between individuals with greater specificity than is obtainable with the large battery of tests based on classic methods (blood group antigens, serum proteins, red cell enzymes, and HLA serology) that routinely have been used for determining parentage. DNA-based test methods for genetic markers can be used on cellular material obtained from many sources stored under a wide variety of conditions, thus eliminating dependence on whole blood or fresh tissue samples. These methods also make it possible to determine differences at a molecular level for HLA markers previously defined as a single entity by serologic techniques. Matching organ and tissue donors and recipients using information based on similarity of critical sequences in the HLA region may have a significant impact on the future of transplantation.

Selection of Assays

Assays for DNA polymorphism vary, from methods to detect a change in a single amino acid in a sequence to changes in the patterns observed in VNTR (variable number of tandem repeats) fragments obtained from minisatellites on several chromosomes (1). In selecting an assay for use in parentage testing it is important that it meet all the usual criteria for reproducibility and reliability. In addition, it is also important that the method and reagents be available in more than one laboratory because independent confirmation of a result must be possible (2). Ideally, any assay used is based on a well-documented principle which has been validated with regard to specificity, sensitivity, sample requirement, and so forth.

A DNA system used for parentage testing should meet several specific requirements, some of which are dictated by the use of the results to report mathematical comparisons with other individuals in a defined population group. The chromosomal location should be known and recorded by the International Gene Mapping Workshop. Family studies using the marker must be done to determine that the inheritance pattern follows expected mendelian rules (2,3). Studies should be done to document the frequency of mutation and/or recombination at the locus. Ideally, the rates of mutation and recombination will be very low, and to be useful should not exceed 0.1.

Many molecular methods are available for typing the various loci coding for HLA specificities. The selection of a procedure will depend on the type of resolution (low, intermediate, or comprehensive) needed to provide clinical data. Molecular methods are helpful for typing of patients and family members for solid organ or bone marrow transplantation, classifying individuals for unrelated donor registries, and in studies of disease association. Although many different techniques are used, including RFLP, gene amplification, and sequencing, the discussion in this chapter will be limited to general quality assurance and quality controls that are applicable, regardless of the specific test format.

Restriction Fragment Length Polymorphism (RFLP) Assays

One of the most useful types of genetic marker for determining parentage is a single locus VNTR or minisatellite region. Made up of 500 to 10,000 base pairs, these chromosomal regions differ in the number of smaller repeat core sequences present in an individual (4). The inheritance of these regions is similar to alleles of functional genes. At defined loci the number of possible alleles is large, so the frequency of any single allele is small. Thus, these marker systems are very polymorphic and have powers of exclusion (chance to prove nonparentage) that range between 0.6 to greater than 0.9. Tests for these markers depend on extraction of non-degraded high-molecular-weight DNA that is then digested with a specific restriction endonuclease. After electrophoresis and Southern blotting, bands are identified with a labeled probe.

If an RFLP system is used for parentage testing, there should be published documentation of the loci, the restriction endonucleases, and the probes used to detect the polymorphism. The range of variable band sizes to be expected in the system and the occurrence of constant bands must be determined. The standard operating procedure (SOP) should detail the conditions used for each step in the test.

After extraction, the amount of DNA in the sample is adjusted and a measured amount is restricted. A test gel or other method must be used to ensure complete digestion of the DNA. Because there may be lot-to-lot variability in restriction enzymes, each new lot of enzyme should be tested with known samples to determine if the number and size of bands is as expected. The preparation of gels, the amount of restricted DNA added and the conditions of electrophoresis should be standardized. Variations in gel concentration, electric field, and time of electrophoresis can change the position of the bands and prevent resolution of two closely spaced bands or result in small bands being lost. To control for these variables, it is essential to run size markers with each group of samples tested (5). Multiple discrete size markers should span the range of the alleles usually found in the system. A human DNA control is also required. Samples from two individuals with different size fragments can increase the utility of this type of control. For many systems NIST-certified K562 sizing markers are available to be used as additional controls. In parentage testing, the samples from the trio (mother, child, alleged father) should be tested together on the same gel. In addition, the AABB Standards require that coelectrophoresis be performed on samples of individuals whose relationship is at issue (2).

The various steps and reagents used in the detection of the restriction fragments should be documented. New lots of membranes used for blotting should be evaluated to be sure all expected bands are present. If the probes are labeled inhouse, it is important to establish criteria to determine if they are sensitive for the amount of DNA in the samples. New lots of probe must be tested to ensure expected bands are detected.

Sizing RFLP Bands and Determination of Paternity Index (PI)

A major concern for a laboratory using RFLP systems for determining if individuals are related is the sizing of the observed alleles (bands). Unlike most genetic systems with discrete alleles, the markers in RFLP systems (designated in kilo bases) are random. In cases of nonpaternity or when two individuals are unrelated, visual inspection of the membranes (colorimetric detection with an enzyme label) or exposed film (isotopic or chemiluminescent label) will usually show an obvious pattern indicating the absence of shared alleles (a non-match). In cases with exclusions, sizing is done mainly to maintain a record of which fragments were observed. In cases where bands are shared between two individuals, sizing becomes critical. It is difficult to determine if an individual who appears to have a single band is homozygous or is heterozygous for two alleles that vary by only one or two core repeats. Evaluation of the lane containing the coelectrophoresed sample is very important when the fragments may be of similar size. In some cases apparent homozygosity may be related to the location of the fragment on the gel. In some individuals the second band is missed because it is above or below the limits of the gel used for doing the Southern transfer. In rare cases when multiple loci are tested on a single membrane, alleles at the extremes of the size range for one loci may overlap with the expected fragments of the other loci. AABB Standards only require that sizing be done once; however, interpretation of results must be done twice (2). Thus, there should be a method in place to have the membranes reviewed or a comparison of the membrane and sizing data by a second individual.

Although parentage testing cannot prove relatedness, comparison of the frequency of the shared allele(s) with random individuals in a population is key to providing mathematical estimates that the tested persons are related. In paternity testing it is this comparison of alleles that is used to determine the paternity index (PI) and likelihood of paternity. The designation of the band size done by any measurement technique (manual, digitizer pad, video imaging, etc.) is subject to error and is not exactly reproducible when samples are retested. Thus, before using an RFLP loci for calculating a PI, each laboratory must determine two values for the test system, sigma (the reproducibility of band size on multiple assays) and delta (the ability of the test system to resolve two closely spaced alleles) (6).

Calculation of the PI depends on comparing the chance (x) of the tested man passing the obligatory paternal genes found in the child with the frequency (y) of similar markers in a random population (1). It is therefore important to select a database for each RFLP marker system that corresponds to the results obtained with the analytic system in use. A database determined from samples tested in your own laboratory is ideal. However, it is often difficult to obtain a sample size that is adequate for establishing a meaningful frequency set. If one chooses to use a database determined in another laboratory, then it is important to exchange samples with the other laboratory to determine that the analytic method used in your laboratory gives band sizes similar to those used to establish the database (5).

Two methods are used to determine the frequency of the observed RFLP band(s) for calculation of the PI. Using the delta value for a marker system, a bin size proportional to the size (kb) of the measured band is used to calculate the frequency (y) of the marker in the population. An alternate to the floating bin just described is to use fixed bins (4). In this approach the expected range of band sizes is divided into several equal bins. Determining y can be a problem when the measured band is located on or very near to a bin limit.

When determining whether individuals are related, samples from the individuals should be tested on the same gel. In cases of disputed parentage it is not unusual to test multiple men and/or children with the same women. Often the samples from additional individuals are obtained after the initial testing has been completed. In such cases the new trio should be tested together. Band sizes obtained on repeat testing of individuals should be compared with the prior tests. These should be close to the same size as observed on the prior test. If the size of the band on the repeat test is outside the bin (+/− delta) of the original test, then testing should be repeated. When an exclusion is observed, retesting (entire trio, tested man only) of the system is advisable to rule out the possibility of a sample mix-up.

Polymerase Chain Reaction (PCR) Amplification

The selection of DNA loci for parentage testing using PCR should meet the same criteria as those used for RFLP: be demonstrated by family studies to follow mendelian inheritance, have low rates of mutation and/or recombination, and be recorded by the International Human Gene Mapping Workshop (2,3). Additional criteria include documentation of the sequences of the primer pairs, the size(s) of the repeat and constant units, and the reaction conditions that ensure optimum and specific amplification.

The sample used for PCR analysis must be collected and processed to ensure that adequate undegraded DNA is available for testing. As minimal quantities of DNA are needed for PCR amplification, samples other than whole blood, such as buccal swabs and dried blood spots on filter paper, have been used for parentage testing. The success of using these small samples depends on having adequate instructions for personnel on the technique used to collect and identify each sample (i.e., multiple swabs from one individual), the method of drying the sample if necessary, and the preparation for shipping. The procedure used should ensure that samples are handled in a manner that will prevent contamination, tampering, or substitution. Each laboratory should validate these processes.

Quality control procedures must be set up for the pre-analytic steps used in PCR, including reagents and methods used for DNA extraction and restriction. Special care must be used to protect pre-amplification samples from contamination with post-amplification products (7).

In techniques used for HLA typing that include more than one amplification step, contamination related to PCR carryover is a potential source of error. The laboratory should be designed so that there are dedicated spaces for the preparation of PCR reagents (primers, buffers, master mix, controls, etc.), for DNA isolation from the specimen, and for preparation of the amplification reaction mixture. The sample amplification, product detection/analysis, and storage of post-amplified material must be done in a separate area.

The American Society for Histocompatibility and Immunogenetics (ASHI) Standards indicates that mandatory use of laminar flow or static air hoods for pre-amplification is an alternative to physical separation (7). They also specify the use of dedicated lab coats, gloves, and disposable supplies. Dedicated positive displacement pipets or filter-plugged tips must be used for each amplification step. There should be procedures established for frequent cleaning and/or treatment of work surfaces. Work areas should be routinely monitored for nucleic acid contamination. In addition to negative controls, open negative control tubes in the work area and wipe tests of the pre-amplification should run under the same assay conditions as the unknown samples (7).

The thermal cyclers used for parentage testing samples must be evaluated to assure wells have minimal variability. A human DNA control of known phenotype should be used to test the well-to-well variability. Periodic review of instrument performance should be documented. ASHI requires verification monthly that thermal cyclers are capable of precise and reproducible temperature maintenance (3). Records of calibration, routine maintenance, and repairs should be kept for each instrument. If more than one thermal cycler is used interchangeably, tests should be done to compare the quantity and quality of the amplified product from each instrument using a standardized set of reagents and samples (5). Similar testing should be done if a new instrument is obtained.

During testing by PCR several specific controls must be run with each batch of samples amplified. A negative control must be processed along with test specimens. This control is used to ensure that there has not been contamination of the PCR product. A human DNA control of known phenotype shall be tested with every amplification run. If the detection of the alleles at a locus requires an electrophoretic step of the amplification product, size markers with discrete fragments similar to the alleles usually observed must be used. Allelic ladders should contain fragments with known numbers of repeats that span the range of sizes expected at the loci. If a loci has alleles with heterogeneity of repeat lengths, resolution of fragments that differ by less than one repeat should be demonstrated by electrophoresis of a mixture of samples containing fragments that differ by less than one repeat. The ideal ladder should be composed of fragments that have been confirmed by sequence analysis or that have been compared to sequenced fragments. Allelic ladders should be placed on the gel so that they flank the unknown samples. The number of size marker lanes run should be sufficient to ensure the correct sizing of alleles in the unknowns. The AABB Standards requires that coelectrophoresis of DNA from individuals whose relationship is at issue shall be a routine part of quality assurance (2).

When doing HLA typing using molecular methods, the locus and alleles must be defined for each template/primer combination. Sequences must be compared with published databases from the WHO Nomenclature Committee for HLA (updated in *Tissue Antigens,* on the ASHI World Wide Web pages, or in *Human Immunology*) (7). Hybridization of probes with designated allele combinations must be established, and controls should be capable of detecting cross-hybridization with closely related sequences. ASHI Standards require that amplification reactions include procedures to detect technical failures (3). Internal controls such as additional primers or templates that result in a product that can be distinguished from the intended allele product will detect most failures caused by inhibitors or interfering substances.

Results from PCR testing, whether a dot blot, a strip membrane, autoradiograph, or a mini gel, shall be read and interpreted twice. Each reading should be done independently. If sequencing is used to obtain the primary data, ASHI suggests that the second independent interpretation could be the reading done using software (7). As with RFLP tests, sizing of the bands on a gel only needs to be done once. The designation of alleles should be based on the observed phenotype. Standardized nomenclature should be used rather than an arbitrary designation of the allele(s). When results are based on short tandem repeats, the allelic description should be based on the number of repeat units, if known.

Forensic testing results to determine if samples are from the same source are commonly reported as genotype. However, in tests evaluating the relatedness of individuals, the report should not indicate homozygosity (i.e., reporting two identical alleles) when it is only implied by the test result. Exclusion of parentage should not be based on findings at a single PCR locus (2). Calculation of the PI from loci determined by PCR should be based on the appropriate population and from data tables containing an adequate sample size for determination of allelic frequencies.

Reporting of Results

HLA typing results must designate the type of assay and indicate the MHC locus using the WHO-defined nomenclature (3). When reporting RFLP results, the name of the DNA locus tested as defined by the Nomenclature Committee of the International Human Gene Mapping Workshop and the restriction endonuclease used must be provided. When a marker is determined by PCR it is also important to use standardized nomenclature. The DNA commission of the International Society for Forensic Haemogenetics has published guidelines that include rules for designating STR alleles (8). Reporting of parentage test results should be based on the phenotype observed, not the implied genotype (2). If it is concluded that there is *not* a relationship between tested individuals, then the basis for the opinion must be provided. When testing fails to exclude a relationship between a child and the tested man, a combined paternity index as well as the individual system indices must be part of the report. A probability of paternity as a percentage and the prior probabilities used must also be included on the report. The methods used to calculate the index values and probability must be validated. If a computer program is used for these calculations or any other aspect of the reading and reporting of test results, it must be appropriately documented and validated.

Quality Management

Standards for parentage testing laboratories and histocompatibility testing have been published by AABB and ASHI. These documents form the basis for the inspection and accreditation (I&A) programs conducted by each organization. The College of American Pathologists (CAP) also inspects and accredits laboratories. Parentage testing using molecular techniques is included under the CAP molecular pathology check list. Participation in external proficiency testing programs is considered essential to obtaining accreditation. The AABB and CAP jointly sponsor a proficiency testing program for laboratories doing parentage testing. Unknown samples from a trio are provided 3 times a year. Test results on classic and DNA systems and calculation of PI, are evaluated based on a consensus of reporting laboratories. Paper problems covering HLA results and estimation of relatedness in special situations are also included. The ASHI and CAP jointly sponsor proficiency testing programs for HLA. These programs include evaluation of serologic tests as well as the use of molecular methods.

Laboratories doing parentage and/or HLA testing must establish programs for quality assessment and improvement. The AABB in addition to requiring documentation of standard operating procedures and policies also requires that an accredited laboratory develop and maintain a quality plan. Methods for ensuring ongoing self-assessment of case documents, performance thresholds, variance reports, and corrective actions taken are considered an essential part of quality management.

REFERENCES

1. Polesky HF. Blood groups, human leukocyte antigen and DNA polymorphism, and parentage testing. In: Henry JB, ed. Clinical diagnosis and management by laboratory methods. Philadelphia: WB Saunders, 1996:1413–1426.

2. American Association of Blood Banks. Standards for parentage testing laboratories. 3rd ed. Bethesda, MD: AABB, 1997.

3. American Society for Histocompatibility and Immunogenetics. Standards for histocompatibility testing. Lenexa, KS: ASHI, 1996.

4. National Research Council (USA). The evaluation of forensic DNA evidence. Committee on DNA Forensic Science: an update. Commission on Forensic Science: an update. Washington D.C., National Academy Press, 1996.

5. Walker RH, ed. Parentage testing accreditation requirements manual of the American Association of Blood Banks. 2nd ed. Bethesda, MD: AABB, 1995.
6. Endean DJ. RFLP analysis for paternity testing: observations and caveats. In: Proceedings of the 1989 International Symposium on Human Identification. Madison, WI: Promega Corporation, 1990:55–76.
7. Baxter-Lowe LA, Hurley C, Maurer D, et al. Responses to comments submitted to the DNA Standards Committee: 1996 revisions to DNA standards (section P). ASHI Q 1997;21: 24–29.
8. Olaison B, Bär W, Mayr W, et al. DNA recommendations 1997. ISFH Newslett June 1997; Annex 2:1–3.

CHAPTER 46

Molecular Assays for Genetic Diseases

WAYNE W. GRODY

The molecular diagnosis of genetic disease, typically accomplished by detection of a heritable germ line mutation or a surrogate polymorphic DNA marker linked to the mutation, presents a number of quality assurance considerations that are quite unique from the other applications of molecular pathology and immunopathology. Moreover, these considerations extend well beyond the technical aspects of test performance to encompass a wide range of pre- and post-analytic problems as well. Basic research findings are advancing more rapidly than in any of the other areas of laboratory medicine—and are being just as quickly translated to clinical application—so there has been scant time for the diagnostic procedures to mature in step with each successive research advance. It is not unusual for directors of diagnostic molecular genetics laboratories to read about the identification of a new, long sought-after disease gene in the pages of *Science* or *Nature Genetics* one week; to have ordered the relevant polymerase chain reaction (PCR) primers for amplification of the gene the very next week; then to start adapting these sequences into diagnostic reagents and begin offering the test to clinicians and patients shortly thereafter. Needless to say, this rapid interval of translation from the research laboratory to the clinical laboratory often does not allow sufficient time for development of reference standards, quality control procedures, or full clinical validation, let alone FDA licensure.

More than any of the other testing areas covered in this book, molecular genetics relies almost entirely on the use of "home brews" rather than manufactured kits, thus placing the onus of assuring quality performance exclusively on the laboratory rather than on a manufacturer or the FDA. The stakes for mishaps remain extraordinarily high. Molecular genetic diagnostic procedures almost always function as stand-alone tests, rather than as adjuncts to more traditional testing methods or as part of a panel as is often the case in immunohistochemistry or molecular oncology. Many of the disorders and carrier states being examined have no known or easily detectable morphologic or biochemical changes, and diagnosis relies wholly on detection of the mutation at the DNA level. Based on that finding alone, a patient may be labeled forever as a carrier of a recessive or dominant mutation, and a drastic and irreversible clinical intervention—such as pregnancy termination or mastectomy—may be exercised.

The incendiary combination of rapid introduction of new and unproved tests, dearth of quality control standards, and difficulty (or, in some cases, impossibility) of clinical validation has drawn concern from a number of medical, legal, psychosocial, and lay constituencies. An advisory body composed of representatives of each of these stakeholders has been established to examine these issues and make recommendations for improvement of the quality of delivery and appropriate use of all genetic tests, of which molecular genetic tests are just one part (the others being cytogenetic tests and biochemical genetic tests). This group, designated the Task Force on Genetic Testing, was convened in 1995 under the auspices of the NIH-DOE Working Group on Ethical, Legal, and

Social Implications (ELSI) of Human Genome Research. At time of this writing, a set of Interim Principles has been published and circulated to a broader professional and lay audience for commentary; finalization and implementation of the recommendations is expected to be an ongoing process for some time.

Rather than develop all of its guidelines de novo, the Task Force has sought input from numerous professional organizations and the FDA, which already have working quality assurance standards in this area. For example, this author serves on the Task Force as a representative of the College of American Pathologists (CAP), which has in place an extensive set of laboratory accreditation guidelines and proficiency testing programs in molecular genetics (see below). In a field moving forward as rapidly as this one, it is probably unrealistic to expect any single set of standards to remain fixed and accepted for very long; they must continue to be modified and updated to incorporate the latest technological developments, scientific discoveries, and legislative directives.

Unique Clinical Applications of Diagnostic Molecular Genetics

One reason diagnostic molecular genetics is so often more problematic than the other areas of molecular testing derives from the nature of its clinical applications. These lie in four main categories (**Table 46-1**), only one of which has any analogy with the other subdisciplines of molecular pathology or indeed with the rest of laboratory medicine in general.

Diagnostic Genetic Testing

Diagnostic genetic testing is the paradigm already most familiar to general laboratorians. It is performed on an individual who shows clinical symptoms or signs of a particular disorder or set of disorders, and the purpose of the testing is to definitively confirm the clinical impression and/or rule out other candidates in the differential diagnosis. Because powerful contemporary molecular analytic techniques such as PCR work on fixed or dead cells, this application can also be used postmortem or on stored biopsy tissues if a fresh specimen from the patient is not available. This application probably carries the least degree of psychosocial risk, and hence ethical concerns, of any in genetics, because patients who are already symptomatic are less likely to be shocked, emotionally devastated, or newly stigmatized by having a diagnostic label placed on their condition (or at least no more so than those undergoing biopsy and standard surgical pathology diagnosis of a lesion).

TABLE **46-1**

Clinical Applications of Diagnostic Molecular Genetics

Diagnosis/Confirmation of clinical impression
Carrier screening
Prenatal diagnosis
Presymptomatic diagnosis/Predisposition testing

Carrier Screening

Carrier screening refers to detection of recessive mutations in healthy individuals for purposes of reproductive planning. This application carries greater psychosocial and societal risk, as healthy individuals may learn that they are somehow "defective." Even though the presence of a recessive mutation will never adversely affect an individual's own health, and it is estimated that all of us carry five or six of them, the consequences of this discovery can be considerable. Cases of such individuals being subjected to insurance or employment discrimination have been documented (1).

Moreover, as will be discussed in more detail subsequently, the quality assurance issues differ, depending on the setting and purpose of the carrier screening. This application can be subdivided into screening of those individuals with a family history of the disorder, and population-based screening of large numbers of individuals who have no family history but may be at risk of the disorder because of its prevalence within their ethnic group.

With family history of a disorder, the screening is generally more straightforward, as the medical need is readily apparent and the a priori risk appreciable (e.g., 50% for the sibling of an affected patient). Furthermore, for a mutationally heterogeneous disease, the availability of the affected index case increases the chance of identifying the particular mutation in that family, making subsequent screening of relatives very easy and virtually 100% sensitive. Nevertheless, numerous studies have shown that many relatives of affected patients do not care to be tested, and may recruit a variety of psychological defense mechanisms for interpreting and dealing with their a priori risk (2). Even without an identified mutation in the index case, the availability of the family unit may permit carrier testing by linkage analysis or chromosome haplotyping.

In population screening, in contrast, one does not know going into the testing which particular mutation(s) to test for, and the absence of affected family members precludes linkage analysis. For disease genes with a large number of mutations, such as the cystic fibrosis transmembrane conductance regulator (CFTR), even screening for many DNA sequence changes using a large panel of allele-specific oligonucleotide (ASO) probes will yield suboptimal carrier detection sensitivity in a general population, making genetic counseling of those testing negative quite complex and problematic (3–5).

Prenatal Diagnosis

Prenatal diagnosis is a particularly unique endeavor to medical genetics. Often the end result of a population carrier screening program, it is performed for many other indications as well. The availability of specific gene probes has allowed for the prenatal detection of many single-gene defects that formerly were difficult or impossible to ascertain in the fetus.

The amniocytes obtained from the most commonly used fetal sampling procedure, amniocentesis, are derived from skin fibroblasts and thus do not express the relevant protein products of a number of organ-specific disorders. For example, diagnosis of Duchenne muscular dystrophy at the protein level using antibodies against dystrophin would require a fetal muscle biopsy, a technically difficult and risky procedure. But as amniocytes, like all nucleated cells, contain the full complement of the fetal genome, they are perfectly adequate substrates for diagnosis at the DNA level. (Note: for tests requiring Southern blotting, the amniocytes will usually need to be cultured first to obtain sufficient DNA for analysis; PCR-based tests can be performed directly on the uncultured amniocentesis specimen.)

However, it should be kept in mind that fetal specimens entail a number of unusual considerations, not least of which is that they represent the cells of one individual isolated from the body of another (the mother), necessitating the incorporation of certain quality control procedures not required in other forms of molecular genetic testing. For example, there should be a protocol in place, using either visual inspection and/or DNA fingerprinting analysis, by which the laboratory can ensure against false results due to maternal cell contamination of amniocentesis and chorionic villus samples.

Prenatal diagnosis raises serious and controversial ethical issues surrounding the indications for abortion based on the results of testing. Thus, the laboratory must be cognizant at all times about the appropriateness of prenatal test ordering in this context.

Predisposition DNA Testing

Presymptomatic DNA testing is applied primarily to late-onset dominant disorders such as Huntington's disease and familial breast cancer. Although this type of genetic testing is relatively straightforward and prognostically valuable for such disorders as multiple endocrine neoplasia (6), when applied to disorders such as Huntington's disease and breast cancer, the psychosocial and ethical problems present the greatest challenge of any diagnostic molecular genetic test. Reporting out positive results can carry substantial risk of severe adverse consequences, including patient suicide (7). Even the ultimate clinical implications of a positive test result may be unclear; major but inappropriate medical and surgical interventions might be undertaken on the basis of the test's results.

Such findings also have important economic implications, especially in the realm of health and life insurance, employment, and general life planning. Discovery of a heritable mutation in an individual can exert these same adverse effects, by proxy, on other members of the tested person's extended family, none of whom may have consented to this type of examination.

On the other side of the coin, for many of these disorders the technology currently available is still not capable of detecting all possible mutations in the involved genes, engendering a new and dangerous kind of "false negative." For all these reasons, presymptomatic testing is subject to some of the most stringent quality assurance procedures in all of laboratory medicine and, for some disorders, should not even be performed at all outside of a carefully designed research protocol (8).

General Molecular Genetics Laboratory Quality Assurance

Several general concerns for quality assurance in the diagnostic molecular genetics laboratory are quite similar to those that should be in place within any DNA diagnostic laboratory (they are discussed at greater length elsewhere in this volume). Among these are the need for adequate physical separation of pre- and post-PCR activities, the use of appropriate positive and negative and sensitivity controls, adherence to standard containment guidelines for work with recombinant DNA, systems for monitoring the completeness of restriction endonuclease digestions, and so on. These procedures are described in detail in the inspection checklists and guidelines for molecular pathology and molecular genetics published by the CAP, the American College of Medical Genetics (ACMG), the National Committee on Clinical Laboratory Standards (NCCLS), and others. One or more of these checklists will need to be used for inspection and accreditation by any laboratory performing DNA-based testing in the genetics area as well as the broader discipline of molecular pathology. The remainder of this chapter will focus on those quality assurance concerns that are more unique to the molecular diagnosis and screening of genetic disease.

Test Validation

As was already mentioned, a substantial proportion of the tests performed in molecular genetics laboratories are of the "home brew" variety, and thus a greater responsibility for demonstrating validity of the procedures falls on the laboratory itself. Many people divide test validation into two types: analytical validation and clinical validation. The former reflects the accuracy, precision, and sensitivity of the technical procedure itself as performed in any particular laboratory, while the latter involves the predictive value of a positive or negative result, assuming it was accurately obtained. Establishing analytical validation requires the robust adaptation of findings in the literature to the individual laboratory bench and comparison of the results with those of some predicate procedure, if available, or with those of an external expert laboratory with which a set of pilot samples are split. Analytical validation of molecular genetic techniques more often takes the form of the latter, as more traditional methods for these analytes are usually not available (i.e., the DNA test is the only way to determine presence or absence of the mutation). In addition, the laboratory may test specimens from patients known to have the disease and from normal control individuals, looking for correlation of mutation detection with the former group only, though this approach can be problematic owing to genetic heterogeneity, reduced penetrance, and presence of benign DNA polymorphisms (see below).

Clinical validation is notoriously difficult in some areas of genetic testing, owing to a number of unusual features in the basic biology of the genes and diseases being examined (**Table 46-2**). These features can compromise both the positive and negative predictive value of the test. Many mutations, especially in dominant disorders, are not fully penetrant: not every person carrying the mutation will actually express the disease phenotype. So even a test that is working perfectly at the technical level, detecting a particular mutation in 100% of individuals carrying it, may not always reliably predict the appearance of disease. Mutations in the BRCA1 gene, for example, show a penetrance of about 80% to 85% (9,10), meaning that even the accurate detection of a mutation will not predict breast cancer in a substantial fraction of those women testing positive. Furthermore, for late-onset disorders, the interval between DNA testing and appearance of symptoms (if they are to appear at all) is measured in years or even decades, so practical clinical validation may not even be possible within a reasonable time-frame of test development.

Even for many early-onset and recessive diseases, determining positive predictive value can be difficult because the genotype-phenotype correlations are not constant. In

TABLE 46-2

Problems in Clinical Validation of Molecular Genetic Tests

Reduced penetrance
Long delay between testing and disease onset
Genetic heterogeneity
Population polymorphisms
Variable genotype-phenotype correlations

cystic fibrosis (CF), for example, while there is some correlation between particular mutations and the presence or absence of pancreatic insufficiency (11), other genetic indicators of disease severity and onset have been inconsistent (12); even some patients homozygous for the classic "severe" mutation, ΔF508, have had minimal lung disease (13). This makes genetic counseling, especially in the prenatal setting, fairly difficult.

The triplet repeat expansion mutation of Huntington's disease (14) and the premutation expansion of fragile X syndrome (15) exhibit "gray areas" of intermediate expansion that may or may not predict disease in patients and offspring, respectively. In fragile X syndrome, and possibly in other diseases as well, even the presence of a definite full mutation may not be sufficient to cause disease; a secondary chemical alteration (methylation) of the DNA region, not reflected in its primary nucleotide sequence, is required (16). Presumably by a similar mechanism, the sex of the parent in whom a mutation is found may confer markedly different risks of its pathologic expression in the offspring, a phenomenon known as imprinting (17,18).

Many large genes, such as CFTR and BRCA1, may also contain nucleotide changes that are not true mutations at all but benign polymorphisms (19). For this reason, validation of a laboratory test for a mutation not previously reported requires either very long clinical follow-up or survey for the DNA change in a large number of normal individuals. And in still other disorders, the correlation between DNA marker and disease remains too loose to ever achieve high positive predictive value, no matter how many individuals are studied or how long the clinical follow-up (e.g., apoE genotyping for Alzheimer's disease risk [20]).

The utility of a negative test result is likewise difficult to evaluate for diseases caused by complex genetic determinants, owing to the phenomenon of genetic heterogeneity. This can be due to more than one gene causing the same disease (e.g., familial breast cancer, tuberous sclerosis) or the presence of more than one (sometimes hundreds) mutant allele of the same gene in the population (e.g., cystic fibrosis). Thus, a woman with a strong family history of breast cancer who tests negative for a panel of BRCA1 mutations may actually carry a mutation in BRCA2 or a mutation in BRCA1 that was not part of the testing panel.

Validation of tests for such diseases must take into account the overall carrier detection rate of the gene or mutation panel being used, and this will often vary dramatically depending on the ethnic origin of those being tested. For example, the ΔF508 mutation accounts for as many as 87% of CF carriers in some northern European groups but <10% in many Asian and Amerindian groups (21). Of course, one can increase the sensitivity of any of these tests to virtually 100% by first requiring testing of a known affected index case to identify a particular family's mutation, which can then be used as a specific test for subsequent screening of unaffected relatives; but, unfortunately, such an approach is not applicable to population screening.

Finally, there are those tests that do not directly detect mutations at all but rather nonpathologic polymorphic DNA markers *linked* to a disease gene. Such tests by definition can never achieve 100% predictive value because of the chance of random crossover events between the gene and marker disrupting the linkage phase.

Internal Test Validation and Quality Assurance

In this section we consider those steps that the individual diagnostic molecular genetics laboratory must take to ensure that its own results are of the highest possible accuracy and reproducibility. These steps will occur *after* the laboratory director has decided to offer a particular test, based on his or her critical reading of the literature regarding the correlation of the DNA marker with the disease (sometimes called *external* validation). As before, only those aspects particularly unique to DNA-based genetic disease testing will be discussed here.

Standards and Controls

As in other areas of molecular pathology, the inclusion of appropriate positive and negative controls is essential for proper performance and interpretation of molecular genetic tests. Obtaining them can be a problem in some cases, however. Because most of the tests are home brews, commercial standards are not always readily available. DNA samples, either genomic or cloned fragments, containing some of the more common mutations of the CFTR and other important disease genes can be purchased from such sources as the Coriell Institute and the American Type Culture Collection; however, securing positive controls for the rarer mutations included in some test panels may be more difficult. Of course, small DNA fragments containing any desired mutation can be prepared by oligonucleotide synthesis, and at least one commercial supplier (BioVentures, Inc., Murfreesboro, TN) specializes in marketing such custom controls. One can also try to procure rare mutant DNAs from research laboratories that have collected and studied patient samples.

For large and varied mutation test panels, it may not be possible to either obtain or include positive controls for every rare mutation in every test run. Indeed, few labs testing for 30 or more CFTR mutations routinely include all such controls. Although this practice may appear to violate a basic tenet of quality control, it may be justified by the impracticality and/or expense of such an approach and because the population frequency of the rarest mutations is significantly below the expected false-negative rate. There is also a danger in PCR-based genetic testing of repeatedly amplifying mutant controls in run after run, as it increases the risk of false-positive results due to amplicon contamination (22).

Some ASO-based testing methods, especially those employing reverse dot blot hybridization, incorporate a sort of internal control for false-negatives in that probes for both the mutant and wild-type alleles are included, and at least one of them should produce a hybridization signal in every carrier screening test (23). Some type of sensitivity control should also be included in every test as a monitor that there was sufficient target DNA, and absence of PCR inhibitors, for amplification to proceed to a detectable level. CAP guidelines further state that, for any test in which absence of a PCR product is one of the possible diagnostic results, coamplification of the specimen with another set of primers specific for some "housekeeping gene" (e.g., actin) should be employed.

Another type of standard important in all gel-based DNA tests is the size marker. Whereas for many applications in molecular pathology the commercially available DNA fragment ladders (e.g., a *Hin*dIII digest of lambda bacteriophage DNA) are adequate for sizing of the test DNA bands, some genetic disease tests require much finer band size determination than is achieved by semilogarithmic plotting against a size standard. For example, it is crucial that the trinucleotide repeat expansion mutations of Huntington's disease, especially those that fall within the range of 30 to 45 repeats, be sized accurately to the exact repeat number (i.e., down to the level of three nucleotides). The smaller premutations of the FMR-1 gene of fragile X syndrome also require accurate sizing for meaningful reproductive genetic counseling. This goal is best achieved not with commercial size standards but by constructing and running in each electrophoresis gel a homemade ladder composed of a series of expansion mutations of known repeat length, derived from previously tested patient specimens.

Clinical Follow-Up

As alluded to above, no one expects each diagnostic molecular genetics laboratory to reinvent the wheel and establish clinical validity of every test it offers; instead, this determination is gleaned from literature review and from the general standard of practice as promulgated by professional organizations. However, the individual laboratory must have an ongoing program to make some reasonable effort at verifying its results by clinical correlation and follow-up whenever possible. This may involve simply noting the findings of ancillary clinical or laboratory findings, such as sweat chloride test results in a patient undergoing CFTR mutation testing. It should be more formalized in prenatal testing, where some effort should be made to confirm positive results in a tissue or blood sample from the abortus or newborn.

Proficiency Testing

An important measure of a laboratory's quality can be derived by comparing its performance with peer laboratories doing the same test. This is the principle behind proficiency testing (PT), in which identical sample unknowns are sent to many laboratories and the results reported and compared. Such programs are especially valuable in revealing consistent, repetitive errors that may otherwise go unnoticed by the laboratory (low accuracy, high precision). In another sense, PT is merely a more formal and widespread version of the strategy of splitting pilot samples with another expert laboratory during initial test validation.

An accepted and widely subscribed national PT program in molecular genetic testing now exists, administered jointly by the CAP and the ACMG (24). It consists of surveys mailed to participating laboratories twice a year, each of which contains several challenges. Because there are so many genetic diseases for which DNA testing is possible, and no two laboratories will offer exactly the same test menu, marketing surveys have been conducted to determine the diseases most widely tested so that challenges for those can be offered on a regular basis. Thus, every PT packet contains unknown samples for at least two of the following diseases: cystic fibrosis, sickle cell anemia, Duchenne muscular dystrophy, fragile X syndrome, and Huntington's disease. The marketing surveys are repeated periodically so that newly emerging disorders that become popular testing targets, such as factor V Leiden, can be added to the PT program in a timely fashion. It is recognized that laboratories may use different techniques to test for the same disease, and the CAP does not specify any particular method to be used in the PT surveys. Indeed, one of the greatest values of the program is to ascertain which methods are most favored and most accurate among all the participating laboratories nationwide, based on the survey results.

CLIA regulations specify that a laboratory must participate in a PT program covering every analyte for which it tests. Unfortunately, unlike the CAP's other molecular pathology surveys for such applications as paternity testing and immunoglobulin gene rearrangements in which every participating laboratory performs the same test, there will always be molecular genetics laboratories offering rare disease tests that are not covered by the PT program. It is simply not practical or cost-effective to construct PT surveys for every rare disease or even every rare mutation in the more common diseases (e.g., CF). Partly for this reason, a generic linkage test has been offered, employing a DNA probe or PCR primers supplied in the packet, which can be performed by those laboratories that do not test for any of the diseases included in that survey. Also included with each of the challenges are a number of interpretive and genetic counseling questions relevant to the test results, reflecting the importance of pre- and post-analytic factors in molecular genetic testing.

Laboratory Accreditation

In addition to PT, molecular genetics laboratories must participate in onsite inspections by a recognized or deemed agency. Inspection checklists developed by the CAP, ACMG, and several individual states are more stringent and more specific to molecular procedures than the federal CLIA regulations. But regardless of which checklist is used, it is important that the inspectors be knowledgeable in both molecular diagnostics and human genetics. The inspectors are expected to pay attention to all aspects of quality control and should examine actual patient electrophoresis and hybridization photos and autoradiograms, report forms (see below), and PT results. Laboratories unable to pass inspection or correct their deficiencies are reported to the Health Care Financing Administration (HCFA) as part of a registry that becomes a matter of public record.

Personnel Qualifications

There has been much controversy over staffing of molecular genetics laboratories at both the technical and directorial levels. Because current medical technologist training programs include little or no exposure to either human genetics concepts or molecular biologic techniques, medical technologist certification has not been considered essential or even necessarily desirable for the staff personnel performing these tests. In actual practice, most of the technical staff in these laboratories have come from molecular biology research backgrounds. Efforts are under way to develop a certification mechanism for molecular genetics/molecular pathology technicians to recognize this special expertise and experience, as has been available for some time in the cytogenetics field.

For laboratory directors, there is already a recognized board certification mechanism in clinical molecular genetics, administered by the American Board of Medical Genetics (ABMG). Controversy has arisen, however, over its exclusion of molecular pathologists who are competent to perform and interpret these tests yet have access to no similar certification mechanism under the American Board of Pathology (ABP) (25). At time of this writing, there is some movement toward development of a joint board examination in this laboratory specialty, coadministered by the ABP and ABMG and open to both geneticists and pathologists who have completed an acceptable period of training in the area.

Appropriateness of Test Ordering and Reporting

Because of the numerous ethical dilemmas raised by molecular genetic testing, impinging on such matters as genetic privacy, abortion, insurability, stigmatization, and eugenics, laboratories must remain cognizant of the reasons for each of their test requests and be prepared to question or reject those that appear inappropriate under recognized practice guidelines. Making such judgments requires seasoned knowledge of the technical, molecular biologic, and psychosocial aspects of each test on the menu.

Even though its performance might be perfectly straightforward at the technical level, a request for Huntington's disease testing on a 10-year-old child, for example, should elicit at the very least a questioning call by the lab director to the ordering physician. Similar calls should be prompted by any other request that appears either genetically inappropriate or ethically dubious; examples include a request for prenatal diagnosis of CF when only one parent's CFTR mutation can be detected, a request for BRCA1 mutation screening in a woman without a strong family history of breast cancer, or a request for CF carrier screening in an asymptomatic child.

Concern has also been raised about the potential for molecular genetic testing being performed without the patient's knowledge or approval, using sensitive amplification techniques to retrieve DNA from archival specimens originally obtained for other purposes (26).

Because of the complexity in molecular genetic test indications and interpretation, requisitions for these tests must contain more information than would be required for most other clinical laboratory tests. For example, a detailed pedigree is needed for any linkage study, and ethnic information is required for deciding the appropriate mutation screening panel to use—or even whether to test at all—for many diseases. For certain emotionally charged predictive tests such as Huntington's disease or BRCA1 and BRCA2, documentation of informed consent may be required.

Report forms for molecular genetic tests must also provide much more information, often in free text form, than more conventional laboratory tests. It is not sufficient to state merely that a particular mutation was found or not; the report must indicate the risk of the mutation being associated with disease or the residual risk of disease if the mutation was not found, all discussed in the context of its inheritance pattern, mutational mechanism, and penetrance. Recommendations for genetic counseling about the result should be included when appropriate. The laboratory must also have a protocol in place for dealing with inadvertent revelation of nonpaternity in a molecular genetic study of a family.

Given the significant potential for adverse psychosocial and economic consequences of molecular genetic testing, serious consideration must be given to maintaining the confidentiality of the test results. In some cases, at the patient's discretion, the results may even be withheld from the medical record and conveyed only to the patient. This is standard practice in Huntington's disease testing, for example. Yet at the same time we must guard against becoming so paranoid over patient privacy that potentially life-saving medical information is no longer accessible to consulting health care providers.

Some of the concerns over genetic discrimination in health insurance may become moot if a more national system of health care evolves; however, the potential for personal stigmatization of those testing positive for mutations will still remain. For all these reasons, the molecular genetics laboratory must maintain an extremely close relationship with referring physicians and genetic counselors, distinguished by frequent communication during the ordering and reporting phases of test performance.

Conclusion

The ethical ramifications of molecular genetic testing are numerous and difficult, arguably exceeding in complexity those of any other area of contemporary medical practice. They have warranted the creation of the ELSI arm of the

Human Genome Project and sparked the recent formation of a President-appointed National Bioethics Advisory Commission. They have given pause to all of us involved in genetic test ordering and performance, and have placed genetics practitioners in the center of the raging national debates over health care reform, abortion rights, and invasion of privacy.

Yet it is safe to say that these challenges, though often contentious, have not dampened our excitement over the tremendous beneficial potential of molecular genetic technology. This powerful new method of diagnosis has already revolutionized the practice of clinical genetics, and should continue to dramatically transform all of laboratory medicine in the years to come.

REFERENCES

1. Billings PR, Kohn MA, de Cuevas M, et al. Discrimination as a consequence of genetic testing. Am J Hum Genet 1992;50:476–482.
2. Fanos JH, Johnson JP. Perception of carrier status by cystic fibrosis siblings. Am J Hum Genet 1995; 57:431–438.
3. Tsui L-C. The spectrum of cystic fibrosis mutations. Trends Genet 1992;8:393–398.
4. Williamson R. Universal community carrier screening for cystic fibrosis? Nat Genet 1993;3: 195–201.
5. Tatsugawa Z, Fox MA, Fang C, et al. Education and testing strategy for large-scale cystic fibrosis carrier screening. J Genet Couns 1994;3:279–289.
6. Lips CJM, Landsvater RM, Hoppener JWM, et al. Clinical screening as compared with DNA analysis in families with multiple endocrine neoplasia type 2A. N Engl J Med 1994;331:828–835.
7. Hersch S, Jones R, Koroshetz W, Quaid K. The neurogenetics genie: testing for the Huntington's disease mutation. Neurology 1994;44:1369–1373.
8. Collins 1996.
9. Easton DF, Bishop DT, Ford D, et al. Genetic linkage analysis in familial breast and ovarian cancer: results from 214 families. Am J Hum Genet 1993;52:678–701.
10. Biesecker BB, Boehnke M, Calzone K, et al. Genetic counseling for families with inherited susceptibility to breast and ovarian cancer. JAMA 1993;269:1970–1974.
11. Kerem B-S, Rommens JM, Buchanan JA, et al. Identification of the cystic fibrosis gene: genetic analysis. Science 1989;245:1073–1080.
12. Cystic Fibrosis Genotype-Phenotype Consortium. Correlation between genotype and phenotype in patients with cystic fibrosis. N Engl J Med 1993;329:1308–1313.
13. Burke W, Aitken ML, Chen S-H, Scott R. Variable severity of pulmonary disease in adults with identical cystic fibrosis mutations. Chest 1992; 102:506–509.
14. Goldberg YP, Kremer B, Andrew SE, et al. Molecular analysis of new mutations for Huntington's disease: intermediate alleles and sex of origin effects. Nat Genet 1993;5:174–179.
15. Fu Y-H, Kuhl DP, Pizzuti A, et al. Variation of the CGG repeat at the fragile X site results in genetic instability: resolution of the Sherman paradox. Cell 1991;67:1047–1058.
16. McConkie-Roswell A, Lachiewicz AM, Spiridigliozzi GA, et al. Evidence that methylation of the FMR-1 locus is responsible for variable phenotypic expression of the fragile X syndrome. Am J Hum Genet 1993;53:800–809.
17. Lerer I, Meiner V, Pashut-Lavon I, Abeliovich D. Molecular diagnosis of Prader-Willi syndrome: parent-of-origin dependent methylation sites and nonisotopic detection of $(CA)_2$ dinucleotide repeat polymorphisms. Am J Med Genet 1994; 52:79–84.
18. Ranen NG, Stine OC, Abbott MH, et al. Anticipation and instability of IT-15 $(CAG)_N$ repeats in parent-offspring pairs with Huntington disease. Am J Hum Genet 1995;57:593–602.
19. Zielenski J, Tsui L-C. Cystic fibrosis: genotypic and phenotypic variations. Ann Rev Genet 1995; 29:777–807.
20. Corder EH, Saunders AM, Strittmatter WJ, et al. Gene dose of apolipoprotein E type 4 allele and the risk of Alzheimer's disease in late onset families. Science 1993;261:921–923.
21. Romeo G, Devoto M. Population analysis of the major mutation in cystic fibrosis. Hum Genet 1990;85:391–445.
22. Kwok S. Procedures to minimize PCR-product carry-over. In: PCR protocols: a guide to methods and applications. San Diego, CA: Academic Press, 1990:142–145.

23. Chehab FF, Wall J. Detection of multiple cystic fibrosis mutations by reverse dot blot hybridization: a technology for carrier screening. Hum Genet 1992;89:163–168.
24. Grody WW. Proficiency testing in diagnostic molecular pathology. Diagn Molec Pathol 1994; 3:221–223.
25. Grody WW. Diagnostic molecular pathology news and comment. Diagn Molec Pathol 1994;3: 71–73.
26. Grody WW. Molecular pathology, informed consent, and the paraffin block. Diagn Molec Pathol 1995;4:155–157.

CHAPTER 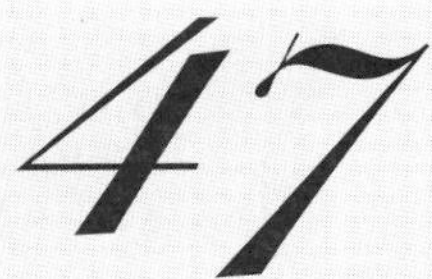

Molecular Assays for Infectious Diseases

YINGZE ZHANG
GARTH D. EHRLICH

History of Molecular Assays for Infectious Diseases

The presence of infectious agents in clinical specimens can be discerned through the detection of their genetic material. All infectious agents (prions excepted) possess a nucleic acid (DNA or RNA) genome, which can be detected through hybridization studies based on the intrinsic complementarity of the two strands in the double helix. Hybridization studies can be performed directly on organismal nucleic acid or on enzymatically amplified DNAs and cDNAs.

Prior to the advent of the polymerase chain reaction (PCR) (1), the first of the in vitro enzymatic DNA amplification methodologies, molecular diagnostics for infectious diseases was based primarily on filter hybridization technologies such as Southern blotting and dot blotting. These assay formats are based on the binding of the target DNA to a nitrocellulosic or nylon filter and then probing the filter with a tagged nucleic acid probe. The reporter group on the probe DNA can be either a radioactive nuclide or some other type of visualization signal, such as a chromogenic substrate or a fluorescent molecule. Southern hybridization, while highly specific, requires massive quantities of target DNA and is not sensitive enough for the detection of low copy number infectious agents or for the detection of residual neoplastic disease. In most cases, it is crucial to make the diagnosis of an infection in the early stages of a disease, prior to the development of a high titer infection. Thus, Southern blotting is inadequate as a diagnostic technique in most cases. Such filter hybridization assays are also very labor-intensive and can require a week for completion. This makes them less than ideal for a clinical setting where high throughput capability and rapid assay turnaround times are important factors in test format selection.

Since its invention, PCR has provided the promise of a solution for issues of sensitivity, specificity, throughput, and turnaround times necessary for the diagnosis of infectious disease agents. Under ideal conditions, PCR can detect a single copy of any given target sequence in a clinical sample; therefore, the primary reason for a false-negative result arising from PCR-based diagnostics is sampling error attributable to Poisson distribution (2).

The specificity of PCR comes from the use of oligonucleotide primers. Primers can be designed to be broadly inclusive, targeting genomically conserved regions, or highly specific, through usage of species- or strain-specific sequences. With the development of robotic pipetting stations and automated thermal cyclers, it is possible for a single individual in the course of a day to perform hundreds of amplification reactions with minimal hands-on effort, permitting rapid reporting of results while minimizing labor costs.

Numerous other in vitro DNA and RNA amplification strategies have been developed in the decade since PCR. In general, most of these techniques are more cumbersome to perform and require more effort for reaction optimization because they use multiple enzymes, multiple primer pairs, or both to achieve amplification. For example, the repair chain reaction (RCR) requires two sets of primers and a thermostable DNA ligase as well as a DNA polymerase. Strand displacement amplification (SDA) is even more involved, requiring two sets of overlapping primers, one of which contains thioester bonds as opposed to phosphodiester bonds in the DNA backbone, a restriction enzyme, and a DNA polymerase (3). Thus, these alternative amplification strategies, which were developed largely to circumvent the PCR patent, do not lend themselves to the design of home-brew molecular diagnostics and will not be further considered here.

Some signal amplification technologies, as opposed to target amplification technologies, have proved to be useful in the quantitation of viral genomes. Assays based on branched-chain DNA (bDNA), developed by Chiron Diagnostics, have proved valuable in monitoring viral titers for chronic pathogens such as human immunodeficiency virus type 1 (HIV-1), and hepatitis B and C viruses. These commercially developed bDNA assays are quite robust, but this technology does not lend itself to use in the design of home-brew assays.

PCR-Based Assays for Specific Pathogens

PCR-based assays have been used for the detection of fastidious infectious agents, both viral and bacterial, for which there are no or inadequate culture methods available (4). It has also been used for the description of novel bacterial agents through the employment of generic 16S ribosomal RNA primers, which target conserved motifs that flank species-specific sequences (5). PCR has proved invaluable in the detection of slow-growing bacteria associated with chronic infections such as tuberculosis and otitis media with effusion (6,7). PCR can also be used for definitive typing of bacterial strains associated with nosocomial outbreaks and for the detection of genotypes associated with various clinically important phenotypes such as antimicrobial or antiviral resistance and toxin production (8,9).

Development of PCR-Based Simplex Assays

Initially, PCR-based assays were limited to a simplex format wherein a single set of primers was employed for the detection of a single pathogenic agent (10,11). As with any type of diagnostic assay, specificity is of paramount importance and the primer selection process determines the specificity.

Primer Selection

A good PCR-based assay has to be specific for the target pathogen and sensitive enough to detect five or fewer genomic equivalents. Depending on the nature of the assay, the primers can be either generic, for a related group of pathogens, or specific, for a particular strain; in either case, it is necessary to empirically determine the assay's characteristics through use of a panel of nucleic acids from related pathogens (7,12).

A generic primer pair, selected from regions of the genome that are conserved among the related pathogens, can be used to detect the presence of any of a wide group of organisms that are distinguishable from other more distantly related pathogenic groups. For example, ribosomal 16S primers can be designed that will detect all Enterobacteriaceae organisms, but will not support amplification of other gram-negative organisms. In contrast, strain-specific gene sequences, such as those encoding surface antigens, can be used to distinguish between highly related pathogens of the same species.

It is not always an easy task to select robust primers pairs, and numerous software programs, such as Oligo and Primer, have been developed to aid in primer design. In general, primers should be selected with minimal intra- and inter-primer complementarity, and the G/C ratio should reflect that of the flanking sequences. For diagnostic purposes primers should be positioned to support amplification of products ranging from 100 to 500 nucleotides in length.

Synthesis of primers should be performed on well-designed and maintained equipment; we have found the Applied Biosystems DNA automated synthesizers to be very reliable. Following synthesis, the oligonucleotides should be purified by reverse phase chromatography, which will select for only full length primers. For long-term storage of primers, it is important that they be vialed at high concentration following lyophilization.

Sensitivity

The sensitivity of a PCR-based assay is usually determined by using a serial dilution of the purified DNA from the specific pathogen (13). In our laboratory, a 10-fold dilution series from 10 ng/PCR to 10 fg/PCR are usually used for bacterial DNAs, and 10 pg to 10 attograms for viral DNA. Because bacterial genomes contain between 1 and 5 fg of DNA, detection of the 10 fg sample is indicative of the assay's ability to detect 2 to 5 genomic equivalents.

Once the sensitivity is determined, the three lowest dilutions that support amplification should be routinely used as the positive controls. It is important to determine the sensitivity of the assay using multiple strains of the target species to ensure that strain variation does not adversely affect detectability.

Specificity

Assay specificity is influenced by several factors (14). In general, the PCR annealing temperature is set at a point that will permit the primers to bind stably to target DNA, but not permit binding to related DNAs. In other words, if mismatches are present, the primer will not support elongation by the polymerase. This is achieved in practice by doing a series of calibration PCRs where only the annealing temperature is changed, selecting the highest temperature at which amplification is not diminished.

The Mg^{2+} concentration of the PCR assay can also affect the specificity; higher Mg^{2+} reduces the specificity of the assay by stabilizing mismatches. A 1 mM increase in (Mg^{2+}) is roughly equivalent to a 100 mM increase in the monovalent cations. The addition of cosolvents such as glycerol, ethanol, and DMSO can also increase the specificity of the PCR assay by destabilizing primers-template mismatches.

The specificity of a PCR-based assay can be determined by amplifying a panel of unrelated and related pathogens with the assay. We routinely use human, a variety of bacterial (or viral), and yeast DNAs as specificity controls for PCR-based bacterial (or viral) assays (12). A huge excess of bacterial and viral control DNAs (1 million genomic equivalents) should be used to ensure the specificity of the assay in the presence of large amounts of irrelevant DNA.

Validation of PCR-Based Assays Using Clinical Specimens

In most cases, PCR-based assays for infectious agents will be employed as diagnostic tests for clinical specimens. It is, therefore, important to validate the PCR-based assay through the performance of a clinical trial wherein its sensitivity and specificity are compared against the current gold standard detection modality. Improvements to be looked for in the PCR-based assay over more traditional methods include:

1. Earlier detection of the pathogen in longitudinal studies (15,16).
2. Greater sensitivity in cross-sectional studies (17,18).
3. Better turnaround time for slow growing and fastidious organisms (19).

All validation testing should be performed in a blinded fashion such that the individual who evaluates the PCR results is not aware of the data generated by the gold standard testing. PCR-based assays should be at least equivalent to standard detection formats before being introduced for clinical testing.

Because of their intrinsic sensitivity, PCR-based assays often will appear to have a lower specificity when compared to current gold standard assays. This is not actually the case in most instances, but is an artifact of evaluating a more sensitive test with a less sensitive one. Therefore, it is necessary to employ other means of evaluation, including clinical findings, histopathology, and additional independent PCR-based assays, to resolve differences (18). In the absence of any additional informative testing modalities, discrepant results can be adjudicated by the application of a second (or third) PCR-based assay targeting a different genomic region of the target pathogen. Thus, if two or three independent PCR-based assays all indicate that an infectious agent is present even in the absence of a positive gold standard result, it can be assumed that the specimen is positive.

PCR-Based Assays for Infectious Agents

The original application of PCR with infectious agents was for the individual detection of the three human retroviruses, HIV-1 and the human T-cell lymphoma leukemia viruses (HTLV-I and -II) (10,20,21). Shortly thereafter, PCR was applied to the detection of cytomegalovirus (CMV) and human papilloma viruses (HPV) (11,22). In the past decade, PCR-based assays have been developed for many infectious agents including gram-negative and gram-positive bacteria, acute pyogenic organisms, chronic bacteria such as mycobacteria, mycoplasma, spirochetes, unculturable bacteria, DNA viruses, RNA viruses, and retroviruses (23,24). These tests have been used in the routine diagnosis of bacterial and viral infections at major medical centers and reference laboratories.

For some agents, quantitative PCR-based assays have been developed and used to monitor viral load. Recently, viral load testing for HIV-infected patients has been demonstrated to be the best predictor for disease progression (25,26). By monitoring the viral load in HIV-1-positive patients who are receiving antiviral treatment, it is possible for the clinician to determine, based on viral titer increase, when the virus begins to become resistant to the current drug regimen and so therapy can be modified appropriately. Similarly, quantitative testing has been introduced for the hepatitis B and C viruses. Quantitative testing can be performed using either a limiting dilution approach where the titration end point is the loss of signal, or by using an internal control of known copy number against which the signal for the experimental organism can be compared. Recently, a commercial assay developed by Roche Diagnostics for quantitative HIV-1 determinations received FDA approval for use in clinical diagnostics.

PCR-based assays can also be used to distinguish between early stage CMV infection and immunologic rejection in transplant patients, as it is often not possible through histopathologic examination to distinguish between the two conditions. De novo CMV infection or viral reactivation following transplant may result from the use of immunosuppressive drugs to control rejection. If CMV infection is incorrectly believed to be of immunologic rejection of the transplant, the clinician will increase the dose of the immunosuppressants, resulting in exacerbation of the CMV disease. Similarly, if a patient is incorrectly diagnosed with CMV infection and really has rejection, the physician may reduce the immunosuppressive drugs and make the rejection worse. Thus, accurate and rapid detection of CMV by PCR-based analyses can provide the critical information necessary for clinical treatment (15,16,27).

Another example of the clinical applicability of molecular diagnostics is the PCR-based detection of bacterial DNA, which can be used in patients suspected of having bacterial infections who have been treated with antimicrobial agents, thereby rendering the bacteria unculturable (12).

PCR-Based Multiplex Assays for Infectious Agents

Like the first simplex assays, the first PCR-based multiplex assays were designed for the detection of the human retroviruses as part of an epidemiologic study of intravenous drug abusers (28). The reason for the development of these assays was to reduce the workload, as it was possible to assay for three retroviruses simultaneously. Multiplex assays were also designed for single pathogens. In one case a multiplex assay was designed to determine if viruses related to a known agent were associated with similar disease entities. In this case, HTLV-1 had been associated with tropical spastic paraparesis, a chronic demyelinating diseases of the central nervous system, and the question was raised as to whether related viruses might be associated with multiple sclerosis. In an effort to minimize the risk of not finding a related virus, a multiplex PCR-based assay was designed to support amplification of four genomic reagents simultaneously (17). Infection with retroviruses, particularly HIV, can be emotionally devastating, so it is important to obtain a confident positive diagnosis of this infection; therefore, it is recommended that an HIV-1 screening assay employ a multiplex format.

In the past several years the concept of multiplex PCR-based assay has been extended to a variety of areas (29). These include assays based on:

- Syndromic illnesses that have a number of differential diagnoses.
- Particular organ systems that can be infected with a number of different pathogens.
- Behavioral parameters such as illicit drug use.
- Antibiotic resistance (determining the presence and type).

Rationale for Multiplex Assays in Molecular Diagnosis

Most infectious illnesses for a given organ system present clinically with the similar symptoms, thereby making it difficult to make a definitive agent-specific diagnosis by examination. This is because many pathogens can produce remarkably similar constellations of clinical features. Culture methods for bacteria and viruses partially address this problem by supporting simultaneously the growth of multiple pathogens without the clinician having to specify each and every candidate agent in the differential diagnosis. In contrast, most currently available molecular diagnostics for infectious disease agents monitor for a single pathogen, and therefore are inadequate in many clinical settings (29).

Multiplex PCR-based assays will provide a golden opportunity for the application of PCR-based diagnostics in the clinical setting. This panel format necessitates that the PCR-based assay be capable of amplifying and analyzing multiple independent amplicons simultaneously while including the ability to discriminate among them. Of equal importance, in most cases, is the maintenance of the sensitivities and specificities of the component simplex assays that comprise the multiplex assay (29). The development of PCR-based multiplex assays and their configuration into automated formats (30) will ensure better and more correctly targeted health care, reduced morbidity, and a reduction in overall medical costs (29).

Development of PCR-Based Multiplex Assay

Multiplex testing is conceptually simple, but it is a labor-intensive laboratory process to develop panel-based assays, as extensive technical and regulatory hurdles must be overcome prior to widespread introduction. The addition of each additional target to the multiplex assay increases dramatically the extent of optimization that is necessary to achieve a robust multiplex assay. This is primarily due to primer-primer interactions, which interfere with the sensitivity of the component assays, particularly when one target is present at much higher levels relative to another.

Within the context of the multiplex assay, each primer-probe set should have near single copy detection capabilities. The component primer pairs should not interfere with the amplification efficiency of primer pairs for other pathogens. Furthermore, the amplification efficiency of one target sequence should not be materially affected by the copy number of the other targets.

A stepwise matrix-style approach works best for the development of multiplex assays. To use this approach, it is necessary to develop several robust PCR-based simplex assays for each target organism to be tested. Care should be taken in the design of the oligonucleotide primers for all of the assays to ensure that the components of the simplex assay will function under the same general thermal cycling temperatures. Generally, more than one test should be developed for each pathogen as it is impossible to predict a priori which assays will work best with which other assays.

Initially, two organisms are chosen from which to build a duplex assay. Then each of the several simplex assays for one organism are tested in combination with each of the several simplex assays for the second organism. All of the pairwise combinations for these two organisms are then compared against one another, as well as against the original simplex assays, for sensitivity and specificity. The most robust duplex assay is then chosen to be used as a single block in the second step, wherein the simplex assays for a third organism are assessed against one another in combination with the extant duplex assay.

If additional organisms are to be tested for after the development of a triplex assay, then simplex assays for the fourth target are added to the existing triplex assay in a manner analogous to that used for the development of the tripartite assay.

Pathogen-Based Multiplex Assays

Cytomegalovirus

Although greater than 40% of the general population in the United States is CMV seropositive, only those individuals who are immunosuppressed experience clinical symptoms associated with CMV infection. CMV infection is responsible for significant morbidity and mortality among both the pharmacologic-induced and pathogen-associated immunodeficient patient populations.

Detection of active CMV infection has traditionally been assessed by viral culture or shell vial assay. The development (31) and testing of a multiplex PCR-based assay for CMV has validated the theoretical advantages of PCR for earlier detection and greater sensitivity while also yielding a surprising finding that those individuals who do not clear their CMV levels below the PCR detectability threshold will suffer a clinical relapse of CMV disease (15,16).

Bordetella pertussis

Whooping cough is caused by the bacterium *Bordetella pertussis*. In recent years, pertussis infection has been increasing in the United States. Traditional diagnosis of pertussis must be performed by direct culture of the bacteria on freshly prepared bacterial media. This technique requires both special media and lengthy incubation time (up to 7 days) prior to read out. Furthermore, because of the fastidious nature of *B. pertussis* it is often not recovered through culture, even when all clinical indications point to its presence. In addition, if a patient has been treated with antibiotics, the probability of obtaining a positive culture result is greatly reduced.

Serological test using direct fluorescence antibody has been used, but it is not very useful for the rapid diagnosis of early onset infection. PCR-based detection of *B. pertussis* was first reported by Glare et al. (32), who designed PCR primers from a repetitive DNA sequence. Since then, several reports have been published on the detection of *B. pertussis*. Wadowsky et al. (18) have reported the development of a multiplex assay for the *B. pertussis*. In this study, nasopharyngeal swab specimens were collected from several hundred clinically suspicious patients, and the DNA was used for the detection of *Bordetella pertussis* with the results compared to culture. A triplex PCR-based assay was used in which two separate pertussis DNA targets were amplified as well as a human β-actin gene sequence which served as an internal control for amplifiability of the specimen. This assay was demonstrated to have 100% sensitivity and was able to detect numerous cases of pertussis that culture missed, but that were confirmed through chart review and convalescent sera.

Syndromic-Based Multiplex Assay

Upper Respiratory Bacterial Infections

Upper respiratory tract infections are the most common infectious malady of mankind and are a particular source of morbidity and mortality for infants and the elderly. Many different types of bacteria, both gram negatives and gram positives, are associated with acute and chronic forms of otitis media, sinusitis, and pharyngitis. Therefore, to be cost- and time-effective, a respiratory screening assay needs to be able to detect multiple pathogens simultaneously.

Among upper respiratory infections, the most common pathogens are *Streptococcus pneumoniae, Moraxella catarrhalis, Haemophilus influenzae*, and *Staphylococcus aureus.* We have designed an assay that can detect three of these pathogens (33) which has been used extensively in several laboratories (34) (Emler et al in preparation) (35) and we are currently integrating *S. aureus* into the assay.

Lower Respiratory Bacterial Infections

Lower respiratory illness can also be caused by a variety of pathogenic bacteria. One of the goals of our laboratory has been to develop molecular diagnostic assays for bacterial pathogens associated with chronic cough, including *B. pertussis* and *Mycoplasma pneumoniae* (18,36). To that end, we have developed single-organism multiplex assays for each of these agents. Future plans are to combine them together, along with assays for *Chlamydia pneumoniae,* for a panel-based test format. Other pathogens such as *Legionella* spp. and *Klebsiella pneumoniae* could also be added to create a more comprehensive screening assay.

Respiratory Viral Infection

Respiratory viral infections are pandemic and are caused by numerous readily transmissible species, including adenoviruses, influenza virus, parainfluenza virus, rhinoviruses, enteroviruses, and respiratory syncytial viruses. All of these viruses, with the exception of the adenovirus, consist of a RNA genome. Therefore, the detection of these RNA viruses can be performed by first converting a section of the RNA genome into a complementary DNA (cDNA). This is accomplished through application of a reverse transcription process catalyzed by a retrovirally encoded RNA-dependent DNA polymerase (reverse transcriptase, or RT). The cDNA is then amplified using a standard PCR-based assay.

A multiplex PCR/RT-PCR-based assay for adenovirus, influenza virus, and parainfluenza virus has been developed and is used for the characterization of middle-ear effusions from humans and the chinchilla animal model of otitis media (37,38).

Bacterial and Viral Meningitis

Bacterial or septic meningitis is a life-threatening illness requiring expensive hospitalization stays, often in an intensive care unit, and intravenous antibiotics. In contrast, aseptic meningitis, associated with enteroviral infection, is a relatively benign self-limiting disease. Unfortunately, it can be very difficult to differentiate these syndromes based solely on clinical findings. Because the consequences to the patient are so dire if the wrong diagnosis is made, most patients that present to a hospital emergency room with symptoms of meningitis are admitted for treatment, even though only a small percentage will actually have septic meningitis.

A PCR-based diagnostic assay that could be used to make the differential diagnosis would be medically important if rapid turnaround times could be achieved. To that end, two bacterial multiplex assays have been developed for the detection of *H. influenzae*, *S. pneumoniae*, and *Neisseria meningitidis* (39) (Gluestein et al., in preparation), with ongoing efforts to incorporate an RT-PCR assay for enteroviruses. Due to the very high degree of conservation in the 5′ untranslated region of the enteroviral genome, it is possible to design primers that will support amplification for virtually all enteroviral species.

Behavior-Based Multiplex Assays

Behavior-based assays are designed for groups of organisms that share a common mode of transmission affected by human actions. When a behavior pattern results in the high probability of transmission of a particular infectious agent(s), behavior-based PCR screening among this population can be used to detect infections and monitor the effectiveness of interventional strategies to minimize further spread of the disease.

The use of behavior-based multiplex PCR assays for infectious agents is not a new concept in the field of molecular diagnostics. In fact, the first multiplex assay introduced by Ehrlich et al. (17) was designed to screen for the various human retroviruses (HTLV-I, HTLV-II, and HIV-I) in behaviorally defined high risk populations. In that study, HTLV-II was demonstrated to be the principle retrovirus being spread among the intravenous drug user population in New York City. Similarly, the early detection of infectious disease agents could be used to monitor sexually active individuals and to provide a guide for antimicrobial therapy during the asymptomatic stage of infection prior to the development of more serious sequelae that can be associated with substantial morbidity.

Summary

PCR-based assays provide the promise of greater sensitivity and specificity when compared to traditional methods of microbiologic detection while simultaneously providing a more rapid turnaround of results. The development and implementation of PCR-based multiplex assays for the simultaneous detection of panels of pathogens associated with various organ systems and behavioral practices will provide a cost-effective means for the introduction of large-scale molecular diagnostics.

REFERENCES

1. Saiki RK, Scharf S, Faloona F, et al. Enzymatic amplification of beta-globin genomic sequences and restriction site analysis of sickle cell anemia. Science 1985;230:1350–1354.
2. Ehrlich GD. Laboratory protocols for the PCR-based detection of infectious disease agents. In: Ehrlich GD, Greenberg SJ, eds. PCR-dased diagnostics in infectious disease. Boston: Blackwell Scientific, 1994:335–340.
3. Walker GT, Fraiser MS, Schram JL, et al. Strand displacement amplification—an isothermal, in vitro DNA amplification technique. Nucleic Acids Res 1992;20:1691–1696.
4. Relman DA, Loutit JS, Schmidt TM, et al. The agent of bacillary angiomatosis. An approach to the identification of uncultured pathogens. N Engl J Med 1990;323:1573–1580.
5. Wilson KH, Blitchington R, Greene RC. Amplification of bacterial 16S rRNA sequences with polymerase chain reaction. J Clin Microbiol 1990;28:1942–1946.
6. Young KK. The detection of mycobacterial DNA using PCR. In: Ehrlich GD, Greenberg SJ, eds. PCR-based diagnostics in infectious disease. Boston: Blackwell Scientific, 1994:537–558.

7. Post JC, Preston RA, Aul JJ, et al. Molecular analysis of bacterial pathogens in otitis media with effusion. JAMA 1995;273:1598–1604.
8. Sakullah S, Pasculle W, Lanning R, et al. Typing of *Legionella pneumophila* serogroup 1 isolates by degenerate (D-)RAPD fingerprinting. Mol Cell Probes 1995;9:405–411.
9. Arlet G, Phillippon A. PCR-based approaches for the detection of bacterial resistance. In: Ehrlich GD, Greenberg SJ, eds. PCR-based diagnostics in infectious disease. Boston: Blackwell Scientific, 1994:665–687.
10. Kwok S, Mack DH, Mullis KB, et al. Identification of human immunodeficency virus sequences by using in vitro enzymatic amplification and oligomer cleavage detection. J Virol 1987;61:1690–1694.
11. Shibata D, Martin WJ, Appleman M, et al. Detection of cytomegalovirus DNA in peripheral blood of patients infected with human immunodeficency virus. J Infect Dis 1988;158:1185–1192.
12. Zhang Y, Issacman D, Wadowsky RM, et al. Detection of *Streptococcus pneumoniae* in whole blood by PCR. J Clin Micro 1995;33:546–601.
13. Ehrlich GD, Greenberg S, Abbott M. Detection of human T-cell lymphoma/leukemia viruses (HTLV). In: Innis MA, Gelfand DH, Sninsky JJ, White TJ, eds. PCR protocols. a guide to methods and applications. San Diego: Academic Press, 1990:325–336.
14. Ehrlich GD, Sirko DA. Parameters for maximizing the sensitivity and specificity of the polymerase chain reaction. In: Ehrlich GD, Greenberg SJ, eds. PCR-based diagnostics in infectious disease. Boston: Blackwell Scientific, 1994:45–56.
15. Mañez R, Kusne S, Aguado JM, et al. The time of infection after transplantation is the best predictor of disease progression in CMV-seronegative liver recipients of CMV-seropositive allograft. J Infect Dis 1996;173:1072–1076.
16. Kusne S, Mañez R, St. Frye BL, et al. Use of DNA amplification for diagnosis of cytomegalovirus DNA amplification for the diagnosis of enteritis after intestinal transplantation. Gastroenterology 1997;112:1121–1128.
17. Ehrlich GD, Glaser J, Lavigne K, et al. Prevalence of human T-cell leukemia/lymphoma virus type II infection among high risk individuals: type-specific identification of HTLVs by polymerase chain reaction. Blood 1989;74:1658–1664.
18. Wadowsky RM, Michaels RH, Libert T, et al. Multiplex polymerase chain reaction-based assay for the detection of *Bordetella pertussis* in nasopharyngeal swab specimens. J Clin Microbiol 1996;34:2645–2649.
19. Emler S, Rochat T, Rohner P, et al. Chronic destructive lung disease associated with a novel mycobacterium. Am J Respir Crit Care Med 1994;150:261–265.
20. Abbott M, Byrne B, Kwok S, et al. Enzymatic gene amplification: qualitative and quantitative methods for detecting proviral DNA amplified in vitro. J Infect Dis 1988;158:1158–1169.
21. Kwok S, Ehrlich GD, Poiesz B, et al. Enzymatic amplification of HTLV-I viral sequences in peripheral blood mononuclear cells and infected tissues. Blood 1988;72:1117–1123.
22. Manos MM, Ting Y, Wright DK, et al. The use of polymerase chain reaction amplification for the detection of genital human papillomaviruses. Cancer Cells 1989;7:209–214.
23. Ehrlich GD, Greenberg SJ. PCR-based diagnostics in infectious disease. Boston: Blackwell Scientific, 1994.
24. Persing DH, Smith TF, Tenover FC, White TJ. Diagnostic molecular microbiology: principles and applications. Washington, DC: American Society for Microbiology, 1993.
25. Gupta P, Ding M, Cottrill M, et al. Quantitation of human immunodeficiency virus type I DNA and RNA by a novel internally controlled PCR assay. J Clin Microbiol 1995;33:1670–1673.
26. Mellors JW, Rinald CR Jr, Gupta P, et al. Prognosis in HIV-1 infection predicted by the quantity of virus in plasma. Science 1996;272:1167–1170.
27. Wilkens L, Werner M, Nolte M, et al. Influence of formalin fixation on the detection of cytomegalovirus by polymerase chain reaction in immunocompromised patients and correlation to in situ hybridization, immunohistochemistry, and serological data. Diagn Mol Pathol 1994;3:156–162.
28. Ehrlich GD, Glaser JB, Maese J, et al. Multiple sclerosis, retroviruses and PCR. Neurology 1991;41:335–343.
29. Ehrlich GD. Syndromic illnesses demand multiplex PCR-based assays. Mol Diagn 1996:83–87.

30. Findlay JB. A containment system for PCR amplification and detection. In: Ehrlich GD, Greenberg SJ, eds. PCR-based diagnostics in infectious disease. Boston: Blackwell Scientific, 1994:97–114.

31. Randhawa PS, Jaffe R, Rinaldo C, et al. Detection of cytomegalovirus in formalin fixed paraffin embedded donor, native and allograft liver tissue using a multiplex PCR-LH assay. Mod Pathol 1994;7:125–128.

32. Glare EM, Paton JC, Premier RR, et al. Analysis of a repetitive DNA sequence from *Bordetella pertussis* and its application to the diagnosis of pertussis using the polymerase chain reaction. J Clin Microbiol 1990;28:1982–1987.

33. Post JC, White GJ, Aul JJ, et al. Development and validation of a multiplex PCR-based assay for the upper respiratory tract bacterial pathogens, *Hemophilus influenzae*, *Streptococcus pneumoniae*, and *Moraxella catarrhalis*. Mol Diagn 1996;1:29–39.

34. Post JC, Aul JJ, White GJ, et al. PCR-based detection of bacterial DNA after antimicrobial treatment is indicative of persistent, viable bacteria in the chinchilla model of otitis media. Am J Otolaryngol 1996;7:1–7.

35. Bakaletz LD, White GJ, Post JC, Ehrlich GD. Blinded multiplex PCR analysis of middle ear and nasopharyngeal fluids from chinchilla models of single- and mixed-pathogen-induced otitis media. Clin Diagn Lab Immunol 1998;5: 219–224.

36. Dolor M, Beyer A, Ehrlich GD, Gupta P, Libert T, Wadowsky RM. Comparison of multiplex PCR-based assay and culture for the detection of *Mycoplasma pneumoniae* in seeded pleural fluid specimens. Annual American Society for Microbiology Meeting, November 13, 1996.

37. Ehrlich GD, Aul JJ, White GJ, et al. Persistence of DNA in middle-ear effusions of chinchillas as determined by the PCR. Sixth International Symposium on Recent Advances in Otitis Media, June 4–8, 1995.

38. Anderson KW, Post JC, Wadowsky RM, Ehrlich GD. The development and application of a multiplex PCR/RT-PCR-based assay for adenovirus, influenza virus and parainfluenza virus to otitis media. (Submitted).

39. Rådström P, Backman A, Qian NY, et al. Detection of bacterial DNA in cerebrospinal fluid by an assay for simultaneous detection of *Neisseria meningitidis*, *Haemophilus influenzae*, and streptococci using a seminested PCR strategy. J Clin Microbiol 1994;32:2738–2744.

CHAPTER 48

Quality Assurance in Forensic DNA Testing

RHONDA K. ROBY
THEODORE D. ANDERSON
VICTOR W. WEEDN

Forensic DNA testing for the identification of evidentiary material involved in the resolution of legal disputes is a powerful technique. However, stating that a semen stain exhibits a profile consistent with that of a suspect and computing the frequency estimate of that profile has very little meaning if any speculation exists that an error has occurred in analyzing those two specimens. Because the results of DNA testing can have such a profound impact on the lives of litigants, those performing this testing must assure all parties that the results are correct and accurate (1). This assurance is founded in the rigorous standards set forth by agencies and advisors from the scientific, legal, and various other communities (**Table 48-1**) providing the basis and foundation for what has become known as quality assurance (QA).

DNA testing procedures were developed by research laboratories during the rapid onset of biotechnology to discriminate between different experimental populations. For this reason, DNA testing as practiced in these laboratories did not emphasize many of the concerns inherent in handling individual samples. Quality assurance aspects of DNA testing are not typically emphasized by research laboratories. Conversely, QA has become a major component of DNA testing in service laboratories. The first commercial applications of DNA testing were in forensic identification and paternity testing. Quality assurance in these fields was inspired by the anticipation of rigorous scrutiny from the courts (2–4).

DNA Testing in Forensic Laboratories

Forensic scientists around the world have introduced basic molecular biologic techniques into their laboratories to conduct DNA testing on biological evidentiary specimens. Each method has been in practice in clinical laboratories or research facilities prior to the crime laboratory. Each method has its own advantages, limitations, and quality assurance and control issues. It is not possible to discuss each test method in length; therefore, references are provided that discuss the various test methods (5–8).

DNA test procedures used in the forensic laboratory concentrate on core genetic loci where the DNA varies among humans—that is, the DNA is highly polymorphic. Currently, crime laboratories around the world are conducting RFLP (restriction fragment length polymorphism) and polymerase chain reaction-based (PCR) DNA test methods.

Unlike clinical diagnostic specimens, forensic DNA testing often involves specimens that are highly degraded, contaminated, or from multiple unknown sources. Forensic DNA specimens have their own inherent problems and require special attention to chain of custody, extraction, and analysis; forensic DNA testing has strict QA requirements.

TABLE 48-1

Recognized Organizations in the Forensic Community

AAFS	American Academy of Forensic Sciences
ABC	American Board of Criminalists
ASCLD	American Society of Crime Laboratory Directors
ASCLD-LAB	ASCLD-Laboratory Accreditation Board
ASCLD-LAB DNA PRC	ASCLD-LAB DNA Proficiency Review Committee
CACLD	California Association of Crime Laboratory Directors
DAB	DNA Advisory Board
ISFH	International Society of Forensic Haemogenetics
NCFS	National Center for Forensic Science
TWGDAM	Technical Working Group on DNA Analysis Methods

QA for Forensic DNA Laboratories

Quality assurance encompasses every aspect of DNA testing. Whether one is discussing the DNA testing necessary to include or exclude an individual as a suspected rapist or to identify remains discovered at a clandestine gravesite, DNA testing that has successfully met or exceeded rigorous QA standards will assure the legal system that the results are accurate and precise (8).

These rigorous standards include proper documentation of all QA measures. This documentation includes detailed attention to all aspects of laboratory functions from sample handling to reporting: education and continuing education; training of all personnel; internal and external audits; quality control (QC); written protocols; proficiency testing; proper corrective action for noted deficiencies; equipment maintenance and calibration; safety; and facilities (9,10).

Laboratory Facilities

Separate areas should be provided, as necessary, for various laboratory functions to prevent possible contamination or sample exchanges. The laboratory bench-space area should be appropriate to accommodate the number of personnel assigned to a specified area. Air handling should be designed to accommodate the testing performed in the facility (e.g., PCR testing). Heating, ventilation, and air conditioning systems should be of adequate capacity to produce environmental conditions that comply with safety standards, and should be designed to prevent cross-contamination. The scientists should be provided with appropriate administrative areas to conduct all paperwork and telephonic communication with investigators and attorneys.

Chain of Custody

The forensic scientist must pay particular attention to the collection and handling of evidentiary material. He or she must exercise procedures that have no deleterious effects on the evidence in both the preservation of the evidence and the identification of the evidence. Challenges in the courts today seem to be focusing not on how the tests were conducted, but from where the sample came and who had possession of the specimen at any one particular moment.

Standard Operating Procedures

Written standard operating procedures, or SOPs, should be available to all laboratorians while conducting scientific analyses. Standard operating procedures provide the step-by-step methods and include proper quality controls to adequately review data generated by the specified test procedure. Scientific literature review citations are important supporting documentation for a procedure and should be included in each SOP, if available. The SOPs should be read by the scientific staff prior to being signed into place by the laboratory director or other official, and should be reviewed annually thereafter. Any deviations from an SOP should be documented in the appropriate case folder. If revisions are needed due to procedural changes or typographical errors found in the SOP, an SOP should be reissued. All outdated SOPs should be placed in archives for a period of time specified by the laboratory.

Quality Control

Quality control involves all aspects of DNA testing that have a direct impact on the final laboratory result. A thorough QC program has several components. One component consists of controls and standards appropriate for each DNA test. In addition, the performance of the reagents and supplies must be tested prior to their implementation into casework. Furthermore, the QC program must provide a means of verifying that the correct specimen is analyzed, is adequate in quantity and quality for that particular test, and is not contaminated. Finally, the results must be correctly interpreted.

Validation Studies

Documented validation studies must be completed prior to implementation of any new test procedure for the purpose of characterizing forensic evidentiary material. For example, studies must be conducted on any new extraction protocol, restriction enzyme, synthetic primers, probes, loci characterized, and multiplex testing. Evaluated data from validation studies should include different populations, mixed samples, nonhuman samples, reproducible profiles using different body fluids and substrates, and effects of environmental insults.

At the conclusion of the study, a report should be written summarizing the data generated and conclusions. All data and documentation should be available for review. The Technical Working Group on DNA Analysis Methods (TWGDAM) has published extensive recommendations for validating forensic DNA analysis methods (11–13).

Equipment

Equipment used in the generation, measurement, or assessment of data must be appropriate in design and located in space for ease of operation, inspection, cleaning, and maintenance. Written records should be maintained of all inspection, maintenance, testing, and calibration. These records shall contain the date and type of maintenance and the initials or name of the operator. Equipment used for the generation, measurement, and/or assessment of data shall be tested, calibrated, and/or standardized before use.

Documentation

A designated individual or individuals should maintain all documentation files. Copies of all validation studies, procedures, and amendments, and written records of internal and external audits should be filed. A report should be generated for all corrective actions. General policies and standard operating procedures must be readily available for the practicing laboratorian.

QA Committee

A QA committee should be formed within a crime laboratory to constantly evaluate the QA measures and practices previously mentioned and to offer mechanisms for improvement and for correction of deficiencies. The QA committee should have oversight of the laboratory's documented QA program to ensure that the work performed follows a total quality program. In this program, the laboratory should conduct periodic self-inspections by review of documentation and discussions with all levels of personnel.

Conclusion

Thorough documentation is paramount for any forensic DNA testing laboratory. Protocols and SOPs, adequate facilities and equipment, identification of evidentiary material tested, identification of scientists performing tests, equipment maintenance, accurate notetaking, and accurate reporting of test results are basic necessities for conducting forensic DNA testing.

Forensic Guidelines and Laboratory Accreditation

The first published sets of QA standards for DNA testing were those set forth by the American Association of Blood Banks (AABB) (14) and TWGDAM (11). The AABB standards, issued in 1990, were created for paternity testing laboratories performing RFLP analysis (see Chapter 45). In 1994, the AABB revised its paternity testing standards (15) by including key provisions for PCR testing.

TWGDAM has been the leading body that provides guidance on QA standards within the forensic DNA community. TWGDAM was established as an independent organization and is funded and hosted by the Federal Bureau of Investigations (FBI). The TWGDAM committee is composed of leading forensic scientists from the United States and Canada and is currently divided into four subcommittees: QA/QC, RFLP, PCR, and Mitochondrial DNA. TWGDAM members discuss recent court challenges, current procedures used in the laboratory, and collaborative research projects. TWGDAM issues specified guidelines (11–13,16–18) that, in the absence of other requirements, have been widely accepted by the courts as the de facto forensic DNA testing standards.

Accrediting Agencies

The American Society of Crime Laboratory Directors-Laboratory Accreditation Board (ASCLD-LAB), which endorses TWGDAM's guidelines, has established inspection criteria and accredits crime laboratories performing all aspects of criminalistics testing, including DNA analysis (9, 19). The College of American Pathologists (CAP) has also established inspection criteria and accredits molecular biology/pathology laboratories (20). The National Center for Forensic Science (NCFS) accredits forensic DNA laboratories.

The first DNA laboratory was accredited in February 1993 by ASCLD-LAB (**Table 48-2**). Many of the CAP and NCFS criteria overlap with those of ASCLD-LAB. Emphasis on specific standards may differ with ASCLD-LAB, CAP, and NCFS. ASCLD-LAB, CAP, and NCFS all require a complete and thoroughly documented QA program. Documentation of all aspects of a laboratory's daily functions is required.

ASCLD-LAB requires participation in approved external proficiency testing surveys. ASCLD-LAB-approved proficiency testing surveys must follow the TWGDAM and ASCLD-LAB DNA Proficiency Review Committee (PRC) published guidelines (16). These guidelines were created in response to apparent problems and weaknesses in the early proficiency testing programs, and are patterned after the Food and Drug Administration's Good Manufacturing Practices.

Inspectors for ASCLD-LAB are themselves from ASCLD-LAB-accredited laboratories. All documentation is submitted to the agency's inspector or inspection team prior to the official audit. The inspection team will then visit the facility and conduct a thorough review of critical QC records, proficiency tests, training files, case folders, and/or any other relevant documentation. Furthermore, these teams may conduct on-site interviews with laboratory personnel.

CAP requires participation in any relevant CAP proficiency testing surveys that are offered (20,21).

TABLE **48-2**

ASCLD-LAB Accredited Laboratories (as of November 1997)

United States	130
Australia	7
New Zealand	4
Canada	1
Hong Kong	1
Singapore	1

Proficiency Test Providers

The AABB introduced an inter-laboratory exchange program in 1982, the Parentage Specimen Program (PSP), for conventional serological tests. In 1987, the California Association of Crime Laboratory Directors (CACLD) distributed the first proficiency samples for DNA analysis to laboratories willing to participate. In 1991, the AABB supplemented the PSP with its first DNA proficiency testing module. Virtually all crime laboratories initially performed external proficiency testing through sample exchanges with neighboring laboratories or through participation in the PSP.

The Collaborative Testing Service (CTS), a private entity that functions in association with the Forensic Science Foundation and under direction from members of ASCLD, offers a variety of proficiency testing programs to forensic laboratories. CTS began to offer DNA proficiency testing services in 1991. In that same year, Cellmark Diagnostics, Inc., launched the International Quality Assurance Scheme (IQAS), a DNA proficiency testing program.

In 1993, the DNA module of the PSP was replaced with the CAP/AABB cosponsored Parentage Identity DNA Proficiency Testing Survey. In that same year, the CAP began to offer the Forensic Identity DNA Proficiency Testing Survey (21).

In 1997 the CAP began offering a proficiency testing program for DNA database analysts. External proficiency testing provides crime laboratories and forensic analysts with the ability to compare results with other crime laboratories.

ASCLD-LAB DNA PRC performs on-site visits of proficiency test manufacturers and providers to ensure compliance with their guidelines. Currently, ASCLD-LAB has approved the Forensic Identity Survey offered by the CAP, the IQAS Scheme offered by Cellmark Diagnostics, Inc., and programs offered by both Serological Research Institute (SERI) and CTS. All of these programs can service ASCLD-LAB-accredited laboratories.

Other Organizations

The International Society for Forensic Haemogenetics (ISFH) and the American Society for Histocompatibility and Immunology (ASHI) have established guidelines with respect to DNA testing. ISFH has published broad guidelines in the area of forensic DNA testing. In addition, ISFH has a QA commission that acts as the main functional body for quality oversight of DNA testing in Europe. A subcommittee known as the European DNA Analysis Panel (EDNAP) coordinates standardization and development of new methods (22).

In the United States, with the passage of the DNA Identification Act of 1994 (42 USC §14131, 1995) which was incorporated into the Omnibus Crime Bill, a DNA Advisory Board (DAB) was established consisting of a chairperson, state and local crime laboratorians, the chairperson of TWGDAM, and other active members in the forensic DNA community. One of the leading aims of the DAB is to publish QA standards for the forensic community. This publication is expected to be released by the time of the printing of this book. The DNA Identification Act authorizes the appropriation of grant monies to states to establish DNA databanks of convicted offenders and nonsuspect crimes. The contingency for receiving these monies is the implementation of a strict QA program based on TWGDAM standards (13). One key component of this QA program involves regularly-scheduled, external proficiency testing.

Audits

Regular audits of forensic laboratory operations are essential components of QA programs (23). An audit of the laboratory by a qualified external examiner provides the laboratory management with an opportunity to determine if its operation meets its established quality assurance program, as well as providing a review of the standards promulgated by various agencies (18).

Training

A DNA analyst must be required, at minimum, to hold an undergraduate degree in the sciences with additional training and coursework in general forensic sciences, law, expert witness training, and statistics. A forensic scientist must understand the potential value of forensic evidentiary material. It is speculated that the DAB will be requiring coursework in genetics, biochemistry, molecular biology, and statistics for DNA analysts.

Currently, most training of forensic scientists occurs in the laboratory and at workshops and conferences. In contrast to the clinical medical laboratories where the director signs all reports (24), forensic scientists are responsible for the analytical work, the interpretation of data, report writing, and courtroom testimony (25). The forensic scientist must be regarded as a professional and must receive the appropriate diversified training to handle evidence, test this evidence, interpret data, and present information to the courts.

Certification

In recent years, the American Board of Criminalists (ABC) introduced a certification examination for criminalists. The ABC is a certifying body/agency of and for professional laboratorians in the field. To obtain certification, a criminalist must meet certain educational requirements, possess experience as demonstrated by years performing casework, and pass a comprehensive forensic science examination. The examination was developed with significant guidance from the Educational Testing Service.

Once a criminalist has passed the general examination, he or she may also be tested and certified in a particular concentration (e.g., trace evidence, forensic biology, drug identification). To maintain certification a criminalist must participate in continuing education, undergo proficiency testing at least twice a year, and forward documentation of requirements to the ABC Review Committee.

Certification has been a much discussed topic at the DAB meetings and will most likely be addressed in its final report. The DAB is expected to require some form of certification, not necessarily that offered by ABC.

Standardization

Standardization in this context does not refer to the implementation of uniform procedures used by laboratories employing a scientific method, but rather to the uniform language of a DNA profile for a specific locus. Standardization "can help to avoid confusion, mistakes, and complications, and . . . encourage efficiency, reproducibility, and quality control" (22). Proficiency tests offered through external proficiency test providers and interlaboratory studies not only offer participants a mechanism by which to compare their individual results to the community's, but also show the importance of standardized nomenclature. Most recently, this need of standardization was demonstrated by the use of inconsistent nomenclature in reporting short tandem repeat results (26).

Legal Issues

The legal system has had significant influence on the implementation of QA standards in forensic laboratories for DNA testing. In *Minnesota v Schwartz*, the judge remarked that the reliability of DNA identity will become the major courtroom issue in future trials (27). In *New York v Castro* (3), Judge Sheindlin ruled that inadequate QA was sufficient to hold DNA evidence as inadmissible. Since that ruling, few cases, if any, have resulted in DNA evidence being held as inadmissible due to insufficient QA. In *U.S. v Jakobetz* (4), the judge commented, "The field is moving so fast that what was criticized a year ago as needing improvement has already been improved." Obviously, forensic scientists are meeting the demands of courtroom challenges by focusing on more stringent QA guidance and practice.

Conclusion

Several organizations have had the opportunity to evaluate the quality of forensic DNA analysis. The Office of Technology Assessment (OTA) was asked to investigate the propriety of forensic DNA testing. The OTA issued a report in 1990 (28) that strongly endorsed the types of DNA testing being used in forensic laboratories: "The Office of Technology Assessment (OTA) finds that forensic uses of DNA tests are both reliable and valid when properly performed and analyzed by skilled personnel." In addition, the report concluded, "The issue of setting standards for forensic applications is the most pressing of the five policy issues identified by OTA."

The National Research Council (NRC) issued a report in 1992 entitled *DNA Technology in Forensic Science* (29). In this report, the NRC stated that governmental regulation is necessary to oversee the voluntary accreditation programs of professional organizations. They recommended that the Department of Health and Human Services in conjunction with the Department of Justice be legislatively mandated to regulate forensic laboratories.

The National Institute of Standards and Technology investigated the performance of the forensic community on the basis of proficiency testing. The results were exceptional. In fact, RFLP analysis yielded allelic sizing variations that did not exceed a few hundred bases and coefficients of variation less than 2% (30).

Standards continue to be set in the DNA testing communities, and technical QA measures are being developed and will continue to evolve. However, innovations are so rapidly occurring in this area of biotechnology that QA measures continue to lag practice.

Jurisdiction and responsibilities of various organizations are being defined, and identification of laboratories capable of performing quality DNA testing will occur as accreditation takes place. Forensic laboratories are in the midst of the natural and inevitable maturation of this growing important field of laboratory testing.

Acknowledgments

The authors wish to acknowledge Carleton T. Garrett, MD, PhD, Susan Johns, Mark A. Lovell, MD, Jeffrey Morris, MD, PhD, Jim Mudd, and Richard Walker, MD.

REFERENCES

1. Stolorow MD, Clarke GW. Forensic DNA testing: a new dimension in criminal evidence gains broad acceptance. The Prosecutor 1992;5:13–28.
2. *State v Andrews*, Case No. 87-1565 (Ninth Judicial Circuit Court, Orange County, Florida, Division 15, November 6, 1987); *Andrews v State*, 533 So. 2d 841 (Florida District Ct. App., 1988).

3. *People v Castro*, 545 N.Y.S. 2d 985 (N.Y. Sup. Ct. 1989).
4. *U.S. v Jakobetz*, 747 F. Supp. 250 (D. Vt. 1990).
5. Weedn VW, Lee DA, Roby RK, Holland MM. DNA analysis. In: Wong SHY, Sunshine I, eds. Handbook of analytical therapeutic drug monitoring and toxicology. New York: CRC Press, 1996:35–49.
6. Weedn VW, Roby RK. Forensic DNA testing. Arch Pathol Lab Med 1993;117:486–491.
7. Weedn VW, Roby RK. Overview of future DNA technologies. In: Proceedings from the 3rd international symposium on human identification. Madison, WI: Promega Corporation, 1992:117–133.
8. Kirby LT. DNA fingerprinting: an introduction. New York: Stockton Press, 1990.
9. American Society of Crime Laboratory Directors. ASCLD accreditation manual. American Society of Crime Laboratory Directors-Laboratory Accreditation Board, 1985.
10. Stiles TR. Quality assurance in toxicology studies. In: Ballantyne B, Marrs T, Turner P, eds. General and applied toxicology. New York: Stockton Press, 1993;1:345–358.
11. Technical Working Group on DNA Analysis Methods. Guidelines for a quality assurance program for DNA restriction fragment length polymorphism analysis. Crime Lab Dig 1989;16:2:40–59.
12. Technical Working Group on DNA Analysis Methods. Guidelines for a quality assurance program for DNA analysis. Crime Lab Dig 1991;18:2:44–75.
13. Technical Working Group on DNA Analysis Methods. Guidelines for a quality assurance program for DNA analysis. Crime Lab Dig 1995;22:2:21–43.
14. American Association of Blood Banks Standards Committee. P7.000 DNA polymorphism testing. In: AABB standards for parentage testing laboratories. Arlington, VA: AABB, 1990.
15. American Association of Blood Banks. Standards for parentage testing laboratories. Bethesda, MD: AABB, 1994.
16. Technical Working Group on DNA Analysis Methods Quality Assurance Subcommittee, ASCLD-LAB DNA Proficiency Review committee. Guidelines for DNA proficiency test manufacturing and reporting. Crime Lab Dig 1994;21:2:27–32.
17. Technical Working Group on DNA Analysis Methods. Guidelines for a proficiency testing program for DNA restriction fragment length polymorphism analysis. Crime Lab Dig 1990;17:3:59–64.
18. Technical Working Group on DNA Analysis Methods. A guide for conducting a DNA quality assurance audit. Crime Lab Dig 1993;20:1:8–18.
19. American Society of Crime Laboratory Directors. Guidelines for forensic laboratory management practices. ASCLD, 1986.
20. College of American Pathologists. Checklist 12: molecular pathology. Northfield: CAP, 1993.
21. Weedn VW, Roby RK. New CAP program to focus on forensic DNA testing. CAP Today 1992;6:48.
22. Bockstahler LE. Overview of international PCR standardization efforts. PCR Methods Appl 1994;3:263–267.
23. National Research Council. The evaluation of forensic DNA evidence. Washington, DC: National Academy Press, 1996.
24. American College of Medical Genetics. Standards and guidelines: clinical genetics laboratories. Bethesda, MD: American College of Medical Genetics, 1993.
25. Bashinski JS. Laboratory standards: accreditation, training, and certification of staff in the forensic context. In: Ballantyne J, Sensabaugh G, Witkowski J, eds. Banbury report 32: DNA technology and forensic science. Cold Spring Harbor, NY: Cold Spring Harbor Laboratory Press, 1989:159–173.
26. Anderson TD, Roby RK, Weedn VW. Analysis of the polymerase chain reaction-based DNA testing data from the College of American Pathologists' forensic identity and parentage identity proficiency testing programs. In: Proceedings from the seventh international symposium on human identification. Madison: Promega Corporation, 1997:207–208.
27. *State v Schwartz*, 447 N.W.2d 422, 427–428 (Minn. 1989).
28. Office of Technology Assessment. Genetic witness: forensic uses of DNA tests. Washington, DC: US Government Printing Office, 1990.
29. National Research Council. DNA technology in forensic science. Washington, DC: National Academy Press, 1992.
30. Mudd JL, Baechtel FS, Duewer DL, et al. Interlaboratory comparison of autoradiographic DNA profiling measurements. 1. Data and summary statistics. Anal Chem 1994;66:3303–3317.

Index

Note: Page numbers followed by f indicate figures; those followed by t indicated tables.